Disease in the Merchant Navy

A history of the Seamen's Hospital Society

Gordon C Cook
MD, DSc, FRCP, FRCPE, FRACP, FLS
Visiting Professor
University College London

CRC Press
Taylor & Francis Group
Boca Raton London New York

CRC Press is an imprint of the
Taylor & Francis Group, an **informa** business

First published 2007 by Radcliffe Publishing Ltd

Published 2019 by CRC Press
Taylor & Francis Group
6000 Broken Sound Parkway NW, Suite 300
Boca Raton, FL 33487-2742

First issued in paperback 2019

ISBN 13: 978-0-367-44617-8 (pbk)
ISBN 13: 978-1-84619-236-4 (hbk)

British Library Cataloguing in Publication Data
A catalogue record for this book is available from the British Library.

Typeset by Phoenix Photosetting, Chatham, Kent

Contents

Preface

Founded in 1821, the Seamen's Hospital Society (SHS) (which was, and remains, entirely dependent on voluntary contributions) became one of the greatest of Victorian charities – supported by Queen Victoria herself, and also by many royal personages throughout Europe and beyond.[1,2]

At the conclusion of the Napoleonic Wars, London's dockland was inundated with unemployed mariners from numerous nations who were without family and friends; many were suffering from a sexually-transmitted, or tropical disease. In 1818, a small group of philanthropists (which included William Wilberforce and Zachary Macaulay) conceived a plan to assist this multi-ethnic group and this was enthusiastically supported by public subscription. This organisation was known as the *Committee for the Relief of Distressed (destitute) Seamen*. The 'plan of campaign' was that *clinical* facilities were to be made available *free* to seafarers of all nations in the Port of London (the Royal Navy already had a well developed welfare system) irrespective of race, religion or nationality, without the necessity of a letter of introduction (which was demanded by most of London's general hospitals). So successful, in fact, was this enterprise that it was decided to found a *permanent* institution (the SHS); the first meeting of the Committee of Management took place on 8 March 1821 (see Appendix I).

Between the date of foundation and 1870, *clinical* facilities were placed on three successive ships which had been hulked – HMS *Grampus,* HMS *Dreadnought,* and HMS *Caledonia* (renamed *Dreadnought)* – all on loan from the Admiralty and moored off Greenwich Reach. In 1832 John Lydekker, a member of Lloyd's and a notable ship-owner, bequeathed to the SHS in his Will (he had died suddenly of Asiatic cholera) a sum which amounted to approximately £55,000; the financial stability which resulted from this benefaction enabled the Society to obtain *incorporation* by Act of Parliament the following year.

In 1870, *clinical* facilities were moved on-shore – in the former Infirmary of the Royal Hospital (also lent by the Admiralty), which had become vacant following the removal (most to their homes) of the Greenwich pensioners.

In order to serve London's docklands more satisfactorily, rapid expansion then took place – first with Dispensaries (outpatient facilities) at the East India Dock Road and Gravesend, and later involving a 'branch' hospital – the Albert Dock Hospital (situated between the Royal Albert and Royal Victoria Docks) (1890) which was in 1899 to become the original site for the London School of Tropical Medicine, also founded by the SHS.[3] So successful was this latter venture that the 'tropical' cases were subsequently provided with a hospital of their own (Hospital for Tropical Diseases [HTD]) in 1920; this was situated at Euston.

The SHS flourished, with inevitable interference by the two World Wars, until the implementation of the *National Health Service Act* of 1946. As a result, in 1948 the hospital passed from the stewardship of the SHS to the hands of the Minister of Health. This marked the beginning of a steady decline in the services provided by this great charity, and although under its charter of 1833 it still supports the welfare of seafarers and their dependents (both physically and spiritually), its only *clinical* facility is to be found at the Dreadnought Unit in St Thomas's Hospital, London. The HTD at Endsleigh Gardens was closed in 1939 and the 'flagship' hospital, the *Dreadnought* ceased to function in 1986. Its Nurses' Home and Pathological Laboratory now forms part of the University of Greenwich; the Albert Dock Hospital has now been demolished, and the associated convalescent home and sanatorium have long ceased to serve their intended and, in their day, vital functions.

My personal interest in the SHS was aroused by the fact that it gave rise to the formal discipline *tropical medicine*. In fact, it has even been termed the 'God-mother' of this specialism – which owes much to the inspirational genius of those (both medical and laymen) in command of the Society in the latter years of the nineteenth century.

G C Cook
The Seamen's Hospital Society,
29 King William Walk,
Greenwich, SE10 9HX
September 2007

References

1 G C Cook. The Seamen's Hospital Society. In: *From the Greenwich hulks to Old St Pancras: a history of tropical disease in London*. London: Athlone 1992: 33–67.
2 G C Cook. History of the Seamen's Hospital Society. *J Greenwich Hist. Soc.* 2005; 3(2): 67–78.
3 G C Cook. The Seamen's Hospital Society: a progenitor of the tropical institutions. 1999; *Postgrad Med J* 75: 715–7.

Prologue

The history of this Society closely reflects the condition of merchant seamen and their medical/social problems in the nineteenth and twentieth centuries; in fact, it represents a microcosm of life (and death) amongst this group of individuals during that period.

Although the major 'thrust' of the Society's activity has involved *curative* medicine, the Society has also done much to improve health in the mercantile marine generally. Much of its work was originally directed at venereal disease and tuberculosis, but arguably its greatest achievement was elimination of scurvy from the merchant navy, in the latter years of the nineteenth century.

In this book, I have therefore described the medical facilities – both preventive and curative – the *raison d'etre* of this Society. I have described, therefore, the diseases afflicting the seafarer, as well as the many distinguished physicians and surgeons who have served the Society over nearly two centuries. I have also, I hope accurately, described the history of the Society from its foundation until the present day.

Two families – the Lydekkers and the Nairnes – have played major rôles in the history of the Society.[1–3]

The early history of the SHS has been succinctly outlined in the *SHS Quarterly Magazine* for 1929.[4] It is unlikely that the Society would have come into existence had it not been for the *Committee for Relief of Distressed (destitute) Seamen* – founded in 1817–18 (*see* Chapter 5). The original Board of Management included many distinguished officers of the Royal Navy, the Honourable East India Company's Service, and Elder Brethren of Trinity House, together with prominent businessmen of the day. In the days of the hospital-ships (Chapter 8), the only access from land was by rowing boat; patients were brought to the ship's side and carried up a steep gangway on to the deck. The cost of removal to land (in 1870) was considerable, and if the SHS had had, as was at one time envisaged, to build a *new* hospital it would have been vast; therefore, the Committee of Management considered that the Society had a claim to assistance from the Chatham Chest (into which it had paid so much, without receiving any benefit) but the Admiralty felt otherwise! Soon after becoming 'land-based', the SHS expanded its services: dispensaries in the East India Dock Road (1880), Gravesend (1887), and Southampton (1929); in-patient accommodation was provided at the Albert Dock (1890), the Angas convalescent home (at Cudham, Kent) (1918), the King George's Sanatorium for Sailors (at Liphook, Hampshire) (1921), Tilbury Hospital (1924), and the Queen Alexandra Memorial Hospital, Marseilles (1929). Sadly, this latter institution survived for a mere five years.

References

1 W R Dawson. John Lydekker: the Memorial at Lloyd's. *Supplement to Lloyd's List and Shipping Gazette* (reissued by the Seamen's Hospital Society in pamphlet form) London: E G Berryman & Sons Ltd 1907: 11 March; 20.
2 Anonymous. The Nairne family. One hundred years' service for the Seamen's Hospital Society. *SHS Quart Mag* 1937; 9 (1): 11–14.
3 C S Nairne. *John Nairne (1711–1795) (minister of Anstruther Easter) and his descendants.* McCorquodale & Co Ltd: private circulation, 1931: 47.
4 Anonymous. Seamen's Hospital Society: early history 1821–1970; history from 1870 to the present day. *SHS Quart Mag 1929*: 1(2, 3): 23–28, 43–47.

PART I

Beginnings (1817–1821)

'And now abideth faith, hope, charity, these three; but the greatest of these *is* charity'

Holy Bible: 1 Corinthians 13.

Chapter 1

Social conditions and disease prevention in early nineteenth century Britain

In relating the history of this great Victorian charity – the Seamen's Hospital Society (SHS) – it is essential to appreciate something of the social conditions prevailing in England in the early nineteenth century. The eminent historian, GM Trevelyan (1876–1962), wrote in 1944: 'Social history might be defined negatively as the history of a people with the politics left out'! It is of course quite impossible to omit politics entirely, but in this first chapter I attempt to give an idea of the social environment in England at the time the Society was founded – in the early nineteenth century.[1]

English social life

Two decades of war with Revolutionary and Napoleonic France (1793–1815) had brought with it the worst possible scenario for the Industrial Revolution and the accompanying social changes which were, in Britain, in full swing. There was violent disruption of economic life, and a mood of 'anti-Jacobin' resentment to (and against) proposals for reform, together with much sympathy with the claims and sufferings of the poor.[2]

Although society in Britain remained, until the mid-nineteenth century, primarily rural, the Industrial Revolution resulted in London and the provincial towns growing into the vast overcrowded and insanitary conurbations of the 1830s.[3] This was therefore a period of urban expansion on a vast scale – ultimately recognised by Government, especially in the context of health and education. As Briggs has stressed, this transformation would have been impossible without the simultaneous development of an improved communications system – canals, and later railways.[4]

Governmental spending on the Napoleonic Wars had created a great deal of price-inflation; furthermore at the time of their termination there were several bad harvests; prices were high, and there was little work for the returning soldiers and sailors from the Wars. The aristocratic (ruling) class furthermore considered that town building, sanitation and factory conditions, although important to the 'masses', were not a direct concern of Government.

England's control of the seas at that time gave her a monopoly over many markets in America, Africa and the Far East, but European ones were either opened or closed to British goods according to the vagaries of diplomacy and war. These violent fluctuations of demand and employment had a profound (and usually deleterious) effect on the English working classes.

The Wars also had the effect of cutting off the supply of European corn – which had become necessary to steady food prices; therefore, between 1792 and 1812 wheat prices escalated. While this put money into the pockets of tenant farmers, freehold yeomen, and the receivers of tithes and rents, the poor (both urban and rural) suffered severely. Owing to the population explosion and a series of poor harvests, there was insufficient home-grown grain. In 1815, the Corn Laws (which governed both import and export of grain) were passed by Parliament; the aim was to restore agricultural prosperity at the expense of the consumer. For a generation to come (in fact, until the Repeal of the Corn Laws by Robert Peel [1788–1850] in 1846), the question of agricultural protection divided England – giving a political focus to differentiation between *urban* and *rural* life – which the ongoing Industrial Revolution was making more marked each year; as a result, town dwellers lost touch with farming, and village inhabitants with manufacture. Bread and cheese, washed down with beer or tea, became the staple diet of the labouring classes. Britain was thus experiencing two great divisions: *town against country,* and *rich against poor.*[5]

The democratic movement, inspired by the French Revolution, and also the writings of Thomas Paine (1737–1809), author of the '*Rights of Man*', was suppressed in the 1790s by both public opinion and Government action.[6] Despite this, the English village during the first half of the *nineteenth* century was still able to provide human '*exports*' (colonists) to overseas countries including Canada, Australia and New Zealand; the situation in post-war England assisted this great colonisation movement.[7] Relative overpopulation was at this time terrifying the contemporaries of Thomas Malthus (1766–1834).[8] However, whilst numerous English villagers were seeking employment overseas, many others had been drifting (especially during the Wars) into the *industrial* areas of Britain. Another large class constituted the unskilled labourers (or 'navvies'); these men were engaged in road and canal building, and shortly afterwards embankments and railway tunnels. At the opposite end of the spectrum (i.e. distanced from the ranks of the labourer) were skilled engineers and mechanics. In the midst of the Napoleonic Wars therefore, unemployment, low wages and starvation had been commonplace.

Many women, who had been deprived of their means of livelihood by the decay of cottage industries, entered fieldwork (alongside their husbands). Large capitalist farmers began employing gangs of women for hoeing and weeding; they had previously only turned out at hay-time and harvest. There was also an escalation of prostitution. At the other end of the social spectrum, 'ladies' (such as Florence Nightingale [1820–1910][9] and the Brontë sisters) were expected to conform to a very restricted life-style; as a result of the increasing wealth of men, their lives were rapidly becoming 'devitalised' and idle.[10]

The 'new age' also produced a substantial leisured class which had no direct relationship to the land, the professions, or to industry and trade. At the beginning of King George III's long reign (1760–1820), 'fund-holders' (who enjoyed an income secured by the national credit) numbered about 17,000; one-seventh of the total debt was held abroad – largely by Dutch investors. However *after* Waterloo (1815), only one twenty-fifth of Britain's colossal debt was in the hands of 'foreigners'.[11]

Religious revival

In Britain, a huge religious revival was taking place at all levels of society; this was initiated (and spread from below upwards) by 'anti-Jacobin panic' – based on a sharp revulsion from French 'atheism and deism'; this both survived the return of peace in 1815, and 'came to terms with the liberal reaction that followed'. The Victorian gentleman and his family were as a consequence more religious in their habits, and sober in their tone of thought, than their predecessors in the more light-hearted days of Horace Walpole (1717–1797) and Charles James Fox (1749–1806).[12] In the 'lower ranks' of society, a horror of French Republican atheism assisted the Wesleyan movement to spread more widely than ever; its founder, John Wesley (1703–91)[13] had died shortly before. The *Established* Church at that time possessed neither organisation nor zeal, especially in the new industrial districts, and this rôle was subsumed by the various Non-conformist sects (which were largely anti-French and generally conservative while the Wars lasted, and afterwards inspired by 'new evangelical vigour'). The Evangelicals of whom William Wilberforce (1759–1833) (*see* Figure 1.1), the 'Clapham Sect' (*see* Chapters 5 and 6), and Fowel Buxton (1786–1845) were to be numbered, cared less about the Church as an institution than about the 'saving of souls'.[14]

Humanitarianism became the order of the day, and co-operation in the name of the 'anti-slavery' movement took place between many diverse groups – including free-thinkers such as Jeremy Bentham (1748–1832)[15] and the utilitarians. In the opinion of Wilberforce, the Established Church 'obstructed the anti-slavery cause'. The bridge between Establishment and Dissident (as well as that between anti-Jacobin and Liberal) was clear in the Evangelical party, which had now assumed a position *within* the Church. Organised public opinion carried legal abolition of the Slave Trade in 1807, and Buxton took on the leadership (in the 1820s) of a campaign which triumphed in 1833; this was of course the year in which Wilberforce, who being a 'cross-bencher' was always ready to work with those of any party to abolish the slave trade, died.[16]

As the first half of the nineteenth century progressed, anti-Jacobin spirit receded, and there was a significant growth in humanitarianism, evangelicanism, and 'respectability' (see below); this change can be traced to the time of the Reform Bill of 1832. The popular prophet of this new phase was Charles Dickens (1812–70)[17]; and the age of Bentham (see above) and Henry Brougham (1778–1868)[18] was dawning; the movement for the abolition of negro-slavery aroused passionate popular approval, and the ill-treatment of children became a dominant theme in the public conscience. In the opinion of Trevelyan, a growth in humanitarianism rather than the massive advances in machinery and engineering was 'the thing of which the Nineteenth Century had best reason to be proud'.[19]

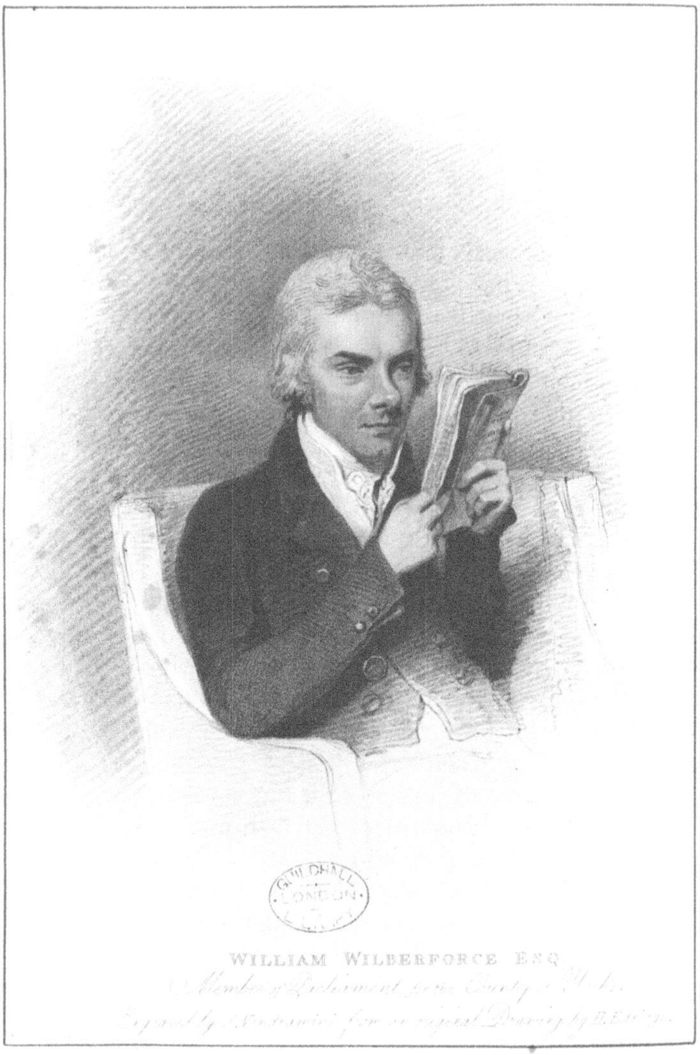

Figure 1.1: William Wilberforce MP (1759–1833): one of the nineteenth century's great philanthropists, prominent anti-slavery campaigner, and active participant in the establishment of the Society. [Courtesy, Guildhall Library, London].

British seafarers in the early nineteenth century

On the broad canvas which I have outlined above there arose a spirit of caring for the Seamen who had served Britain well during the Napoleonic Wars (*see* Chapter 2). The British Mercantile Marine, which together with the Royal Navy (RN) had thwarted the ambition(s) of Napoleon, was 'incomparably the greatest in the world'.[20] During the reign of King George IV (1762–1830) 2.5 million tonnage was still 'moved by wind and sail', but the era of iron and steam was dawning (see below). Between 1800 and 1830, *Trinity House* (*see* Chapter 5) established lighthouses and floating lights around the coasts of England, while docks were 'built in every considerable port town'.[21]

The Thames estuary still held unchallenged supremacy as the centre of trade for both Britain and the World; on the eve of the Reform Bill (see above), one quarter of the World's tonnage (including the great East Indiamen) was owned and registered in London; next were Newcastle (202,000 tons) and Liverpool [chiefly for the American trade (162,000 tons)], followed by Sunderland and Whitehaven. In war-time, the relationship of the RN with the merchant marine and the remainder of the seagoing population (including fishermen, whalers and smugglers), was all important – the major link being the 'press-gang' system (*see* Chapter 3) – a chaotic and iniquitous development! Bands armed with cutlasses were led by the King's officers from the RN to 'crimp' mariners and landsmen from ships 'in harbour or at sea, [and] from ale-houses and streets, or even at the church-door whence the bridegroom and members of the congregation were sometimes carried off'! This led to numerous problems – including the breaking up of families, and frequently recruitment of the most unsuitable individuals. Then, once on board the King's ship, the 'pressed' man was poorly paid, and subsisted on an unsatisfactory diet. The men, for all their ill-treatment, knew that the nation regarded them as 'its bulwark and glory'! This continued until the end of the century.[22]

The British Army in the early nineteenth century

In the last few years of the Napoleonic struggle(s) (from about 1810–15) the British army (greatly strengthened by Wellington's victories) became for a short time more popular than the navy. The British army, unlike her navy, consisted very largely of aristocrats who commanded privates (the 'scum of the earth'); few of them, however, looked to the army as their real means of livelihood and would return to their former lifestyle(s) after the battles. There was of course also an intermediate class – the non-commissioned officer. The French equivalent consisted very largely of conscripts. Major reasons for enlistment included: alcoholism, unemployment, and personal problems (involvement with a woman, or the law of the land). Following Waterloo, a small standing army was maintained; however, its popularity declined rapidly immediately the war was won! Overall, the nation felt that provided her navy was efficient, the army (which was essentially an aristocratic institution) could be safely neglected![23]

Growing importance of preventive medicine

By the mid-nineteenth century, hospitals in England had become well established, and medicine was largely community-based. But, the value of the hospital was generally recognised to be limited, *prevention* (on land as well as sea) being the overwhelming objective (*see* Figure 1.2), a fact which clearly dominated the scenario in the early days of the SHS.[24] Epidemic disease was extremely important (imported cases of smallpox, cholera and typhus were, for example, by no means unusual on hospital ships), but quarantine procedures (*see* Chapter 4) were operative against some of them; furthermore, sailors suffered from problems which also afflicted the non-maritime community, e.g. scurvy and sexually transmitted disease.

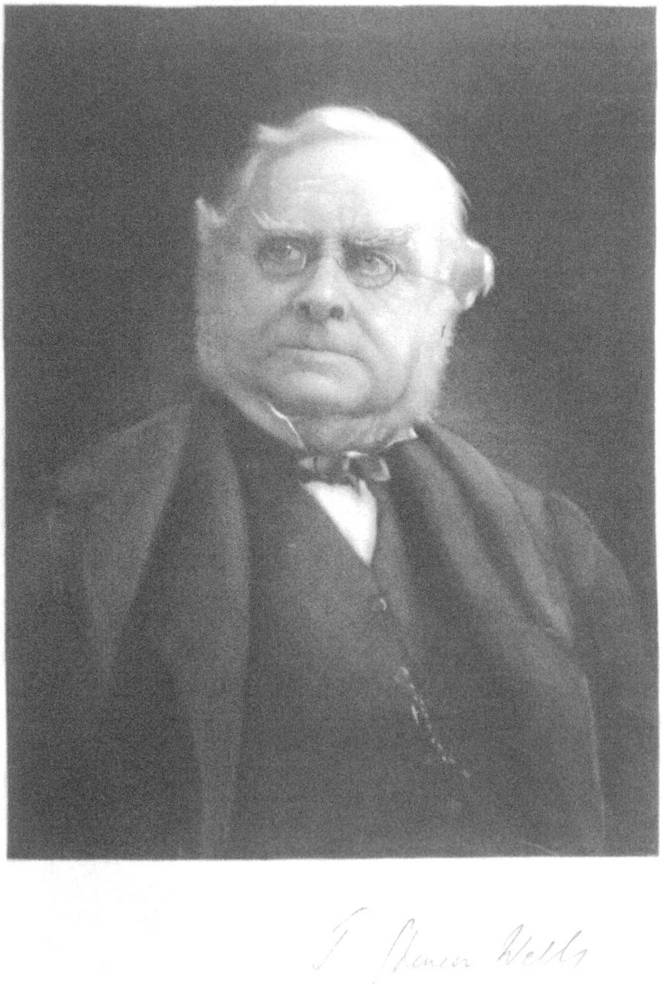

Figure 1.2: Sir Thomas Spencer Wells, Bt, FRCS (1818–1897) who during his naval career did much to improve the condition of the sea-farer. [*See also* J E Sewell. Wells, Sir Thomas Spencer, first baronet (1818–1897). In: H C G Matthew, B Harrison (eds). *Oxford Dictionary of National Biography*. Oxford: Oxford University Press 2004; 58 72–4]. [Courtesy, the Wellcome Library, London].

Epidemics were still regarded as 'Acts of God'; He sent them to 'Chasten and punish a wicked people'. The miasma-contagion controversy persisted. There was increasing concern about the rôle of environment on disease causation and this had a profound effect on imperial enterprises; James Lind (1716–94)[25] (*see* Figure 1.3) of the RN, who had experienced many tropical diseases in the warm climate of the West Indies, and John Pringle (1707–82)[26] (*see* Figure 1.4) of the army, were convinced that living in close proximity to other individuals, in an unsophisticated environment, encouraged disease transmission.[27] Therefore, good sanitation and ventilation were considered imperative; this view assumed monumental signifi-

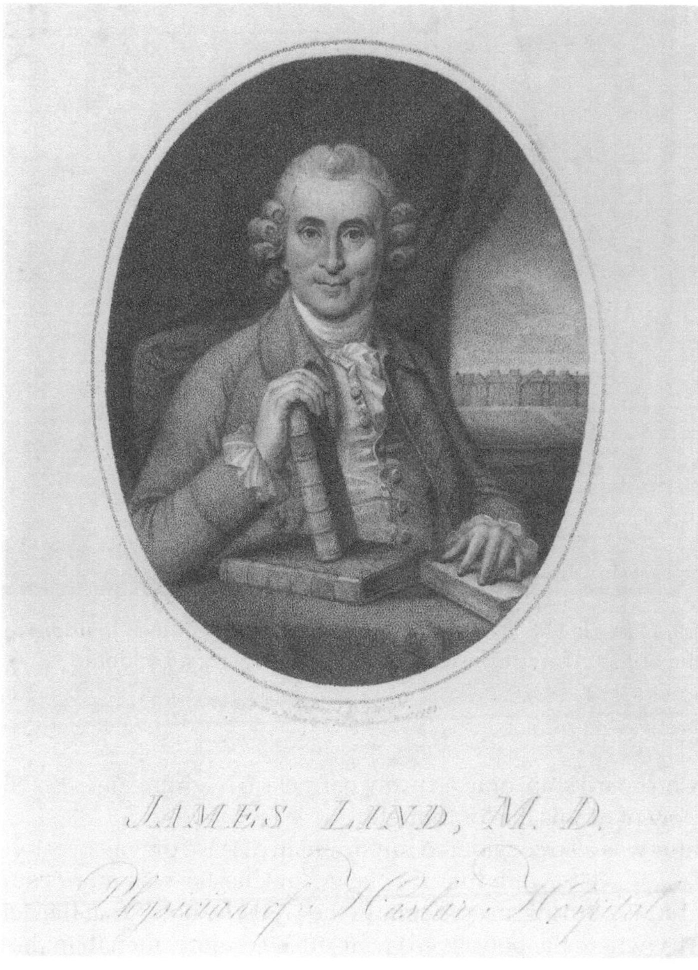

Figure 1.3: James Lind (1716–1794), of the RN, who established naval hospitals, and did much to improve health conditions in the RN [reproduced with permission, the Wellcome Library, London]. (*See also*: M Bartholomew. Lind, James (1716–1794). In: H C G Matthew, B Harrison (eds). *Oxford Dictionary of National Biography*. Oxford: Oxford University Press 2004; 33: 810–3. [Courtesy, the Wellcome Library, London].

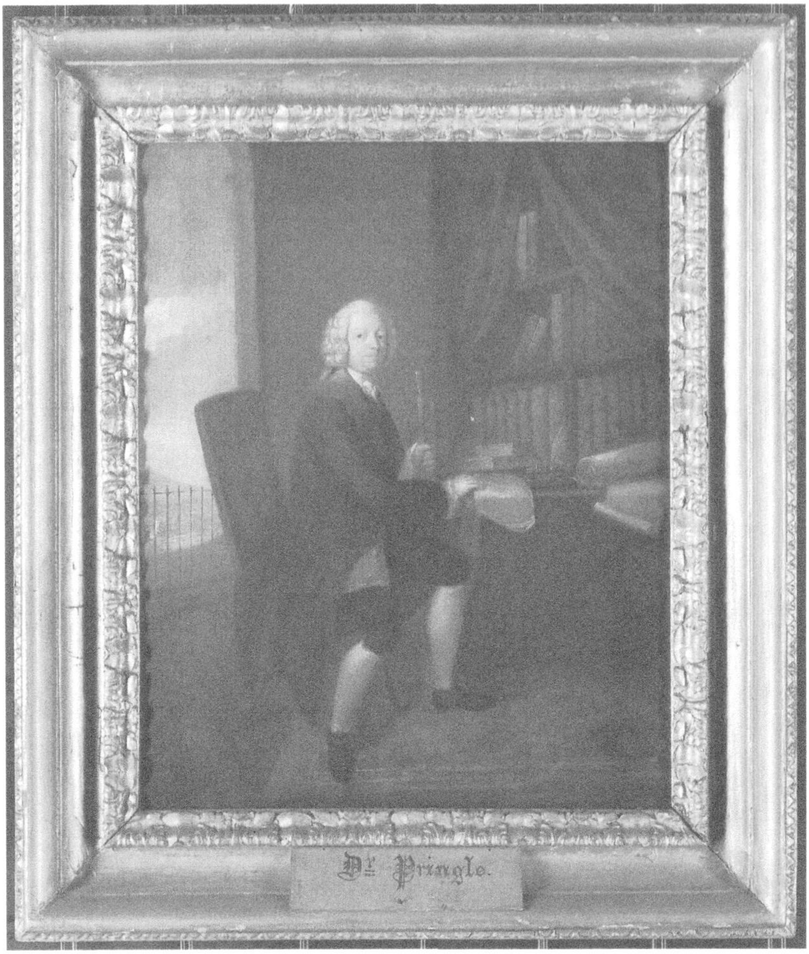

Figure 1.4: John Pringle FRS (1707–82) of the Army, who did much to improve the state of hygiene in the British Army. [Courtesy, the Wellcome Library, London].

cance in life on board ship, or in an army barracks[28]; Nightingale (see above) became a major exponent of this line of thought.

Social status was also considered important in disease prevalence. John Haygarth (1740–1827) was well aware that the 'fever' in Chester was more common in the lower social strata; during an epidemic in the 1770s, he noted that the densely populated suburbs (where the poor lived) were affected more often than the prosperous areas in the centre of the town.[29] Others (in addition to Haygarth) also started fever hospitals ('Houses of Recovery') in the 1790s and early 1800s; any contagious fever, with the exception of smallpox, qualified for admission, and early removal of the patient prevented his/her becoming a focus for the spread of infection. Patients did *not* require a formal recommendation from a hospital governor for these institutions, nor did they have to pay for admission; these facts made the *fever hospitals* totally different from the *general voluntary hospitals*.[30]

The fever hospitals were supported by the middle and upper-classes. The *Society for the Betterment of the Condition of the Poor* (SBCP) was one of numerous philanthropic societies founded during the early days of the Industrial Revolution. Although the SBCP had strong medical interests, it was also concerned with: education, living and working conditions, and above all moral 'purity'; such organisations (which were largely paternalistic) to which Wilberforce (see above) belonged, had Christian evangelical (Evangelical Anglicanism) zeal as their underlying *raison d'etre*. Wilberforce was in fact a Vice-President of the London Fever Hospital, and the seventh Earl of Shaftesbury (1801–85)[31] (see below), who was also profoundly evangelical in his outlook, became an active member of the General Board of Health (GBH) created in 1848. The major *medical* input to the GBH came from Thomas Southwood Smith (1788–1861).[32] Both Wilberforce and Shaftesbury (see above) were active Parliamentarians and helped pass much early social legislation – beginning with the Factory Act of 1802 (which dealt principally with child labour).

But there was another, very different, motive for the social reform of this period, i.e. to improve the Nation's efficiency; Bentham (see above) was the apostle of utilitarianism – a gospel of 'the greatest happiness for the greatest number'. He, amongst others, was aware that the Old Poor Laws were both ineffective and inappropriate for the new economic circumstances of the age; the Law attempted to distinguish between the 'worthy' (orphans, widows, injured or ill) and 'unworthy' (beggars, vagabonds and the wilfully unemployed) poor. *Paupers* could only be 'relieved' in a poorhouse (workhouse) of the parish of their birth. A major problem with this form of relief was that most parishes were too small to afford a workhouse – where it was expected that paupers should be accommodated. Many parishes hired the part-time services of a local doctor to provide medical care – because it was by then recognised that much poverty was health-related (see above). In 1832, Parliament at last ratified an enquiry into the operation of the Poor Laws; the nine Commissioners included three clergymen (all with an evangelical leaning) and two lawyers – one of whom, Edwin Chadwick (1800–90),[33] wrote the *Commissioners' Report* of 1834 which led to the Workhouse Amendment Act of that year. They felt that poverty was fundamentally a *moral* problem resulting from laziness, vice and moral decay which could be solved by simple Christian virtues.

Since the late sixteenth century, the English Poor Laws had sought to provide a 'net' to catch the deserving poor who, through death of a breadwinner, sickness, unemployment, inadequate wages or sheer misfortune, were unable to secure the bare necessities of life; the Poor Law embodied a rudimentary acceptance of responsibility for those who had fallen on hard times – many decades before creation of the Welfare State. To receive a meagre level of maintenance, removal to a poorhouse, or workhouse – where the able-bodied were expected to work – was necessary. Medical services of course provided only a fraction of the 'survival kit' for the unfortunate, but many Poor Law Guardians, hired the part-time service of local doctors to care for the sick and injured.[34]

Under the New Poor Law of 1834, the old Parish system was abolished – and replaced with larger units (or Unions) each of which incorporated a workhouse – with an associated infirmary and a Poor Law Medical Officer. Poor Law Commissioners were appointed (on a permanent basis) with the object of ascertaining that the Law was uniformly administered throughout the country. Chadwick was appointed Secretary, and in conjunction with medically qualified men – Southwood Smith (see above) and James Kay (later Sir James Kay-Shuttleworth 1804–77)[35] – became increasingly convinced of a clear relationship (a vicious circle) between poverty and poor living conditions, and disease. Chadwick became a firm believer (largely under the influence of Smith) that miasmata (before the 'germ theory' of disease was accepted) were the major cause(s) of illness resulting from: squalor, dirt and excrement. As a result he wrote: *Report on the Sanitary Conditions of the Labouring Population of Great Britain* (1842); 'filth diseases' could, he rightly felt, be prevented by social improvement(s) and engineering advances, rather than by medical means alone. Chadwick's *Report* was in fact published during a decade of intense political and social unrest; a series of bad harvests (see above) (there was a serious potato famine in Ireland between 1845 and 1849),[36] and this coupled with continuing operation of the Corn Laws (see above) led to widespread hardship amongst the poor. The anti-Corn Law League and Chartism (a working-class movement aimed at securing a legal right to form trade unions) occupied much public attention – greater in fact than the public health movement.[37]

There was thus at the time the SHS was founded in 1821 growing concern about deterioration of living conditions and increasing ill-health in the larger (industrial) towns and cities of Britain; 'consumption', 'convulsions', typhus, pneumonia, small-pox, dropsy, and 'debility' had become significant medical problems. Although the SHS was therefore set up to care for the sick or distressed seafarer, conditions on land were also very far from satisfactory.

References and notes

1 G M Trevelyan. Cobbett's England. I (1793–1832) In: *English Social History: a survey of six centuries, Chaucer to Queen Victoria.* London: Longmans, Green & Co. 1944: 463–485. [*See also:* A Briggs. The experience of industrialization. In: *A social history of England.* 3rd ed. London: Penguin 1999: 205–228].

2 The *Jacobin* period occupied the years from about 1792 until 1822, during which the SHS had its origin. The term denoted a sympathizer with the principles of the French Revolution, an extreme radical in politics or in social organisation. It had originally been used in a descriptive sense of a French political club (or society) established in Paris in 1789, in the old convent belonging to the Jacobins, to maintain and propagate the principles of extreme democracy and absolute equality. Around 1800 it became a nick-name for any political reformer. [*See also:* J A Simpson, E S C Weiner (eds.) *Oxford English Dictionary* 2nd ed. 1989; 8: 173–174].

3 W F Bynum. Medicine in the community. In: *Science and the practice of Medicine in the nineteenth century*. Cambridge: Cambridge University Press 1994: 55–91.

4 *Op cit.* See note 1 above (Briggs).

5 *Op cit.* See note 1 above. [*See also:* J Prest. Peel, Sir Robert, second baronet (1788–1850). In: H C G Matthew, B Harrison (eds). *Oxford Dictionary of National Biography.* Oxford: Oxford University Press 2004; 43: 406–18].

6 **Thomas Paine** (1737–1809) was both an author and revolutionary. [*See also:* M Philp. *Paine.* Oxford: Oxford University Press 1989; J Keane. *Tom Paine: a political life.* London: Bloomsbury 1996; M Philp. Paine, Thomas (1737–1809) In: H C G Matthew, B Harrison (eds). *Oxford Dictionary of National Biography.* Oxford: Oxford University Press 2004; 42: 398–413].

7 R Hughes. *The fatal shore: a history of the transportation of convicts to Australia, 1787–1868.* London: Collins Harvill 1987: 688.

8 J Bonar. *Malthus and his work.* London: Macmillan 1885: 432; P James. *Population Malthus: his life and times.* London: Routledge & Kegan Paul 1979: 524. [*See also:* J M Pullen. Malthus, (Thomas) Robert (1766–1834). In: H C G Matthew, B Harrison (eds). *Oxford Dictionary of National Biography.* Oxford: Oxford University Press 2004; 36: 365–370].

9 E T Cook. *The life of Florence Nightingale.* Vols 1 (1820–1861) and 2 (1862–1910). London: MacMillan & Co 1913. [*See also:* C. Woodham-Smith. *Florence Nightingale 1820–1910.* London: Constable 1950; M E Baly, H C G Matthew. Nightingale, Florence (1820–1910). In: H C G Matthew, B Harrison (eds). *Oxford Dictionary of National Biography.* Oxford: Oxford University Press 2004; 40: 904–912].

10 *Op cit.* See note 1 above. (Trevelyan).

11 *Op cit.* See note 1 above (Briggs); C Hibbert. *George III: a personal history.* London: Viking 1998: 464.

12 *Op cit.* See note 1 above (Trevelyan). [*See also:* P Langford. Walpole, Horacio [Horace], fourth earl of Orford (1717–1797). In: H C G Matthew, B Harrison (eds). *Oxford Dictionary of National Biography.* Oxford: Oxford University Press 2004; 57: 49–63; L G Mitchell. Fox, Charles James (1749–1806). *Ibid;* 20: 609–622].

13 H D Rack. Wesley [Westley], John (1703–1791). In: H C G Matthew, B Harrison (eds). *Oxford Dictionary of National Biography.* Oxford: Oxford University Press 2004; 58: 182–193. [*See also*: J Wesley. *Primitive physick: or an easy and natural method of curing most diseases.* Bristol: William Pine. 1770: 156; S Ayling. *John Wesley.* London: Collins 1979: 350; R Hattersley. *John Wesley: a brand from the burning.* London: Little Brown 2003: 457].

14 **William Wilberforce** (1759–1833) was MP for Hull and an outstanding philanthropist. He possessed strict religious views (he took part in the foundation of the Church Missionary and the Bible Societies), and was an ardent campaigner for the abolition of slavery – especially in the West Indies. He was also a founding member of the Seamen's Hospital Society and its predecessor. [*See also*: J Pollock. *Wilberforce.* London: Constable 1977: 368; J Wolffe. Wilberforce, William (1759–1833). In: H C G Matthew, B Harrison (eds). *Oxford Dictionary of National Biography.* Oxford: Oxford University Press 2004; 58: 879–87; W. Hague. *William Wilberforce: the life of the great anti-slave campaigner.* London: Harper Press 2007: 582.] [*See also*: G C Cook. *The Incurables movement: an illustrated history of the British Home.* Oxford: Radcliffe Publishing 2006: 58–9]. **Sir Thomas Fowell Buxton** (1786–1845) was a noted philanthropist who advocated the abolition of slavery in the British dominions (1822–33) [*See also:* O M Blouet. Buxton, Sir Thomas Fowell, first baronet. (1786–1845). In: H C G Matthew, B Harrison (eds). *Oxford Dictionary of National Biography.* Oxford: Oxford University Press 2004; 9: 292–4].

15 **Jeremy Bentham** (1748–1832) was a barrister, whose major contributions were in ethics, jurisprudence, logic and political economy. He was a champion of utilitarianism, a movement, the underlying principle of which was 'the greatest happiness for the greatest number'. [*See also*: F Rosen. Bentham, Jeremy (1748–1832). In: H C G Matthew, B Harrison (eds). *Oxford Dictionary of National Biography.* Oxford: Oxford University Press 2004; 5: 221–34].

16 N Grant. *The Savage Trade.* Harmondsworth, Middlesex: Kestrel Books 1980; H. Thomas. *The Slave Trade. The history of the Atlantic Slave Trade: 1440–1870.* London: Picador 1997.

17 **Charles Dickens** (1812–1870) was arguably the foremost of nineteenth century British novelists. In addition, he was also one of the great social reformers and philanthropists of the nineteenth century. P Ackroyd. *Dickens* London: Sinclair-Stevenson 1990: 1195; M Slater. Dickens, Charles John Huffam (1812–1870). In: H C G Matthew, B Harrison (eds). *Oxford Dictionary of National Biography.* Oxford: Oxford University Press 2004; 16: 59–78.

18 **Henry Brougham** (1778–1868). *See* M Lobban. Brougham, Henry Peter, first Baron Brougham and Vaux (1778–1868). In: H C G Matthew, B Harrison (eds). *Oxford Dictionary of National Biography.* Oxford: Oxford University Press 2004; 7: 970–80.

19 *Op cit.* See note 1 above (Trevelyan).

20 *Ibid.*

21 *Op cit.* See note 1 above. [*See also* K Wheatley. *National Maritime Guide to Maritime Britain.* Exeter: Webb & Bower 1990: 208; A Burton. *The Daily Telegraph Guide to Britain's Maritime Past.* London: Aurum Press 2003; 174; Anonymous *Trinity House.* London: Trinity House (undated): 12].

22 *Ibid;* T Smollett. *The adventures of Roderick Random* Oxford: Oxford University Press 1979: 481. [*See also:* J Schneer. *London 1900; the Imperial metropolis.* London: Yale University Press 1999: 336].

23 **Arthur Wellesley** (later, the first Duke of Wellington) (1769–1852) had an outstanding military career culminating in his victory at Waterloo in 1815. He was Prime-Minister from 1828 until 1830. The Battle of Waterloo (18 June 1815) was fully reported by an anonymous writer in *The Times* for 22 June 1815. [See also: N Gash. Wellesley [*formerly* Wesley], Arthur, first duke of Wellington (1769–1852). In: H C G Matthew, B Harrison (eds). *Oxford Dictionary of National Biography.* Oxford: Oxford University Press 2004; 58: 1–27; D Gates. The transformation of the Army. In: D Chandler, *The Oxford Illustrated History of the British* Army. Oxford: Oxford University Press 1994: 133–59. *Times, Lond* 1815; 22 June: 2–4).

24 *Op cit.* See note 3 above; G C Cook. Thomas Spencer Wells, Bt, FRCS (1818–97) and his contributions to Naval Medicine. *J Med Biog* 2007; 15: 63–67. [*See also* J E Sewell. Wells, Sir Thomas Spencer, first baronet (1818–1897). In: H C G Matthew, B Harrison (eds). *Oxford Dictionary of National Biography.* Oxford: Oxford University Press 2004; 58: 72–4].

25 M Bartholomew. Lind, James (1716–1794). In: H C G Matthew, B Harrison (eds). *Oxford Dictionary of National Biography.* Oxford: Oxford University Press 2004; 33: 810–3.

26 J S G Blair. Pringle, Sir John, first baronet (1707–1782). In: H C G Matthew, B Harrison (eds). *Oxford Dictionary of National Biography.* Oxford: Oxford University Press 2004: 45: 398–400.

27 *Op cit.* See note 3 above. [*See also* G C Cook. *From the Greenwich Hulks to Old St Pancras: a history of tropical disease in London.* London: Athlone Press 1992: 338].

28 *Op cit.* See notes 24, 25, 26 above.

29 **John Haygarth** (1740–1827) who had Quaker origins, was a physician to the Chester Infirmary; S Harrison. Haygarth, John (1740–1827). In: H C G Matthew, B Harrison (eds). *Oxford Dictionary of National Biography.* Oxford: Oxford University Press 2004; 26: 44–5.

30 H Richardson (ed) Hospitals for Infectious Diseases. In: *English Hospitals (1660–1948): a survey of their architecture and design.* Swindon: Royal Commission on the historical monuments of England 1998: 132–53; C B Carruthers, L A Carruthers. *A history of Britain's Hospitals.* Lewes: The Book Guild 2005: 430.

31 J L Hammond, B Hammond. *Lord Shaftesbury.* 4th ed. London: Longmans, Green & Co. 1936: 323; G Battiscombe. *Shaftesbury: a biography of the seventh earl 1801–1885.* London: Constable 1974: 365; GBAM Finlayson. *The seventh earl of Shaftesbury 1801–1185.* London: Eyre Methuen 1981: 639; J Wolffe. Cooper, Anthony Ashley – seventh earl of Shaftesbury

(1801–1885) In: H C G Matthew, B Harrison (eds). *Oxford Dictionary of National Biography.* Oxford: Oxford University Press 2004; 13: 223–7.

32 R K Webb. Smith (Thomas) Southwood (1788–1861). In: H C G Matthew, B Harrison (eds). *Oxford Dictionary of National Biography.* Oxford: Oxford University Press 2004; 51: 310–3. [*See also:* GC Cook. Thomas Southwood Smith FRCP (1788–1861): leading exponent of diseases of poverty and pioneer of sanitary reform in the mid-nineteenth century. *J Med Biog* 2002; 10: 194–205].

33 **Edwin Chadwick** (1800–90) was by profession a lawyer. He visited many parishes in order to observe the Old Poor Laws in operation. Chadwick wrote the 22-volume *Commissioners' Report* (of 1834) which was an in-depth social survey, and showed that under that system, relief for able-bodied individuals was too easy to acquire. He wrote his classical *Report on the Sanitary Conditions of the Labouring Population of Great Britain* in 1842. [*See* P Mandler. Chadwick, Sir Edwin (1800–1890). In: H C G Matthew, B Harrison (eds). *Oxford Dictionary of National Biography.* Oxford: Oxford University Press 2004; 10: 836–40].

34 D Fraser. *The Welfare State.* Stroud, Gloucestershire: Sutton Publishing Ltd. 2000: 120; T May. *The Victorian Workhouse.* Haverfordwest, Pembrokeshire: Shire Publications Ltd. 2002: 32. [*See also Op cit. See* note 30 above (Richardson, 54–75)].

35 **James Kay** (1804–1877). R J W Selleck. Shuttleworth, Sir James Kay-, first baronet (1804–1877). In: H C G Matthew, B Harrison (eds). *Oxford Dictionary of National Biography.* Oxford: Oxford University Press 2004; 50: 473–6.

36 C Woodham Smith. *The Great Hunger: Ireland 1845–1849.* London: Penguin Books 1991. p510.

37 A Briggs. *Chartism.* Stroud, Gloucestershire: Sutton Publishing Ltd. 1998: 112.

Chapter 2

Britain's major maritime organisations, shipyards, and London's docks

Historically, sea-transport can be summarised under three headings: (i) man-power, (ii) wind-power, and (iii) mechanical power. Although Britain's *merchant navy* had existed since the 'dawn of history', and from its origin(s) had been involved in the trading of goods (both for everyday and luxury use) (see below), the Royal Navy (RN) – a fighting force – can trace its origins only as far back as King Henry VIII (1491–1547) or conceivably Henry V (1387–1422), although '... romantics claim it dates to King John (1167[?]–1216)', or even to the fleet that King Alfred (849–899) assembled to fight the Danes. Although a definitive date for its origin is therefore impossible (it slowly *evolved* from the King's Ships without the formality of a Royal charter). A more acceptable date is probably 1660, i.e. during the reign of King Charles II (1630–85).

The *Oxford English Dictionary* merely defines the RN as 'the navy of the UK and its predecessors'.* Its prestige and power in Victorian times was largely based upon its success(es) during the Napoleonic Wars, and in particular Admiral Lord Nelson's (1758–1805) (see below) victory at Trafalgar on 21 October 1805. Until the formation of the RN, lifestyles at all levels of maritime existence lacked organisation; 'officers' were appointed (usually on a short term basis) by the Navy Board, while the ordinary seamen, who were often compelled to serve by 'press gangs', were usually hired for a single voyage only – as was the case in the Merchant Navy.[1]

The Mercantile Marine (Merchant Navy)

Britain has, since time immemorial, been heavily dependent on her Merchant Navy. Since Neolithic times, it has harvested fish (from the sea) and traded goods abroad. As early as 1500 BC, boats were ferrying goods across the Humber estuary, while tin was exported to Europe in ingots. During the Roman occupation (c. 50–400 AD), the British Isles formed one component of a large trading network, centred on the Mediterranean; Roman vessels brought goods to London, and took away raw materials. After the end of the Roman empire, trade with Frisian ports continued; it attained renewed momentum with the Viking settlements from late in the ninth century, bring-

*J A Simpson, ESC Weiner (eds). *Oxford English Dictionary* 2nd ed. 1989; 14: 183.

ing Britain into close contact with: Scandinavia, Russia, Iceland, and beyond. In 1066, the Norman Conquest brought trading links with France and the Mediterranean.[2] In medieval England, an increase in trading evolved; for example, wool was exported to the Low Countries via London, Hull and Southampton, whilst wine was imported from Bordeaux. Meanwhile, Venetian galleys visited English ports. The Baltic and North Sea trade was dominated by the Hanseatic League, which was a mercantile association of German ports – with branches in Scandinavia, England and the Netherlands. The English Navigation Acts date back to the late fourteenth century.[3]

As a result of important Spanish and Portuguese discoveries (the age of the great explorers), a totally new trade pattern emerged after about 1550; English merchants became interested in long distance trade routes – to the Orient and Russia. Three important voyages were made at this time by Sir James Lancaster (1554/5–1618): (i) to Achin (on the Sumatran coast) (1592); (ii) a plundering expedition to the West Indies (1594); and (iii) the first expedition of the English East India Company (EIC) (1601–3) (see below) (of which Lancaster was leader) which established a trading post at Achin.[4]

In the seventeenth century, the EIC (with its distinctive pink and white striped flag – see below) chartered large ships, and imported valuable cargoes of porcelain, silk and tea from China. Also, in the north Atlantic, the 'triangular trade' developed: slaves were carried from Africa to the Americas, the ships returning to England laden with tobacco, timber, sugar and rum, and thence to Africa with textiles, etc.[5] As her American colonies grew more wealthy, Britain exported both luxuries and manufactured goods.

By 1750, approximately 50% of British registered shipping was involved in the American trade. Overall, the combined effect(s) of the Navigation Acts and monopolies of the great chartered companies, led to a great increase in English commerce and shipping. Throughout the eighteenth century, the wars with France had seriously disrupted commercial transactions between the two countries; a positive result was, however, uncontested control of the Indian and American routes. As coastal and European trade(s) expanded, shipbuilding (see below) flourished. By the late eighteenth century, British industry sought even more substantial opportunities, and began to break up the older chartered monopolies.[6]

In the nineteenth century (a period widely known as 'Pax Brittanica') the merchant service reached its zenith; there was increasing 'free trade' worldwide. This century also saw a transition from wood to steel, and from sail to steam. The merchant navy was carrying much mercantile material, but it also began transporting passengers to the 'new world'. From the 1850s also, cable-laying ships conveyed the international electric telegraph system; which produced immediate links with most parts of the world.[7] Prior to the increased efficiency of steamships for long voyages, the design of sailing ships evolved to meet new demands for: increased speed, greater cargo space and smaller crews. Iron (followed by steel) sailing ships were built – many at Clydeside, Tyneside, and Teeside. The fast sailing vessels (including 'tea clippers' – typified by the 'Cutty Sark') sailed round the world – utilising the trade-winds; these took emigrants to Australia (via the Cape of Good Hope) and returned with wool (via Cape Horn). It was not until 1885, that steam tonnage actually overtook sail![8]

Functions of the Merchant Navy in recent times

During the late nineteenth century and up to the 1960s, the mercantile marine has therefore undertaken three major tasks: (i) *industrialisation*, (ii) *fishing*, and (iii) the organisation of *passenger lines*. Development of the steam-ship in the mid-nineteenth century revolutionised world trading; as a result of her vast resources of coal and iron, Britain led the field.

INDUSTRIALISATION

By 1830, British shipping tonnage was estimated at 6.5 million (40% steam-driven), but by 1914 this figure had leapt to 22.5 million (95% steam). The markets of the British Empire and Europe were linked by fast and regular liners operated by major shipping countries and using fixed routes – no longer dependent on winds and seasons. The SS *Agamemnon* – built for Alfred Holt of Liverpool in 1865 – together with her sister ships, was, for example, able to travel (by steam) for 8,000 miles without a refuel. Perishable foodstuffs were for the first time carried under refrigerated conditions. New enclosed docks were constructed at major ports, and these were serviced by both railways and roads. Smaller companies merged to form larger organisations, and seamen and dockers formed unions seeking improved pay and better conditions of service. Today, the bulk of the world's merchandise continues to be carried by sea; however, most is transported in container ships and bulk carriers; although these require far fewer sailors, and specialised port facilities are necessary.[9]

FISHING

Fishing was always a major function of the merchant navy. The North Atlantic has been the most important cod fishing ground since the fourteenth century; hand-lines and baited hooks were originally used. The North Sea herring grounds have been exploited by the Dutch (using large deep sea drift nets) from the fifteenth century. From the sixteenth century, the Grand Banks off Newfoundland have been fished for cod, which were gutted, salted and dried on shore, before being transported as 'stockfish' to Europe. Large herring fleets were established in eastern coastal ports of Britain (including Great Yarmouth and Lowestoft) during the eighteenth century; the 'drifting method' (curtains of netting were suspended below the sea's surface to enmesh shoals of fish by their gills) was increasingly used. An increasing demand for cod during the nineteenth century led to the development of trawling at, for example, Brixham, Fleetwood, Hull and Scarborough; this procedure involves dragging sack-like nets along the sea-bed to entrap great quantities of fish.[10]

PASSENGER LINES

The merchant service has over the last century or so, also possessed *passenger liners*; these subsequently provided links across the world – for businessmen, emigrants, tourists, and mail – before the advent of air transport. First passenger liners had in fact operated along US rivers in the early nineteenth century; by 1825, paddle-steamers were sailing along the coasts of Britain, and in 1826, the *General Steamship Navigation Company* began operating a route from London, to Lisbon and Gibraltar.

By 1850, services to India and Hong Kong, and across the Atlantic had been established; these were financed by British and US mail contracts. The Peninsula and Oriental (P&O) system carried mail to Hong Kong, and the Royal Mail Steam Packet Company secured the West Indies route.

From these early beginnings the great passenger liners, which before the advent of extensive air travel (in the 1950s and 60s) were the sole links across the oceans: the Cunard and White Star Lines for example, competed for the fastest Atlantic crossing (the 'Blue Ribband'); both size and luxury features increased steadily until the *Queen Elizabeth,* with a tonnage of 85,000, was launched in 1940.[11] Although luxury liners still exist, the vast majority of travellers currently use air transport.

The East India Company (EIC)

Intimately associated with the development of Britain's merchant navy was the EIC.[12] It was founded in 1600 by Queen Elizabeth I in order 'to set forth on a voyage to the East Indies and other islands and countries'; the Company was presented with a monopoly on all trade with the East Indies. The initial plan was to set up a trading station to secure pepper and spices from the great market at Bantam (now Jakarta), in south-east Asia. The Portuguese had already traded with that area for about a century, and the Dutch had arrived in Bantam six years earlier.

Five vessels sailed from the Thames on 2 April 1601 (see below), reached the East Indies in 1602, and returned home, with 'valuable cargoes of pepper and other exotic commodities' on 16 June 1603. They were:

- the '*Malice Scourge*' (*Red Dragon*) of 600 tons, with 202 men and captained by John Davis;
- the '*Hector*' (300 tons, 108 men);
- the '*Ascension*' (260 tons, 82 men);
- the '*Susan*' (240 tons, 88 men);
- the '*Gift*' (a 130 tons, victualling ship).

They carried goods of an estimated worth of £7000, and a cargo consisting of £28,472 worth of bullion. By the time they reached Table Bay, 105 men had died, most from scurvy (*see* Chapter 4). The second expedition set out from England in 1604; an EIC dockyard was opened at Deptford in 1609, a factory at Surat, India (which was transferred to Bombay in 1662) in 1612, and 'trading stations' at Fort George (Madras – now Chennai) and Bengal in 1639 and 1640, respectively. In 1784, the duty on tea was reduced from 100 to 12½%; this led to a vast increase in the British popularity of tea – one of the largest commodities.

The Company became extremely powerful and remained in control of trade to the East until 1833; any ship wishing to sail to the East had to obtain a licence from the Company, whose headquarters were at East India House, and all goods imported from that region had to be landed at the Company's wharves in the Port of London (see below). The EIC ships (or East Indiamen) were the largest, best built, most expensive and most heavily armed merchant ships of their day; they had crews of up to 130 men.[12]

The officers wore uniforms not unlike those worn by sailors in the Navy, and were trained to defend their valuable cargoes from pirates. Life at sea was, however, harsh and dirty, and the work – which was very physical – often dangerous; one of the most difficult tasks was the adjustment of the sails in rough weather. Much illness (including scurvy [*see* Chapter 4]) resulted, and many sailors died of tropical diseases – especially whilst in the East. To make up crew numbers on the return voyage(s), Indian Seamen (Lascars) many of them from Bengal, the Punjab or western India, were recruited; the EIC was, or should have been, responsible for their well-being whilst in London (*see* Chapter 3).

By the late eighteenth century, the EIC controlled all opium grown in Bengal; insidiously, the illegal export of opium from India to China grew (despite the fact that the Chinese Emperor had outlawed its import). Private traders took the drug to China; their ships anchored off the Chinese coast and Chinese smugglers bought it in exchange for silver. The British fought several opium wars with China (beginning in 1840) in order to secure trading rights along the south-east coast of China.[13] In 1858, English and French soldiers marched on Peking – where on the orders of the eighth Earl of Elgin (1811–63) (the British Commander) they plundered, looted and burned the Emperor's Summer Palace.[14]

It was very largely due to the EIC that the British mercantile ship-building industry became well established on the River Thames; following failure of their private yard at Deptford, most ship-building was carried out at Blackwall. When the SHS was founded in 1821, several retired commanders from the EIC (in the Honorable Company's Service [HCS]) took an active rôle in management; furthermore, in the early SHS minutes (*see* Appendix I), EIC personnel are to be found amongst its staff and patients.

The Royal Navy (RN)

It will now be clear to the reader that the Merchant Navy had evolved over several millennia. However, in the latter years of its existence, the RN provided a closely allied profession. In fact, the RN has become over the last few centuries, the 'functioning instrument for the purpose of maintaining Great Britain's safety, wealth and strength'. It also, in the eighteenth and nineteenth centuries, became popular with the British masses; in 1740, for example, the patriotic song 'Rule Britannia' was first sung.

During the eighteenth century, the RN rapidly increased in size; in 1713 it numbered some 48,000, and by 1813, 142,000. Not surprisingly, annual expenditure rocketed – surges usually being restricted to times of war. Most of the administration – both afloat and in the dockyards – was carried out by the Commissioners of the Navy (the Navy Board); this body was responsible for victualling as well as for the welfare of naval personnel.[15] Between 1740 and 50, care of the sick sailor came to the fore, and work began on permanent naval hospitals, that at Haslar being pre-eminent.[16]

History of the RN

Naval-power was essential (until the advent of the aeroplane) for the survival of this 'island race', a fact that can be traced back to Roman, Saxon, and Medieval times.[17] Roman naval power (based on the galley) had been founded in the Mediterranean. Towards the end of Roman rule, 'Courts of the Saxon shore' were set up on the east coast in order to resist raids by Angles, Saxons and Jutes. Anglo-Saxon kingdoms – which had been founded by sea-raiders – were attacked by Viking longships (from Scandinavia), from around 800 AD. King Alfred (see above) responded by building similar warships. However, the shores of Britain were always vulnerable to sea-borne attack, and invasions by Norwegians and Normans took place in 1066 AD. The Norman and Plantagenet kings ruled on both sides of the Channel, relying on a fleet of hired and converted merchant ships – most provided by either London or the Cinque Ports. The earliest necessity for an *organised* Navy probably dates to the Hundred Years War (1338–1453); victories over France prevented invasion, and allowed Kings Edward III and Henry V to invade (and conquer) substantial parts of France.

King Henry VIII had, as one of his numerous ambitions, to make England a major world power. He established dockyards (see below) to build royal ships, and to repair old ones. Although hired merchant-ships still made up the bulk of the fighting force, a small permanent Royal fleet was established during his reign.

By 1520, an embryonic *admiralty* was formed. Britain's navy provided escorts for the 'merchant adventurers'. Deptford was and remained for many years the most important dockyard in the UK. By 1540, Henry VIII possessed 45 ships – all but 10 of which had a tonnage >100; between 1543 and 45, three more (all with a tonnage >400) were constructed. In 1545 the navy was granted a new name: 'The King's majesty's council of his marine', and the following year, the Navy Board was established to organise supply, and financial aspects of the RN. By Elizabeth I's time, English privateers (with Royal approval) were attacking Spanish ships, and returning from the newly discovered Americas with plundered silver. This, together with English help for the Dutch (in their revolt against Spain) led in 1588 to the dispatch of ships to oppose the Armada, the English fleet consisting of 34 Royal and 192 hired (merchant) ships. Following this, the Royal fleet remained small; privateering continued as the major war-like force.[18]

By about 1600, England and Holland began challenging Spain and Portugal for the opening of the *long distance* trade-routes (see above); rivalry developed in the North Sea, and also in the Mediterranean and Far East – where English and Dutch East India Companies competed. Under the direction of Samuel Pepys (1633–1703) of the Navy Board and James, Duke of York (1633–1701) (Lord High Admiral) the English navy slowly emerged.[19] A permanent force of warships and professional officers, with established fighting instructions, was established during the Dutch Wars (1652–74). Following the 'Glorious Revolution' of 1688, Britain and the Netherlands united under William and Mary, and the major enemy immediately became France.

The first *admiralty* building dated from 1699; this modest establishment was replaced by the present building (to the south of Trafalgar Square) in 1725. From there, messages were conveyed via a system of hilltop telegraphs linked to all major ports of England. The First Lord of the Admiralty was automatically a member of the Cabinet.

During the eighteenth century, both Britain and France established colonial outposts in India and North America and rivalry between them intensified. By the middle of the century, the RN had become in effect, a 'standing navy'.[20] Major administrative reforms had by then taken place: (i) the Board of Admiralty (with a large secretariat) had been formed, (ii) the advent of an efficient victualling department was effected, (iii) well developed overseas bases (see below) were created, and (iv) the evolution of a system of seniority took place. By 1748, there was a standard uniform for officers in the RN. A system of 'half-pay' for those serving on land also came into operation, and superannuation for sea-officers was established.[21]

The Seven-Years War (1756–63) marked the summation of a strategy designed to damage both French trade and colonial links (in addition to protecting their own) – by Britain's colonial policy. French fleets were blockaded at Brest and Toulon – and chased when they attempted to exit; this in turn left the French forces in Canada, India and the West Indies unsupported from Europe. The conquest of French Canada was dependent on amphibious operations against Louisbourg (1758) and Quebec (1759). Martinique and Grenada fell to Britain, whilst French forces were driven from India. Meanwhile, British Naval power prevented the loss of India and the British West Indian Islands during the French Revolution (1775–83); France and Spain supported the Americas. In consequence the Deptford, Woolwich, Chatham, Sheerness, Plymouth and Portsmouth dockyards (see below) were enlarged in order to implement a massive shipbuilding programme; this involved a vast amount of timber as well as many thousands of men.

The RN in recent times

British efforts were, in the late eighteenth and early nineteenth centuries directed to preventing invasion, and safeguarding trade, revolutionary France (*see* Chapter 1) being the major threat. Britain rose to new heights of military might – supported by her own *industrial revolution*. From the late eighteenth century, naval officers had adopted more flexible battle tactics compared with the rigid ones laid down in the early days of the century. British victories were gained at the 'Glorious First of June' (1794), Camperdown and St. Vincent (1797), the Nile (1798), Copenhagen (1800) and of course Trafalgar (1805) itself. Decisive victories at the latter three battles had been won by Nelson. In fact, Britain's naval strength led to the defeat of Napoleon's attempts to close Europe to British trade; meanwhile, an army was sent to Portugal to open a new war front. Approximately 60% of Britain's budget for the armed services went to the RN (by then the 'Senior Service'). Levies were placed on imported malt, tobacco and candles.

In the late nineteenth and twentieth centuries, vast changes took place in the RN: wooden hulks became redundant; new classes of warship evolved, and older ones changed their function. Torpedo-boats, submarines and mines were introduced; later the aircraft carrier was developed, making the battleship largely obsolete. Britain had emerged from the great wars with France as the greatest worldwide naval power; for a century (from 1805) Britain policed the seas (the 'Pax Brittanica'), its major activity being protection of her *maritime* trade. In 1854, war with Russia broke out (the Crimean War); tension arose with France (provoked by colonial rivalry and attempts to modernise the French navy). The Fisher-Selbourne initiative of 1903 laid the foundations of the principle that all officers, seamen, engineers, and Royal Marines should be of one company.[22] Finally, a naval arms race with the growing might of Germany led to the Great War of 1914–18. Following the 1939–45 war, the USA and USSR emerged as 'supernations', nuclear submarines and guided missiles transforming naval warfare.[23]

Shipbuilding in Britain

In 1690, all Royal dockyards (with the exception of Portsmouth) were sited in the Thames basin. Two others were situated at Blackwall and Rotherhithe. Deptford and Woolwich were, however, unsuitable for rapid refits. During the eighteenth century, facilities at both Portsmouth and Plymouth were greatly improved and enlarged. Also, at this time a great deal of shipbuilding was taking place at Buckler's Hard shipyard – situated at a small village on the Beaulieu River.[24]

Before 1815, most ships had in fact been built in private yards (where regular inspections, ventilation and repairs were also undertaken), although the naval authorities would have preferred *all* building to have taken place in the Royal dockyards. During the eighteenth century overseas bases were established at: Gibraltar, Minorca, Malta, Jamaica, Antigua and Halifax.[25] Dry-docks were essential for cleaning the keels of ships, repairing masts, and replacing worm-eaten sheathing.

When the Deptford Master-shipwright, Sir Thomas Slade (1713/14–1771), had been appointed Surveyor of the Navy, in 1755 (as a result of Admiral Lord Anson's influence)[26] the quality of British ships improved rapidly, copper sheathing, for example, being introduced between 1779 and 1781. During these years England's *dry-docks* gave her an enormous advantage over most other countries. In 1750, the EIC had built a dry-dock at Bombay, and another in 1806; these were of enormous value to the Navy in 'maintaining its squadrons in the Indian Ocean'.[27]

Between 1710 and 1810, the average tonnage of 'ships of the line' grew steadily, approximately doubling during this period.[28] After 1714, shipwrights were no longer 'impressed' for dockyard service, but demands for their services escalated in times of war. Although there was little change in the numbers of journeyman shipwrights in the Royal dockyards during the eighteenth century, the most industrious of them was then ready to transfer to the 'merchant yards'.

The Port of London and its Docks

The Port of London came into being approximately two millennia ago. A trading settlement emerged at the first location above the sea where it was possible, at low tide, to bridge the tidal River Thames; as a result, *Londinium* rapidly became the largest city in England. 'During the greater part of its existence ... London [has] remained primarily a riverside port, a long narrow city hugging the Thames from which it drew its nurture'. In order to avoid the great loop of the Thames, a 'short cut', connecting Blackwall with Limehouse, was planned (but never executed) by the architect and engineer Willey Reveley (1760–1799) in 1796.[29] Therefore, the lower reaches of the Thames constitute arguably, historically speaking, the most important highway in the world. For centuries, when roads were few and of poor quality, this was the *major* route (for princes and pilgrims alike) in their passage to and fro from the City of London. The merchandise of the world entered by this route, and it was for many centuries the principal highway *within* London, as well as being the setting for all state occasions.[30]

During the eighteenth century, London became the world's busiest port; the quays and warehouses were extremely congested. Ships had often to wait weeks, and sometimes months, before their cargoes were unloaded. Cargoes were thieved and plundered from ships, barges, and more often the quayside. Pilfering (largely a result of gross congestion) was commonplace; one estimate is that in the early nineteenth century, one in five East Indiamen was plundered, and the dutiable merchandise ferried ashore to elude the Customs Officers. Smuggling was rife; the larger ships were forced to anchor downstream – at Limehouse or Blackwall.[31]

By the end of the century, it became clear that the 'Legal Quays', which lay along the river, were inadequate to deal with London's vast maritime traffic. Figure 2.1 gives an indication of gross overcrowding in the Pool of London in 1804. Until the early nineteenth century, every ship entering the Port of London was compelled to unload all dutiable cargo at these quays which were situated on the north shore between London Bridge and the Tower.

The dock system

Although the River Police had originated in 1801, the only real solution to this problem was to build large docks down river so that ships could be unloaded on the quays, where well-protected warehouses existed. Therefore, William Vaughan FRS (1752–1850) published an important book in 1793: a treatise '*On Wet Docks, Quays and Warehouses for the Port of London, with hints respecting Trade*'.[32] As a result, enclosed dock systems were constructed; these not only reduced congestion, but also drastically reduced the number of thefts from ships moored on the Thames. By the 1790s the Brunswick or Perry's Dock, at Blackwall (*see* Table 2.1), was able to accommodate '28 large East Indiamen, and from 50 to 60 ships of smaller burthen'. In the early nineteenth century, work began on large new dock systems, which were London's first purpose-built handling docks: the West India Dock (on the Isle of Dogs) dealt with all traffic from the West Indies and was opened in 1802; the London Dock (at Wapping) (1805), and the East India Dock (at Blackwall) (1806); this latter was incidentally heavily bombed during the 1939–45 war, while the Export Dock was obliterated in 1946. Figure 2.2 shows an unloading scene at the East India Dock in 1867. The Regent's Canal Dock (which linked with England's canal network) opened in 1820, and St Katherine's (which had the advantage of being close to the City) in 1828. Figure 2.3 shows the situation regarding London's Docks in 1821 – the year in which the SHS was

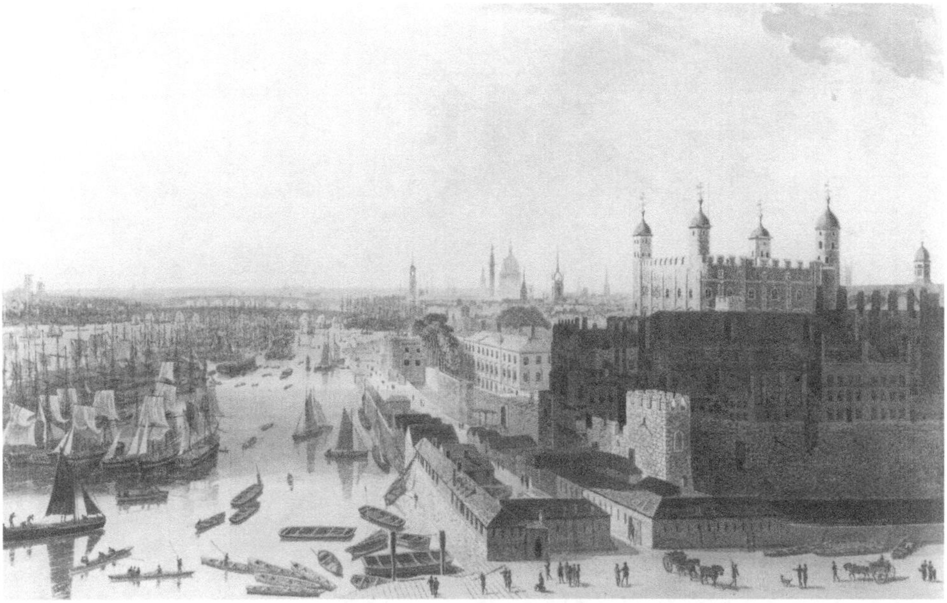

Figure 2.1: Aquatint of the Pool of London in 1804 [by W Daniel] showing ships lying off the Legal Quays. There was gross over-crowding, and many ships had to wait in midstream for weeks until they were unloaded; this inevitably led to mass pilfering by riverside gangs. [Reproduced with permission, The Guildhall Library, London].

Table 2.1: The Port of London's Docks.

Name	*Location*	*Date of:*	
		Opening	*Closure*
Perry's, Brunswick	Blackwall	1789	[absorbed by East India Dock in 1806]
West India	Isle of Dogs	1802	1980
Surrey and Commercial	Rotherhithe	1804	1970
London	Wapping	1805	1968
East India (& Perry's Dock)	Blackwall	1806	1967
Greenland	Rotherhithe	1807	1971
St Katherine's	Wapping	1828	1968
Royal Victoria	Newham	1855	1981
Millwall	Isle of Dogs	1868	1980
Royal Albert	Newham	1880	1981
Tilbury	Tilbury	1886	–

[*See also* A. Bryant. *Liquid history: to commemorate fifty years of the Port of London Authority 1909–1959.* London: The Curwen Press 1960].

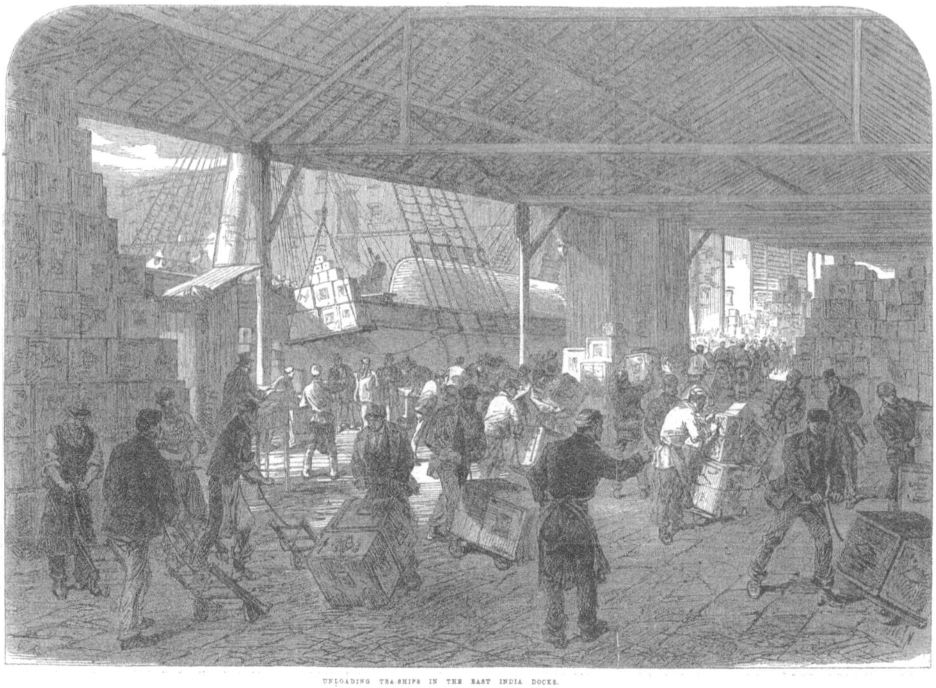

Figure 2.2: The East India Dock in 1867: unloading tea-ships (reproduced from the *Illustrated London News*, 1867: 26 October).

founded. Despite these new systems, the river remained exceedingly busy and congested, much crowding resulting from colliers carrying coal from the north-east of England to London. The East India Dock Company, which already owned secure warehouses in the City of London, subsequently bought Perry's Dock (*see* above and Table 2.1). In 1833, the East India (modernised in the latter 1880s) and West India Dock Companies merged; the former maintained a Sailor's Home – in East India Dock Road.[33]

The heart of London's 'sailor town' therefore became centred on Wapping and Limehouse; this area was thus crowded with sailors returning home, mostly after long voyages, which had lasted several months. Most Chinese seamen settled in Limehouse and Pennyfields – which became known as Chinatown – and was infamous for its gambling and smoking rooms. They stayed in lodgings and spent much time and money in public houses and brothels until another ship could be found. When penal colonies were established in Australia (*see* Chapter 1), many convicts boarded ships in the East India Dock. Emigrants – bound for the colonies and America – also left from these docks. Many immigrants landed here, and subsequently settled in the East End of London. More Docks were built in the late nineteenth century: Royal Victoria (1855), Royal Albert (1880), and Tilbury (1886); these were designed specifically to accommodate large ocean-going steamships. The vast riches housed in the warehouses contrasted starkly with the poor

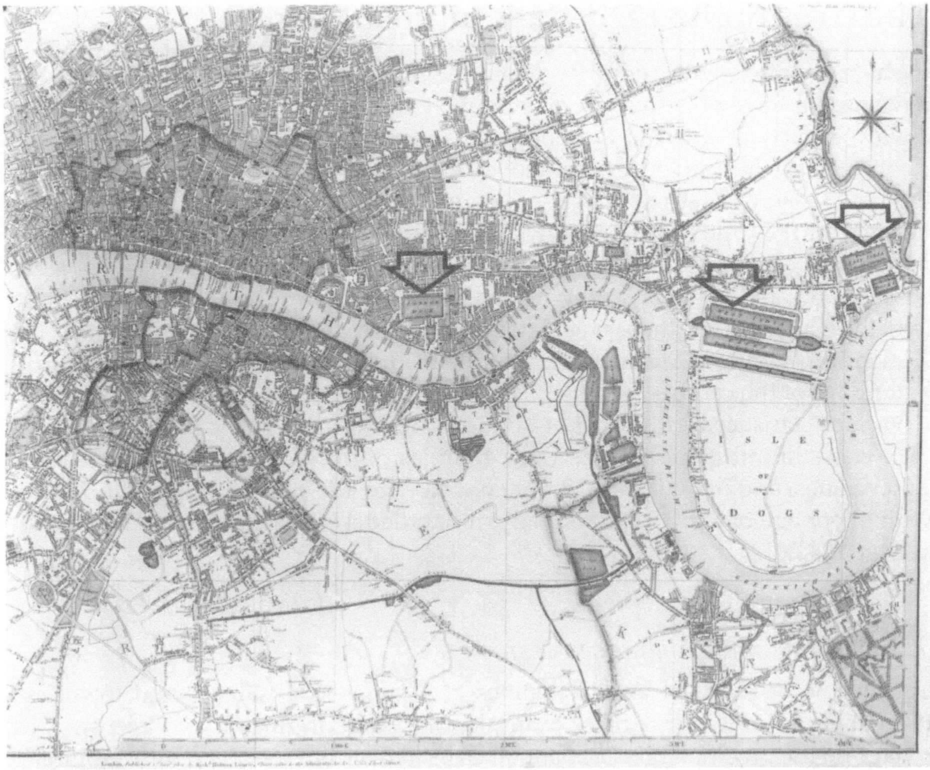

Figure 2.3: Map, showing the location of London's Docks when the SHS was launched. The London, West India, and East India Docks are arrowed. [From: Richard Holmes Laurie, '*New Plan of London*' 1821 – based on a survey by Outhett].

living conditions of most port workers and their families – especially the casual dockers.

In 1909, the Port of London Authority (PLA) (its main building was situated on Tower Hill) was established to supervise London's docks, and manage the River Thames generally; it opened the King George V dock in 1921. By the 1930s, 100,000 individuals were employed in the world's largest port (which encompassed 700 acres of enclosed dock water, and 1700 riverside wharves), and 35 million tons of cargo were dealt with annually. In the 1950s and 60s, the East India Docks handled short-sea and coastal traffic.

By the 1960s and 70s new technology (i.e. large container ships) had made the Port of London Docks virtually obsolete. The Old Port of London had therefore been rendered moribund in the space of a mere 20 years. There were soon many closures: the East India Dock (in 1967), St Katherine's (1968), London (1968), Surrey (1970), West India (1980), and the 'Royal Docks' (1981). At present, London's docks are situated 25 miles downstream – at Tilbury Container Port.[34]

The river in the early days of the SHS

In the early nineteenth century – when the SHS was founded – the Thames must have been a 'hive of activity'. For example tea, (the new season's crop which was always eagerly awaited in London) (see above) was at that time sold at the Sale Room of East India House (see above). In the 1850s a race developed to obtain the new season's first tea; 'clippers' were built (see above) – based on American designs. In 1849, the navigation laws were repealed – thus permitting foreign ships to compete on British trade routes. In 1869, the Suez Canal was opened;[35] steamships – powered by coal – now reached London more rapidly than the clippers (e.g. the 'Cutty Sark'); these were later used to carry wool from Australia and New Zealand, to London. Steam ferries, tunnels and river craft were common in the latter days of the century.

Various statistics for the Port of London have been given for 1936 (i.e. when the SHS was still influential): there were 45 miles of dock quayage, 517 warehouses, 1,500 cranes, and 6,550,000 cu. ft. for cold storage; the port received 61,132 vessels with a tonnage of 62,151,310 annually; it handled 43,000,000 tons of goods valued at £466,724,261.[36]

Thames-side names, and sea-terms

Tracing the origin(s) of familiar names of Thames-side villages and towns is in itself an interesting pursuit. For example, *Greenwich* originated as 'Green-wic' (the village on the green), while *Deptford* takes its name from the 'deep ford'.[37] Similarly, a study of sea-terms is of interest. Examples are: 'pews or coffins' (bunks), 'donkey's breakfasts' (mattresses), 'Fanny Adams' or 'Harriet Lane' (salt port), 'cracker hash' (baked broken biscuit and salt pork), and 'gubbins' (scraps from the captain's table).[38]

References and Notes

1 R Natkiel, A Preston. *Atlas of Maritime History.* London: Bison Books 1988; W J Bassett-Lowke. The progress of transport by water – I & II. *SHS Quart Mag* 1939; 11 (2): 17–19 and 11 (3): 19–22; Anonymous. *The National Maritime Museum: the story of Britain and the Sea.* London: National Maritime Museum: undated.
2 *Op cit.* See note 1 above; H M Bartlett. *A history of the merchant navy.* London: Harrap & Co. 1937: 302; Anonymous. *SHS Quart Mag* 1937; 9 (2): 23.
3 *Ibid;* [*See also:* FC Bowen. The Navigation Acts. *SHS Quart Mag* 1937; 9 (1): 18–20].
4 **Sir James Lancaster** (?–1618) was a pioneer of English trade with the East Indies, and participated in the Spanish Armada (1588). In 1592 he sailed in the first English voyage with the East India Company to the East Indies, returning with a rich booty; *Op cit.* See note 2 above. [*See also*: C F Beckingham. Lancaster, Sir James (1554/5–1618). In: H C G Matthew, B Harrison (eds). *Oxford Dictionary of National Biography.* Oxford: Oxford University Press 2004; 32; 358–9].
5 *Op cit.* See note 1 above; N Grant. *The Savage trade.* Harmondworth, Middlesex: Kestrel

Books 1980; N Tattersfield. *The forgotten trade.* London: Jonathan Cape. 1991: 460; H Thomas. *The Slave Trade: the history of the Atlantic Slave Trade 1440–1870.* London: Picador 1997.

6 *Op cit.* See note 2 above.

7 G Cookson. *The cable: the wire that changed the world.* London: Tempus 2003: 160.

8 *Op cit.* See note 2 above; [*See also*: J. Morris. *Pax Brittanica: the climax of an empire.* London: Penguin Books 1979; B Lubbock. *The log of the "Cutty Sark".* Glasgow: James Brown & Son. 1924; R Hughes. *The fatal shore.* London: Collins Harvill 1982: 688].

9 *Op cit.* See note 2 above (Bartlett).

10 *Ibid.*

11 *Ibid.*

12 [MFT]. Eastward ho! *SHS Quart Mag* 1934; 6 (1): 18; A Werner, N Lane. *Gateway to the East: history of East India trade.* London: Museum in Docklands 1991; J Keay. *The Honorable Company: a history of the English East India Company.* London: HarperCollins 1991: 475; A Wild. *The East India Company: trade and conquest from 1660.* London: HarperCollins 2000: 191; J Sutton. *Lords of the East: The East India Company and its ships (1600–1874).* London: Conway Maritime Press 2000: 160; A Farrington. *Trading Places: The East India Company and Asia 1600–1834.* London: The British Library 2000: 128; A Farrington. Trading Places: The East India Company and Asia. *History Today.* 2002 (5): 40–41. [*See also:* A Bryant. *Liquid history: to commemorate fifty years of the Port of London Authority 1909–1959.* London: Curwen Press, Plaistow 1960].

13 *Ibid;* [*See also* V Berridge, G Edwards. *Opium and the people: opiate in nineteenth century England.* London: Yale University Press 1987: 370; M Booth. *Opium: a history.* London: Simon and Schuster 1996: 381; M Binyon. Fruit of gunboat diplomacy and opium. *Times, Lond* 1997; 28 June: 14].

14 *Op cit.* See note 12 above, and note 1 above (Bassett-Lowke); O Checkland. Bruce, James, eighth earl of Elgin and twelfth earl of Kincardine (1811–1863). In: H C G Matthew, B Harrison (eds). *Oxford Dictionary of National Biography.* Oxford: Oxford University Press 2004; 8: 307–11.

15 D A Baugh. The eighteenth century navy as a national institution 1690–1815. In: J.R. Hill (ed). *The Oxford Illustrated History of the Royal Navy.* Oxford: Oxford University Press 1995: 120–160.

16 A L Revell. *Haslar: the Royal Hospital.* Gosport: The Gosport Society 1984; H. Richardson (ed.). Naval Hospitals. In: *English Hospitals 1660–1948: a survey of their architecture and design.* Swindon: Royal Commission on the Historical Monuments of England. 1998: 76–86.

17 *Op cit.* See note 12 above (Bryant).

18 D Loades. From the King's ships to the Royal Navy 1500–1642. In: J R Hill (ed). *The Oxford Illustrated History of the Royal Navy.* Oxford: Oxford University Press 1995: 24–55.

19 *Op cit.* See note 2 above; C S Knighton. Pepys, Samuel (1633–1703). In: H C G Matthew, B Harrison (eds). *Oxford Dictionary of National Biography.* Oxford: Oxford University Press 2004; 43: 644–52.

20 *Op cit.* See note 15 above.

21 *Op cit.* See note 12 above (Bryant).

22 **John Arbuthnot Fisher** OM GCB, GCVO (1st Baron Fisher of Kilverstone) (1841–1920) had a distinguished naval career, eventually becoming First Sea Lord (1904–10). He was responsible for many reforms in the Royal Navy, including many new technological innovations, e.g. the *Dreadnought* battleship and the submarine. [*See also*: J. Morris. *Fisher's Face.* London: Penguin Books 1996; P G Halpern. Fisher, John Arbuthnot, first Baron

Fisher (1841–1920). In: H C G Matthew, B Harrison (eds). *Oxford Dictionary of National Biography.* Oxford: Oxford University Press 2004; 19: 695–702]. **William Waldegrave Palmer** KG, PC, GCMG, (1859–1942) became the Second Earl of Selbourne in 1895. He was a prominent politician who later became First Lord of the Admiralty (1900–04); Selbourne was made an Elder Brother of Trinity House in 1904. [*See* also D G Boyce. Palmer, William Waldegrave, second earl of Selborne (1859–1942). In: H C G Matthew, B Harrison (eds). *Oxford Dictionary of National Biography.* Oxford: Oxford University Press 2004; 42: 548–52].

23 J Winton. Life and education in a technically evolving navy 1815–1925. In: J R Hill (ed). *The Oxford Illustrated History of the Royal Navy.* Oxford: Oxford University Press 1995: 250–279; N A M Rodger. Nelson, Horatio, Viscount Nelson (1758–1805) In: H C G Matthew, B Harrison (eds). *Oxford Dictionary of National Biography.* Oxford: Oxford University Press 2004; 40: 396–410; B Lavery. *Nelson's fleet at Trafalgar.* London: National Maritime Museum 2004; 208; R Harding (ed). Bicentenary of Trafalgar. *Mariner's Mirror* 2005; 91: 129–384.

24 *Op cit.* See note 15 above; *[See also*: A Cleeve. An historic dockyard. *SHS Quart Mag.* 1935; 7 (2): 17; P Kemp. *The history of ships.* Rochester: Grange Books 2002: 224].

25 *Ibid.*

26 **George Anson**, Admiral Baron Anson (1697–1762) had a distinguished naval career, and served as First Lord of the Admiralty from 1751–6, and 1757–62. He circumnavigated the globe (1740–44) but in so doing lost approximately three-quarters of his men – most from scurvy. [*See also*: J R Hill (ed). *The Oxford Illustrated history of the Royal Navy.* Oxford: Oxford University Press 1995; *Op cit.* See note 15 above; N A M Rodger. Anson, George, Baron Anson (1697–1762). In: H C G Matthew, B Harrison (eds). *Oxford Dictionary of National Biography.* Oxford: Oxford University Press 2004; 2: 260–6; B Lavery. Slade, Sir Thomas (1703/4–1771). In: H C G Matthew, B Harrison (eds). *Ibid*; 50: 900–1].

27 *Op cit.* See note 24 above.

28 *Ibid.* [*See also*: L Dunn. *Thames Shipping*, 2nd ed. London: Carmania Press 1994: 112].

29 C W Hind. Reveley, Willey (1760–1799) In: H C G Matthew, B Harrison (eds). *Oxford Dictionary of National Biography.* Oxford: Oxford University Press 2004; 46: 512–3.

30 *Op cit.* See note 12 above (Bryant); F Barker, P Jackson (eds). *London: 2000 years of a city and its people.* London: Cassel & Co Ltd. 1974: 255–257.

31 *Op cit.* See note 12 above (Bryant).

32 **William Vaughan**, FRS (1752–1850) was prominent in the mercantile and commercial life of the City of London, and in 1783 was elected a director of the Royal Exchange Assurance Corporation. He took prompt measures to restore tranquillity during the naval mutiny at the Nore in 1797. Vaughan subsequently became one of the leading authorities on docks, and between 1793 and 97 published a series of pamphlets and tracts on the construction of docks for the Port of London. Recognition of the importance of London's docks was in fact, largely due to Vaughan. He wrote: *'On Wet Docks, Quays and Warehouses for the Port of London, with hints respecting Trade'* in 1793. [*See also*: note 12 above (Bryant): 21–22. See note 30 above (Barker, Jackson). E I Carlyle, A McConnell. Vaughan, William (1752–1850) In: H C G Matthew, B Harrison (eds). *Oxford Dictionary of National Biography.* Oxford: Oxford University Press 2004; 56: 211–12].

33 *Op cit.* See note 12 above (Bryant); A Palmer. *The East End's four centuries of London life.* 2000: 200; C Weightman. *London's Thames.* London: John Murray 2004: 150.

34 *Ibid*; [*See also*: S Humphries *The call of the sea: Britain's maritime past 1900–1910.* London: BBC books 1997: 191].

35 Z Karabell. *Parting the desert: the creation of the Suez Canal.* London: John Murray 2003: 310.

36 Anonymous. The Port of London. *SHS Quart Mag* 1938; 10 (3): 19; D J Owen. Seaports. *SHS Quart Mag* 1938; 10 (3): 17–19.
37 H E Hobbs. The origin of Thames-side names: a fascinating study. *SHS Quart Mag*. 1935; 7 (4): 18–19.
38 R M Reynolds. Some old sea terms. *SHS Quart Mag* 1937; 9 (3): 18.

Chapter 3

Conditions of service in Britain's maritime organisations

During the *fifteenth* century, roads in Britain were almost non-existent; therefore, many communities sprang up in and around ports; only there was it possible to obtain seafood, and trade with other ports. Sailors, who had inevitably moved away from this environment, were usually viewed as rogues and vagabonds. Although life at sea was at that time pretty miserable, it was probably no worse than life on land!

The men

British merchant seamen of this era were apparently easily recognised by their clothes and walk; most came from humble homes, and the majority were uneducated, being brought up at sea the hard way. One British shipmaster described them as: 'designing and unforgivable beasts whose life and habits made them unfeeling and unprincipled [and], when ashore, [they] spent their time in the company of the lowest people that could be found, more or less in a state of intoxication'. One estimate at that time was that 'excessive alcohol consumption accounted for more than half the shipwrecks and tragedies at sea'.[1] In the year ending 31 January 1807, 2,413 seamen died abroad; of these only 143 were over 40, and a mere 34 over 50 years old! As late as 1865 mortality from drowning accidents amongst British seamen was 2,607; at the same time, deaths from 'disease' amounted to 2,259 (433 due to cholera, 255 dysentery, 146 yellow fever, 326 undefined 'fever', 7 alcoholism, and only 39 deaths were recorded as 'natural') (*see* Chapter 4). Most crews of foreign-going ships were in fact in poor health by 35–40 years of age, and life-expectancy rarely exceeded 45 years.[2]

Before 1850, *crimps** had a virtual monopoly in the supply of seamen. They were a major problem for seamen of this era; they might be boarding-house Masters, or their servants or agents, who offered intoxicating liquors (usually cheap spirits) and loose women to those newly arrived in port; they also shanghaied seamen for outward-bound ships – taking an advance in wages. Crimps often took charge of a

*'to impress (seamen or soldiers); to entrap, to decoy'. [J A Simpson, ESC Weiner (eds). *Oxford English Dictionary* Oxford: Clarendon Press 1989 ; 4: 22].

sailor from the time he was paid off from a homeward-bound ship until he joined an outward-bound one.

Soon after mooring, the seamen were frequently so inebriated that they had to be carried to a lodging house(s), and several days later they might be 'lying almost naked in the gutter having been robbed of their pay and even their clothes'.[3] As a result, many were left 'to perish from cold and hunger in the streets'.[4] In many cases, the sailor was already ill on arrival at the Port of London and after a few hours lying in the gutter he died unless treatment was rapidly instituted.[5]

When the Napoleonic Wars finally ended in 1815, about 125,000 seamen were discharged from the merchant service; they were then unemployed. Coupled with this, wages had plummeted; before the wars a merchant seaman earned 25/= (shillings) to 35/= monthly, while in 1804, a figure of £6/6s has been quoted for some merchant ships.[6] When unemployed, many found it difficult to establish a place in which to settle; furthermore, many suffered from illnesses contracted during their service, but there was 'no provision for the alleviation of their sufferings'.[7] Many unemployed seamen were therefore: '... to be found in the streets of London, friendless, homeless and without work'; this was the *raison d'etre* behind the philosophy of the philanthropists who founded the SHS (*see* Chapter 6) and its predecessor (*see* Chapter 5).

Life in the Merchant Navy

Webb has given two examples of incidents in the life of merchant seaman in the Port of London as recently as the early *nineteenth* century. There was apparently an underground Dock Office opposite the Royal Mint, where sailors received their pay; as they climbed the stone steps into the street, many were met by criminals and prostitutes from the East End of London – who enticed or hustled them to their dens of iniquity, where either peacefully or forcibly they were separated from their money. They ended inevitably by being shanghaied* and were soon afterwards at sea again. His second illustration involves a bar in a particularly evil tavern, where after a great deal of alcohol, the sailor would be lured behind the bar by attractive girls, and fall through a trap-door into a cellar – where he was rendered unconscious and taken senseless on board a ship moored in the river. Life in other ports, e.g., Liverpool and Cardiff, was equally grim.[8]

At this time, the Royal Navy (RN) was heavily dependent on the 'press gang' (see above); it was not until 1853 that *continuous* service began in the RN, and as recently as 1917 that a proper recruiting system, and a National Wage was introduced into the *Merchant Navy*.

*'to drug or otherwise, render insensible, and ship on board a vessel wanting hands' (*nautical slang*). [J A Simpson, ESC Weiner (eds) *Oxford English Dictionary*. Oxford: Clarendon Press; 15: 169].

Conditions on board ship

A description of living conditions on board ship in 1890 claims: 'At all times the forecastle was a foulsome and suffocating abode; here 14 sailors and apprentices slept, washed and dressed and had their food [which consisted] almost entirely of inferior salted pork, unpalatable beef and brown biscuits, too often mouldy and full of maggots ... the forecastle was full of rats which found their way into the hammocks in which the crew slept'. There was also the foul stench of bilge water, and the drinking water was also heavily contaminated.[9]

In a book written as recently as 1922, the author wrote in a chapter entitled *Life on board a merchant steamer,*

> ... conditions of the daily life of seamen on board their ships are quite unapprehended by the general public ... or a public indignation would have been aroused that would have swept their evils away.

After explaining improvements at that time, in living conditions 'on land' he continued, 'unseen forecastles [which were where the average sailor lived, unlike the officers and their servants who were accommodated in comfortable cabins were] still ... much as they were ... in 1894, when a campaign for their improvement ... began'. He also emphasised the vast overcrowding of a century before; as well as a lack of ventilation and lighting, food was often bad, drinking water was in short supply, and there were no water-closets. The air-space for 12 sailors in 1894 was 864 cubic feet, or less. If 'little cargo could be carried [he pointed out] ships would no longer be an economic proposition'.[10] Not until 1835 was the carrying of medicine(s) by all ships made obligatory.

Life in the Royal Navy

Far more has been written about day-to-day life in the RN than the Merchant Navy. By the nineteenth century, conditions in the RN, when compared with those in the Mercantile Marine, were moderately good. This had however, not always been the case; under James I (who reigned from 1603 to 1625), the fighting Navy had been allowed to decline. British superiority at sea was, it is said, during the eighteenth century, more dependant on men than ships.[11] Both Lloyd and Rodger have outlined shipboard life during this period: 'The RN had access to the largest reservoir of seamen of any nation', the maritime population having grown rapidly during the seventeenth and eighteenth centuries – this being dependant both on recruitment, and the *impressment* of landsmen (see below); '... if the government had commanded a systematic power to transfer large numbers of men from merchant ships to the [RN], [the best seamen were those obtained afloat], the main burden of the shortage would have fallen on the merchants'; however, the latter had sufficient support in the House of Commons to prevent this happening. By an Act of 1740, 'no landsman could be *pressed* [my italics] during his first two years at sea'.[12]

We shall probably never know how many men on board the King's ships were true volunteers (there were undoubtedly more in times of war), but 'pressed' men probably accounted for 20–30% of the overall complement. Also, in wartime eighteenth century governments had largely suspended a clause in the navigation laws requiring merchant crews to be composed entirely of *British* nationals; during the Napoleonic wars (see below) the RN had enlisted many foreigners (perhaps 15% of a ship's complement) as crew. 'In view of the possibility of suffering under harsh discipline in the [RN], and … higher pay in the merchant service, it seems incredible [today] that any seafarer would *volunteer* [my italics] for naval service in time of war'. Those who did, experienced another dimension to naval recruiting and retention; an officer joined the *RN* as a profession, whereas *volunteer* seamen merely joined a ship for a short time (being 'paid off' at the end of the voyage); an entire crew might, for example, move if a new captain took over.[13]

At a personal level, there were then no arrangements for drying wet clothes; however, from 1623 it became possible to exchange damaged clothing. The slop chest contained a variety of ill-assorted garments, an attire which lacked uniformity. Only in 1810 was soap provided to sailors of the RN.[14] Desertion was commonplace.

After long service abroad (e.g. war service), many Captains asked the Admiralty to offer their men leave of absence – trusting in their loyalty. They were expected to watch newspaper announcements for sailings and to return when summoned to serve under them again, often in a different ship.

The late Georgian navy

The Seamen's Hospital Society (SHS) was founded (*see* Chapter 6) in the latter days of the Georgian era; George IV (1762–1830) was on the throne, and his reign was to continue for the first nine years of its existence; therefore, the structure and social conditions in the maritime service was fundamentally Georgian. Rodger has given a valuable insight into living conditions on board ship in those days. Sailors on a warship reflected land-based society in a microcosm, a battle was a relatively rare occurrence, and between times, life was routine and on the whole relatively humdrum – spent either in port(s), or in blockading enemy strongholds. On board, there was a sharp division of labour: seamen hauled ropes, handled sails, or raised the anchor (by turning the capstan); carpenters worked on repairing the hull or other wooden fittings; the cook prepared food in the stove or cauldron; and the chaplain said prayers and conducted religious services. Various warrant and petty-officers carried out a multitude of tasks – from issuing clothes and rations, to administration of punishment(s).

The seaman's living conditions were exceedingly cramped; he slept in a hammock for a four-hour stretch. His diet consisted of bread (baked like a biscuit), beer, salt pork/beef, cheese, and occasionally stockfish and brandy. Discipline was strict; the sailor was flogged for drunkenness or theft. Despite all this, a generally good relationship apparently existed between the officers and men.[15]

RN personnel

Most successful officers in the RN started their careers in boyhood, aged 12–14 years; for example, Admiral Lord Anson (1697–1762) (*see* Chapter 4), and at a much later date Lord Fisher (1841–1920) (see Chapter 2) who joined the navy in 1854 at the early age of 13 years. They were frequently sons or nephews of captains, and were examined by three captains under direction of the Navy Board. The minimum age of a lieutenant was 20, and the required length of sea-service (from 1728) six years. But, they had to be appointed to a lieutenant's berth in a *commissioned* ship – a feat much easier in war than peace-time. The career ladder was then: post-captain or captain (commander was a rank which appeared later) and then rear-admiral; there were very few Admirals of the line. This was therefore a system of patronage – with much political and aristocratic influence, although a great deal of sea-service was generally valuable! Following appointment, a period on shore on *half-pay* was acceptable.[16]

Overall, insufficient attention had been paid, in the past, to the needs of sailors in the RN; Sir Gilbert Blane (1749–1834) claimed that the lives of sailors 'were so unnatural, both as regards lodging and diet, as to lead readily to the prevalence of disease'.[17]

Rates and pay

The earliest record of a classification of shipping 'rates' dates from 1546 (the term had probably been introduced to refer to the *rate of pay* of the officers and men serving on board); ships comprising '*the fleet*' were described as: 'shyppes', 'galleases' (long low vessels propelled by oars and a sail), 'pynnaces' (smaller versions of galleases) and 'roo-baergers' (rowing barges). In 1612, they were classified as: 'Shipps Royal' and 'Middling Shipps' (with a tonnage of 600–800), 'small shipps' (350 tons), and pinnaces (250–80 tons). Division of RN ships into different 'rates' (six in all) is first recorded in 1626 in a table drawn up by order of King Charles I (1600–49). From 1651, the number of guns carried, also entered the equation. A First Rate for example, carried > 100 guns, a crew of 850–950 men, and possessed a tonnage of 2,000–2,600; a fourth rate had 50 guns and 350 men. Descriptions were, for example: a 'Third Rate of 80 guns' or a 'Sixth Rate of 24 guns'. Another classification involved the number of decks. However, several miscellaneous types were not rated at all, e.g. sloops, yachts, fire-ships, and bombs (i.e. vessels carrying 6–8 light guns, with heavy cannon or mortars of wide bore, for bombarding shore-based forts).[18]

As regards actual rates of pay, acceptable standards had been laid down in the reign of King Henry VIII (1491–1547): four shillings monthly for seamen and gunners, with two pence a day extra as a victualling allowance. In Stuart times, the navy often went unpaid! Pepys (1633–1703), for example, wrote in his diary that he was very unhappy with the situation regarding naval pay; on 7 October 1665 he wrote: 'Did business, though not much, at the office because of the horrible crowd and the lamentable moan of the poor seamen that lie starving in the streets for lack of money ...'.[19] In 1803, Lloyds was to set up a 'Patriotic Fund' to honour heroic deeds involving all ranks, and to provide aid for sailors who had been crippled by wounds, or slain – thus leaving widows and orphans.

Men were often paid a year or more late – as soon as the ship arrived in England however, her books were deposited with a Commissioner of the Navy, and the men were paid within two months – however, the last six months' pay was always held. Numerous money lenders and traders would 'help' an impoverished sailor in return for a letter of attorney.

Recruitment to the maritime service: the volunteer and the 'Press Gang'

There were points for and against joining the RN. If a man in fact joined, he was certain to serve on a ship, but he would not, in all probability, obtain leave until the end of a war. If, however, he signed on as a *merchant* seaman, he would be paid far more, and could leave a ship at the end of every voyage; however, to do this he had to avoid the 'press gangs' (see below).

The origin(s) of 'impressment' remains unclear. Shakespeare's Sir John Falstaff had a commission to *impress* soldiers for the King's Service. But, the origins were probably bound up with feudalism. The 'press gang' was no respecter of persons and it was liable to seize any unprotected person who came its way! The victim (preferably a seafarer rather than a landsman) would then be carried off to sea for a period of service – usually at least two or three years. Many of the 'victims' were diseased and/or infected; it is likely that this led to a great increase in disease (see Chapter 4). James Lind (1716–94) considered that impressed men (in the RN) were generally 'such idle fellows as are picked upon the streets, or prisoners'. These men had therefore been enmeshed in a dangerous/distasteful service against their will; discipline had however, since Tudor times, been of a high order and the pressed men were severely punished for any misdemeanour.[20]

The strength of the RN lay in its *volunteers*: 'Better one volunteer than three pressed men' was a familiar cry, but, the captain of a ship had to *pay* for advertisements (including posters) to attract *volunteers*. After volunteering, each man received conduct money as well as two months' wages (in advance) and with this he had to purchase: warm clothes, a hammock, blanket and slops from the purser.

Before the Napoleonic Wars, the strength of the RN was about 25,000, but by 1800, there were 110,000 seamen and 20,000 marines. In consequence, the supply of volunteers failed to keep up with requirement(s); therefore, every captain had to rely on the *Impress Service* to boost numbers of recruits; even then many ships were forced to sail with fewer men than their complement. Until 1757, owners of property were responsible for the supply of men and arms; however, this system was changed by William Pitt the elder (1708–78) so that each county had to supply a certain number of men depending on the size of its population, and the number of seaports it possessed (the Quota system). By introducing this system, Pitt had incidentally initiated *conscription* in Britain. At the beginning of the Napoleonic Wars, London had to find 5,704 men between the ages of 15 and 55 years! County authorities, in conjunction with justices of the peace, reduced the sentences of men who were already in jail on condition that they would *volunteer* for the Quota; transgressors about to be sentenced were often given an option: either go to sea *or* jail! This system did not apparently flood the Navy with scoundrels, but it brought typhus (*see* Chapter 4) to previously healthy ships!

Many years before England had a standing Navy, the Cinque Ports – Sandwich, Dover, Hythe, Romney and Hastings (Rye and Winchelsea were added later, by King Richard I [1157–99]) had provided ships for defence of the realm. The seaman was not covered by Magna Carta and thus had no clear rights; from King John onwards, every time a monarch considered that England was threatened or he intended to go to war with another nation, press warrants were issued. Initially failure to allow oneself to be 'pressed' was punishable by hanging; as time went on, however, the penalty became less severe.

Merchant ships provided a convenient target for crimps and Press Gangs; with the exception of officers and apprentices they could take any man they wanted. 'One man out of a merchant ship was better [it was said] than three lieutenants got in town'! Many merchant ships had small secret hiding places where two or three of the most valued men evaded the sharp-eyed press gang. Using the Honourable East India Company's own soldiers (the only ones serving in India in the late eighteenth century) to press men for a ship belonging to the company was theoretically illegal – but there was no one there to argue the case! There was one aspect of 'pressing' about which the RN officers were punctilious – i.e. ascertaining that seamen from *merchant ships* received the pay due at the moment of *pressing*.[21]

End of Impressment and emergence of the modern merchant navy

During the first half of the nineteenth century, between the Napoleonic Wars and the outbreak of the Crimean War (1851–54) this pernicious practice was to cease. In 1813, 99 ships of the line and 49 cruisers (manned by 130,127 men) were in service; by 1817, the numbers were 13, 89 and 22,944, respectively. During 30 years of peace, hostility between the *merchant* seamen and the *RN* diminished – largely because the two services were growing further apart, and men were no longer pressed from one service into the other. The Admirals fought a rear-guard action to maintain impressment in principle because they felt that it was necessary for the well-being of the RN, but it could no longer be enforced in practice![22]

On 17 March 1835, the First Sea Lord (Sir James Graham [1792–1861]) introduced a Bill whereby all masters of ships were required to keep crew lists which were compulsorily lodged with the Customs authorities before sailing; registration was regarded as an *alternative* to impressment. Thus, this year marked a significant landmark in the history of the British Seaman – namely, a final distinction between the *RN* and *Merchant Navy*. In a crisis, the possibility that Coastguards and Fishermen could be recruited was examined. For the first time in her history, Britain therefore possessed a well-trained *standing navy* without the need for impressment; a standard uniform was introduced in 1857.

Those who did not care for the way-of-life essential to a man of war (RN), could thus find employment in an expanding mercantile marine. There, the chances of promotion were better, even if conditions improved more slowly; men like Plimsoll (1824–98) (the 'sailors friend') represented public opinion, and compelled Government to intervene in order to protect the interests and lives of the seamen. Flogging however, died a long slow death; it was still extant, albeit at a much reduced rate, in 1852. In summary, the 1860s saw the end of the old navy (under sail) with emergence of a modern *RN* and *Merchant Service*.[23]

Maritime developments in the nineteenth century

During the nineteenth century, in which the SHS was founded, maritime supremacy was an essential factor in enabling the British to 'throw their armies into action upon the colonial frontiers, or warn off the predations of rival Powers'; the RN (the 'Nelson fixation' still prevailed) was in fact 'the genius of the Pax Brittanica' which had 'enjoyed a prestige so mystic that its power was taken for granted'.

By the mid-*nineteenth* century, most of the Navy's battleships were still 'heavy wooden three-deckers [the last, HMS *Victoria* with 120 guns – which also possessed auxiliary steam engines – was launched in 1859], which were fully rigged, and rated by the numbers of their guns' (see above). Shortly afterwards, the keel of the steam iron-clad HMS *Warrior* (currently preserved as a hulk at Portsmouth Dock Yard) was laid. The admirals 'regarded a warship less as a weapon of war than [as] a floating pageant, or perhaps a work of art'.[24]

Socially, the RN escalated during Queen Victoria's long reign (1837–1901); its officers, who were formerly drawn from the middle classes, now included many men of 'title and means'; naval ratings too, were men of a higher standing than formerly – being 'volunteers pursuing a regular and relatively well-paid career'. Impressment was in abeyance (see above), although never legally abolished. The RN increasingly became an *imperial* force – and was more concerned with 'protection of the imperial sea-lanes, the suppression of subversion, showing the flag, and overawing the natives'! Powerful lobbies were set up (the Navy League playing a prominent rôle) with the object of preserving and expanding the RN. The 'Empire' and the RN were to become virtually synonymous! Naval bases overseas (coaling was one of their major functions) were of vital importance (most were directly involved with the 'raj' in India). Most 'strategic island[s] had by then been acquired by the British' and the safety of shipping routes assumed the chief preoccupation of London's strategists'.

'Sea-power was [then] the basis of Empire, but Empire … was essential to sea-power'. In 1869, the Suez Canal (a French enterprise – inspired by the engineer Ferdinand de Lesseps [1805–94]) was opened; this meant that Egypt (as foreseen by Napoleon) became crucial to the 'Eastern Question' (i.e. the passage to India). By 1875, it became obvious to the rulers of the British Empire that the Suez Canal was strategically extremely important (almost 50% of ships sailing from Britain to India now took this route). 'Suez [had in effect] replaced the Cape of Good Hope as a synonym for the beginning of the east'. So important was the Canal to Britain that the British prime-minister, Benjamin Disraeli (1804–81) bought the Canal (on behalf of the Government) from the Khedive for nearly £4 million.[25]

Ventilation, sanitation and health

Although compared with early times, external appearances of ships had changed significantly, there was no substantial alteration to their interior design until the mid-nineteenth century – i.e. when steam was introduced. The more 'healthy' ships were considered to be the older ones – whose timbers did not exude moisture; newly constructed ships 'sweated' in cold and damp weather – giving off moisture, and were associated with epidemics. Bilge water was considered to be a source of disease; therefore, a leaky ship – which took in salt water to dilute the bilge – was considered more healthy.

The crew slept in hammocks – suspended from bolts attached to the beams of the deckhead – which were extremely cramped; a width of only 16 inches was allowed for each. Ventilation also was unsatisfactory up to the eighteenth century, being provided solely via the gunports on either side, and through the hatchways leading from the lower to upper decks. When the weather deterioriated, the gunports had to be closed – leaving *no* ventilation whatsoever! Windsails had been used to assist ventilation; Stephen Hales (1677–1761), an inventive clergyman, had introduced a system (the ship's lungs) which consisted of bellows – operated by hand. In 1756 the Lords Commissioners of the Admiralty ordered Hale's ventilators to be fitted to several ships, but they were not widely used due to operational difficulties.[28]

Epidemic disease was far more likely to involve large ships compared with small ones, a fact that has been the case until comparatively recently. Vermin were commonplace, as were cockroaches; Thomas Swaine, who styled himself the 'Ratcatcher to His Majesty's [RN]' wrote a book entitled: *The Universal Directory for Taking Alive, or Destroying, Rats and Mice …'* (1773); he apparently used white arsenic powder as a rat-killer.[27]

Health at sea, differs from that on land from several points of view:

(i) the community is a closed one; the same food is cooked in a single galley; several men sleep in the same cabin; and opportunities for recreation/exercise are limited,
(ii) ships can pass rapidly through extremes of temperature, and,
(iii) exposure to disease is more common in the tropics than in temperate climes.

Diseases (*see* Chapter 4) include: gastroenteritis (and typhoid), tuberculosis, malaria, yellow fever, plague and typhus. Whereas 30 years ago, the 'glory hole' housed 100–150 men, it now contains 4–6! Bunks/wardrobes are now made of metal, and *not* wood; therefore there are no cockroaches. Ventilation is now far superior; some ships even have air-conditioning. Baths/showers are now incorporated, and food/dining facilities are infinitely better! In addition, ships carrying 100 individuals *must* carry a surgeon, and *all* must carry the *Ship Captain's Medical Guide* originally written in 1856 by Leach of the SHS.[28]

Victualling

Victualling in the RN through the ages has often left much to be desired. In Elizabethan times (1533–1603), a pound of biscuit-bread, and a gallon of ale were allowed daily for every boy and man in the ship's company; to this was added:

> one pound of salt beef, *or* a pound of salt pork and pease ['four days in the week'] and on the other three days: salted fish (either hake, ling, or cod), 7 oz. of butter and 14 oz. of cheese. On Fridays, fish was eaten and half rations . . . served.

There was little change in the seventeenth and eighteenth centuries. Allison has given numerous examples of defective victualling in the seventeenth and eighteenth centuries. Diets usually contained no fresh foodstuffs; although there were traces of ascorbic acid in beer, the diet was otherwise lacking in anti-scorbutic activity. Much food had in fact already perished (beef, pork and bread particularly did not keep well), and often the ship put to sea before the true quality of the food on board had been tested. The Victualling Board was not established as a special department of Admiralty administration until the end of the eighteenth century.[29]

Safety and welfare of seafarers – throughout the ages

For many centuries, the welfare of the seafarer was an issue addressed by numerous British charitable foundations; it is probably true that at present Dutch and German ships have accommodation which is superior to that on English vessels.

Trinity House, an elegant listed Georgian building in Trinity Square – overlooking the Tower of London – is the present headquarters of a unique maritime institution (*see* Chapter 5). It is thus one of the oldest charitable maritime organisations. Founded by a Royal Charter of King Henry VIII in 1514, it has throughout almost five centuries cared for the safety of shipping, and was largely instrumental in establishing lighthouses around the coasts of Britain as well as caring for the welfare of seafarers and their dependents. The Corporation was initially established at Deptford; it moved to Ratcliffe (in East London) in 1618, and 42 years later to Water Lane in the City. Destroyed by fires in 1666 and 1714, its house was rebuilt and served as the 'home' of the Corporation until removal to its present venue in 1796; in December 1940 the building was seriously damaged during an air raid attack. Amongst its charitable functions today is the maintenance of 19 almshouses at Walmer, Kent (Chapter 5), as well as port welfare facilities for seamen of all nationalities. Former Masters of Trinity House have included the diarist, Pepys.[30]

Another charity which preceded the foundation of the SHS was the Marine Society (see Chapter 5).

Board of Trade Regulations

Board of Trade regulations for construction of crews' quarters on ships now include the following stipulations: (i) *All* seamen in ships of >2,500 tons will sleep aft or amidships, (ii) each watch will have its own sleeping-quarters, and (iii) accommodation will be larger and better ventilated [than previously].[31]

The National Maritime Museum and the Museum in Docklands

This museum, at Greenwich, houses a vast amount of maritime history. Although the RN figures predominantly, there is also inclusion of information, including exhibits regarding conditions experienced by sailors of the *mercantile marine*. The Queen's House was built in 1632, having been designed by Inigo Jones (1573–1652). It was for many years used by the Greenwich Hospital School; The National Maritime Museum subsequently took it over, and it was first opened to the public in 1936.[32]

The recently opened *Museum in Docklands*, an off-shoot of the Museum of London, houses a great deal of merchant naval history.[33]

References and Notes

1 A G Course. *The merchant navy: a social history.* London: Frederick Muller Ltd. 1963: 300.
2 *Ibid.*
3 *Ibid.*
4 R Harley. *First [annual] report of the Seamen's Hospital Society.* In: *Under the Patronage of His Majesty. The first and second Reports of the Committee of Management of the Hospital Ship Grampus, for sick and diseased seamen arriving in the Port of London. Supported by donations and voluntary contributions. Established in 1821.* London: W. Gilbert 1822: 12–19.
5 G Webb. *Some notes on five hundred years of seamen's welfare.* Gillingham, Kent: King George's Fund for Sailors. 1959: 168–87; W R N Bowers: *Naval adventures during 35 years service.* 1833: 2 (appendix 2): 301.
6 *Ibid* (Webb).
7 *Ibid* (Webb): 188–207; *Op cit.* see note 4 above: 16–17.
8 *Ibid* (Webb): 168–87.
9 A Werner, N Lane. *Gateway to the east.* London: Museum in Docklands: 21.
10 W E Home. *Merchant seamen: their diseases and their welfare.* London: John Murray 1922: 15–25; R Hope. *Poor Jack: the perilous history of the merchant seaman.* London: Chatham Publishing 2001: 376; T B Shaw. *Naval hygiene.* London: Oxford University Press 1929; 28: 215.
11 D A Baugh. The eighteenth century navy as a national institution 1690–1815. In: J.R. Hill (ed) *The Oxford Illustrated History of the Royal Navy.* Oxford University Press 1995: 120–160.
12 C Lloyd. *The British Seaman 1200–1860: a social survey.* London: Collins 1968: 267–284; *Op cit.* [*See also* note 11 above].
13 *Op cit.* See note 11 above: 138–9, 146.
14 R S Allison. *Sea Diseases.* London: John Bale Medical Publications Ltd. 1943: 61–62. [*See also*: M Lewis. *England's Sea-Officers: the story of the Naval Profession.* London: George Allen & Unwin Ltd. 1939: 55–121].
15 N A M Rodger. *The wooden world: an anatomy of the Georgian Navy.* Glasgow: Fontana Press 1986. [*See also* P Earle. *Sailors: English Merchant Seamen 1650–1775.* London: Methuen

1998: 85–106; Anonymous. *The National Maritime Museum: the story of Britain and the sea.* Greenwich: National Maritime Museum: 18].

16 *Op cit.* See note 11 above.

17 *Op cit.* See note 14 above: (Allison, 68–69); J Wallace. Blane, Sir Gilbert, first baronet (1749–1834). In: H C G Matthew, B Harrison (eds). *Oxford Dictionary of National Biography.* Oxford: Oxford University Press 2004; 6: 172–5.

18 *Op cit.* See note 14 above: (Allison): 51–52.

19 *Ibid*: 62–53.

20 *Ibid.* 58–61.

21 D Pope. The Press Gang. In: D. Pope. *Life in Nelson's Navy.* London: Chatham Publishing 1997: 93–106. [*See also* note 11 above (133–139); note 15 above (Earle): 29–38; M Peters. Pitt, William, first earl of Chatham [*known as Pitt the elder*]. (1708–1778) In: H C G Matthew, B Harrison (eds). *Oxford Dictionary of National Biography.* Oxford: Oxford University Press 2004; 44: 452–70].

22 *Op cit.* See note 12 above: 267–284. [*See also*: P Padfield. *Maritime Supremacy and the opening of the Western mind.* London: Pimlico 2000: 340].

23 *Ibid*; J Parry. Graham, Sir James Robert George, second baronet (1792–1861). In: H C G Matthew, B Harrison (eds). *Oxford Dictionary of National Biography.* Oxford: Oxford University Press 2004; 23: 204–10; A McConnell. Plimsoll, Samuel (1824–1898). In: H C G Matthew, B Harrison (eds). *Ibid.* 2004; 44: 583–5.

24 J Morris. *Heaven's command: an imperial progress.* London: Penguin Books 1979: 410–421. [*See also: Op cit.* See note 1 above: 240–267].

25 *Op cit.* See note 1 above. [*See also* Z Karabell. *Parting the desert: the creation of the Suez Canal* London: John Murray 2003: 310; J Parry. Disraeli, Benjamin, earl of Beaconsfield (1804–1881). In: H C G Matthew, B Harrison (eds). *Oxford Dictionary of National Biography.* Oxford: Oxford University Press 2004; 16: 270–97].

26 *Op cit.* See note 14 above (Allison): 53–57. [*See also*: *Op cit.* See note 11 above; D G C Allan. Hales, Stephen (1677–1761). In: H C G Matthew, B Harrison (eds). *Oxford Dictionary of National Biography.* Oxford: Oxford University Press 2004; 24: 553–6].

27 *Op cit.* See note 10 above (Hope): 57–58; [*See also Op cit.* See note 10 above (Shaw): 276–288].

28 H M R Jones. Health in the merchant navy. *Health Horizon* 1956 (autumn): 12–17; G C Cook. Leach, Henry (1836–1879). In: H C G Matthew, B Harrison (eds). *Oxford Dictionary of National Biography.* Oxford: Oxford University Press 2004; 32: 950–1.

29 *Op cit.* See note 14 above (Allison): 63–68.

30 Anonymous. *Trinity House: Trinity Square, Tower Hill, London EC3.* London: Trinity House. Undated: 12.

31 A Bone. Before the mast. *SHS Quart Mag* 1937; 9 (4): 19–20.

32 A Burton. *The Daily Telegraph Guide to Britain's Maritime Past.* London: Aurum Press 2003: 174; J Newman. Jones, Inigo (1573–1652). In: H C G Matthew, B Harrison (eds). *Oxford Dictionary of National Biography.* Oxford: Oxford University Press 2004; 30: 527–38.

33 C. Ellmers. *Museum in Docklands: highlights.* London: Museum of London 2003: 72.

Chapter 4

Diseases afflicting sailors before 1821

'For the number of seamen in time of war who die of ship wreck, capture, famine, fire or sword, are but inconsiderable in respect of such as are destroyed by the ship diseases, and by the usual maladies of intemperate climates.'

James Lind (1716–94) – 'the father of nautical medicine'.

The history of disease and mortality in seafarers, from ancient times, has been well documented. One estimate, for example, is that during the Seven-Years-War (1756–62), only 1500 men serving in the Royal Navy (RN) were killed in action, whereas nearly 15,000 died as a result of disease. Morbidity and mortality from disease was in fact a major problem of the seafarer in the sixteenth to eighteenth centuries. Blane (see below) wrote of his West Indian experiences:

> It appears by my returns, that there died in the course of the twelve months preceding July last, on board of ships, seven hundred and fifteen seamen and marines, of whom only fifty-nine died in battle and of wounds. There died at the same time in hospitals eight hundred and sixty-two: that out of twelve thousand one hundred and nine men, which is the sum total of the complement of twenty ships of the line, there have perished in one year one thousand five hundred and seventy-seven, that is nearly every seventh man.

Between 1793 and 1813 about 100,000 naval personnel died: 6.3% were killed by enemy action, 12.2% as a result of shipwreck (or another disaster), and 81.5% as a direct result of disease, or accident. During Ogles' voyage to the West Indies in 1742, only about 3,000 out of 6,000 men were fit for duty. Major health problems were: scurvy and typhus ('ship fever' or 'gaol fever'). Yellow fever ('yellow jack') was a further problem; in 1697, for example, 50% of men (and all of the captains) died during Neville's expedition to the West Indies.[1]

Scurvy was the major problem of long distance voyages; during Admiral Lord Anson (1697–1762)'s (*see* Figure 4.1) disastrous circumnavigation of 1740–44, 1,051 out of 1,955 men died as a direct result of this disease. The value of fruit in warding off scurvy had, however, been well known to Elizabethan sailors; in 1593, for example, Sir Richard Hawkins (1562?–1622)[2] wrote: '... that which I have seen most fruitful for this sickness is sour oranges and lemons'. Although James Lind (1716–94)'s much publicised controlled trial of lime juice as a *preventive* agent (see below)

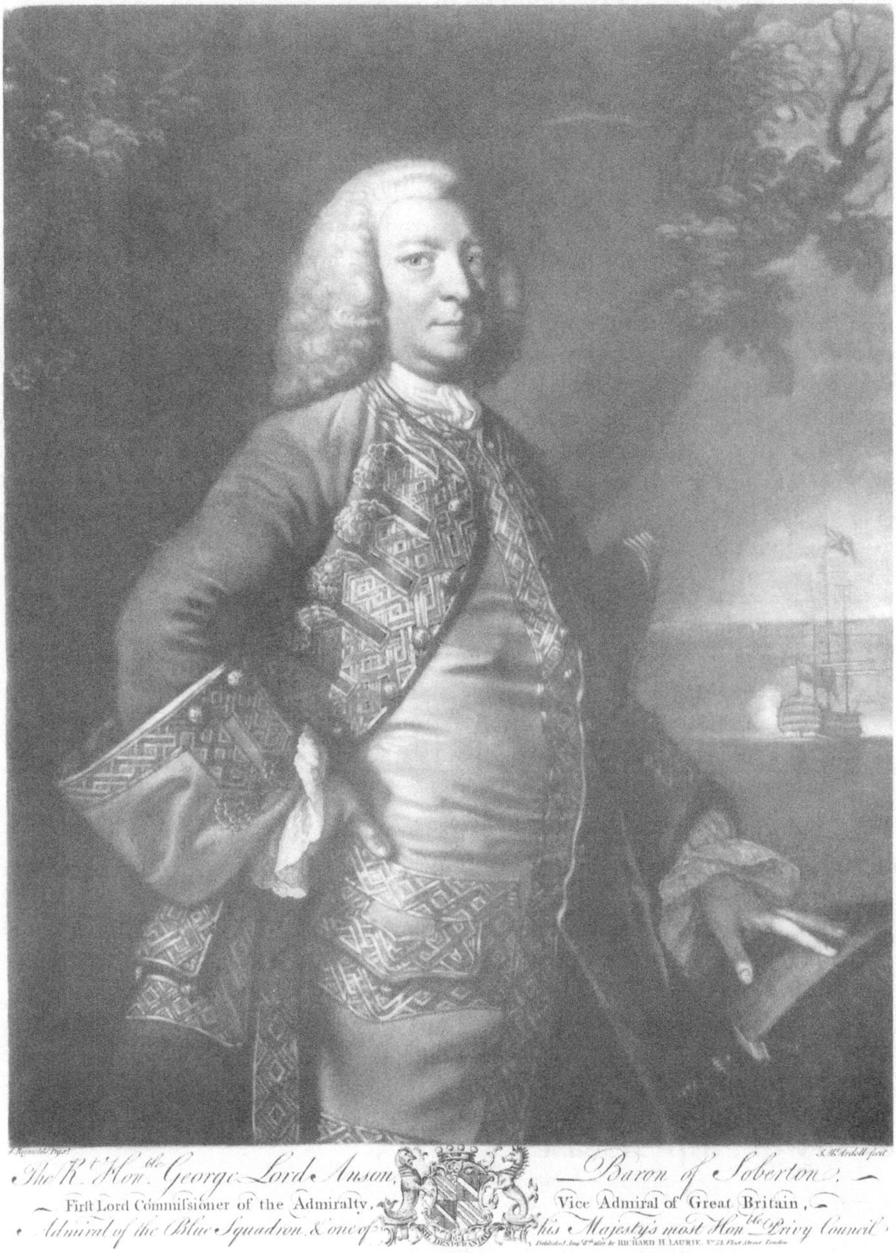

Figure 4.1: This engraving (in the SHS archive) is inscribed: Admiral Lord Anson, Baron of Soberton (1697–1762). 'First Lord Commissioner of the Admiralty. Vice Admiral of Great Britain. Admiral of the Blue Squadron and one of His Majesty's most Honble Privy council.' Published by Richard H Laurie, No. 53 Fleet Street, London. [SHS Archive]. [*See also*: N A M Rodger. Anson, George, Baron Anson (1697–1762). In: H C G Matthew, B Harrison (eds). *Oxford Dictionary of National Biography*. Oxford: Oxford University Press 2004; 2: 260–66.]

was carried out in 1747 (and published in 1753), cases continued appearing in the Mercantile Marine until the early days of the twentieth century (*see* Chapter 11); in the RN, scurvy had been largely tamed by the mid-1790s. From 1740 onwards, *fresh meat* was requested by the Admiralty for the Channel and Western Squadrons. In 1747, fresh greens and beef were specified, and in 1757 (while Anson was first Sea Lord) efforts were made to supply the Western Squadron with these items whilst *at sea*. It is estimated that between 1780 and 1813 deaths from scurvy in the RN were halved, much of this progress having occurred between 1740 and 80. But problems lay with the Victualling Commissioners – who often displayed 'complacency and conservatism'.[3]

'The Surgion's Mate' (for many years an official manual – and used by most surgeons' mates) was published as early as 1617; this had been written by John Woodall (1569–1643), a surgeon at St Bartholomew's Hospital, London, and Surgeon-General to the Honourable East India Company (Chapter 2). He had been a sea-surgeon and surgeon to the military forces in France, Germany, Poland and East Prussia; and was also Master of the Company of Barber-Surgeons in 1633. In his *magnum opus*, he clearly outlined the cure for scurvy (see below) a century before Lind's publication of 1753:

> 'The juyce of Lemons is a precious medicine and well tried being sound and good. It is to be taken each morning two or three spoonfuls and fast after it for two hours and if you add one spoonful of Aqua Vitae thereto to a cold stomach it is the better. Some Chirurgeons also give of this juyce daily to the men in health as a preservative, which course is good, if they have store, otherwise it were best to keep it for need.'[4]

In retrospect, it is perhaps ironic that limes were considered the best cure for scurvy; in 1918, fresh lemons were shown by Chick and her team to possess approximately four-times the vitamin C content of limes.[5] In 1757, Lind also wrote a classical monograph on typhus.

In 1744, at the Admiralty's request, hospitals for the RN were established at several leading ports; The Royal Hospital, Haslar opened in 1746 (the first patients were admitted in 1754) and that at Plymouth in 1761. From 1780 onwards, evaluation of health was required before boarding a 'man of war'.

History of ship-diseases

Ancient writings

As Allison has emphasised, there are few references to sea (or ship) diseases in ancient writings (it is just possible that these mariners already appreciated the *cause* of scurvy), although they were commonplace in the sixteenth to eighteenth centuries. Allison has argued that the rarity of scurvy in ancient times was largely a reflection of shorter voyages; both the English and Dutch East India Companies experienced scurvy on long voyages, 3–4 months being the optimum 'incubation period', and that the 'fevers and fluxes' did not become a problem until 'impressment' became widely practised; the pressed individuals frequently came from poorer social strata, and were often exposed to epidemic disease *before* joining a ship (*see* Chapter 3). The relative rarity of sea diseases in early days was possibly also connected with the simplicity of ship design (with the consequent absence of overcrowding).

The sixteenth to eighteenth centuries

In the Spanish Armada of 1588, the might of England's sea-power (moored off Plymouth) was used against Portugal and Spain. One hundred and thirty galleons (with tonnage varying from 700 to 1300) manned by 30,000 fighting men (together with their slaves and servants) appeared in the English Channel, and threatened invasion of Britain. According to Blane (see below), England had a mere 49 vessels – most in private service, and with a minority belonging to the RN. The Spanish fleet carried 180 priests, but a mere 85 surgeons and/or surgeons' assistants; their food and drinking water also left much to be desired, and dysentery was rife. But the English fleet also had its problems; this sixteenth-century account, for example, appeared in the Acts of the Privy Council:

> 'Whereas a dysease and sickness began to encrease in Her Majesties Navye, for remedie of the dysease and for a staie of further contagion, their Lordships thought meet that some learned and skilful physicians should presently be sent thither; and for that their Lordships hard that good reporte of the sufficiency learning and care of Dr. Gilbert [see below], Dr. Marbeck, Dr. Browne and Dr. Wilkinson, as they were thought very fytt persons to be employed in the said Navye and to have care of the helthe of the noblemen, gentlemen and others in that service.'[6]

William Gilbert (1544–1603), an adviser to the Privy Council, was born at Colchester, and educated at St John's College, Cambridge; he took the MD degree in 1569. Gilbert subsequently became a Fellow, Censor, Treasurer and President (1600) of the Royal College of Physicians. He was also personal physician to Queen Elizabeth I, and his major claim to fame rests on his contributions to the science of electricity (including properties of the magnet). He died (probably of plague) in 1603.[7]

Similar advice to Lind's had been offered by Sir James Lancaster (1554/5–1618)[8] (*see* Chapter 2) – who also served with the East India Company. Lancaster's work has been largely neglected. A pioneer of English trade with the East Indies, he performed a therapeutic experiment, which *prevented* scurvy – some two centuries before Lind. Historically, a major problem with this disease was lack of diagnostic clarity from other disease entities; Sir Gilbert Blane (1749–1834)[9] wrote that confusion reigned amongst medical authorities as to what exactly constituted scurvy, and further how it should be treated.[10]

During Pepys (1633–1703) period as Secretary of the Navy Department, the fleet was manned by 3,000–4,000 men. King Henry VIII instigated expansion of the RN (Chapter 2), and by 1813, numbers of naval personnel had escalated to around 140,000. It was difficult and/or impossible to attract adequate number of volunteers, and therefore *impressment* (*see* Chapter 3) became an important means of filling the vacancies. The great pioneers (the *fleet physicians*) of naval social medicine – Lind, Blane, Trotter, and Burnett – did much to lower the prevalence of scurvy, 'yellow jack', dysentery, and typhus. When these diseases had been brought under control, their superiority waned, and they were replaced by mere *ship's surgeons*.[11] Lloyd has outlined the diseases which afflicted the Fleet (commanded by Lord Hawke) at the Battle of Quiberon Bay in November 1759. Ship fever (typhus) was spread by the 'infected clothing of pressed men', and scurvy ('the scourge of the sea'), both proved to be significant problems.[12]

Disease in Nelson's navy in the late eighteenth century

Admiral Viscount Nelson (1758–1805) considered that '... it is easier for an officer to keep men healthy, than for a physician to cure them'. During the Revolutionary and Napoleonic Wars (*see* Chapter 1) – which lasted, with only a short break, for 22 years – the RN lost 72,000 men from disease or accident on board ship, and only 1,875 in battle; a further 13,600 died in ships lost by accident or bad weather. By 1799 (the sixth year of war), the navy employed 10,000 seamen, 20,000 marines and 634 surgeons; 646 ships were in commission (with 17 receiving-ships in service), but only 400 of these carried surgeons; the remainder merely had a surgeon's mate. Geographical distribution of the ships is of interest:

119	Home waters
81	West Indies
15	American coast, and Newfoundland
39	The Cape of Good Hope Station
69	Portugal, Gibraltar and the Mediterranean
2	The West African Coast
273	In port and refitting
48	Guard, hospital and/or prison ships.[13]

The most important 'naval diseases' at this time were therefore: scurvy, typhus (which had then become commonplace as a result of the Quota System and the press gangs) and yellow fever (which continued to be a major problem in the West Indies).

The nineteenth century

In the late eighteenth and early nineteenth century, disease at sea remained one of the greatest problems facing a ship-owner. The major health hazards then were: tuberculosis, typhoid, cholera, dysentery or one of the tropical diseases (see below); other problems were: hernia, scurvy, and syphilis. The sailor had no formal terms of service, and no sickness benefits; the only hope, if he was severely ill or wounded, was assistance from the Chatham Chest. In the early nineteenth century, of the diseases encountered at sea only smallpox was preventable, by vaccination which had been introduced in 1796 by Edward Jenner (1749–1823). It was not until 1840 that William Budd (1811–80) demonstrated that typhoid (enteric) fever was spread by human excreta. Transmission of typhus by lice was not established until 1909. Proof of mosquito-transmission of *Plasmodium* spp was made in 1897 (by Ronald Ross [1857–1932]); four years later (in 1901) the role of the mosquito (*Aedes aegypti*) in transmitting yellow fever was unravelled.[14]

By the late *nineteenth* century, the prevalence of the most important 'Sea Diseases' in the RN was in decline. This had begun with Lind's recommendations of 1781; all newly pressed men were placed in a receiving (or slop) ship where they could be washed and provided with clean clothing before being drafted to other vessels. From then on, the incidence of typhus in the RN plummeted. However, in the *Mercantile Marine*, these diseases were to continue for several more decades.

The first annual report of the SHS (1822) highlighted some of the health problems facing the Mercantile Marine:

> '... It frequently happens, that vessels coming into the Thames from long voyages, have most distressing cases of sickness, disease, or accident on board; the subjects of which are now sent to [HMS] Grampus [the first of the SHS Hospital-ships], where timely application being afforded, many have been restored with astonishing rapidity, who but for this institution, must have waited some days before admission could have been procured for them into hospitals on shore, and with the hazard of being rendered incurable, from the effect of delay in applying a remedy. This is a feature peculiar to the Seamen's Hospital; the importance and great advantage of which must be obvious to every feeling and reflecting mind.
>
> The rules and regulations by which other hospitals are governed, limit the period which the patients are permitted to remain in them, to that of their receiving medical treatment, which is generally sufficient, as the objects to whom their beneficence is extended have homes to receive them after cure; and friends to support and comfort them; whilst, on the contrary, a sailor who has gained admittance into an hospital is, after being relieved from his complaint, discharged in a weak condition, without a home to go to, or a place to yield him a night's repose, and is compelled to wander about the streets; whereas, in the Seamen's Hospital, every person is allowed to remain on board in a state of convalescence, until he has completely regained his health and strength; and, in the interim, an opportunity is afforded him of obtaining employment, by his own endeavours, in which he is aided by the personal intercession of the Committee among their friends connected with the shipping interests; by which means many men are embarked almost immediately for those climates most congenial to their constitutions.'[15]

Alcoholism was also a major problem at this time; like 'tropical fevers' it affected all classes – from senior officers to the bosun's mate. Tobacco chewing was another habit prevalent amongst seamen.[16]

The major sea-diseases

What then were these diseases which destroyed so many sailors? In the appendix to his work: *An Essay of the Most Effectual Means of Preserving the Health of Seamen in the Royal Navy,* Lind gave a list of the illnesses experienced by 5,743 seamen admitted to the Royal Hospital, Haslar, during a two-year period, 1 July 1758–1 July 1760:

Fevers	2174
Scurvy	1146
Consumptions	360
Rheumatisms	350
Fluxes	245
Total:	4275

He then proceeded to record other complaints among the remaining 1468 seamen admitted to that hospital (*see* Table 4.1). The most devastating 'fever' at sea at that time was undoubtedly typhus, which Lind felt was related to the filthy vermin-infested clothing worn by most of the men seized by the press gangs for compulsory service in the navy. Typhoid fever and plague were also common; in the tropics, ships' companies suffered heavily from malaria and yellow fever (see above).[17] In the early eighteenth century, typhus was prevalent and carried a high mortality; the first English fleet sent to America in 1756, for example, lost two thousand men from this disease alone. Until comparatively recently the causal organisms responsible for all of these diseases were of course unknown; for a large part of the period under review, therefore, they were undifferentiated and grouped together as 'fevers'* or 'calentures' (the latter term from the Spanish word '*calentura*' having no special significance). Though the essential part played by the louse in transmission of typhus was not recognised until the last century, health reforms introduced in 1781 had done much to reduce its incidence in the RN.

Malaria came under the 'umbrella' of 'ague' ('malignant fever of the remitting or intermitting, but most frequently of the double tertian kind') and yellow fever, or the 'black vomit', were responsible for numerous deaths, especially in the West Indies. It was not until the close of the nineteenth century, when their mode of transmission had been delineated, that these two diseases were brought under control. Strictly speaking, they were not 'sea diseases' at all, but early observers considered that they were due to the 'noxious land breeze'. They are included here because the conditions under which the seamen of the RN had to live and fight to secure Britain's interests and possessions abroad, made them relevant.

A high proportion of sailors was vaccinated against smallpox after about 1800, although religious scruples prevented anything like a 100% up-take. Like scurvy, venereal disease contributed to 'the basis of marine practice from its frequent occurrence, and the various forms it assumes'.

William Turnbull (1729?–96) considered that consumption was frequently the consequence of smallpox and dysentery, and that chronic rheumatism, which

*This term had a much wider context than in the present day.

Table 4.1: Diseases, excluding major ones, (arranged on a *symptomatic* basis) leading to 1468 admissions to the Royal Hospital, Haslar, in a two year period – 1758–60.*

Angina	10
Apoplexy	3
Asthma	40
Ague and Intermittent Fever	67
Pains of 'Old Hurts'	80
Cachectic	20
Dropsy	24
'Chincough'	5
Colics	10
Deafness	6
Epilepsy	30
Eye Disorders	30
Gout	3
Gravel	20
Headaches	17
Spitting Blood	30
Hypochondriacs	10
Jaundice	15
Incontinence Urine	25
For the Lethargy	3
For the Lientary	7
Leprosy	30
Lumbago	20
Madness	14
Melancholy	5
Measles	31
Palsy	20
Strangury	5
Scrofula	15
Scalded Hands	20
V.D.'s chirurgical – Itch chiefly	680
The 'True Peripneumony'	29
The True Pleurisy	11
Cutaneous Diseases	73
Sciatica	7
Smallpox	53

*Figures represent, after exclusion of the *major* 'ship diseases' (see p. 52), numbers of cases suffering from each entity.

affected a 'younger part of the crew', was associated with 'A long train of rainy and stormy weather in the Channel ...'. The West Indies station was, in Turnbull's opinion, 'avowedly the most unhealthy'. He also wrote on yellow fever, considering it to be most common in individuals 'lately [arrived] from Europe'. In addition, he described tetanus, and fish-poisoning. In a 'break-down' of the causes of disease in three voyages to the West Indies, Turnbull noted 290 with 'fevers', 141 with 'dysenteries or fluxes' and the remainder of the 506 were 'scorbutic patients'. He offered good advice generally, although obviously he could not have suspected the causative role of the mosquito (or any other vector) in transmitting disease. He considered that men should not sleep on shore, being more concerned with 'night vapours' than mosquitoes) and that ships should anchor some distance from the coast – 'so far as not to smell the land air'.[18]

The 'fluxes' or diarrhoeas made their appearance especially when men were debilitated after long periods at sea, or were convalescent from 'fevers' and other acute illnesses. The larger outbreaks, which often attained epidemic proportions, were probably caused by *Shigella* spp resulting from a contaminated or impure water supply.

Accounts by Authorities on Sea Diseases

Both Brugis and Aubrey wrote contemporary texts in the seventeenth and eighteenth centuries, respectively, on various aspects of nautical medicine; the latter's book was especially concerned with the management and care of negro slaves.[19] William Cockburn (1669–1739)[20] was probably the first writer to produce a text exclusively devoted to the medical aspects of sea diseases (*Sea Diseases, or a Treatise of their Nature, Causes and Cure* [1736]). Educated at Edinburgh and Leyden (where he obtained an MD), he later became a fellow of the Royal Society and of the (Royal) College of Physicians. He was also Physician to the Fleet (accompanying Sir Cloudsley-Shovell in a squadron of ships which served in the Mediterranean in 1704). In 1731 he became Physician to the Royal Hospital, Greenwich (*see* Chapter 13). The principle diseases at sea, he wrote, were 'scurvy, fevers, and fluxes'. He was also an expert on 'pressed' men (Chapter 3) and of the diseases which resulted from this practice.[21]

Another pioneer of Sea Diseases during this period was Thomas Dover (c1660–1742) ('the quicksilver doctor'); as well as being the inventor of Dover's Powder (for gout), he wrote an important book '*The Ancient Physician's Legacy to his Country, being what he has collected himself in forty-nine years of practice*' (1733), which went to seven editions – the last being published in 1762.[22]

In his text *The Naval Surgeon,* first published in 1806, Turnbull (see above) listed the diseases prevalent at various stations, as well as those more common in winter ('fevers and inflammatory complaints' including typhus, 'intermittent fevers or agues', and rheumatism) and summer (which assume a 'chiefly nervous and putrid form'). Dysentery, he wrote, was especially liable to appear 'after a long [period] of stormy or rainy weather, and when the ship [had] been for a considerable time at sea'; it was more common in the tropics, and 'often [appeared] at the same time with scurvy'.[23]

Pope has recalled in detail the impact that 'fevers' – especially yellow fever and scurvy – had on John Markham's expedition to the West Indies in *Hannibal* in 1795; he lost 200 men from yellow fever during a 6-month period.[24] But this experience was by no means unique; almost every expedition ended with a similar tragedy!

Early twentieth century

Home (see above) has given details of disease prevalence in the *Mercantile Marine* immediately prior to the Great War (1914–18), i.e. when the SHS had been in existence for nearly a century; he emphasises that there was no official documentation, as was the case in the RN, and furthermore, that many diagnoses were made by laymen (i.e. ship's captains) unlike those in the RN and Army in which they were made by qualified medical practitioners.

The most striking difference in death-rates in the merchant navy, compared with the RN and Army was the high injury-rate (4.14 per 1000 men, compared with 1.07 and 0.62, respectively, in the other groups). Alcohol-associated deaths were also higher – 0.69 compared with 0.03 and 0.01. The respective figures for cardiovascular disease and suicide, were 0.44 (compared with 0.20 and 0.25) and 0.30 (compared with 0.11 and 0.18). When heat-stroke, injuries and suicide were combined 4.56 men per 1000 died, compared with 1.18 and 0.86 in the RN and Army. Of interest is that Lascars* had a death-rate from pneumonia which was three-times that of the other groups; Home attributes this to overcrowding and/or defective ventilation. Death-rate associated with tuberculosis (attributed to similar factors) was over twice as high in Lascars compared with the other groups. The *space* allocated to the Lascars was little more than half that granted to British and 'foreign' seamen.

Dysentery and malaria were also more common in the *Merchant Service* compared with the other groups; in Home's opinion though, this was mainly due to less efficient diagnosis (by laymen). He concluded:

> The Ministry of Health takes care of the health of every one in England outside the fighting services, why [then] do we discriminate against the merchant service?[25]

Naval medical officers of the eighteenth and nineteenth centuries

The difference between a naval *surgeon* (essentially a craftsman) and a *physician* was enormous; the latter (there were only three on the Navy List of 1799) was appointed either to the Fleet or to a specific hospital, and he was essentially a gentleman – who was bound by a strict ethical code – and always possessed a medical *degree*; he had previously served as a ship's surgeon for five years or more. A *surgeon* however, had to pass, following an apprenticeship, an examination at Surgeon's Hall, Lincoln's Inn Fields. Regulations stated that a prospective surgeon

*An East Indian sailor [*see*: J A Simpson, E S C Weiner (eds). *Oxford English Dictionary* 2nd ed. Oxford: Clarendon Press 1989; 8: 666].

(or surgeon's mate) had to apply to the *Navy Commissioners of the Sick and Hurt* at Somerset House for a letter to the Surgeons' Company; he then had to pass a second examination organised by the Surgeons' Company, and if successful, a third which was organised by the Commissioners. Despite this seemingly rigorous system, many naval surgeons were far from being of the highest calibre. A surgeon was paid £5.00 per month, and two pence per man per month by the ship in which he served, and £5.00 for every 100 men he treated for venereal disease; there was also the 'Queen Anne's Free Gift to Surgeons' which was paid annually; this depended on the size of the ship. Surgeon's mates were also entitled to this award albeit at a lower level! 'Half pay' for surgeons depended on seniority; the first 20 (provided they had served for nine years) received 5s, and the next 100 (with seven years service) 3s daily; surgeon's mates and others received lower rates of pay.[26]

In Turnbull's judgement (see above), the first step towards keeping a ship's company healthy was to 'diminish the quantity of salted food administered to them'. He also believed that flannel worn next to the skin was 'one of the best preservations of health'; therefore, (he wrote) all seamen serving in the West Indies should be issued with two *thin flannel shirts* – which absorb perspiration. Surgery in the early nineteenth century was rudimentary, amputation being performed without an anaesthetic, or any antiseptic cover. Hernia (from which numerous sailors suffered) was treated with a 'well constructed truss' and *not* surgery.

Overall, the life of a sailor was probably only 'slightly more unhealthy than that of his 'brother living in a town or city'; drinking water (a ration of small beer was a substitute) was often smelly, but unlikely to be contaminated by sewage! A farm labourer had, by and large, as strenuous a life as that of a seaman – and just as much chance of getting a hernia! When ill, the sailor could report sick and consult the ship's surgeon, unlike his land-based 'brother' who was unlikely to be able to afford medical treatment.[27]

Hospital and health-care facilities

The benefits of the Royal Hospital, Greenwich were *strictly* reserved for those who had served in the RN. Despite this, sixpence was deducted every month from the salaries of *all* seamen (including those of the Merchant Navy) in the British Empire – whether they belonged to the RN or not![28] Hospital facilities at Haslar, Plymouth and Chatham – with their splendid buildings were also restricted to those who had served in the RN.[29] These factors obviously provoked a great deal of bad feeling in the *Mercantile Marine*. That is one major reason why the emergence of the SHS in 1821 (*see* Chapter 6) brought such welcome news for the sailors in the *Merchant Service*.

References and notes

1 R S Allison. *Sea diseases: the story of a great natural experiment in preventive medicine in the Royal Navy*. London: John Bale Medical Publications Ltd. 1943; J J Keevil. *Medicine and the navy 1200–1900*. Vol 1, 1200–1649; vol 2, 1649–1714. Edinburgh & London: E &

S Livingstone 1957 and 1958: 255 and 332; C Lloyd, J L S Coulter. *Medicine and the navy 1200–1900.* Vol 3, 1714–1815; vol 4, 1815–1900. Edinburgh & London: E & S Livingstone 1961 & 1963: 402 and 300; D A Baugh. The eighteenth century Navy as a national institution 1690–1815. In: J R Hill (ed). *The Oxford Illustrated History of the Royal Navy*. Oxford: Oxford University Press. 1995: 120–60. [*See also*: P Earle. Mortality and medicine. In: *Sailors: English Merchant Seamen 1650–1775.* London: Methuen: 129–142; G C Cook. Influence of diarrheal disease on military and naval campaigns. *J Roy Soc Med* 2001; 94: 95–97.]

2 D Loades. Hawkins [Hawkyns] Sir Richard (c1560–1622). In: H C G Matthew, B Harrison (eds). *Oxford Dictionary of National Biography*. Oxford: Oxford University Press 2004; 25: 934–6.

3 *Op cit*. See note 1 above (Keevil); J Watt. The medical bequest of disease at sea: Commodore Anson's circumnavigation 1740–44. *J Roy Coll Phys Lond*. 1998: 32: 572–579. [See also: G Williams. *The prize of all the oceans*. London: HarperCollins 1999: 264.]

4 J H Appleby. Woodall, John (1570–1643). In: H C G Matthew, B Harrison (eds). *Oxford Dictionary of National Biography*. Oxford: Oxford University Press 2004; 60: 155–7; Anonymous. John Woodall. 1570–1643. *Br J Surg* 1617–17, 4; J Woodall. *The surgions mate: a complete facsimile of the book published in 1617*. Bath: Kingsmead Press: 1978; C M Longfield-Jones. John Woodall, Surgeon General of the East India Company. Part I: Events leading to Woodall's appointment. *J Med Biog* 1995; 3: 11–19. *Ibid*. Part II: A consideration of the provision made for treating injuries and diseases at sea. 71–78.

5 J Watt, E J Freeman, W F Bynum (eds). *Starving sailors: the influence of nutrition upon naval and maritime history.* Bristol: National Maritime Museum: 1981; G C Cook. Scurvy in the British mercantile marine in the 19th century, and the contribution of the Seamen's Hospital Society. *Postgrad Med J*. 2004 80: 224–9.

6 *Op cit.* See note 1 above (Allison).

7 S Pumfrey. Gilbert, William (1544?-1603). In: H C G Matthew, B Harrison (eds). *Oxford Dictionary of National Biography*. Oxford: Oxford University Press 2004; 22: 195–202; C Singer. Dr William Gilbert (1544–1603). *J Royal Nav Med Serv*. 1916; 2 (4): 495; M Smith. William Gilbert (1544–1603): physician and founder of electricity. *J Med Biog*. 1997; 5: 137–145.

8 C F Beckingham. Lancaster, Sir James (1554/5–1618). In: H C G Matthew, B Harrison (eds). *Oxford Dictionary of National Biography*. Oxford: Oxford University Press 2004; 32: 358–9.

9 J Wallace. Blane, Sir Gilbert, first baronet (1749–1834). In: H C G Matthew, B Harrison (eds). *Oxford Dictionary of National Biography*. Oxford: Oxford University Press 2004; 6: 172–5; G Blane. *Selected Dissertations on Several Subjects of Medical Science*. London (2 vols): 1833.

10 *Op cit.* See note 1 above (Allison).

11 *Ibid*: 49–69 and 88–112; C Lloyd (ed). *The health of seamen: selections from the works of Dr James Lind, Sir Gilbert Blane and Dr Thomas Trotter*. London: Navy Records Society. 1965. [See also: G C Cook. Richard Dobson Kt MRCS FRS (1773–1847) and the inferior status of naval medicine in the early nineteenth century: end of the fleet Physicians. *Notes Rec R Soc* 2005; 59: 35–43.

12 C Lloyd. *Hearts of Oak: the battle of Quiberon Bay November 20th, 1759*: 744–751.

13 D Pope. The Real Enemy. In: D. Pope. *Life in Nelson's navy*. London: Chatham Publishing 1997: 131–148.; [See also: B Lavery. *Nelson's fleet at Trafalgar*. London: National Maritime Museum 2004: 208.]

14 V Corstorphine. *Some aspects of the history and development of the Dreadnought Seamen's Hospital between 1821 and 1870*. 1968 [SHS Archive]; J Winton. Life and education in a

technically evolving navy 1815–1925. In: J R Hill (ed). *The Oxford Illustrated Dictionary of the Royal Navy*. Oxford: Oxford University Press 1995: 254; [See also: G C Cook. Disease in the nineteenth century merchant navy: the Seamen's Hospital Society's experience. *Mariner's Mirror* 2001; 87: 460–471; G C Cook. Medical disease in the Merchant navies of the world in the days of sail: the Seamen's Hospital Society's experience. *Ibid*. 2005; 91: 46–51; G C Cook. *Tropical medicine: an illustrated history of the pioneers*. London: Academic Press 2007.]

15 R Harley. First (annual) report of the Seamen's Hospital Society. In: *Under the Patronage of His Majesty. The first and second Reports of the Committee of Management of the Hospital Ship Grampus, for sick and diseased seamen arriving in the Port of London. Supported by donations and voluntary contributions*. Established in 1821. London: W. Gilbert 1822: 11–18.

16 W E Home. The Diseases of the Merchant Seamen. In: *Merchant Seamen: their disease and welfare needs*. London: John Murray 1922: 82–97.

17 *Op cit*. See note 11 above (Lloyd). *Op cit*. See note 1 above (Allison). xv-xxiii; J Lind. *Essay on the most Effectual Means of Preserving the Health of Seamen in the Royal Navy*. 3rd ed. London: 1774.

18 E I Carlyle, A McConnell. Turnbull, William (1729?-1796). In: H C G Matthew, B Harrison (eds). *Oxford Dictionary of National Biography*. Oxford: Oxford University Press 2004; 55: 595; G C Cook, A J Webb. Perceptions of malaria transmission before Ross' discovery in 1897. *Postgrad Med J* 2000; 78: 738–740.

19 T Brugis. *Vade Macum, or A Companion for a Chyrurgion for Land or Sea Service*. London: 1652; T Aubrey. *The Sea Surgeon or the Guinea Man's Vade Macum*. London: 1729.

20 C Creighton, A Guerrini. Cockburn, William (1669–1739). In: H C G Matthew, B Harrison (eds). *Oxford Dictionary of National Biography*. Oxford: Oxford University Press 2004; 12: 346–7; *Op cit*. See note 1 above (Allison).

21 W Cockburn. *Sea Diseases; or a Treatise of their Nature, Causes and Cure*. 3rd ed. London: 1736; *Op cit*. See note 1 above (Allison). [See also: G C Cook. Robert Robertson, FRS (1742–1829): physician to the Royal Hospital, Greenwich, 18th century authority on 'fever', and early practitioner in care of the elderly. *J Med Biog* 2006; 14: 42–45.]

22 S P Menefee. Dover, Thomas (bap 1662 d 1742). In: H C G Matthew, B Harrison (eds). *Oxford Dictionary of National Biography*. Oxford: Oxford University Press 2004; 16: 759–61.

23 *Op cit*. See note 18 above.

24 *Op cit*. See note 13 above (Pope).

25 *Op cit*. See note 16 above.

26 *Op cit*. See note 11 above (Cook); T Smollett. *The adventures of Roderick Random*. Oxford: Oxford University Press 1979: 481.

27 *Op cit*. See note 1 above (Allison).

28 P Newell. *Greenwich Hospital: a Royal Foundation 1692–1983*. London: The Trustees of Greenwich Hospital 1984, 16–19, 121–122, 150.

29 *Op cit*. See note 1 above (Allison): 150–167; H. Richardson. Naval hospitals. In: *English Hospitals 1660–1948: a survey of their architecture and design*. London: Royal Commission on the Historical Monuments of England: 76–86.

Chapter 5

The SHS's *precursor*, early meetings aimed at London's homeless: 'Most of the Destitute seem to be Sailors'

The history of care for British seafarers since 894 is set out in a letter dated 1821 (i.e. the year of the foundation of the SHS) to the Chairman of the Society [Committee] for Destitute Sailors. In a preamble, the author records:

> Having observed in the public papers of March 19th 1821, the Committee of the Seamen's Hospital for managing the funds subscribed in the winter of 1817–18 I beg leave to lay before them all the provision for Seamen their wives, widows and orphans. The fundamental maxim of our Country is [the author continued], that Trade is the nursery of Sailors, that Sailors are the Soul of the Navy, that the Navy is the Security of Commerce and that these two united produce the richest Power and Glory of Great Britain. [After giving credit to King Henry VIII for founding the Royal Navy (RN), he continued]: Queen Elizabeth was zealous in providing for the British Merchant Seaman, her grant to the *Trinity House* [and] how willing Her Majesty was to promote the funds of this great and benevolent establishment'.[1]

As early as 1785, a letter published in the *Daily Advertiser* had proclaimed: 'I am shocked at the number of miserable objects, lascars, that I see shivering and starving in the streets'.[2]

History of sailors' health

Historically, welfare of the sailor is shrouded in antiquity. The *Hull Seamen's Guild* (later *Trinity House*) was established in 1456, and five years later an almshouse was opened 'for the sustentation and relieving of thirteen persons who by misfortune of the sea shall happen to fall into poverty by loss of goods'. About 200 years later the almshouse was enlarged to accommodate thirty seamen's widows in little chambers or cells, to which, at a later date casements were fitted 'for sweetening the lodgings'.[3] Some 50 years after this initiative (in 1514) (Hull had been the first port to take practical steps towards seamen's welfare) *Trinity House* began its charitable work for sailors in London (*see* Chapter 3); founded by Royal Charter, a Hall and Almshouse were established at Deptford. Captain Sir Arthur Clarke KBE (a former President of the SHS) has outlined the history of this famous institution. Despite loss of much archival material in two fires, there is evidence of the existence of *Trinity House* (as a *Guild or Fraternity of Mariners* at Deptford) in Tudor times. The first Charter (granted by Henry VIII) and confirmed by Elizabeth I, enlarged the privileges and duties of a body which was already actively engaged in safeguarding the interests of mariners, and the Thames-borne trade of England. The relief of poor seamen and their relations has always been a high priority of this institution. Elder Brethren (elected from the Younger Brethren) of the past have included: Drake, Hawkins and Frobisher.[4]

Between 1514 and 1694, hospitals (i.e. homes for the aged and *not* hospitals in the modern sense) were opened in six ports: the *Merchant Venturers' Almshouses* (Bristol) (1550), the *Sir John Hawkins Hospital* (Chatham) (1594), *Scarborough Trinity House and merchant seamen's hospital* (1602), the *Whitby merchant seamen's hospital* (1675), the *Fisherman's Hospital* (Great Yarmouth) (1668), and the *Royal Hospital (Greenwich)* (1694). Elsewhere, little or nothing was done for sailors for over a century.

During the eighteenth century, an almshouse for merchant seamen was instituted in Sunderland (1750), and in 1756 the *Marine Society* (see below) was founded by the London-based philanthropist Jonas Hanway. Its immediate aim was to encourage poor men and boys of good character to join the RN at the beginning of the Seven Years War (1756–63); by the end of that war, the Society had recruited 5,451 men and 5,174 boys. In 1772 it was incorporated by Act of Parliament to apprentice poor boys to the RN and Merchant Service, to equip them with clothing, and to provide a pre-sea education. In 1786, the 350-ton sloop *Beatty* (which became the first pre-sea training ship in the world) was commissioned; this was in the charge of a Superintendent assisted by a Mate, Schoolmaster, Boatswain and Cook. The ship was succeeded by a succession of training ships, most moored off Deptford and Greenwich. In more recent times, the Society has supported other maritime organisations, including the SHS, *King George's Fund for Sailors*, the *Sea Cadet Corps*, the *Outward Bound Schools*, the *Sail and Training Association*, the *Nautical Institute*, and the *Annual National Service for Seafarers*. Between 1974 and 76, the Society either merged with, or established links, with: *The Sailors Home* and *Ensign Club*, the *Seafarers Education Service*, the *College of the Sea*, the *British Ship Adoption Society* and the *Merchant Navy Comforts Service Trust*.[5]

By the nineteenth century roads were improving and increasing numbers of people were becoming aware of ships and sailors; the nation's conscience had been aroused, and many other voluntary organisations with the object of caring for seamen's welfare were founded. Many of these were primarily missionary societies (including the *British Sailors Society* [1833] and *The Mission to Seamen* [1856]), the major purpose of which was to attend to the sailors' *spiritual* requirements. At this time also, Sailors' Homes were established at several ports, some on hulks; here the sailor could get a decent bed and meal, and be free from touts and prostitutes. However, the first institution to provide *medical* and *surgical* aid (specifically for the sailor) was the Seamen's Hospital Society (SHS), preceded by about three years by the *Society for the Relief of Destitute Seamen* (CRDS).

Other nineteenth century initiatives

Several benevolent funds for the mercantile marine had been launched *before* the SHS was founded – *Lloyds Patriotic fund* (1803), and *The shipwrecked fishermen and mariners Royal Benevolent Society*, with Queen Victoria as the Patron, and Admiral the Right Hon. Sir George Cockburn as the first President, which had its origin in 1839. It was founded 'for the purpose of forming a fund for the relief of Mariners and Fishermen, or in the case of loss of life, for the Widows and Orphans'. In 1850, this Society was *incorporated* by Act of Parliament, and in 1865, its title was changed to *'The Belvedere Hospital for Worn-out and Disabled Merchant Seamen'*; in 1868 this was again altered to *'The Royal Alfred Aged Merchant Seamen's Institution'*. In its first 100 years, 1839–1939, it assisted a total of 895,000 persons.[6] *The Royal Patriotic Fund Corporation* was founded in 1854.

But not all organisations were *bone fide*. For example, the *Royal Naval Asylum* for the education and maintenance of orphan and other children of HM sailors and mariners originated in a fraudulent pretence of establishing in 1798, an institution (the *British Endeavour*) of this nature in Paddington. The Duke of Sussex and others having their suspicions aroused, investigated the project, and the projector or manager was subsequently committed to prison for fraud. As the utility of the design was apparent, a naval asylum was however subsequently founded, and flourished for some time at Paddington, the Duke of Cumberland being the first president.[7]

Welfare of sailors in the nineteenth century

Care of destitute individuals amongst Britain's rapidly growing population (especially in London) was therefore by no means original. Various philanthropists (William Wilberforce MP [1759–1833] and Zachary Macauley [1768–1838] included – see below) focused their thoughts and actions on servicemen who had served Britain during the Napoleonic wars – and had no fixed abode on land![8]

At a time when the British Industrial Revolution was getting into full swing (Chapter 1) there was therefore, already a growing interest (and concern) about the health of the Merchant Seaman. Some six years before the battle of Trafalgar (21 October 1805)[9], the *Gentleman's Magazine* quoting a letter from a Southwark surgeon – Alexander Stewart – who had made recommendations concerning the health of serving staff employed on the Honourable East India Company's Ships, i.e. '...those valuable men, the British seamen'. The areas to be targeted included: 'Cleanliness, Air, Diet, Water, Liquor, Rest, Exercise, and Clothing', matters which had been emphasised (on land) by John Wesley (1703–91) and Simon Tissot (1747–1834) in the eighteenth century, and by Thomas Southwood Smith (1788–1861) and Florence Nightingale (1820–1910) amongst others in the nineteenth. But the concern was not specifically 'medical'; it involved the overall well-being of the sailor – including his 'soul'. In a letter (based on a book) addressed to 'The Honourable the Court of Directors', Stewart considered that when death seemed inevitable, pastoral care should be available; '... there are [he wrote, currently] no *chaplains* on-board the East India ships.'[10]

A 'refuge for the destitute'

The state of seamen in the Port of London immediately after the Napoleonic Wars has been well described by John Ashton in: *Social England under the Regency*. There was at that time a great 'trade depression' in England, and thousands of men-of-war's men were paid off – without receipt by a pension.[11]

As early as May 1807, *The Times* reported on a meeting of the Committee of a newly formed charity, '*Refuge for the destitute*' based in Lambeth – which had as its president the Duke of York (1763–1827). An abstract of its report was 'made public, in the confident persuasion, that this Institution need only be known, in order to insure it the liberal support of the benevolent'. The Committee was impressed with the necessity of 'affording moral and religious instruction to the inmates of the Refuge'. They had therefore 'engaged a Clergyman of the Church of England to read Prayers, and deliver a Discourse, on a Sunday, and attend twice in the week besides for the instruction of the ignorant'. Up to that date, 58 persons had applied for admission, and of these 20 had been successful: 'The males [were] employed splitting fire-wood, and occasionally working in the garden. The females [were] employed in spinning, making house-hold and body linen, washing, &c.'. Several 'liberal donations' had been received, and the 'Funds of the Charity' already stood at approximately 2500/(£). The report continued ' ... most of the difficulties [facing the inauguration of this institution], are now done away, and, a Refuge is actually opened, where the penitent Criminal, the deserted Female, the helpless Labourer, and the famished Stranger, may find employment, support, and instruction.' A further meeting (the 'Annual Dinner') of 'that excellent Institution' was held at the City of London Tavern on 28 January 1808, under the presidency of the Duke of York. This was, apparently, also valuable and augured 'favourably of its future success'.

Nearly a decade later, little more than a year after the Battle of Waterloo (18 June 1815)[12] another meeting was held – again at the City of London Tavern. This took place on 29 July 1816. During this post-war period, there was great unemployment in some areas (*see* Chapter 1) and it was accompanied by 'great individual distress'. On this occasion, the Duke of York was supported by the Dukes' of Kent and Cambridge, and accompanied by 'the Archbishop of Canterbury [Charles Manner-Sutton (1755–1828)], the Bishop of London, the Duke of Rutland, Lord Manvers, the Chancellor of the Exchequer, . . . William Wilberforce (*see* Chapter 1) and other distinguished individuals'. However, in the ensuing discussion, Lord Cochrane considered that the 'existing distress could *not* [my italics] be truly ascribed to any sudden transition from war to peace' as had already been proposed. Despite these comments, opposed by Wilberforce, several supportive resolutions were passed:

1. That there does exist a stagnation of employment, producing many instances of great local distress.
2. That it may be confidently expected, that those who are able to afford the means of relief will contribute their utmost endeavours to alleviate these sufferings.
3. That though it be impossible for any Association to attempt the general relief of such difficulties, yet that it has been proved by experience, that extensive benefits may be derived from the co-operation and correspondence of a

Society in the Metropolis, encouraging the efforts of individuals associating in different districts, for the relief of their several neighbourhoods. [and]

4. That a subscription be immediately opened, and contributions generally solicited.[13]

The '*Refuge for the Destitute*' celebrated its 11th anniversary in 1818 with a dinner, also at the City of London Tavern. A brief report in *The Times* of this event recorded that 'Above 1,000 *l.* were subscribed, 50 *l.* of which came from the Royal Duke who presided, and 25 *l.* from Lord Sidmouth. The only curious thing [*The Times* continued] was, that 'Mr Protheroe [a Vice-President of the *Refuge for the Destitute*], the Whig Member of Parliament, gave the health of Lord Sidmouth on public grounds'. This immediately brought forth a reply from Protheroe: 'I added, that this tribute of applause did not proceed from a political adherent of the noble Lord's but one who had frequently felt it his duty to oppose the minister, but had never ceased to respect the man'[14].

This charity was *not* however, concerned essentially with the wants of sailors; it had been founded with the idea of assisting London's destitute in general.

'Most of London's destitute seem to be sailors'

By 1818 there seems to have been increasing recognition of the fact that the majority of the 'mendicants' were or had been merchant seamen: 'Of the many objects who are now standing in the streets, the greater part [a leader-writer in *The Times* declared] are in what have once been sailor's jackets: these might, we should suppose, be removed on board some vessel, which should be prepared for their reception, in the River, where their wants might be relieved, and their disorders attended to …'. 'Where parishes become oppressed by the excess of beggars, [he continued], and do not possess the means of suppressing them, let them call meetings, and appeal to the general humanity of their countrymen'. This leading article also outlined the *status quo*. 'The law ordains, that after a confinement of seven days [mendicants] should be sent to their parishes' and that if '… the workhouses are insufficient to contain them, other houses ought to be engaged, either by a general subscription … or by parochial subscriptions.' The writer then recalled (although he considered the action 'anti-christian [and] anti-human') '… that on a former occasion, when a meeting was convened for the purpose of providing some method of relieving the starving manufacturers, a set of political philanthropists stepped in and said, that relief only prolonged their miseries; it was better to let them starve'! Despite this opposition, 'subscriptions were still raised, and much good done'.[15]

The identity of the individual who first saw an urgent need to assist this group of seafarers will in all probability never be known with certainty. However, the following 'cutting' signed by 'WBR' apparently taken from a 'London newspaper of 1863' (during the time of the third SHS Hospital-ship) although somewhat confused, might throw some light on this dilemma:

> In the year 1817–18, at the end of the long war, when large numbers of the seamen who had been discharged from their several vessels were lying about the streets of London sick and destitute, a committee of

naval officers and others was appointed by the "Society for the Aid of Destitute Seamen" to consider what was best to be done for these poor men. This committee used to hold its meetings at the King's Head. Mr. Bob Blake, R.N.[16] (his name was "Bob", not Robert), who was at that time Examining Surgeon to the port of London, and attached to the ship Perseus, lying off the Tower, was appointed by the committee, as their surgeon, to go round and look up the destitute seamen for the purpose of affording them some assistance. Mr. Blake, fulfilling his function as well as he could, placed the sick men in different workhouses and hospitals; but found it so difficult to deal with them, scattered in that way, that he turned his mind to considering what could be done that would be better. He came to the conclusion that the best thing was to recommend the committee to petition the Government for a vessel, which should be devoted to hospital purposes. …

Mr. Bob Blake – *Dr.* Blake he is called in the memorandum lying before me – was, therefore, the originator of the "Dreadnought" as an institution. I believe the fact to be entirely unknown, except to his descendants and their connections; but do not think it should remain so. I may add that the services of Mr. Blake as surgeon to these seamen were entirely gratuitous, and received no further acknowledgment than is contained in the vote of thanks of which the following is a copy:-

> 'At a meeting of the committee of the "Society for the Aid of Destitute Seamen," held on the 16th of January, 1818 – John Deacon, Esq., in the chair:-
>
> Resolved, that the thanks of this committee be given to Dr. Blake for his unwearied, assiduous, skilful, and gratuitous services in attending to the sick destitute seamen. – Committee Room, Jan. 16, 1818.'
>
> Sir, – I am desired to communicate to you the above resolution, and am, Sir, your obedient servant, (Signed) JAMES EDWD. GORDON, R.N., Hon. Sec. To Dr. Blake.

Also in the SHS archive is a letter (which fails completely to throw any further light on this matter) written by Surgeon Bob Blake (on board H M Hospital-ship *Gorgon*), to his parents, during the siege of Copenhagen, on 3 October 1808. This was apparently presented to the SHS by Mr E O Capon (whose uncle was Mr C T Orford, a member of the Board of Management, 1898–1914), in December 1935.[17]

In its issue for 2 January 1818 *The Times* (see above) carried an advertisement:

> 'Proposed Public Meeting to take into consideration the dreadful situation of Discharged Sailors &c. Gentlemen who are willing to cooperate with the advertiser in an endeavour to alleviate the sufferings of those wretched objects who daily crowd the principal streets of the Metropolis are earnestly requested to forward their names and addresses to 'Philanthropos' at the Chapter coffee-house St Pauls who will immediately call them together for the purpose of making the necessary arrangements for a public meeting on this interesting subject'.[18]

The following day, *The Times* published both a Letter to the Editor (from G.L.N. – probably G L Nelson of the Navy Board) and also a further leading article on the destitute state of these poor people … in the streets of London. It is clear that a feeling of urgency had now been implanted in the public's mind. The writer of this letter considered that *most* [my italics] of the individuals under consideration were not vagrants at all, but were sailors and foreigners seeking employment. … in the mean time [he wrote] the winter has begun, and the poor wretches in the streets may die while we are preparing to legislate for their relief'. His master plan was to establish (by subscription) a 'refuge for the destitute' – preferably more than one – in 'different parts of town'. He proposed that 'some large outhouse, stable, or workshop [divided into male and female compartments] should be hired for the winter months, and provided it keep out the weather, it does not signify how old it be'. 'The aged and sick should be made as comfortable as possible; but the relief afforded to temporary distress should always be kept … below what a man is ordinarily able to procure by his own labour …'. He suggested that some individuals frequented certain sites in order that 'some accidental passer by [to save them from perishing], will give them more money than they would gain by a hard day's begging'. This correspondent concluded that his plan, if adopted, would also 'increase the safety of the town'!

The Times leader also referred, 'with unfeigned satisfaction', to a meeting, attended by the Lord Mayor, which had been held the previous day at the Kings Head Tavern,* 25 The Poultry (*see* Figure 5.1)[19]the object(s) of which was 'the suggestion and adoption of some speedy means of affording relief to the destitute objects (chiefly seamen) with whom the streets are crowded'. A topic of considerable moment (highlighted in the leading article) was how to distinguish between 'worthy and unworthy objects' (see below); in this context '*willingness* to work' came to the fore – 'If employment and pay were offered, those who refused them should be punished as vagrants and imposters'. The Lord Mayor 'took notice of the foreign seamen, whom he had sent in vain to their respective Consuls; since they preferred mendacity in England to a free return to their native homes'. Another individual present at the meeting stressed that the problem was only of a temporary nature because 'at an early period of the spring, the departure of the East and West India fleets must provide at once for the seamen now in want of employment'; he proposed that 'a house or vessel should be hired immediately for those who might, on examination, be deemed worthy of support'. Another question asked was, 'why the West Indiamen, on coming into the West India dock, should be compelled immediately to discharge the whole crew …?'. The answer to this seems to have been that retention of even a minority of sailors would have increased the price of sugar! The meeting finally resolved to:

> (i) engage a vessel as an asylum for sailors, and (ii) to investigate (by certain members of the committee) 'all seamen found begging in the streets' of London.[20]

---

*This tavern had existed since the reign of Charles II; the King, it is said, on learning that the wife of the land-lord was in labour, . . . had expressed a wish to see him, duly called 'and saluted her'[18]

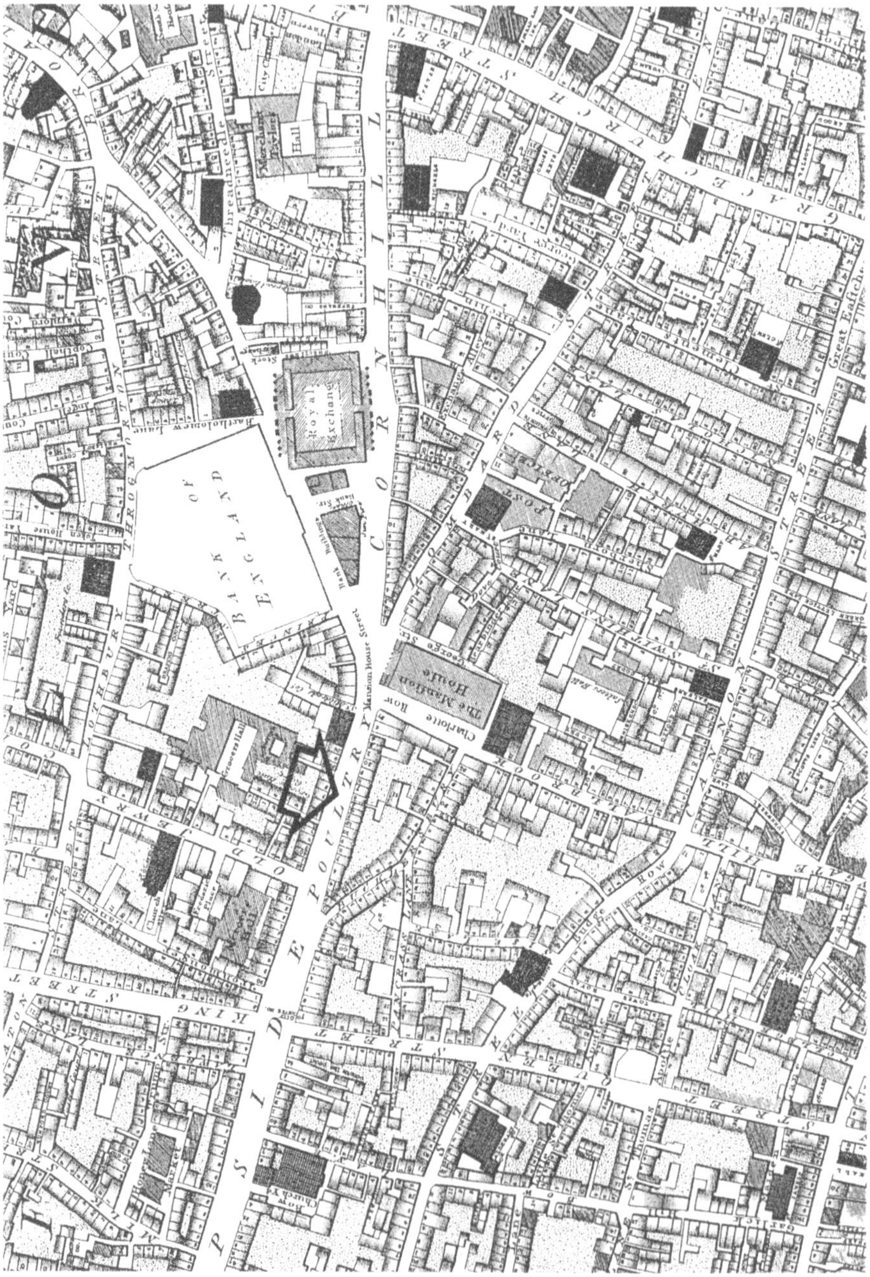

Figure 5.1: Map showing the situation of the King's Head, 25 Poultry – which was to become the headquarters of the Committee for the Relief of Distressed Seamen (CRDS). R Horwood – 1799.

Foundation of the precursor of the SHS

An advertisement in *The Times* (signed by the future Honorary Secretary James Edward Gordon (see below) – later to play an important rôle in the foundation of the SHS – referred to a forthcoming meeting of 'Merchants, Ship-owners, and others to be held at the City of London Tavern (*see* Figures 5.2–5.4) on Monday the 5th instant [in order to discuss the means of] affording relief to unemployed and distressed Seamen, and to aid in the enforcement of the laws against imposters assuming the appearance of Seamen for the purpose of begging'. This meeting, which was reported the following day, was chaired by William Wilberforce:

> Monday, Jan. 5 [1818],
>
> At a GENERAL MEETING held this day, at the City of London Tavern, for the purpose of taking into consideration the means of relieving the Distresses of the wretched Seamen now exposed to want and misery in the streets of the metropolis, the following Resolutions were unanimously adopted:-
>
>> W. WILBERFORCE, Esq. M.P. in the Chair;
>>
>> Resolved, That within the few last weeks the streets of the metropolis have been unusually crowded with Mendicants, in the character of destitute Seamen.
>>
>> Resolved, That the case of a Seaman in distress is one which, at all times, presents a forcible appeal to British feelings and British benevolence.
>>
>> Resolved, That it is therefore expedient, that the situation of the mendicants alluded to be examined, in order that the deserving may be relieved, and impostors dealt with according to the law.
>>
>> Resolved, That a subscription be immediately opened, and the amount placed at the disposal of a Committee of Management.
>>
>> Resolved, That a Committee be now appointed for the purposed above-mentioned – that it have power to add to their number – to elect a Treasurer-nominate Bankers, &c., and that five be a quorum.
>>
>> Resolved, That James Edward Gordon, Esq. Lieutenant in his Majesty's Navy, be requested to accept the Office of Honorary Secretary.
>>
>> Resolved, That the committee sit daily, at the King's Head Tavern, Poultry, at 12 for 1 o'clock precisely …
>
> Many subscriptions were then received:-

The Rt. Hon. The Ld. Mayor, M.P	21	0	0
Sir J. Shaw, Bart, M.P	10	10	0
Lord Cochrane	5	5	0
William Wilberforce, Esq .	21	0	0
Charles Francis, Esq	5	5	0
James Stephen, Esq	21	0	0

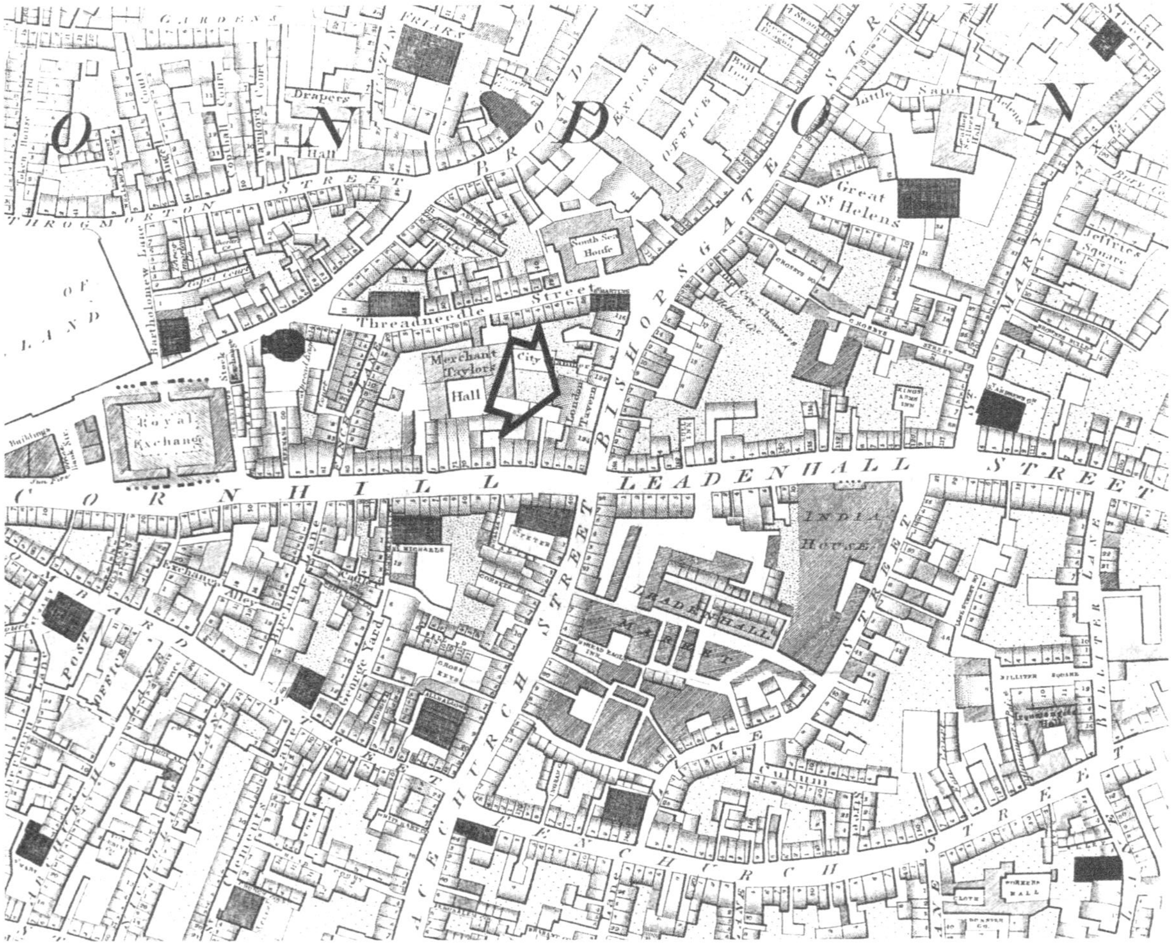

Figure 5.2: Map showing the position of the *London Tavern*, Bishopsgate. This venue was used for early meetings of the *Committee for the Relief of Distressed (Destitute) Seamen*, and subsequently the *Seamen's Hospital Society*. R Horwood – 1813 [original 26 inches ≡ 1 mile].

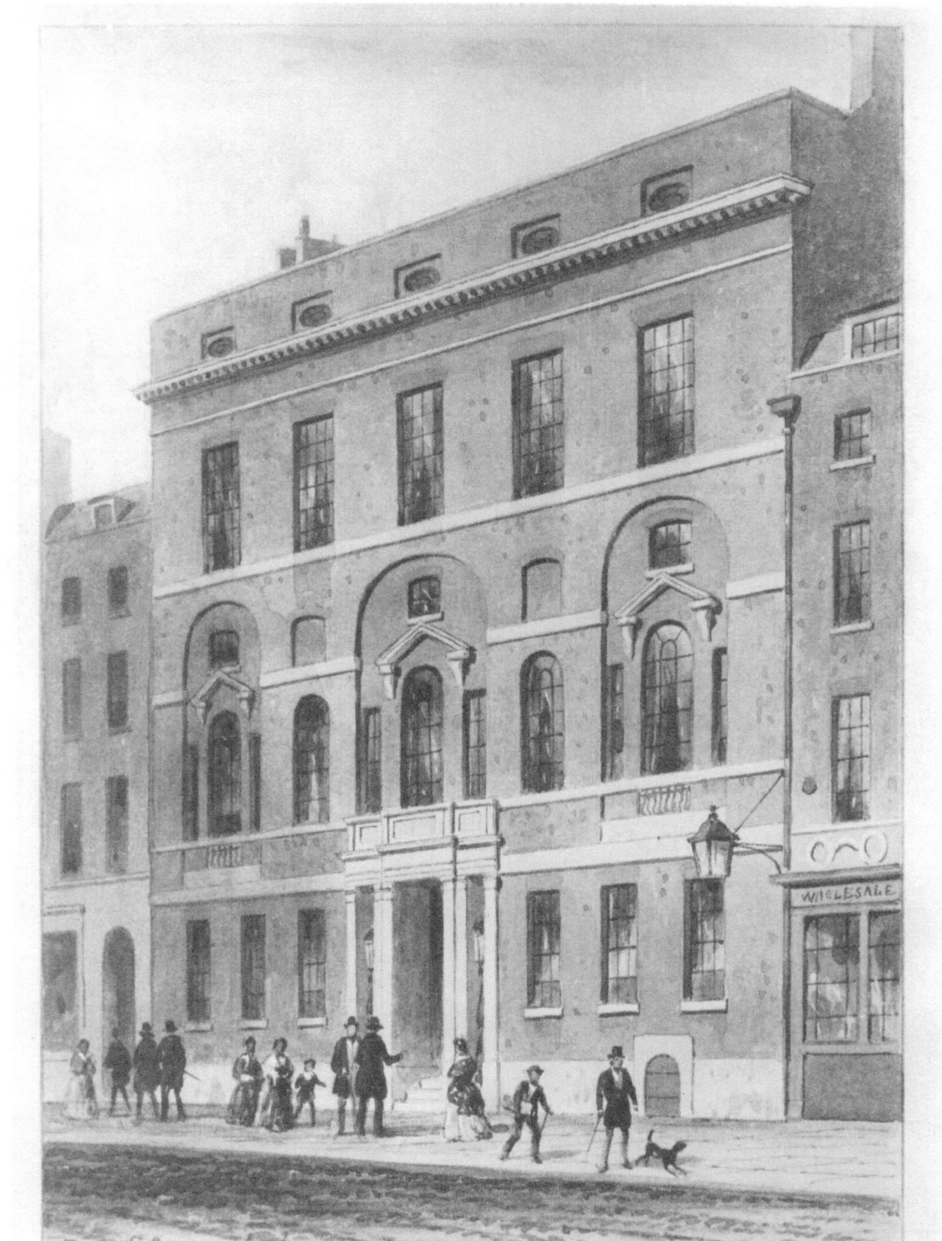

Figure 5.3: Exterior of the *London Tavern*, Bishopsgate (c 1830). T H Shepherd. [Reproduced with permission, the Guildhall Library].

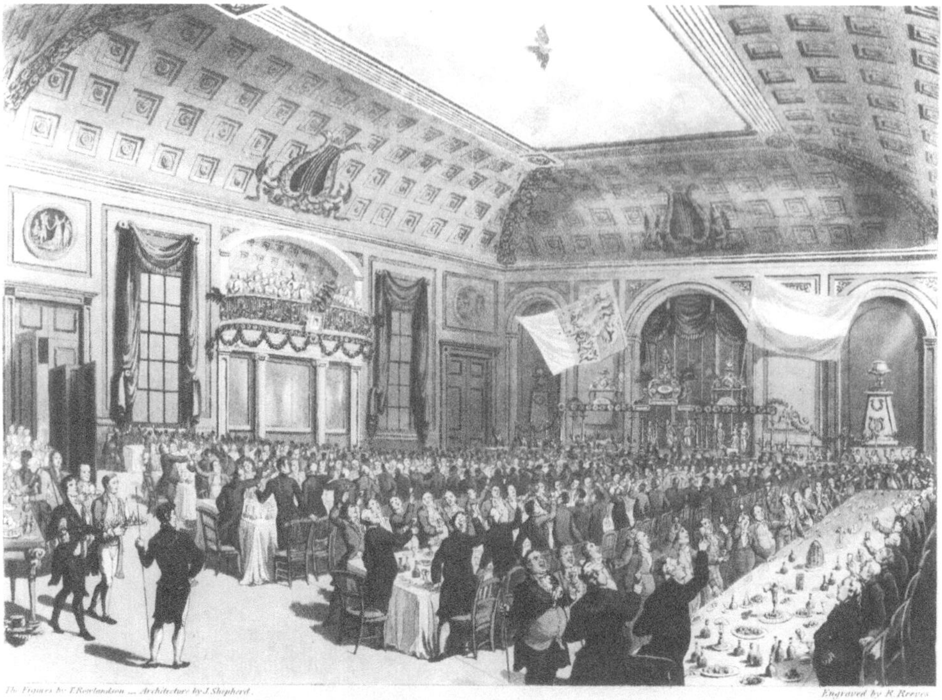

Figure 5.4: Interior of the *London Tavern*, Bishopsgate – during a banquet (1814). Engraving by R Reeves (After T Rowlandson/J Shepherd). [Reproduced with permission, the Guildhall Library, London].

John Dougan, Esq	25	0	0
Sir Ed. Hamilton	5	5	0
John Deacon, Esq	10	0	0
E. Ommaney, Esq	10	0	0
Z. Macauley and Babington	15	15	0
James Kemp	1	1	0
Miss Theodore Newson	2	0	0
James Shears and Son	10	10	10
Buckles, Bagster, and Buchanan	10	10	10
Smith, Martin, Smith, & Co.	10	10	10
Ed Benton, Capt. RN	1	1	0

And others, amounting to about 300 *l*. Subscriptions received at the City of London tavern; by the Committee, at the King's Head tavern, Poultry; and by the following Bankers:– Sir W. Curtis, Bart. and Co., Lombard-street; Sir J. Lubbock, Bart. and Co., Mansion-house-street; Messrs. Hankeys, Fenchurch-street; Messrs. Williamson, Son, Moffatt, and Co.; Sir John Perring. Bart.; Shaw, Barber, and Co., Cornhill.'

In addition, 'The Trinity House [see above] subscribed 200 guineas, and the East India Company 200 *l*'.

The secretariat for the CRDS had appointed J W Buckle as Chairman. An appeal launched on behalf of the newly formed charity rapidly brought positive results from private individuals. The Elder Brethren of Trinity House had already forwarded two hundred guineas. A later letter, dated 20 January, from West India Dock House indicated that the Court of Directors of the West India Dock Company had also voted 'Two hundred Guineas' as a further subscription. 'The Marine Society [see above] agreed to clothe 100 destitute seamen, and quantities of shoes and stockings were also received'. By 8 January, 'upwards of 200 distressed seamen had been relieved with food, and supplied with temporary lodgings'.[21]

The Provisional Committee

The 'Provisional Committee' which had now been set up consisted of nine men:

- Joseph Dowson, jun, Esq.*
- John Drinkald, Esq.*
- Charles Francis, Esq.*
- Captain C.C. Owen, R.N.
- Captain William Young, R.N.*
- George Lyall, Esq.
- Thomas Sturges, Esq.*
- John Deacon, Esq.*
- John William Buckle, Esq.†

They recommended that 'a *Permanent Hospital* should [ultimately] be provided for relief [of Distressed Seamen]' which should take the form of 'a Permanent Floating Hospital … on the River Thames'. This was to be 'for the use of Sick and Diseased Seamen only', and '… supported by voluntary subscriptions, and under the Management of a Committee.'

On 8 January 1818 *The Times* was able to inform its readership that the 'Committee of the Association for the relief of destitute Seamen' had met on 5 and 7 January, when 'Numbers of the mendicants … were examined by a Sub Committee consisting chiefly of nautical men …' [when] about 110 applicants, whose claims to relief as seamen were satisfactorily ascertained, were sent over the water to a house hired for their reception at Newington, until receiving vessels can be got ready'. Cases not by that time examined were given some refreshment, and were to be interviewed on 8 January – when a 'further selection [would] be made to be forwarded to Newington, where arrangements [had] been made for feeding and lodging between two and three hundred, at the moderate expense of 1s[hilling] per day'. Having received razors, 'they proceeded immediately to divest themselves of one mark of their wretched condition, with an eagerness which showed that 'their poverty and not their will consented' to their wearing them. Captain Wake, the harbour-master, told the Committee that 'Lord Melville[22] had given orders to place

*Later to serve on the founding Committee of Management of the SHS.
†Buckle was to become one of the original Vice-Presidents of the SHS.

at their disposal three sloops* of war, at Deptford ...and stationed in such parts of the river as the Committee might think fit [see below]'. *The Times* article concluded: 'It is understood that one [of the ships] will be stationed off the Tower, and another off the entrance to the London Docks. The other, it is supposed, will be fitted up as an hospital ship'.[23]

Support for the new venture

A few days earlier, another correspondent to *The Times* (J.B. – possibly J W Buckle, who was to become chairman of the CRDS), had heartily welcomed the newspapers' initiative(s) in this matter, and cited two case-reports to substantiate his claims; the potential beneficiary, he wrote, constituted a body that ' ... so lately formed the strongest arm of our power, and the greatest terror of our foes ...'.

> I fear [he continued] that a very great number of *foreign seamen* have recently been reduced to the last and lowest extremity of human misery, by having been denationalised and disowned by their native Governments, on account of having served during the late wars, a considerable part of the prime of their lives in the [RN] of Great Britain. Justice and state-policy equally require, that this country should naturalize every foreign seaman or soldier who could prove that he had been denationalized and rejected by his native government, through the length of his servitude in our fleet or army. [He also alluded to] many native seamen who [were] entitled to pensions on account of wounds, hurts, or length of servitude; and whose claims would be at once admitted by the Admiralty Board, if properly laid before the Lords Commissioners. [A further deserving group consisted of] many of our first-rate thorough – based seamen, who having fallen into rags and poverty, [and who] have not, *as they should have been*, received into the present reduced establishment on account of *their want of clothing*; whilst men [of inferior worth, but who were reasonably well clothed had on the other hand] been admitted. [He was aware, he claimed, of] many destitute seamen [who had] been discharged in the *fourteenth* year of their servitude; and in some cases, even within *three months* of the expiration of that term! Pensions, [J.B. ended], should be paid *weekly* rather than *quarterly*![24]

---

*The term *sloop* is derived from a Dutch term first used in 1629 [J A Simpson, ESC Weiner (eds) *Oxford English Dictionary* 2nd Ed 1989; 15: 730]. It denotes a small, one-masted, fore-and-aft rigged vessel; this differed from a *cutter* in that it had a jib-stay and standing bowsprit. Alternatively, the term was used to describe a relatively small ship-of-war – carrying guns on the upper deck only.

'The Society for the Aid of destitute Seamen' (CRDS) is established

Table 5.1 summarises some individuals who were prominent in the formation of the CRDS.[25] Important individuals in the early days of the CRDS were the Secretary (John Wilson Croker [*see* Figure 5.5][26]) and Second Secretary (John Barrow [*see* Figure 5.6][27]) of the Admiralty.

By 10 January 1818, *The Times* writer was extremely enthusiastic about the progress of this new initiative: 'officers in the Royal navy are with much patience and unwearied assiduity examining the various objects as they present themselves. The greater number are *men of war's men* [my italics]'. The article continued by informing the readership that about 250 seamen had by then been housed (and already had 'an improved appearance') in a temporary lodging. The *Abundance* store-ship (see above) was then lying 'off the Tower', and it was hoped that the other ships which were promised by Government would be forthcoming in the immediate future – enabling 'the seamen [to be taken] from the streets and on board by the end of the next week'. 'Applications [the article continued] were so numerous yesterday [9 January 1818], that the Committee, with much regret, [had] been obliged to suspend granting temporary relief, for a day or two, to give time for investigations of the cases already before them'.

The same newspaper published extensive lists of Subscribers (amounting to several hundred names) in its issues dated 14 and 16 January 1818 (see above). In what was in effect an appeal letter, JD (who described himself as 'one of the [Provisional] Committee' and was therefore presumably John Deacon) gave some details of the composition of the Committee which had been set up to administer the Charity:

Table 5.1: *Dramatis personae* of senior personnel involved in the formation of the Committee for the Relief of Destitute (distressed) Seamen (CRDS).

Organisation	*Personnel*
Admiralty Office:	Viscount Melville – First Lord Viscount Sidmouth – Prominent politician J W Croker LlD, FRS – Secretary to the Admiralty John Barrow, FRS, FLS – Second Secretary H Hobhouse
Navy Board (Office):	R L Nelson – Secretary
Deptford Dock Yard:	Resident Commissioner: Capt. C Cunningham, RN. W Stone – Master Shipwright
Committee for the Relief of Destitute Seamen (CRDS):	J W Buckle – Chairman J E Gordon – Honorary Secretary
Royal Hospital, Greenwich:	J Dyer

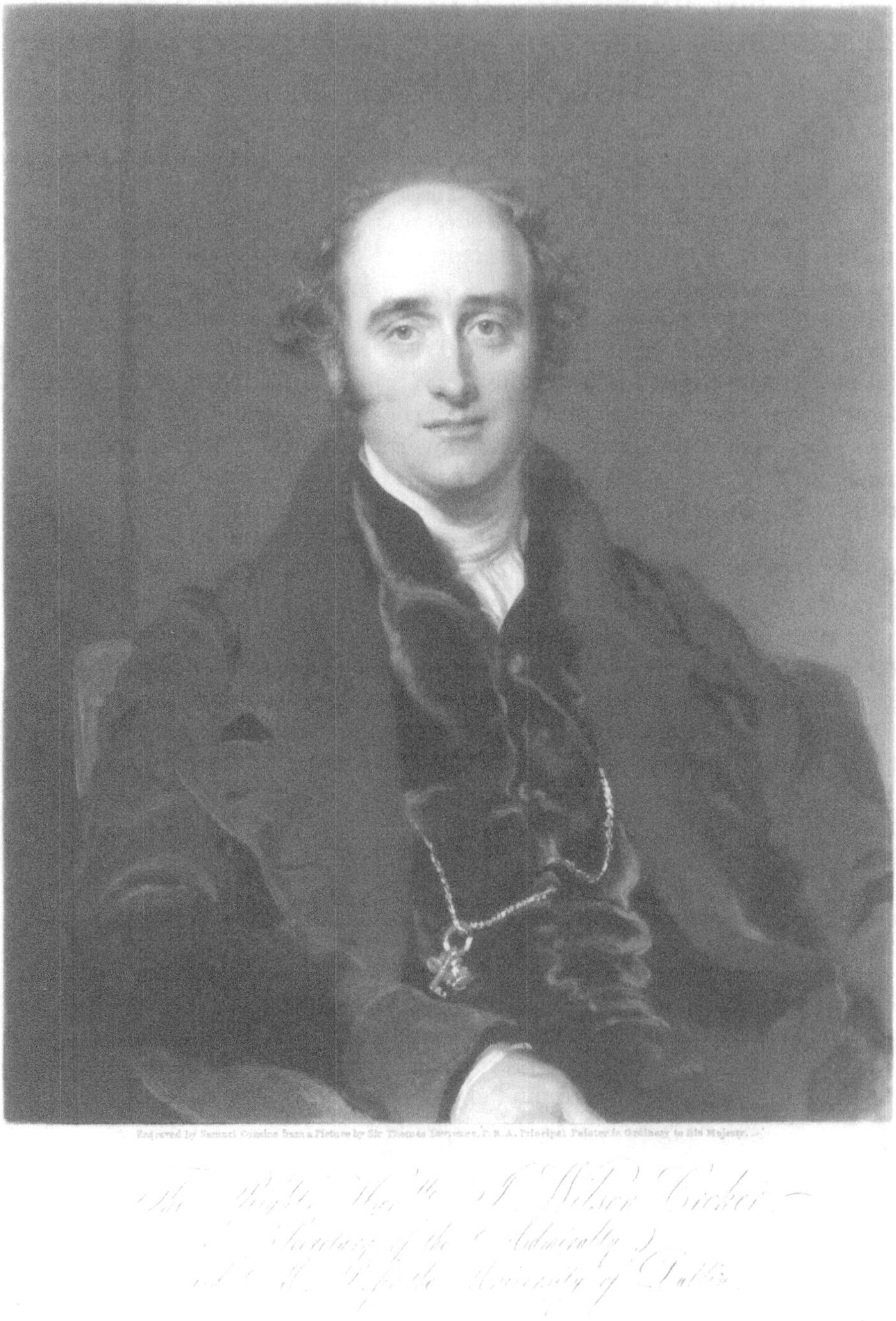

Figure 5.5: John Wilson Croker (1780–1857) – Secretary to the Admiralty. [Reproduced by courtesy of the National Portrait Gallery, London].

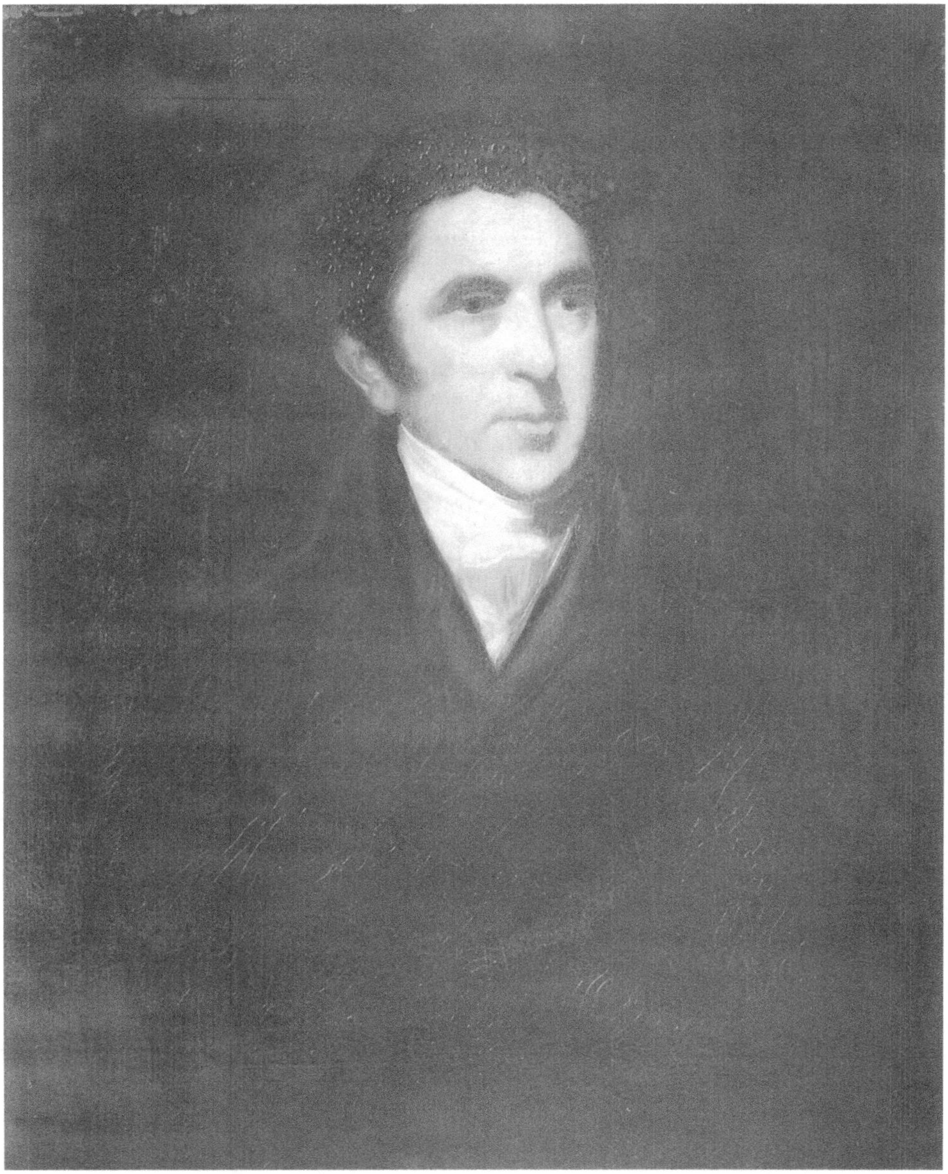

Figure 5.6: John Barrow (1764–1848) – Second Secretary to the Admiralty. [Reproduced by courtesy of the Wellcome Library, London].

'… several naval Captains, and officers and commanders in the merchants' service, men of known integrity, and well calculated to discriminate between the real British seaman and impostor [very few of whom had presented to the Sub-committee of Examination]'. Not all of those 'considered a fit object of commiseration' behaved in a grateful manner! *The Times* of 27 January 1818 recorded the case of one ungrateful wretch, of about 5 feet 3 inches in height, with 'dark eyes and hair' who had been 'humanely provided with food, clothes, and other necessities, and finally sent on board the *Sapphire* receiving ship' had stolen two silver tablespoons, two silver teaspoons, two silver salt spoons and a cellar from the officers' cabin (which belonged to the RN Commander of the ship) and then 'quit the ship'.[28]

Although the scheme (to improve the welfare of destitute seamen) had therefore been accepted in principle, there was a great deal of sorting out of minutiae to be done; the project was therefore by no means 'up and running' yet!

Willing and immediate assistance from the Admiralty

SUITABLE SHIPS

Table 5.2 summarises details of seven ships which the Admiralty duly provided. The rapidity with which they answered urgent requests was, by any standard, remarkable. A letter dated 8 January 1818 (in reply to a request dated the previous day) written on behalf of the Lords Commissioners of the Admiralty (to Buckle – Chairman of the Committee) had offered 'three sloops of war fitted in ordinary, with their Warrant Officers'; these were to be placed 'in such situation of the River as shall be agreed upon with the Harbour Masters, for the reception of Seamen requiring temporary relief.[29]

Table 5.2: Ships (hulks*) loaned to the Committee for Distressed Seamen (CRDS) in 1818.

Name	*Date built*	*Description*	*Tonnage*	*Role for CDS*	*Site of Mooring*
Abundance	1799	Store-ship	674	Accommodation ship	Deptford
Dasher	1797	Sloop (flush-decked)	401	–	Deptford
Dromedary	1799	Store-ship	1048	Hospital-ship	Deptford
Nautilus	1806	Sloop (brig)	185	–	–
Perseus	1812	Sixth-rate (22 guns)	522	Receiving-ship	Tower of London
Plover	1796	Sloop (with quarter-deck & forecastle)	422	–	Deptford
Sapphire	1806	Sloop (with quarter-deck & forecastle)	426	–	Deptford

*P Kemp. *The history of ships*. Kingsnorth, Rochester: Grange Books 2002: 120–121.

A letter from H Hobhouse headed Whitehall (dated 9 January) and written on behalf of Lord Sidmouth[30] referred to the use of the *Helder* and *Batavia* during the previous winter for the reception of 'Foreign sick and distressed Seamen'; this move had apparently been 'fixed by the Admiralty, without the intervention of the Secretary of State' and Hobhouse suggested that application for the use of the *Abundance* and the *Plover* should 'be made directly to the Admiralty'.[31]

Another letter, dated 12 January, indicated that the 'Lords Commissioners of the Admiralty [had that morning already given] orders to the Navy Board* to have three additional ships ready to be brought forward', and one from the Navy Office (dated the same day) confirmed this offer, indicating that the Officers of Deptford Yard had been requested to have '... three additional Sloops in readiness to be delivered to the Committee for Distressed Seamen if necessary ...'.[32] A letter from the Navy Office (dated 14 January in reply to one of 13 January) indicated that directions had been given to the Officers of Deptford Yard to send another 'Sloop of War' to the Tower for the use of the Committee for the relief of Distressed Seamen 'as soon as possible'. A follow-up letter stated:

> Navy Office
> 17th January 1818
>
> Sir
>
> I am commanded by the Commissioners of the Navy to acquaint you, in answer to your letter of the 16th instant, that the Bulkheads† of the Abundance were left up from a consideration that they would afford better accommodation and more comfort to the persons who were to be put on board her, but if the Committee still think it is necessary that they should be taken down, it will be done.
>
> I am
> Sir
> Your humble servant,
> R L Nelson
>
> Lieutenant Gordon
> Secretary to the Committee for the Relief of Distressed Seamen.
> [King's Head, Poultry][33]

A further request was made to the Lords Commissioners of the Admiralty for the loan of the *Dromedary*, in 'addition to the Vessels already placed at their disposal as an Hospital Ship'; this application too was successful.[34]

The following letter dated 12 January was received from the Admiralty:

---

*The *Navy Board* was at this time independent of the Admiralty, but later became absorbed into this institution.

†One of the upright partitions serving to form the cabins in a ship or to divide the hold into water-tight compartments.

Admiralty Office 12 Jan 1818

Sir

Having laid before my Lords Commissioners of the Admiralty Mr Gordon's letter of 9 Inst. enclosing a Resolution of the [CRDS] 'that their Lordships be requested to order a Ship at each of the principal Out Ports for the reception of destitute Seamen' I am commanded to acquaint you that their Lordships have referred the Committee's proposal for Lord Sidmouth's consideration.

I am
Sir
Your very humble Servt.
J. W. Croker

The Chairman of the [CRDS][35]

A follow-up letter dated 21 January from Croker, indicated that Lord Melville had undertaken a 'verbal communication' with Lord Sidmouth on the matter of providing a ship at each of the principal Out Ports for 'the reception of such destitute Seamen as may present themselves'; this request was however, rejected on the ground of expense. The SHS Committee was also reminded that ships 'might be obtained at the different Ports at much less expense ...' than 'navigating them from His Majesty [King Geoge III]'s Dockyards'.[36]

A letter from Commandant C Cunningham RN of the Deptford Dock Yard (dated 2 February) addressed the question of constructing cabins (for the Mate and Clerk on board) in the various ships 'appropriated for the reception of destitute Seamen'. He had no authority to do this, he wrote; however, he enclosed a statement from the Master Shipwright at Deptford giving details of 'the number of Cabins already fitted'. This information was provided (by a colleague) as an appendix:

Deptford Yard
Feb 2 1818

... I have the honor to state below, the Number of Cabins now in the several Ships lent to the Committee for the relief of the distressed Seamen

	Deck	
	Lower	*Upper*
Dasher	6	2
Sapphire	4	2
Perseus	4	4
Nautilus	7	–
Plover	4	3
Abundance	–	13
Dromedary	11	8

I am
Honoured [to be]
Your obedient Servant
W Stone

Commissioner Cunningham[37]

A letter from the Navy Office dated 24 February (signed by Nelson) informed the Committee that Deptford Yard would supply each of the receiving ships with a windsail in order 'to cause a free circulation of air on board …'.[38]

A later letter from the Admiralty Office dated 7 March indicated that directions had been given to the Navy Board to 'cause the Nautilus to be received into charge'.[39] A letter from the same office dated 30 March, confirmed that *Dasher* also, could be used by the Society: 'My Lords Commissioners of the Admiralty having directed the Navy Board to receive the Dasher into charge on the 31st Instant …'.[40] Similar news concerning the *Sapphire* was contained in a letter dated 13 April,[41] and on 23 April identical news was also received regarding the *Plover* and *Perseus*.[42] In a letter from the same source dated 28 May it was clearly stated that HM Ship *Abundance* had been received 'into charge'; the Commissioners of the Admiralty had given this directive to the Navy Board.[43]

As well as fund-raising and arrangements to take over the Admiralty's ships, for the necessities of the newly formed Charity, provision had to be made for clothing the mendicants, and equipping and victualling the vessels. It has already been made clear, that early on, the newly-formed Charity had no difficulty in raising support from the Admiralty, and other Government Departments. However, over the ensuing two years, co-operation became distinctly less positive.

IRON BED CRADLES

A request from Gordon on 4 February 1818 for an additional 100 Iron Cradles was forwarded by the Navy Office to the 'Victualling Board' for attention. This request was granted, and the Storekeeper General was asked to supply 100 cradles with sacking bottoms.[44] The latter had to be obtained from the Royal Hospital, Haslar, and 100 Sacking bottoms and lashings were duly transported to the *Dromedary*.[45]

JUNK

A letter dated 4 February 1818 to 'The Chairman of the Committee for the relief of distressed Seamen' from the Admiralty Office, and signed by Barrow, indicated that 'the Navy Board [had] been directed to furnish a supply of Junk* requested in a letter dated the previous day]'. And in a follow-up letter (12 February) from the Navy Office, Gordon was informed that 'they [had] directed their Officers at Deptford, to furnish 20 cwt of Junk to each of the ships therein mentioned.[46]

BLANKETS, HAMMOCKS AND CLOTHING, ETC

In a letter from Henry Hobhouse (based in Whitehall) to Simon Cock (Esq) (who was to become the Secretary of the SHS [*see* Chapter 6]), dated 12 January 1818, the writer indicated that he had 'laid before Lord Sidmouth [his] letter of 10th instant' and that he needed to know for His Lordship's Information 'the Number

*Old rope and cable [see: J A Simpson, ESC Wiener (eds). *Oxford English Dictionary* 2nd ed. 1989; 8: 315–6].

of Suits of Slop Clothing* which the Committee [was] desirous of receiving from His Lordship for the use of the distressed Seamen whose circumstances they [were] at present Employed upon administering relief to'. A further letter, dated four days later (this time to Gordon) in reply to one of 13 January requesting '700 Blankets, 500 Hammocks [and] 700 Suits of Clothing' indicated that there were 'no Hammocks at [Lord Sidmouth's] disposal, and that he was placed in a 'Difficulty in acceding to the [remainder] of the Request as there was a relative shortage of clothing; he suggested that in any case, future application should be addressed to 'Their Lordships' directly.[47]

Meanwhile, the previous day John Newby had replied to a letter, on behalf of the *Marine Society*, indicating that the following clothing was available for each of 100 men:

- 1 Jacket
- 1 Pair of trousers
- 2 Shirts
- 1 Pair Stockings
- 1 Pair of Shoes
- 1 Silk Handkerchief [and]
- 1 Hat[48]

Following a meeting with Lord Melville, Lord Sidmouth (on behalf of the Admiralty), also approved the donation of the following items of Slop Clothing:

- 300 Flannel Waistcoats
- 300 Flannel and Worsted Drawers
- 150 Kerry [sic] Jackets
- 150 Guernsey D$^{\underline{o}}$
- 150 Frocks
- 300 Shirts
- 150 Blue Cloth Trousers
- 150 Duck D$^{\underline{o}}$
- 300 Pairs of Stockings
- 300 P_____ Shoes
- 300 Hats [and]
- 300 Blankets

This information was contained in a letter from Hobhouse to Gordon dated 20 January. Meanwhile, a letter from the 'Storekeeper General's Office' dated 24 January, pledged: '500 Blankets and 500 Pr. Of Shoes'.[49] This was, however, followed up with an invoice for the 500 pairs of Shoes, and on 18 February for a request for payment of 'the total amount … as soon as convenient.[50]

Blankets were clearly in great demand; for example, letters, some months later, from the 'Storekeeper General's Office' indicated that 100 used Blankets, at 5 shillings each, were available for use on the Dromedary.[51]

---

*The *Oxford English Dictionary* 2nd ed defines 'slop(s)' as: Wide baggy breeches or hose … loose trousers, esp. those worn by sailors, hence ready-made, cheap, or inferior garments generally. [J A Simpson, ESC Weiner (eds) 1989; 15: 731].

It remains far from clear from the correspondence, as to the extent of similar donations (apart from the loan of ships) to the CRDS. A letter, dated 13 March 1818 from Treasury Chambers, addressed to Gordon as Secretary of the CRDS regretted that 'My Lords regret that they cannot feel themselves justified in considering the Clothing and Stores in question as a gratuitous Donation without creating a most inconvenient Precedent'.[52]

OTHER REQUESTS

A request that 'Books for Subscriptions ... may lay in [the Custom House]' was rejected on the grounds 'that the practice of the Department will not admit your request being complied with'.

The Society for Promoting Christian Knowledge was approached (letter, 15 January 1818) regarding a supply of 'suitable books'. Edward Suter, Secretary of the Merchant Seamen's Bible Society (Jerusalem Coffee House) wrote in reply to a request (12 March) for bibles (letter, 18 March 1818), '... ordered one hundred Bibles and one hundred Testaments to be placed at the disposal of the [CRDS] ...'. The writer enclosed available Bibles accompanied by Testaments [in English, Welsh, Gaelic, Irish, French, German and Dutch], and Bibles only [in Spanish, Portuguese, Danish and Italian] supplied by the Society, with a request that selections be made from that list.

Not all requests, however, were successful (see above). A further plea (9 February) to increase the furnishings of the *Dromedary* met with a sharp rebuttal from Commander Cunningham (at the Deptford Dock Yard): '... I have no authority to furnish the Dromedary with anything more than I have done'. He also asked that future requests be made to either the Admiralty or the Navy Board, and *not* directly to the Deptford Dock Yard![53]

Who was entitled to 'relief'?

According to *The Times* of 31 January 1818 'a very numerous meeting of the Gentlemen who have been actively engaged in dispensing relief to the distressed seamen, with whom the metropolis was a few days ago crowded ... took place [yesterday] at the King's Head, in the Poultry'. The important matter of who was a *bone fide* candidate for beneficence was raised; reassurances that impostors would be dealt with 'according to the law' were received from the Chairman, the Lord Mayor, no less. The article continued: 'There are now in the river six ships for the use of the healthy seamen and one hospital ship. They are capable of receiving 1,400 men'. By then 1,041 had been *received* 'on board', and 197 had been effectively disposed of – 'some in merchant's service and others [were leaving] the navy'. The sick were [*The Times* readership was told] attended by 'a physician, a surgeon, and two assistant-surgeons, paid by the Committee'; in addition Dr Rankin (East India Company) also attended gratuitously.

Further details were provided: there were at that time 859 on board who with the exception of about 10 had served [at some time] in the navy; those 'certainly fit for service' amounted to 'less than 500'. About 120 had been 'cured of the itch [scabies], and four had died since 'the ships were fitted out for the reception of the men'. Sufferers from an infectious disease had not been admitted. 'Those applicants ... whom it was impossible to accommodate during [the initial] influx of seamen in the ships, the work-house, and other places, were supplied with threepence each and a fourth of a quartern loaf every day'. For several days past however, 'Orders [had] been given ... to the officer of the *Abundance* receiving-ship to take all seamen who apply on board for examination.' The article added that there had been a mischievous (and inaccurate) account in a Sunday newspaper indicating that the Committee had excluded 'a black man for relief'; the meeting was assured, that foreign seamen were by no means forgotten or excluded: 'there were 59 foreigners, *besides those* [men] *of colour* [my italics], who amounted to 48'; 'those who could not be provided with ships ... in consequence of having fought for England, should be considered in the light of Englishmen'.

Overall, the Committee 'congratulated themselves ... that they were instrumental to the relief of many poor fellows, who were now almost safely over the winter ...'. 'After all necessary investigation, those who were unable to re-enter the service should be sent home, in the event of the refusal of Government to take them under its immediate protection'. Many attending the meeting felt that 'all of those ... able to engage in active service [would] be disposed of in six weeks'. The Committee also determined 'to apply to the Admiralty to grant relief to such of the seamen as were unfit for service ...'. It was also resolved that a Special Committee would 'consider the most proper means of employing the seamen while on board the reception ships'.[54]

A further General Meeting, this time under the chairmanship of Wilberforce (who claimed that 'no objects could appear more worthy of their bounty than those who on so many trying occasions, and in so many hard-fought battles, had contributed to the defence and glory of the country'), was held at the City of London Tavern on 5 February, when only 200 were present – due to the 'unfavourable state of the weather, and the shortness of the notice ...'. This meeting also obtained extensive coverage in *The Times*, and it was announced that the following Thursday (12 February) a further General Meeting would address the far broader issue (not solely the plight of destitute seamen) of 'mendacity of the metropolis'. John Drinkald (a member of the Provisional Committee) informed the meeting that 'if one ship should be insufficient, two might easily be had. There was one at Woolwich and another at Deptford, which by an application to the Secretary of State for the Home Department, might be rendered available for the purposes in view in 24 hours'. The following speaker at this meeting (Mr Stephen) was recorded as saying that 'In consequence of representations, ... an official letter had been received from the Secretary, Mr Croker, stating that the Lords Commissioners were willing to supply a ship for the reception of such seamen as should be selected by the society, on the condition that they should engage for the safety of the vessel'. An offer had (in reply) been made to the Committee, 'at a very reasonable price, of the use of a large ship called the *Ganges*, fitted up for the express purpose of conveying Lascars to the East Indies, and capable of accommodating from 700 to 800 men, and which offer the Committee thought was fit to be submitted to a general meeting'.

Later at that meeting (on 5 February), a Mr Methuen pointed out that 'many of the distressed seamen ... were already receiving pensions'; these included many who had served onboard men of war, but excluded: '... the crews of merchantmen, and those who had been in the East India Company's service'. It was Drinkald's view that 'unless something considerable was done for this destitute class of men, Government would find it difficult, in the event of another war, to man their vessels'. Discipline of the seamen was also the subject of concern to the meeting. Stephen ended another speech: ' ... it was pitiable in itself to see men who had fought and bled for their country perishing of want in the streets of its metropolis, and that the removal of such a pitiable sight was a strong call upon charity [Great applause]. Lord Cochrane [see above] indicated that 'many [of the beggars] had gone to America [where they gave] their services to the Americans who were now become the carriers of Europe. Why [Cochrane asked] were not soldiers in the same distress? They saw none of them on the streets'; a viewpoint which was later challenged by Stephen. Zachary Macauley (*see* Figure 5.7),[55] who was to become a member of the founding Committee of the SHS, was also present and 'expressed much satisfaction that the assistance of the Admiralty would be

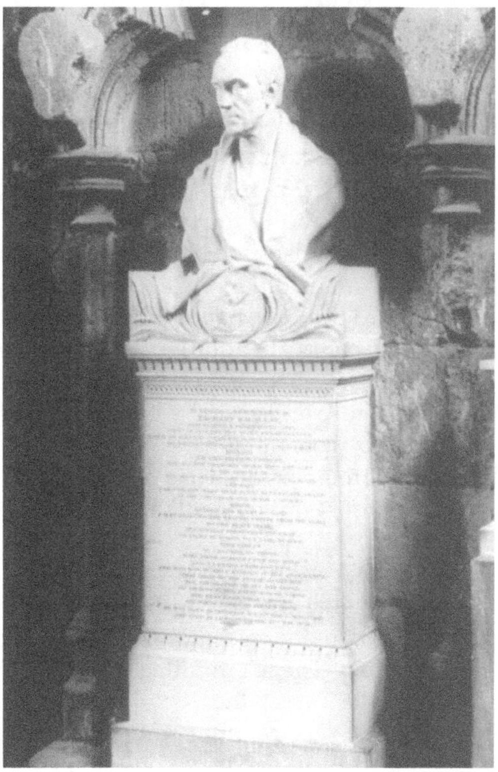

Figure 5.7: Zachary Macaulay (1768–1838). Contemporary bust, [reproduced with permission, Westminster Abbey, London].

obtained'. Rowcroft informed the meeting that there were 'already 39,000 seamen on the books of Greenwich Hospital'. The meeting carried unanimously, a motion for the opening of a subscription.[56]

On 10 February, *The Times* recorded further details of the meeting held at the City of London Tavern on the 5th of that month (see above); this article quoted liberally from a report prepared by J E Gordon (see above). It had already been decided that 'the 14th of February [1818, should be] the last day of admission, except in those who labour under bodily defect or infirmity'. The writer of the introduction considered '... sufficient time having been afforded to all the proper objects of this charity to come in and apply for relief, *those who still infest the streets of the metropolis may generally be deemed impostors*'.

The Charity in operation

The following day (6 February) a group which had been nominated at the meeting held on the 5th, met at the King's Head Tavern, Poultry, to bring 'into immediate effect the intention of the meeting'. This group, numbering 70, was divided into three sub-committees, i.e. *examining, shipping,* and *finance*. They referred to the house rented from a Mrs Hayes of Newington – in which '200 could be received, and sheltered from the weather'. A further 100 men were admitted to the London Workhouse. For those *not* accommodated, bread and money were provided. In '... as short a time as it was possible to get the *Dromedary* prepared for their accommodation, the sick men were lodged on board her, under the care of Dr. Robertson, and the necessary assistants'.

The report stated further that '1,230 men [had] been received on board of the seven vessels granted by the Admiralty for that purpose, and supplied with the necessary clothing: 349 'have been disposed of in the Navy, the merchants' service, or otherwise provided for; and many others are expected to be provided with ships in a few days'. '162 are on board the *Dromedary* [which was used exclusively for the sick]; of whom 61 [were] *serious cases*'. In addition, three had been sent on shore for misconduct, five had died and a further 711 remained on the receiving ships. Of the latter, 351 were considered fit for service, 180 were healthy but unfit for the merchant service, 66 were infirm, 47 were foreigners (only 30 of whom were considered fit for employment), 12 were foreigners desirous of being sent home, 47 were black men (only 20 of whom were fit for employment) and eight 'Men wanting to be sent to their parishes'.

Details of the diet (and also soap, razors, combs, brushes, etc) were then provided, and it was recorded that the cost to maintain each man was 5d daily. On board each ship was a Commander, mate, and clerk, together with Warrant Officers to preserve discipline. The Committee had 'not been unmindful of the moral improvement of the men'; the Rev J Rudge and Mr Maule [had] 'repeatedly performed Divine service on board the several receiving ships; Bibles [had] been distributed, and the general conduct of the men during Divine service [was] mostly exemplary'. The writer continued: 'Dr Blake, R.N. [see above] and Dr Rankin, of the Hon E.I.C.S. have gratuitously contributed their medical aid'. After 14 February (an extended date), 'no application for relief [would] be attended to, *except from such seamen as shall be actually diseased, or disabled from labour by age, bodily defect, or infirmity* [my italics]'. Monthly expenditure amounted to approximately 1000 *l*; subscriptions already received amounted to 11,938 *l* 14s 10d.[57]

A rival institution to care for the spiritual condition of the mendicants?

There were, of course, 'rivals' to the CRDS's strategy but most sought to improve the *spiritual* and not the physical state of the sailors. For example, *The Times* recorded on 19 March 1818 that a meeting had taken place the previous day (also at the City of London Tavern) to found 'an establishment for the extension of religious instruction' for 'seamen in the port of London'. The underlying idea was to 'fit out a large vessel [to be called 'The English Ark'] capable of containing 700–800 persons who might assemble to hear preaching and prayer'.[58]

Examinations for worthiness

As already related, the CRDS had already notified the Admiralty that they intended to close their examinations for worthiness on 14 February 1818 (see above); they had also emphasised the 'measures being taken for the apprehension of such Persons as may appear begging in the Streets after that period, in the Character of distressed Seamen'. It was reported (by Hobhouse from Whitehall) that Lord Sidmouth had duly 'given Instructions to the Magistrates at the respective Police Offices ... to direct their Officers to apprehend all Vagrants and Beggars of the description alluded to, and to proceed against them according to Law'.[59]

On 17 February *The Times* duly announced that the subscription had indeed been closed:

> Although the subscription for the relief of distressed seamen is satisfactorily closed, we must not omit to mention the exertions in aid of that subscription by the town of Sheerness. A meeting was held at that place in the garrison on the 5th inst., at which the utmost zeal was manifested, and the deepest sympathy felt, in 'the sufferings of the gallant and intrepid, but thoughtless and unfortunate British "seamen"'. These were the words used on the occasion; and the sum of 82 *l*. 15s. was forthwith transmitted to town, at a time when it was not known that the other subscriptions were so numerous.

The Charity was, for the moment at least, 'financially viable'.[60]

Overall therefore, from the point of view of accommodation on the River Thames, the institution was well established. But work still remained to be done regarding the provision of supplies, the victualling of the ships, and very importantly the 'disposal' of the mendicants.

What, precisely, was the 'raison d'être' of the CRDS?

There was still a lack of clarity as regards the precise function(s) of the newly formed body; was it solely for providing health care, or was future employment an objective? A letter from the Assistant Secretary of the East India Company (13 January 1818) for example, requested clarification as to whether ' ... a certain number of the [Mendicants] may be received on board of the Company's outward bound Ships' which would be in accordance with the objective(s) of the newly created organisation, i.e., 'the *employment* [my italics] of these Men'. The 'Court do not consider it expedient or advisable to increase the compliment of the Crews of the Company's Ships'. Also, Croker, in a letter from the Admiralty Office dated 26 January, asked on behalf of the Commissioners of the Admiralty if any men on two of His Majesty's Ships, the *Spartan* and *Drake* were fit for service, 'and if there be, to enter them accordingly'.[61]

Problems and controversies in the early days of the Committee for the Relief of Destitute Seamen (CRDS): 1818–1820

Fund-raising was now in 'full swing' – from both small and large contributors, but more was required in order to put the newly formed Charity on a firm financial footing.

Support from the Royal Hospital, Greenwich?

The following letter from the Royal Hospital to Gordon gave solid support to the concept and the necessity to form a Society for destitute seafarers, but refused financial backing (there was a great deal of bureaucracy involved in the care of the *Merchant* sailor):

> Royal Hospital for Seamen
> 6th February 1818
>
> Sir,
>
> I received and laid before the Directors [of the Royal Hospital, Greenwich] at their last Meeting, your Letter to them of the 8th ultimo, representing that the Committee for the relief of the distressed Seamen finding upon enquiry, that a very large proportion of the unfortunate Mendicants who present themselves for relief, are really Seamen in great distress, and that the greater part of them have served on board King's Ships, and expressing the hope of the Committee that the Directors will not find it inconsistent with the due application of the Funds of the Hospital to subscribe in aid of the purposes of the Society; and I have their commands to acquaint you, that by Act of Parliament, and His Royal Highness the Prince Regent [the future King George IV

(1762–1830)]'s Order in Council, they are only authorized to grant relief to such Seamen and Mariners *belonging to His Majesty's Fleet*, as may have received Hurts, or Wounds, or been discharged for Sickness or Debility, or for Service after certain periods of Time; and that all Persons coming within these descriptions are constantly relieved on the production of satisfactory testimonials, & therefore under these restrictions they do not consider themselves at liberty to appropriate any part of the Hospital's Funds to be applied by other Persons than the Commissioners and Governors of the Hospital, or for the relief of Persons not coming within the several descriptions abovementioned.

I am commanded further to observe, that in consequence of the reduction of the Fleet by the termination of the late War [the Napoleonic Wars], the Out Pensioners of the Hospital have rapidly increased to about 34,000, and the Expenditure on account thereof, to £400,000, Per Annum; a Sum far exceeding its Revenues, and that even admitting the Directors were at liberty to exercise their discretion by contributing to the Society's Funds for the indiscriminate relief of *Merchant Seamen* as well as those who have served in His Majesty's Fleet, any sum so subscribed, would in fact be contributed by the Public, by whom it must ultimately be made good.

I am
Sir,
Your most obedient humble servant
J Dyer[62]

More 'teething problems'

A letter dated 4 February 1818 from the Consul of the USA for the Port of London referred to Henry Williams, who had applied at his Consulate 'for relief'. In fact, this man had been born at 'Halifax, in His Britannic Majesty's Province of Nova-Scotia' and was 'not [therefore] entitled to relief from the Consulate'. The Consul referred the matter, therefore, to the 'Examining Committee [of the CRDS] on board the Abundance Receiving Ship …'. In another letter (also dated 4 February), the Consul referred to another individual, Benjamin Barton (whose nationality is *not* stated); this man, he claimed 'was formerly relieved, supplied with food, clothing, and medical aid by me. In consequence of his selling his Clothes, I withheld his allowance for the sake of example to others in his situation'.[63] A letter from the Navy Board (signed by Nelson) outlined the passage of two Austrian Seamen (Hender and Martin) on a 361 ton ship to Malta. The nature of their misdemeanour is not stated, but they were ordered to report to Woolwich immediately.[64]

According to the Admiralty Office, there were 'generally thirty to fifty Seamen [who could be usefully employed] on board the Dromedary' receiving gratuitous treatment at Deptford (letter, 12 January 1819). Gordon was informed that 'the Navy Board [had] been directed to avail themselves of this offer if they [saw] no objection thereto …'.

Pensions and desertion

A letter, also from the Admiralty Office, a week later stated the length of service of one John Beverett *alias* Beverage; he had served at sea for 20 years and six months, and 'in consequence [had] been awarded a Pension of one shilling a day or £18.4.0 per Annum'. A somewhat disquieting letter shortly after that, stated that:

> Since I acquainted you that John Beverett [or Beverage] a Black Seaman was allowed a Pension of £18.4.0 per Annum, the Paymaster of Pensions at Greenwich Hospital has reported … that in 1816 he was allowed a Pension of £15.4.0, since which under the pretence that he was about to return to his Native Country he was allowed to commute his Pension for £30.8.0, which he has since spent. Notwithstanding that he denies having done so (or conduct still more reprehensible) the facts have been fully substantiated, and as he has only served 3 months since the first Pension was granted, he cannot be allowed any further relief, and in point of fact is liable to prosecution for the Fraud he has attempted.[65]

Later that year, the Paymaster of the Royal Hospital, Greenwich wrote indicating in reply to a request, that he could find no record of Daniel Wilson – probably because 'the Man in question goes by some other Name on the Pension List'.[66]

Two further letters (8 April and 20 May 1819) from the Admiralty Office (written by Dyer) also referred to Pensions. The first concerned Joseph Harry *alias* Harvey; he had apparently 'not served 14 years when paid off from the Navy' and was *not* therefore entitled to a Pension. Secondly, James Stone *alias* Hugh Jones was also not eligible for a Pension because he had apparently already received ones from *Marda*(?) and *Devastation*. Yet another letter written by Dyer, on behalf of the Admiralty, concerned a Pension granted to Robert Carvin [sic]; he had been discharged from the Navy when he was allowed £6=00 'in full satisfaction'; and in view of that, no further relief could be offered![67]

In a letter on behalf of the Paymaster of Pensions at the Royal Hospital Greenwich, a question was asked regarding the date of death of one of the Out Pensioners – one Alexander Sinclair; he had died, on board the *Dromedary*, sometime during February or March 1818. There was no evidence of a reply to this request. A somewhat bureaucratic letter (4 December 1818) from Trinity House, informed the Committee that 'until the requisite certificates [including proof of the Petitioner's age] are filled up, and signed by the proper Persons' it was impossible for Trinity House to admit the Petitioner to the Trinity House Pension List.[68]

The Secretary of the Scottish Corporation joined the correspondence to the Society; in a letter to Winnard the case of two poor people recommended by the Board had been 'taken into consideration'; they had apparently refused a passage to Scotland, which had been offered – and council received 'a little temporary aid'. A letter (February 1818) from a Clerk in the Prize Department of the Royal Hospital, Greenwich informed the Committee that Daniel Harkin of the *Domingo* had £1=00 owing to him; in order to claim this he should attend (with proof of identity) any day from 10 to 4 o'clock.[69]

Desertion was also a problem. A letter from the Navy Office (dated April 1818), stated that 'Henry Meecher (Boy) appears by the Books of HMS Forth to have deserted from that Ship on 23 June 1817 at Portsmouth'. An interesting correspondence surrounded Edward Harnett – a 'seaman who had acknowledged [that he was] a *deserter* [my italics] from the Phaeton'; their Lordships (according to a letter received from the Admiralty Office) had 'no intention of claiming him'.[70]

Problems with 'foreign' mendicants

'Disposal' of 'men of colour' proved to be a contentious matter. For example, the following letter was received by the CRDS:

> Downing Street
> 16 June 1818
>
> Sir,
>
> I am directed by Lord Bathurst[71] to acknowledge the receipt of your letter of yesterday's date requesting that the seven persons of color [sic] who state themselves to be Natives of the Island of Jamaica, may be permitted to return thither and to land as free subjects of Great Britain, and to acquaint you in reply that Lord Bathurst thinks it very desirable to obtain further information respecting the Individuals before he can consider himself justified in giving encouragement of their being sent to Jamaica.
>
> If there is reason to believe that any of them has run away from their Masters in Jamaica Lord Bathurst entertains great doubts whether their Masters might not have a right to reclaim them on their return to the Island and . . .;– If the Committee are not enabled to secure to them a maintenance on their arrival in the Island Lord Bathurst is afraid that they will be exposed to temptations which it would be difficult for them to resist; and the opinion very prevalent in the Colonies that freedom cannot be with safety extended to the coloured population would be fortified by the unhappy result of this Experiment.
>
> I am,
> Sir,
> Your most obedient
> humble servant
> Henry Goulburn[72]

Two days later, a further letter from Goulburn (Downing Street) also addressed the matter of the 'Coloured People'; Lord Bathurst had given his approval for 'the four first named Men in the [enclosed] list … proceeding to Jamaica'. Goulburn continued: 'His Lordship has accordingly directed me to send you herewith a duplicate of the letter which he has written to the Governor of Jamaica directing him to afford these people all necessary protection, to be given in charge to the Individuals themselves'.[73]

Also, a letter dated 9 July 1818 from the Admiralty Office (signed by Barrow) concerned three [African] 'Men of Colour'; it had been suggested by the CRDS that they 'may be granted a passage in a Kings vessel to Africa', but the writer had been commanded by the Lords Commissioners of the Admiralty to find out the names of the ships on which they had previously served – before a passage could be ordered for them! In a further letter from Croker (also from the Admiralty Office), a passage was ordered for these three 'Men of Colour': George Ryan, John Lewis and Thomas Pierce (or Pearce). The order was directed to Rear Admiral Sir John Gore of Chatham, and the ship was named as the 'Tartan'.[74]

Further correspondence (dated 5 August) from the Admiralty Office, concerned the 'case of John Prinnett, an Insane Ceylonese Negro', as well as 'two Lists of Men [whose names were appended], who are desirous of returning to their respective homes'. Admiral Sir George Campbell of Portsmouth was directed to provide passages 'in His Majesty's Ship Salisbury for all the West Indians, excepting Joseph Groves who appears to have been Six Years out of the Service, and that the Navy Board are directed to provide Passages, in the Weymouth Storeship, for the two Men Natives of Gibraltar [William Well] and Venice [John Acorn]'. A follow-up letter (dated 7 August) came from Admiral Sir George Campbell on board *Queen Charlotte* in Portsmouth Harbour; the seven seamen were indeed to 'have a passage to their native country in His Majesty's Ship Salisbury' and ... were to 'present themselves at the Admiral's office'.

'With regard to John Prinnett the Navy Board [was] directed to report his Servitude before their Lordships [could] decide on the recommendation of the Committee for his admission into the Naval Lunatic Asylum'. More correspondence was to follow on the unfortunate Prinnett; a letter (dated 12 August 1818) from Barrow at the Admiralty Office indicated that 'this Person has not any claim on the Naval Service'; he could *not* therefore be accommodated at the Naval Lunatic Asylum.[75]

Seven months later, Barrow (at the Admiralty Office) informed Gordon (letter, 11 March 1819) that in reply to a request 'their Lordships would be pleased to order passages for the Six Seamen therein mentioned [in a letter written two days previously] to their respective Countries, in consideration of their Servitude in His Majesty's Navy'; their Lordships had ordered a passage for George Savage in His Majesty's Ship *Newcastle* (then at Chatham), but 'declined to give passages to the five other seamen'.[76]

An ambiguous attitude of the London Hospital

For various reasons the London Hospital was somewhat ambivalent concerning the CRDS's initiative(s). A letter (14 January 1818) from John Jenkinson (Superintendent of the [Royal] London Hospital) indicated that they could not 'accommodate any more of the Distressed Seamen' that week, and 'in fact [the Hospital had] received the last seven without any authority whatsoever'. Furthermore, he wrote: 'The House Committee sits only from 12 to 2 o'Clock on Tuesdays, & till then it is useless to send us any more of the Sailors: in fact our Bedsteads &c are already fully occupied'. A further letter (21 January) from Jenkinson (who on this occasion termed himself an *apothecary*) recorded that the London Hospital could:

> receive two or three cases *tomorrow*, if you could have the goodness to withdraw as many of those already sent in with no discoverable disease

> about them at the same time. *By Friday morning the room we are preparing will be ready*: it will hold 8 very well, *but not more than 10*. Several of the twelve we now have are miserably off for clothing, so we should be obliged by your sending three or four shirts, & as many pairs of shoes & stockings, for their use, by the Bearer.

Jenkinson continued by saying that they were obliged to return a man sent from the *Abundance*. He was clearly unhappy that some of the Seamen sent to the London Hospital did not have an organic disease: 'it is only filling our beds uselessly to take in persons who have no material ailment', he wrote.[77]

A day before this, another letter had been received from the London Hospital, this from the *Secretary* (J Jones) writing on behalf of the Chairman of the House Committee; it stated that they would admit 'into the Hospital as many of these Persons who might be sick or hurt as the Hospital could possibly receive'. Jones was however somewhat concerned about the large numbers of persons in that category, and he concluded by writing that 'the House Committee will continue to do all they can to co-operate with the benevolent views of your Committee – and have given directions to make further accommodation for the reception of an additional number in the Attic story of the building. The House Committee have therefore to request that no more may be sent until your Committee hear from the Superintendent Mr Jenkinson that such arrangements are completed ...'.[78]

A further letter (28th of the same month) recorded that one of the men, John Demay, had died that morning, and he wanted 'to know what is your pleasure respecting his burial'. He furthermore reported that several of the men were still lacking 'Jackets, Flannels &c'; this he felt should be rectified. In a postscript he mentioned that '[the hospital has] been obliged to furnish several of them even with Shirts at our own expense'.[79]

On 3 February a more positive letter (signed by J Jones, Secretary) and again written on behalf of the London Hospital's House Committee, indicated that three men who had been under their care were now considered fit, and had been sent to one of the receiving ships at Deptford; 'following up the humane intentions of your committee [and he continued, the House Committee] will forgo any charge for subsistence'![80]

In a final letter (4 February) from Jenkinson, news was received that three more men (David Jones, John Jackson and John Robertson) had recovered and had been sent (on the previous day) to the *Perseus*, but 'owing to some informality on our part, they were not received. We therefore send them directly to you, for disposal, except Jones who has absconded since'. 'The slops sent here by Mr Drinkald [a member of the provisional committee] were all distributed according to your directions'. 'We have now six of your men [he continued] who will all be ready to leave us in the course of the present month; two or three of them in a very few days'.[81]

A suggested surgeon for the CRDS

In early 1820, Newby, Secretary of the Marine Society (see above) wrote an entirely uninvited letter to the Committee recommending 'Samuel Browne [sic] as a

Candidate for the situation of Surgeon, to be employed ... at Deptford ...'. The writer was convinced that if chosen, he would 'exercise the same assiduous and constant attention to the Objects placed under his care which he has invariably shewn [sic] towards those which have been under his notice as Surgeon to the Marine Society'. This 'additional Duty [the writer continued] is most perfectly compatible with his present one, as the Ships lay contiguous to each other in the River'.[82]

References and Notes

[Folio numbers refer to those in 'Letters received. 1818–1820' (SHS Archive)]

1 Anonymous to J W Buckle. 1821 [SHS archive].
2 Anonymous. *Gateway to the East.*
3 G Webb. *Some notes on five hundred years of Seamen's Welfare.* Gillingham, Kent: King George's Fund for Sailors 1959: 30.
4 A W Clarke. Trinity House, London: safeguard of the Mariner and cradle of the Royal Navy. *SHS Quart Mag* 1929; 1: 7–10.
5 Anonymous. *The Marine Society: annual report and accounts 2001.* London: The Marine Society 2001: 2.
6 F E Thorn. The Shipwrecked fishermen and mariners' Royal Benevolent Society: a brief history of the first hundred years. *SHS Quart Mag* 1939; 11(3): 16–18.
7 H H Drad (ed). *Halsted's History of Kent.* 1886 [SHS Archive].
8 G M Trevelyan. Cobbett's England. In: *English Social History: a survey of six centuries. Chaucer to Queen Victoria.* London: Longmans, Green & Co. 1944: 463–508.
9 The London Gazette Extraordinary. Wednesday, Nov. 6, 1805. Admiralty Office, Nov 6. *Times, Lond.* 1805; 7 November: 1–2; Anonymous Action off Cape Trafalgar. *Times, Lond.* 1805; 12 November: 3; O Warner *Trafalgar.* London: BT Batsford 1959; D Howarth. *Trafalgar: the Nelson touch.* London: Collins 1969; J Terraine. *Trafalgar.* London: Sidgewick & Jackson, Ltd. 1976.
10 Anonymous. *Gentleman's Magazine.* 1799; i; 53.
11 J Ashton. *Social England under the Regency.* London: Chatto and Windus, 1899; Anonymous. Refuge for the destitute. *Times, Lond.* 1807; 23 May: 3.
12 Battle of Waterloo. *Times, Lond.* 1815, 4 November: 3; Howarth D. *A near run thing: the day of Waterloo.* London: Collins,1968.
13 **Charles Manners-Sutton** (1755–1828) was Archbishop of Canterbury from 1805–1828. [See also: W M Jacob. Sutton, Charles Manners – (1755–1828) In: H C G Matthew, B Harrison (eds). *Oxford Dictionary of National Biography.* Oxford: Oxford University Press 2004; 53: 377–8]; Anonymous. *Gentleman's Magazine* 1816; ii: 174–175; William Wilberforce (1759–1833) (*see* Figure 1.1) was one of Britain's greatest philanthropists, and an instigator of the anti-slavery movement. [See also: J Wolffe. Wilberforce, William (1759–1833). In: H C G Matthew, B Harrison (eds). *Oxford Dictionary of National Biography.* Oxford: Oxford University Press 2004; 58: 879–87; [MFT]. *SHS Quart Mag* 1933; 5 (4): 7 & 9; G C Cook. *SHS Annual Report* 2001: 10. Thomas Cochrane, (1775–1860) tenth Earl of Dundonald had a distinguished naval career. From 1848 until 1851, he was Commander-in-Chief on the West Indian and North American stations. His entry in the ODNB considers that he was 'one of the greatest of our admirals, whose name must be ranked with those of Nelson, Hawke, Rodney [and] Blake'. [See also: A Lambert. Cochrane, Thomas, tenth

Earl of Dundonald (1775–1860) In: H C G Matthew, B Harrison (eds). *Oxford Dictionary of National Biography*. Oxford: Oxford University Press 2004; 12: 315–22].

14 Anonymous. Refuge for the destitute. *Times, Lond*. 1807, 23 May: 3; Anonymous. *Times, Lond*. 1808, 23 January: 3; Anonymous. *Times, Lond*. 1808, 1 February: 3; Anonymous. *Times, Lond*. 1818, 6 February: 3; E Prothero. *Times, Lond*. 1818, 7 February: 3.

15 Leading article. Times, Lond. 1818; 2 January: 2; Anonymous. Times, Lond. 1818; 2 January.

16 **Bob Blake** RN (1783–1857) was appointed Surgeon to the RN on 1 April 1809. He had obtained the MRCS four years before (on 12 January 1805). [See also: Anonymous. *A list of the Medical Officers of His Majesty's Navy. With the dates of their respective appointments*. London: Henry Teape 1823: 45; Anonymous. *An alphabetical list of the medical officers of Her Majesty's Fleet with dates of their first Warrants*. London: W Clowes and Sons 1839: 14, *Ibid*. 43; Anonymous. *List of the Fellows and Members of the Royal College of Surgeons of England*. London: Richard and John E Taylor 1850: 42].

17 WBR. *Origin of the Dreadnought Hospital-ship*. From a London paper – dated 1863 [SHS Archive]; B Blake (HM Hospital-ship *Gorgon*) to his parents. 1808: 3 October: 3 [SHS Archive].

18 *Op cit*. See note 15 above.

19 J H Jesse. *London and its celebrities. A second series of literary and historical memorials of London*. London: Richard Bentley 1850; 1: 249; Anonymous 'At the King's Arms in the Poultrey': The Bookshop Emporium of Dorman Newman 1670–1694. *The London Journal* 1998; 23: 1–20.

20 [G.L.N.] *Times, Lond*. 1818: 3 January: 3; Leading article. *Times, Lond*. 1818; 3 January: 2.

21 Anonymous. Distressed Seamen. *Times, Lond*. 1818, 5 January: 2; Anonymous. *Times, Lond*. 1818, 6 January: 2; Anonymous. *Times, Lond*. 1818, 6 January: 3; Anonymous. *Gentleman's Magazine* 1818; i: 79; *DISTRESSED SEAMEN. Times, Lond*. 1818, 14 January: 2; *COMMITTEE in AID OF DISTRESSED SEAMEN. Times, Lond*. 1818, 16 January: 2; J Court (sic) to J E Gordon (Secretary, The Committee of the Association for the Relief of destitute Seamen). *Seamen's Hospital Society Archive; letters received 1818–1820*. 1818: 8 January, (folio 1); J. Dart (sic) (Assistant Secretary, East India House) to The Committee for conducting the subscription for the relief of Distressed Seamen 1818: 8 January; *Ibid*. (folio 2); G. Longlands (sic) to J.E. Gordon, Hon. Sec. to the Committee for Relieving Distressed Seamen. 1818: 20 January, *Ibid*. (folio 16). Sir John William Lubbock, Bt (1774–1840) was the second baronet. His son, of the same name, was to become treasurer and vice-president of the Royal Society, and first Vice-chancellor of the University of London.

22 **Robert Saunders Dundas**, Second Viscount Melville, FRS, KT (1771–1851) succeeded to the title in 1811; the following year he was appointed (by Lord Liverpool) first Lord of the Admiralty – a post which he held for 15 years. He was reappointed (having resigned when Lord Liverpool's government was defeated) to the Admiralty by the Duke of Wellington in 1828; when that administration fell (in 1830) he resigned from political life altogether. [See also: M Fry. Dundas, Robert Saunders, second Viscount Melville (1771–1851). In: H C G Matthew, B Harrison (eds). *Oxford Dictionary of National Biography*. Oxford: Oxford University Press 2004; 17: 292–4].

23 Distressed Seamen. *Times, Lond*. 1818: 8 January: 3; [See also: G C Cook. The Committee for the Relief of Distressed Seamen: correspondence from the Admiralty in 1818–19. *Postgrad Med J* 2006; 83: 54–58.

24 [J.B.] *Times, Lond*. 1818, 5 January: 3.

25 *Op cit*. See note 23 above (Cook).

26 **John Wilson Croker** LID, FRS (1780–1857) was a prominent politician, writer, and Secretary to the Admiralty. [See also: W Thomas. Croker, John Wilson (1780–1857). In: H

C G Matthew, B Harrison (eds). *Oxford Dictionary of National Biography*. Oxford: Oxford University Press 2004; 14: 273–8].

27 **Sir John Barrow**, Bt, FRS, FLS (1764–1848) was Second Secretary (and later Secretary) to the Admiralty. [See also: J M R Cameron. Barrow, Sir John, first baronet (1764–1848) In: H C G Matthew, B Harrison (eds). *Oxford Dictionary of National Biography. Oxford*: Oxford University Press 2004; 4: 102–4.]

28 Anonymous. Distressed Seamen. *Times, Lond.* 1818; 10 January: 3; [J D]. Distressed Seamen. *Times, Lond.* 1818; 16 January: 3; Anonymous. Distressed Seamen. *Times, Lond.* 1818: 27 January: 2.

29 J W Croker (Admiralty Office) to J W Buckle (Chairman of the Committee for the relief of distressed Seamen) 1818: 8 January, I (folio 3).

30 **Henry Addington** (1757–1844) was created first Viscount Sidmouth in January 1805. He was educated at Cheam, Winchester, and Brasenose College, Oxford. He studied law (and became a close friend of William Pitt prior to embarking on a political career) and became MP for Devizes, Speaker of the House of Commons (11 years), Lord privy seal, Lord President of the Council, and Secretary of the Home Department (for 10 years). He was involved in the proceedings against Warren Hastings. Sidmouth was a staunch opponent of Catholic emancipation. In 1812, the labouring classes were suffering greatly from the depression in agriculture and trade. He apparently 'had a full share in the shame and unpopularity which the proceedings against Queen Caroline brought upon the government'. [See also: J E Cookson. Addington, Henry, first Viscount Sidmouth (1757–1844). In: H C G Matthew, B Harrison (eds). *Oxford Dictionary of National Biography*. Oxford: Oxford University Press 2004; 1: 303–11].

31 H Hobhouse to Captain Gordon R.N. 1818: 9 January (folio 4).

32 J W Croker to The Chairman of the Committee for the relief of distressed Seamen. 1818: 12 January (folio 5); H Legge, RG Middleton, J Bumble to Captain Waite, Harbour Master, Deptford Yard. 1818: 12 January (folio 7).

33 R L Nelson (Navy Office) to Captain Gordon, Secretary to the Committee for distressed Seamen 1818: 14 January, *Ibid*, (folio 9); R L Nelson to Lieutenant Gordon, Secretary to the Committee for the relief of distressed Seamen 1818: 17 January, *Ibid*. (folio 13).

34 J W Croker to the Chairman of the Committee for the relief of distressed Seamen 1818: 17 January (folio 15).

35 J W Croker to the Chairman of the Committee for the relief of distressed Seamen 1818: 12 January (folio 6).

36 J W Croker to J W Buckle 1818: 21 January (folio 17).

37 C Cunningham R.N. to the Committee for the relief of destitute Seamen, London 1818: 2 February (folio 21).

38 R L Nelson to Lieutenant J E Gordon 1818; 24 February (folio 35).

39 J Barrow to the Chairman of the Committee for the relief of destitute Seamen 1818: 7 March (folio 36).

40 J Barrow to the Chairman of the Committee for the relief of distressed Seamen 1818: 30 March (folio 39).

41 J Barrow to The Chairman of the Committee for relief of distressed Seamen 1818: 13 April (folio 40).

42 J Barrow to the Chairman of the Committee for the relief of destitute Seamen, 27 Poultry. 1818: 23 April (folio 41).

43 J Barrow to the Chairman of the Committee for relief of destitute Seamen 1818: 28 May (folio 42).

44 R L Nelson to Lieut. J E Gordon 1818: 4 February (folio 25); [?] to Lieut. Gordon, RN, 1818: 9 February (folio 28).

45 Victualling Office to (?), 1818: 12 February (folio 66); [?] to Lieut. Gordon, 1818: 12 February (folio 33); R L Nelson to Lieut. Gordon, 1818: 12 February (folio 31).
46 J Barrow to the Chairman of the CRDS, 1818: 4 February (folio 24); R L Nelson to Lieut. Gordon, 1818: 12 February, (folio 32).
47 H Hobhouse to S Cock, 1818: 12 January (folio unnumbered); H Hobson to Captain Gordon RN, 1818: 16 January (folio 11).
48 J Newby to R D Isbell, 1818: 15 January (folio 14).
49 H Hobhouse to Capt. Gordon, RN, 1818: 20 January (folio 18); J Trotter (sic) to CRDS office, 1818: 24 January (folio 63).
50 [?] to CRDS Office, 1818: 29 January (folio 64); J Trotter (sic) to Secretary, CRDS, 1818: 18 February (folio 34).
51 [?] to J E Gordon, 1818: 25 December (folio 74); J Trotter (sic) to J Winnard (Assistant Secretary, CRDS), 1819: 15 January (folio unnumbered); [?] to J E Gordon, 1819: 27 January (folio 53); [?] to J Winnard, 1829: 18 January (folio 58).
52 [?] to The Honble J E Gordon, 1818: 13 March (folio 37).
53 [?] to J E Gordon Esq, 1818: 17 January (folio 12); G Gaskin to J E Gordon, Esq, 1818: 15 January (folio 61); E Suter to Lieut. J E Gordon, 1818: 18 March (folio 38); C Cunningham to J E Gordon Esq, 1818: 9 February (folio 29).
54 Disposal of the distressed seamen. *Times, Lond*. 1818: 31 January: 3.
55 **Zachary Macaulay** (1768–1838) was one of Britain's greatest philanthropists, who whilst manager of an estate in Jamaica was greatly dismayed at the miserable state of the slave population. He later became Governor of Sierra Leone and Secretary to the Sierra Leone Company and the African Institute. He did much for the abolitionist cause, being a member of the 'Clapham Sect'. [See also: J R Oldfield. Macauley, Zachary (1768–1838). In: H C G Matthew, B Harrison (eds). *Oxford Dictionary of National Biography*. Oxford: Oxford University Press 2004; 35: 51–3. Anonymous. *SHS Quart Mag* 1934; 6 (2): 16].
56 Public meeting for the relief of distressed seamen. *Times, Lond*. 1818: 6 February: 3.
57 Distressed Seamen. *Times, Lond*. 1818: 10 February: 3.
58 Anonymous. British Merchant Seamen. *Times, Lond*. 1818; 19 March: 3.
59 H Hobhouse to Capt. Gordon R.N. 1818: 11 February (folio 30).
60 Anonymous. *Times, Lond*. 1818: 17 February: 3.
61 J Dart to J E Gordon, Esq, 13 January 1818 (folio 8); J W Croker to The Chairman of the Committee for the relief of Seamen in distress, 1818: 26 January (folio 19).
62 J Dyer to Lieut. J E Gordon, 1818: 6 February (folio 26); G C Cook. Correspondence relating to the Committee for the Relief of Distressed (destitute) Seamen. *Mariner's Mirror*; 2007: 93: 209–211.
63 W Aspinwall to the Examining Committee on board the Abundance Receiving Ship for Destitute Seamen 1818: 4 February; *Ibid*, (folio 22); W Aspinwall to C Boucher Esq., 1818: 4 February (folio 23).
64 R L Nelson to J Winnard. [date unclear] (folio 77).
65 [?] to Lieut. J E Gordon 1819: 12 January (folio 50); J Dyer to J Winnard 1819: 19 January (folio 52); Dyer to J Winnard 1819: 25 January (folio 71).
66 L. McLean to John Winnard 1819: 14 October (folio 55).
67 J Dyer to Mr Winnard 1819: 8 April (folio 72); [?] Dyer to Mr Winnard 1819: 20 May (folio 73); J Dyer to Mr Winnard 1819: 29 July (folio 75).
68 Paymaster of Pensions, Royal Hospital, Greenwich to J Winnard 1819: 10 November (folio 76); Deputy Master, Trinity House to J E Gordon 1818: 4 December (folio 69).
69 [?] to John Winnard 1819: 12 July (folio 74). [?] Smith to J Winnard 1818: 24 February; *Ibid*, (folio 67).

70 H Goulburn to J E Gordon Esq. 1818: 16 June; *Ibid*, (folio 43); [?] to J Winnard 1818: 21 April (folio 68); J Barrow to Mr John Winnard 1819: 4 November (folio 56).
71 **Henry Bathurst** KG (1762–1834); the third Earl Bathurst, was a prominent conservative statesman. He had been MP for Cirencester (1793–4), Lord of the Admiralty (1783–9), Lord of the Treasury (1789–91), and commissioner of the Board of Control (1793–1802). He was a personal friend of Pitt. He became president of the Board of Trade (1807–1812) holding concurrently the mastership of the mint. From October to December 1809 he was Foreign Secretary. He also became Secretary for War and the Colonies, and was Lord President of the Council (under Wellington). He took part in the Slave Trade debates, and also supported the Roman Catholic cause. [See also: N Thompson. Bathurst, Henry, third Earl Bathurst (1762–1834). In: H C G Matthew, B Harrison (eds). *Oxford Dictionary of National Biography*. Oxford: Oxford University Press 2004; 4: 354–5].
72 **Henry Goulburn** MP (1784–1856) was an eminent statesman who later became Home Secretary (1834–5) and Chancellor of the Exchequer (1841–46). [See also: G F R Barker, D Eastwood. Goulburn, Henry (1784–1856). In: H C G Matthew, B Harrison (eds). *Oxford Dictionary of National Biography*. Oxford: Oxford University Press 2004; 23: 62–6]. *Op cit*. see note 62 above (Cook)]
73 H Goulburn to J E Gordon Esq 1818: 16 June (folio 43); H Goulburn to J E Gordon Esqr. 1818: 18 June; (folio 47).
74 J Barrow to Lieut. J E Gordon 1818: 9 July (folio 44); J Croker to Lieut. J E Gordon 1818: 13 July (folio 45); [See also: J K Laughton, R Morriss. Gore, Sir John (1772–1836). In: H C G Matthew, B Harrison (eds). *Oxford Dictionary of National Biography*. Oxford: Oxford University Press 2004; 22: 982–3.]
75 J Barrow to J E Gordon 1818: 5 August (folio 46); Admiral Sir George Campbell to Lieut. J E Gordon R.N. 1818: 7 August (folio 49); J Barrow to Lieut. J E Gordon 1818: 12 August (folio 48).
76 J Barrow to Lieutenant J E Gordon 1819: 11 March (folio 54).
77 J Jenkinson to the Committee for Distressed Seamen 1818: 14 January (folio 10); J Jenkinson to Chairman of the Committee for Distressed Seamen 1818: 21 January (folio 60). [See also: A E Clark-Kennedy. *The London: a study in the Voluntary hospital system*. London: Pitman Medical Publishing 1962; vol 1; p210.]
78 J Jones to J E Gordon 1818: 20 January (folio 62).
79 J Jenkinson to the Committee for Distressed Seamen 1818: 28 January (folio 20).
80 J Jones to the Committee for Distressed Seamen 1818: 3 February (folio 27).
81 J Jenkinson to the Secretary of the Committee 1818: 4 February (folio 65).
82 J Newby to the Committee for Distressed Seamen 1820: 21 January (folio 59).

Chapter 6

'This laudable Institution': the *permanent* Society is launched in 1821

By 1820, the 'Committee for the Relief of Destitute Seamen' (CRDS) (Chapter 5) had, since its launch in the severe winter of 1817–18, accumulated significant funds to assist the 'objects' under their care. Rightly, the members of the Committee felt that a *permanent* society was by then indicated. It had been well ascertained that 'in the course of the year, many hundred Seamen in the Port of London [were] destitute of Medical or Surgical aid'. One estimate was that 700–800 seamen were involved. In the first instance, a 'Provisional Committee' of what was to become the *Seamen's Hospital Society* (SHS), was set up. The objectives were: 'framing rules and regulations for the government of the Hospital, with authority to fix a day for the General Meeting of Subscribers, [and] for the election of a Committee for the promotion and management of the interests and concerns of the Charity'. The meeting was to be held at the City of London Tavern. A 'provisional committee' (see below) consisted of: Sir John William Lubbock, Bart. (Chairman); J W Buckle, Esq; Aaron Chapman, Esq; Captain C C Owen, RN; John Deacon, Esq; and George Lyall[1], Esq; William Williams, Esq MP was named as treasurer.[2]

Origin of the SHS – on 8 March 1821 ('Founders day')

Details of the first general meeting of the SHS can be found in the opening pages of the first SHS Minute Book: it was determined 'that a PERMANENT FLOATING HOSPITAL be accordingly established on the River Thames, for the use of Sick and Diseased Seamen only'. The following day, *The Times* published an account:

> At a MEETING at the City of London Tavern, this Day, the 8th of March, . . . for the purpose of ESTABLISHING, by Public Voluntary Subscription, a FLOATING HOSPITAL, for the Assistance and Relief of Sick and Helpless Seamen, under the patronage of His Majesty [King George IV (1762–1830)[3]].
>
> 'The right Rev. the Lord Bishop of CHESTER in the Chair:
> The Report of the Committee, for the Relief of distressed Seamen, was read, on which

It was moved by William Wilberforce, Esq., M.P. [*see* Chapters 1 and 5], and seconded by the Earl of Rocksavage,[4]

1. That the establishment of an Institution for the particular purpose of Relieving Sick and Diseased Seamen, in the Port of London, in those cases in which relief cannot be obtained for them in the existing hospitals, or until they can be admitted into those receptacles, (whose objects are more general,) has become necessary to succour them in that distress and misery to which seamen, from their unconnected and helpless situations, are peculiarly subject: and would, at the same time, be a just and humane tribute to the merits and services of that useful class of men, and highly honorable, as well as beneficial, to the country.
2. Moved by Lord Ellenborough,[5] and seconded by Rear-admiral Sir Edward Codrington,[6]

   That a Floating Hospital [The 'Grampus (formerly a 50 Gun Ship, was to be) moored off Deptford Creek'] be accordingly established on the River Thames, (in conformity with the recommendations of the Report of the Committee of the Society for Distressed Seamen) such Hospital to be supported by voluntary contributions and subscriptions.
3. Moved by Thomas Wilson, Esq., M.P., and seconded by Willm Taylor Money, Esq., M.P.,

   That the following gentlemen be a provisional committee for framing rules and regulations for the government of the said Hospital, with authority to add to their numbers: who shall fix a day for a general meeting of subscribers for the election of a committee for the promotion and management of the interests and concerns of the charity:– John W. Buckle, Esq., chairman of the committee of ship owners; Aaron Chapman, Esq., elder brother of the Trinity-house; Captain C.C. Owen, R.N.; Sir John Willm Lubbock, Bart; John Deacon, Esq.; and George Lyall, Esq.
4. Moved by the Honble Sir George Grey Bart,[7] [and] seconded by Rear-Admiral Spranger,

   That William Williams, Esq., M.P., be Treasurer, and that subscription be received by him, and at the several banking-houses of the metropolis.

   It was moved by the Right Honble The Earl of Darnley,[8] [and] seconded by the Honble Capt. Waldegrave, R.N.,[9]

   That the most grateful thanks of this Meeting are due to His Majesty, for his most gracious kindness and condescension in becoming the illustrious Patron of this charity.

   It was moved by Thos Rowcroft, Esq., and seconded by Sir George Keith,

   That the thanks of the Meeting be given to the Committee of the Society for the Suppression of Mendicity, for the cordial and efficient assistance afforded at all times to the Committee of the Society for the Relief of Distressed Seamen.

> The thanks of the Meeting were given to the Right Rev. Chairman for his excellent conduct of business of the Meeting.

A document (in the SHS archive) makes clear that:

> As the extent of the Plan must depend upon the amount of the Funds contributed, the Provisional Committee are desirous of drawing the serious attention of the Public to the motives and object of the intended establishment, and anxiously solicit the favor of their early Subscriptions for its support.

Appendix II shows a notice appealing for funding, issued following the 8 March 1821 meeting.

The first duty of the provisional committee was therefore, to raise funds for the new Charity and it was 'resolved unanimously' by them, on 13 March, that letters be sent to twelve possible donors. A minute of 20 March summarises some of the early subscribers: J Dart (Secretary to the East India Company) – 100 guineas, W Smith (Deputy Secretary to the Court of Directors of the Bank of England) – /(£)100, The Earl of Hardwicke – 20 guineas; and Captain Alexander Murray – a list of 8 subscribers for 'One Guinea, each Annually'. At the following meeting (23 March), it was further announced that the Elder Brethren of Trinity House were to subscribe £200, and the Directors of the Royal Exchange were donating one hundred guineas to the Charity.

A later minute of the Committee of Management (17 January 1823) leaves no doubt, should there still be any in the mind of the reader, that the SHS arose directly from the CRDS (*see* Chapter 5): '... the distressed Seamen's Society from which the Seamen's Hospital may be said to have originated'.

As temporary accommodation, the Mendicity Society had initially offered premises. On 20 March, however, a somewhat disturbing letter was read from the Secretary (W H Bodkin) of that Society indicating that the SHS should obtain an alternative temporary 'office', as 'it would be impossible to grant the assistance of [his Society's premises] beyond the Week ending the 17th Instant ...'. Captain Owen (a member of the provisional committee) was instructed to look into the possibility of housing their Sick Sailors (then residing at the Mendicity Society) at a house belonging to the London Dock Company, opposite the Dundee Arms, Wapping – at that time used as an 'Asylum for the Houseless Poor'.[10]

The first General Meeting

The rules of the Society, and composition of the definitive 'Committee of Management' were laid down at a General Meeting (also held at the City of London Tavern) on 11 April 1821. *The Morning Post* for 12 April 1821 reported the details:

> A Public Meeting was yesterday held at the city of London Tavern, to adopt Rules and Regulations for the government of the *Permanent* [my italics] Floating Hospital for Seamen, lately established upon the River Thames. The Right Reverend the Lord Bishop of CHESTER was in the Chair, supported by Lord KENYON,[11] Lord GAMBIER,[12] Lord

> CALTHORPE,[13] the Hon. Capt. WALDEGRAVE [see above], Mr. W. WILLIAMS, M.P., and many other Gentlemen who have been forward in establishing this laudable Institution.
>
> The Secretary read the Report of the Provisional Committee.
>
> It was moved that the Rules and Regulations [see below] which it recommended be adopted by the Meeting.
>
> Mr URQUHART objected to them upon the ground that they could not have received sufficient attention from the Subscribers. They ought to have been printed, and submitted to those who were interested in the establishment some days previous to the meeting. The question was put, and the motion carried with one dissentient voice.
>
> It was then agreed that Lord MELVILLE [*see* Chapter 5] should be invited to act as President of the Institution [he accepted in a letter dated 3 May], and his Royal Highness the Duke of CLARENCE [later King William IV[14]], with his Serene Highness Prince LEOPOLD,[15] as Vice-Patrons [they accepted on 18 and 12 April, respectively].
>
> The SECRETARY then said, that at a previous meeting he had announced the gracious intention of his Majesty [George IV] to give 50 guineas as a donation, and 50 guineas annually, to the Institution. But when the cheques came they proved to be for 100 guineas each. Amongst the other subscriptions which had been newly received, was *50 l* [£] from Lord Melville, and the same sum from a Nobleman, who wished that his name should remain unknown. The amount of money now in the hands of the Treasurer amounted to *2,200 l*, and *272 l* annually. Subscriptions which had been received that day would raise the funds to *2,500 l* and the annual income to *500 l*. It was calculated that an annual income of *3,000 l* would effect every object which the supporters of the Institution had in view.
>
> Upon the motion of Lord CALTHORPE, a committee of 24 was then appointed to direct the affairs of the establishment.
>
> A MEMBER of the late Provisional Committee then said, that it was due in justice to the Government to state, that in all its branches the utmost attention and zeal had been manifested to promote the objects which the Committee had in view.
>
> The Right Rev. CHAIRMAN then congratulated the Meeting upon what they had done to relieve the sufferings of a class of men who were justly the pride, as they had proved themselves the strength of this country. He was sure they should all look back to that day with the sincerest pleasure and satisfaction.
>
> The Thanks of the Meeting having been voted to his Lordship, the business of the day was declared to be at an end. … .

A *formal* statement was also included on the front page of the same issue of this newspaper:

> SEAMEN'S HOSPITAL – At a GENERAL MEETING at the City of London Tavern, on Wednesday the 11th instant.

The BISHOP of CHESTER in the Chair:

The Provisional Committee laid before the Meeting the Rules and Regulations for the government of the Society, prepared by them conformable to the Resolution of the General Meeting of the 8th of March; which having been read,

It was moved by Rear-Admiral Sir Edward Codrington, and seconded by Thomas Sturge, jun. Esq. and Resolved with one dissenting voice –

That the Plan and Regulations recommended by the Provisional Committee be adopted.

Resolved unanimously, upon the motion of Admiral Lord Gambier, seconded by the Hon. Capt. Waldegrave, R.N.

That his Royal Highness the Duke of Clarence and his Royal Highness Prince Leopold be invited to become Vice-Patrons of the Institution.

Resolved unanimously, upon the motion of the Right Hon. Lord Selsey, R.N., seconded by Capt. Bowles, R.N.

That the Right Honourable Viscount Melville, First Lord of the Admiralty, be invited to be the President of this Institution.

Resolved unanimously, upon the motion of the Right Hon. Lord Calthorpe, seconded by Wm. Williams, Esq. M.P.

That the following Gentlemen be the Members of the Committee [which contained representatives of the Royal Navy and Trinity House]:–

John Blackett, Esq.
Capt. Bowles, R.N.
John Blackburn, Esq.
Aaron Chapman, Esq.
Wm. Cotton, Esq.
Wm. Curling, Esq.
John Deacon, Esq.
Joseph Dowson, jun. Esq.
Stewart Erskine, Esq.
Charles Francis, Esq.
Wm. Frend, Esq.
Lieut. J.E. Gordon, R.N.
Capt. Gooch, H.C. service*
George Lyall, Esq.
Capt. Lochner, H.C. service*
Capt. Loch [sic], H.C. service*
Zachy. Macaulay, Esq.
Capt. C.C. Owen, R.N.
Rev. Dr. Rudge
Thomas Sturge, Esq.
Daniel Stephenson, Esq.
Wm. Venables, Esq.
John Woolmore, Esq.
Capt. Wm. Young, R.N.

The unanimous Thanks of the Meeting were voted to the Right Rev. Chairman. The Treasurer then reported the following state of the Funds:–

*H C Service indicates the Honourable Company's Service (the East India Company).

	Contributions			Annual Subscriptions		
Remaining from the Fund, and raised for the Relief of distressed Seamen, in the Winters, 1817 and 1818	£601	3	1			
Donations to this Charity, as published	1652	17	6	272	9	6
	£2,254	0	7			
Further Subscriptions:						
Captain Harby	–			1	1	0
Thos. Oldfield, Esq.	10	10	0	–		
John Wilson, Esq.	–			1	1	0
Capt. J.F. Maples, R.N.	–			1	1	0
The Right Hon. Lord Gambier	10	10	0	–		
Jasper Taylor Hall, Esq.	5	5	0	–		
Captain H. Shitner, R.N.	2	0	0	1	1	0
Captain C.R. Biden	2	0	0	1	1	0
Geo. P. Simpson, Esq. H.C.S.	–			1	1	0
A Nobleman, per R. Wilmot, Esq. M.P.	50	0	0	–		
Captain J. Richards, R.N.	–			2	2	0

The Committee will sit at the King's Head Tavern, in the Poultry, daily, from Eleven till Four, to receive Subscriptions.

Books are also left at the several Bankers in London.

W. WILLIAMS, Treasurer

Several sums having been received from Persons whose names are not known, it is requested that Gentlemen whose names have been omitted in the List of Subscribers, will enable the Treasurer to rectify the omission.[16]

It is of interest that the proposed Committee of Management (which is accompanied by other SHS appointments) published in the first SHS Annual Report differs in a number of details from that list. Eight men are *not* included, whereas nine names have been added:

JOHN BLACKBURN, Esq. CHAIRMAN
JOHN BLACKETT, Esq.
Captain BOWLES, R.N.
Captain Sir JAHLEEL BRENTON, R.N. K.C.B.
Captain EDWARD P. BRENTON, R.N.

William Stanley Clarke, Esq.
Harry Cook, Esq.
John Deacon, Esq.
Joseph Dowson, jun. Esq.
John Drinkald, jun. Esq.
Stewart Erskine, Esq.
Charles Francis, Esq.
Lieut. I (sic). E. Gordon, R.N.
Captain Gooch, H.C.S.
Captain Lochner, H.C.S.
Captain John Locke, H.C.S.
Zachary Macaulay, Esq.
Captain Philip Ripley.
Rev. Dr. Rudge, F.R.S.
James Soper, Esq.
Thomas Sturge, jun. Esq.
Thomas Snodgrass, Esq.
William Venables, Esq. Alderman.
Captain William Young, R.N.

Early developments

In February 1821, H Hobhouse (writing from Whitehall) was able to reply to Simon Cock (the SHS Secretary) that His Majesty the King (George IV) had officiously accepted Patroncy of the new Society.[17] And on 1 March, Goulboun wrote that Lord Bathurst had 'much pleasure in accepting the Office of Vice President of the Institution'. Amongst other letters of acceptance from future Vice-Presidents were letters (to Simon Cock) from Captain Joseph Cotton (Deputy Master of the Trinity board) (5 March), William Money (5 March), the Bishop of Chester (6 March), Thomas Wilson (7 March), Lord Liverpool (8 March), The Earl of Hardwick (12 March), William Manning (21 March) and Lord Torrington (31 March). The completed list of Vice-Presidents (and other office-holders) was included in the first SHS report.

Patron,
His most Gracious Majesty the King [George IV]
Vice-Patrons,
His Royal Highness Duke of Clarence, K.G.
His Royal Highness Prince Leopold, K.G.
President,
The Right Honorable Lord Viscount Melville
Vice-Presidents,
Right Rev. Lord Bishop of Durham
Right Rev. Lord Bishop of Chester
His Grace the Duke of Bedford

The Right Hon. EARL SPENCER, K.G.
The Right Hon. EARL BATHURST, K.G. [*see* Chapter 5]
The Right Hon. EARL DARNLEY
The Right Hon. EARL OF ABERDEEN
The Right Hon. EARL OF HARDWICK, K.G.
The Right Hon. EARL OF LIVERPOOL, K.G.
The Right Hon. EARL ROCKSAVAGE.
Right Hon. LORD VISCOUNT TORRINGTON
Right Hon. LORD VISCOUNT EXMOUTH*[18]
Right Hon. LORD ELLENBOROUGH [See above]
The Right Hon. LORD CALTHORPE
The Right Hon. LORD GAMBIER
ALEXANDER BARING Esq. M.P.
JOHN WILLIAM BUCKLE, Esq. [*see* Chapter 5]
Captain JOSEPH COTTON
Sir JOHN WILLIAM LUBBOCK, Bart.
WILLIAM MANNING, Esq. M.P.
W.T. MONEY, Esq. M.P.
THOMAS REID, Esq.
THOMAS WILSON, Esq. M.P.
W. WILLIAMS, Esq. M.P.
WILLIAM WILBERFORCE, Esq. M.P. [*see* Chapters 1 and 5]

Chaplain,
The Rev. DAVID JONES

The names of Rocksavage, Gambier, and the Hon. Sir George Grey had *not* been included in the original published list of Vice-Presidents, although they had apparently all accepted nomination; this embarrassing situation was rapidly solved by increasing the number of Vice-Presidents from the original number of 24![19]

Rules and regulations of the SHS

The *Rules* and *Regulations* (see above) which had been accepted by the General Meeting on 11 April, were clearly laid down in the first and second Annual Reports (published simultaneously) of the SHS:

1. THE qualification of a Member of the Committee, to be a Donation of Ten Guineas, or an Annual Subscription of One Guinea.
2. Vacancies in the Committee to be filled up by the Committee within two months after they shall occur.
3. All the Officers and Servants of the Establishment to be appointed by the Committee.

---

*When Lord Collingwood died (in 1810), Lord Exmouth (formerly Admiral Sir Edward Pellew) became the most distinguished officer in the RN. In 1811 he had become Commander-in-Chief in the Mediterranean, and five years later he was successful in subduing the pirates of Algiers; he hoisted his flag on the *Impregnable* (later the *Caledonia* – see Chapter 8).

4. President, Vice-Presidents, and Treasurer, to act as Committee-men.
5. General Courts of Subscribers to the Charity, to be held on the first Wednesday in February in every year.
6. That of the twenty-four Members of the Committee, the six who shall be found to have attended the fewest number of times in the course of the year, shall be deemed ineligible to serve as Committee-men for the following year; and be replaced by six others, to be elected by the Subscribers.
7. A Donation of Ten Guineas or upwards to be the qualification of a Member for Life, and to entitle him *or her* [my italics] to one Vote at General Meetings.
8. A Donation of Twenty Guineas to two Votes, and Fifty Pounds and upwards to three Votes.
9. An Annual Subscriber of One Guinea to be entitled to one Vote after his second year's subscription shall have become due, and been paid.
10. The Committee, or any ten Members of the Society, to have power to call extraordinary General Meetings, on giving fourteen days public notice.
11. The Rules of the Society not to be changed, except by the Resolution of a General Meeting of Subscribers especially convened; confirmed by a subsequent Meeting especially convened.
12. Meetings of the Committee to be holden [sic] once in every week at least, at which any three Members shall be competent to act.
13. The Committee to have power to make Bye Laws.
14. All questions in Committees to be determined by the majority of Members present. In case of the numbers being equal, the Chairman to have the casting Vote; but who, otherwise, is not to vote.
15. The transactions of the Society to be recorded, with the names, and a minute description of all persons relieved, and the nature of the relief afforded them.
16. The Chairman of the Committee, (or any Member who may act as Chairman *pro tem.*) with one other Member, to sign all Drafts upon the Treasurer, and which are to be counter-signed by the Secretary or the Honorary Secretary.
17. No Debts to be contracted, or payments made, but by the authority of the Committee.
18. An Account of the Receipts, Disbursements, and Funds of the Society, to be laid before every Annual Meeting of Subscribers.
19. Two Members of the Committee (to be chosen by them) to act with the Treasurer as Trustees.
20. All Investments in the Public Funds to be made in the names of the Trustees; and, on the demise or removal of any one of them, the Committee to appoint another.
21. All Legacies, and Donations of Five Guineas and upwards, to be

> invested in Government Securities, whenever and as often as they shall amount to the sum of One Hundred Pounds.
>
> By Order of the Committee
> RICHARD HARLEY, *Sec*

It should be noted that rule no. 6 was *not* minuted at the General Meeting, but had been in the first Annual Report.[20] In the first report, the signatories were not Harley, but Williams, Buckle, Deacon, Owen and Lyall.

A venue for the newly founded institution

An all-important stage in the evolution of the project was of course to obtain a *permanent floating base*. The logical strategy (there was clearly a great deal of sympathy from the Lords Commissioners of the Admiralty – *see* chapter 5) was to request the permanent loan of a hulk – to be used as the *clinical* base of the Society. Negotiations had begun in earnest as early as January 1820 (i.e. some 15 months before the official launch of the SHS).

John Bold has pointed out that since the seventeenth century, ships had been in use as hospitals in the armed services. The advantages were: (i) the conversion of a hulk to accommodate the sick was relatively cheap, (ii) a ship was itself an advertisement – which could attract funding, (iii) most patients arrived at the hospital by boat, and (iv) ships could provide effective isolation for various disease entities. The relative disadvantages are alluded to in Chapter 11.[21]

In reply to a letter from JW Buckle, who had been Chairman of the Committee for the Relief of Distressed Seamen (and was to become one of the original Vice-Presidents of the SHS – *see* above and Chapter 5), the following had been received from the Navy Office:*

> Navy Office 6th Jany 1820
>
> Mr [J.W.] Buckle
>
> Mr Barrow [the second Secretary] having by direction of the Lords Commissioners of the Admiralty transmitted to us your letter to Mr Croker [the Secretary, dated 31 December 1819] requesting that an old Ship may be appointed for the *permanent* [my italics] use of the Society for the Relief of Distressed Seamen as an Hospital Ship, we desire you will let us know what sized ship the Society requires, and her draught of water.
>
> We are
> Your affectionate Friends
> (?) Peake, (?) Legge,
> Mark Lane[22]

The following correspondence bore the desired result:

*The *Navy Office*, which controlled all naval material between 1545 and 1832 was a Department of State and totally separate (and independent) from the Admiralty.

Admiralty Office 13th Jany 1820

Sir,

Referring to your letter of the 31 ulto requesting that a two Decked Ship may be appropriated to the use of the Society for the relief of distressed Seamen as an Hospital Ship, I am commanded by their Lords Commissioners of the Admiralty to acquaint you that they have directed the Navy Board to appropriate His Majesty's Ship Grampus [*see* Figures 6.1and 6.2] to this purpose.

I am
Sir
Your very humble servt.
J. Barrow

J.W. Buckle Esq.
Mark Lane.[23]

A later letter (dated 1 June 1820) from the Trinity Board referred to the question of removal of mud from the proposed mooring site of HMS Grampus:

Trinity House London
1st June 1820

Sir,

Having laid before the Elder Brethren of this Corporation your letter of the 31st Ultn., signifying that His Majesty's Ship Grampus lately granted to the Institution for the relief of Sick Seamen [for use as an] Hospital Ship, and requesting that two lighters may be [employed] to clear away the mud ... where she is to lay: I [desire] to acquaint you, that this Corporation's Ballast-Lighters are never employed in cleaning

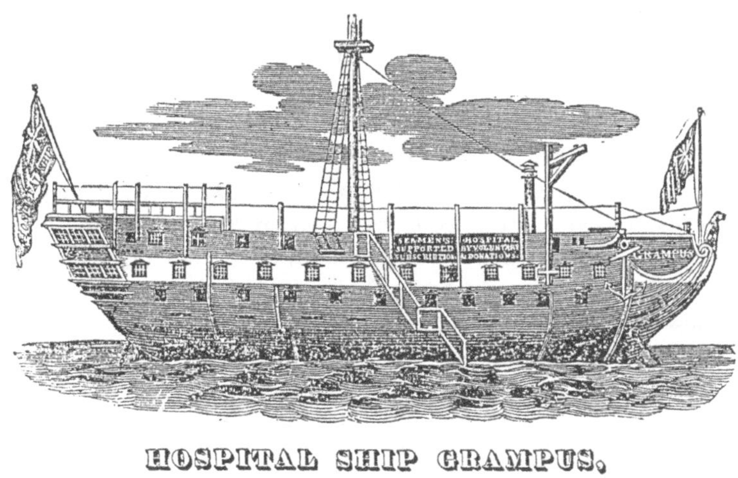

HOSPITAL SHIP GRAMPUS,
LYING OFF DEPTFORD CREEK.

Figure 6.1: Engraving of HMS *Grampus.* [SHS Archive].

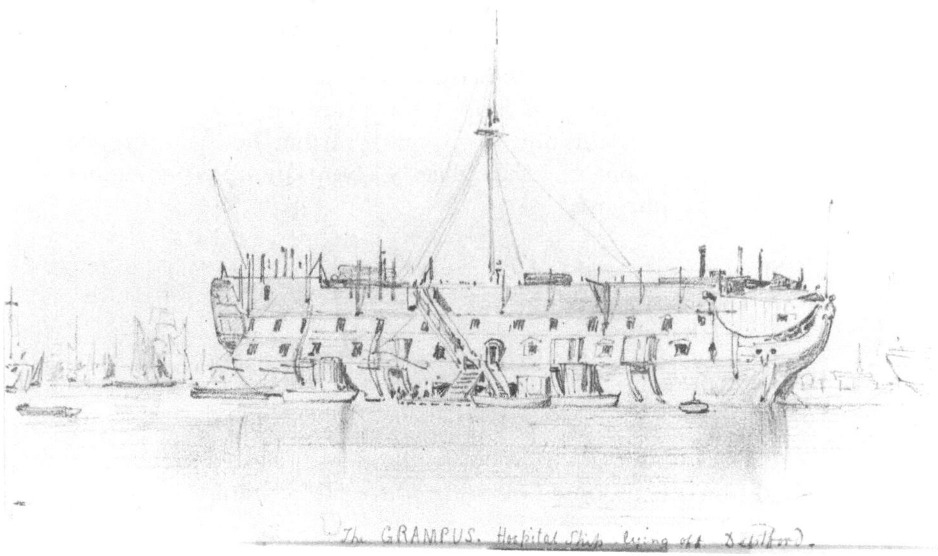

Figure 6.2: Graphite sketch of HMS *Grampus* – attributed to E W Cooke RA, FRS [courtesy of the National Maritime Museum, Greenwich].

away Mud not being fit for such purpose; But Messrs [?] of Canton Place, Blackwater has [suitable] Machinery, adapted for that sort of Work, which he executes for the Dock Companies in the Rivers and to whom I am desired to refer you for the removal of the Mud in question.

I am
Sir
Your most humble Servt. [?]
C. Cunliffe Owen Esqr.[24]

ALTERATIONS TO HMS GRAMPUS

Certain modifications were necessary before HMS *Grampus* was in a suitable state for use as a Hospital-Ship; these were approved on 30 March. A minute of a meeting held on 8 June states: 'The Committee examined a sketch of the Grampus with the proposed alterations, produced by Mr Somerville which was ordered to be referred to the Ship Committee on Wednesday next'. Figure 6.3 shows the profile of an almost identical vessel to HMS Grampus; a similar sketch was probably used in these recommendations. Captain Bowles and John Blackburn Esq '… were requested to confer with Lord Melville respecting the repairs necessary for the completion of the Ship'. In a letter dated 17 July, from Barrow to Blackburn, the committee was informed that: '[their Lordships had] directed the Navy Board to cause … the alterations and repairs to be forthwith carried into effect'. At a meeting held on 10 August it was resolved unanimously, that:

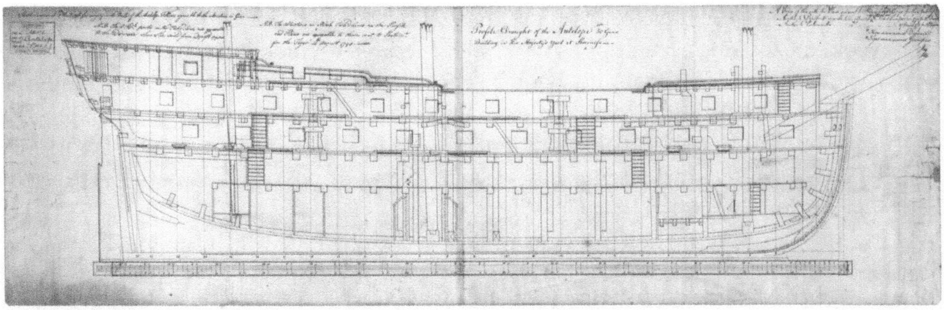

Figure 6.3: Profile of HMS *Antelope,* which was virtually identical with HMS *Grampus* – the plans of which are no longer extant [courtesy of the National Maritime Museum, Greenwich].

> the following inscription be painted in large characters upon each side of the *Grampus* viz:
>
> **Hospital for Sick Seamen**
> **Supported by Voluntary Subscriptions**

And at a later date (20 October) it was:

> ordered that five hundred cards of the following form be printed for distribution, viz:
>
> **Grampus Hospital Ship**
> **'for seamen'**
> **lying off Greenwich**

A further minute (12 October) reads: 'Resolved unanimously: that the Patients be sent on board the Grampus on the 22nd Instant, provided the Ship be then ready'.[25]

Early days of the SHS

Whilst the *Grampus* was being 'fitted out' at Deptford, and as suggested by the Secretary (Bodkin) of the *Mendicity Society* (*see* Chapter 5), a house in Wapping which had been loaned by the London Dock Company, Farm House, Stepney Green, was used for the sick sailors. On 2 May, therefore, the 'secretary [of the SHS] was instructed to take the necessary measures for removing the remaining Twenty One Patients from the depot to the house of Mr J Deacon, Stepney Green by whom the super-numerary sick of the London Hospital were received and taken care of, and to engage that the expenses shall not exceed 5s/6d per Week each'. At a later meeting (11 May), 'The Secretary further reported that the [22] Patients had been removed from the Depôt in Wapping to the Farm House kept by Mr Deacon of Stepney Green who had engaged to subsist them at the rate of 5^{s}/6^{d} each per Week.

Their Allowance [was] as follows. viz. 14 Oz. Bread each per Day, ½ lb. Butter each per Week, 6 Oz Cheese each per Week, Meat 3 days a Week ½ lb dressed with vegetables, Gruel for Breakfast and Beer 2 pints per Day'. Each patient was provided with: 2 shirts, a knife and fork, plates, basins, mugs and 'chamber utensils' under the Rules of Mr Deacon's Establishment'... 'A Medical Gentleman [was in attendance] 3 days a Week, and oftener if necessary. Dangerous cases [were to be] referred to the London Hospital.'[26]

A minute of a meeting held on 11 May states further, that: 'Mr [John] Harkness who [had] gratuitously attended the Sick since they were placed at Wapping, attended the Committee to represent that the distance to which they are now removed puts it out of his power to visit them regularly, but that his Brother [William] also a Medical Man, is willing to attend them at Stepney Green, Gratuitously'. The Chairman (William Williams) communicated to Harkness: 'the warmest thanks of the Committee for his benevolent attention to the Patients up to the present time, and [further] that the Committee will be most happy to avail themselves of the services of his brother so long as the Patients shall remain at Stepney'. A letter was read the following month from the Chairman of the ... *Homeless Poor Committee*, (Nathaniel Gould) 'requesting to know whether the premises at Wapping are unoccupied. The Secretary was desired to say that 'the Beds ... belonging to this Society [and] deposited in them should be forthwith removed, after which this society would have no further occasion for them'.[27]

HMS Grampus *is ready at last, and the first formal reports (1821)*

The early days of the SHS, were by no means, therefore, without teething problems, some of which were summarised in the first Annual Report:

> When His Majesty's Government most liberally provided the society with the ship Grampus, the conveniences of this vessel were supposed to admit of the immediate reception of the objects of the charity; but much further accommodation being found necessary, a statement of the requisite alterations was submitted to the Lords Commissioners of the Admiralty; and their Lordships, actuated by the same spirit which had prompted them to appropriate the vessel to the purposes of the Institution, were pleased to give directions that the same should be forthwith carried into effect.
>
> These additional conveniences were not completed till the month of October [1821]; in the interim, assistance and relief were afforded to such sick and distressed objects as presented themselves, either by obtaining admission for them into the hospitals on shore, with an allowance, in addition to that of such hospitals; or by maintaining them at a temporary hospital, hired for the purpose at Stepney.[28]

The Times published an account of the May meeting of the SHS: Now the *clinical* venue is ready, 'A naval surgeon will reside on board [the *Grampus*, a two-decker]; it will also be attended by visiting physicians and surgeons, who have kindly offered their gratuitous services ...'. In this account, Urquart (see above) (who was 'called to order') is quoted as complaining 'of the manner in which the seamen had [previously] been left destitute both by government and the Trinity House'.[29]

With HMS *Grampus* now, at last, virtually ready to receive patients, the Committee it was decided (on 24 August) '...will meet on board the [ship] on the first Friday in every month, and at the office on all other Fridays at 1 O'Clock precisely'. Following the first meeting (on board HMS *Grampus*) on 17 August, the 'Gentlemen [apparently dined] afterwards at the Ship Tavern [Greenwich]'.[30]

The first annual report of the SHS also highlighted some of the more *general problems* – both strengths and weaknesses – facing the newly-formed society (see also: Chapter 9). Most were associated with caring for this somewhat erratic sort of individual, i.e. the seafarer:

> ... the Committee deem it important to observe, that the very peculiar character of seamen can be known to those only who have passed much time amongst them; Sailors, in general, are bred up to their occupation from early youth, and retain few of the habits of persons employed on shore. Their great failing, and the principal occasion for their misfortunes is, an almost total absence of foresight, and of consideration for the morrow. They appear to have no conception of the possible approach of misery until it is too late to escape it; and when at length they become subject to its visitation, they are appalled, and sink beneath the weight. If informed of, or directed to, Hospitals, Asylums, or other places of relief on shore, which do not bear the title of "Seamen's," they are unwilling to approach them, and will submit to be driven to such receptacles only by extreme anguish and misery.
>
> A sailor, rather than repair to a Hospital on shore, will strip almost the last rag from his back, for the means of obtaining a cure; and it is well known to every person acquainted with the habits of these peculiar beings, that they will at any time prefer to remain on board their ship, even on approaching death, rather than consent to be taken to an hospital on shore, although with a prospect of returning health. This strong predilection will no doubt appear unaccountable, but it is nevertheless general and powerful.

This report continued on a somewhat adulatory note:

> It is not easy to express, or to conceive the situations of hundreds of poor fellows, who, having lived upon the ocean, and braved its perils from their earliest youth, totally estranged from all domestic ties, afflicted with the diseases incident to the climes they have visited [tropical diseases], when at length they reach their native land, instead of finding relief for their sufferings, know nothing of the means by which it is to be obtained; but, on the contrary, see the miserable prospect of a protracted sickness – without a home to receive their exhausted frames, or a relative or friend to compassionate their forlorn condition, and welcome them to the common offices of kindness. How different must be their feelings now, and how gratifying to observe the change wrought in their

> favour by their generous countrymen, by the provision of an asylum, suited to their habits and dispositions, for their reception in the hour of sickness, pain, and want! Their country will henceforth be hailed by them as the harbour, in which they may find a balm for their afflictions; and, they must feel, that they have reason to bless the country that gave them birth.

The lot of a seaman was (this report emphasised) thus very different from that of an individual on shore (a 'landsman'):

> That the situation of seamen is in many respects most helpless, as compared with landsmen, is certain: In common with them, they labour hard for small rewards; but, with this difference, that they have to face many dangers, and to pass through hardships unknown and unfelt by people on shore; and for a less consideration: what little they earn, is, in many instances, disposed of before it is due, either for the relief of aged parents, or for the maintenance of some tender branch of their family, whom their generous hearts will not allow to want while they have any means of assisting them.
>
> That such is the disposition of British seamen is well known; shall then such men, the glory and the defence of their country in war, and the patient and hardy conductors of her commerce with distant countries, be neglected by their benevolent countrymen in the trying hour of their extreme distress? . . .
>
> The [*Grampus*, the report continued] is moored off Greenwich, the most central and eligible situation that could be found, most approximate to the bulk of the shipping in the docks and in the stream, where accidents of every description are continually happening to seamen; it is the only place provided for the reception of sick men arriving from abroad, or to whom accidents may happen on the water, between the mouth of the river, and London Bridge. The Royal Humane Society have presented a complete apparatus for the recovery of suspended animation [drowning], which is kept in constant readiness.

The account then stressed that 'Every sick seaman' was *immediately* received 'without the necessity of any recommendatory letter'. It proceeded to dwell on the excellence and rapidity of the treatment provided:

> It frequently happens, that vessels coming into the Thames from long voyages, have most distressing cases of sickness, disease, or accident on board [*see* Chapters 4 and 11]; the subjects of which are now sent to the Grampus, where timely application being afforded, many have been restored with astonishing rapidity, who, but for this institution, must have waited some days before admission could have been procured for them into hospitals on shore, and with the hazard of being rendered incurable, from the effect of delay in applying a remedy. This is a feature peculiar to the Seamen's Hospital; the importance and great advantage of which must be obvious to every feeling and reflecting mind.

Owing to the fact that many of the target clientele did *not* have a home at which to convalesce, '... every person [the report continued] is allowed to remain on board ... until he has completely regained his health and strength ...'. Harley (presumably the author of this report) followed this up with the following comments (see also Chapter 9:

> It may also be mentioned, that seamen [returning home unwell not infrequently fall into bad company and are turned out] half naked, and in a worse condition than when they [arrived], to perish with cold and hunger in the streets.

Religion (very prominant in early nineteenth century Britain – *see* Chapter 1) was very much to the fore in the minds of the 'founding fathers' of the SHS; the report (see also Chapter 9) emphasised that the purpose of the organisation was *not* only to provide *medical* requirements:

> During the period of their remaining under the care and protection of [the SHS], every effort is used, to impress upon [them] the great importance of religion; to which end they are amply furnished with such religious tracts as are suited to their several capacities . . .

Taking the opportunity of supporting its cause, therefore, the *Blackheath District Society for Promoting Christian Knowledge* generously supplied 50 Bibles and a 'number of Religious Tracts' to the newly formed Institution.

If more detail(s) were required to stress the enormous value of this new endeavour, the first *Annual Report* (see also Chapter 9) provided it:

> Shipwrecks, on various parts of the coasts of England, which unhappily have been so frequent of late, have subjected the constitutions of many Seamen to the severest injury, from long privations and excessive fatigue. In all such cases, when medical assistance can no further avail, a conveyance is provided for them to their homes, with every comfort necessary for the journey.
>
> Instances occur daily, of seamen driven into a life of vagrancy by diseases [he stressed] originating in distress and privation;– men of this description are nevertheless received [by the SHS], if deserving. In these cases it is often found necessary to destroy the raggs which cover them, to prevent infection; and they are then provided with new clothing, and thus enabled to resume their avocations.

It was patently obvious therefore, that some organisation (it was now clear that the SHS had taken on that rôle) must assume the *permanent* task of caring for these destitute seafarers. Until the SHS was founded, there had been a mere handful of almshouses and homes for aged and disabled sailors scattered around the major ports of Britain (*see* Chapter 5) but clearly they were totally inadequate to cope with this massive influx of unemployed seafarers. Neither were any of these organisations equipped to deal with the *medical* problems (often complex) of this group of men; they cared for other aspects of their welfare *only*.[31]

Evidence that the newly formed Society was serving a valuable function

Fig 6.4 summarises numbers of patients treated in the early days of the SHS. An appendix to the first report refers to the number of seamen 'received' during the first year (8 March 1821 to 22 February 1822):

Total Number received	413
Of which,	
Cured, and discharged at the request of the Parties	168
Do. having obtained Ships	79
Do. Ships, found for them by the Committee	30
Do. conveyed to their Homes	4
Absented themselves	20
Expelled, after being cured, for misconduct	10
Died	13
	324
Under Cure and Convalescents [sic]	89
Total	413
Completely Clothed, after being Cured	32
Supplied with Shoes and Stockings only	51

A Committee of Management minute dated 17 August [1821] records the numbers of Seamen 'under care' at that time: 'victualled at Mr Deacon's Farm Stepney 21 – accommodated at the different Hospitals 24 – total 45', and in an update on 31 August, the numbers were 26 and 23, respectively, producing a total of 49. By 26 October, the respective numbers had fallen to 14 and 15; however, there were now 10 'seamen under care on the Grampus – producing a total of 39'. Figure 6.4 also summarises numbers of individuals undergoing in-patient treatment (under the aegis of the SHS) *before* and immediately after HMS *Grampus* became available on 22 October 1821.[32]

Staffing HMS Grampus

The first Annual Report gives the initial staffing of the SHS as follows:

Treasurer
Wm. WILLIAMS, Esq. M.P.

Auditors
JOSEPH DOWSON, Esq.
CHARLES FRANCIS, Esq.
THOS. STURGE, Jun. Esq.
Wm. VENABLES, Esq. Ald.

Physicians
Sir ANDREW HALLIDAY, M.D.
Dr. D. MACKINNON,
Dr. C.J. ROBERTS.

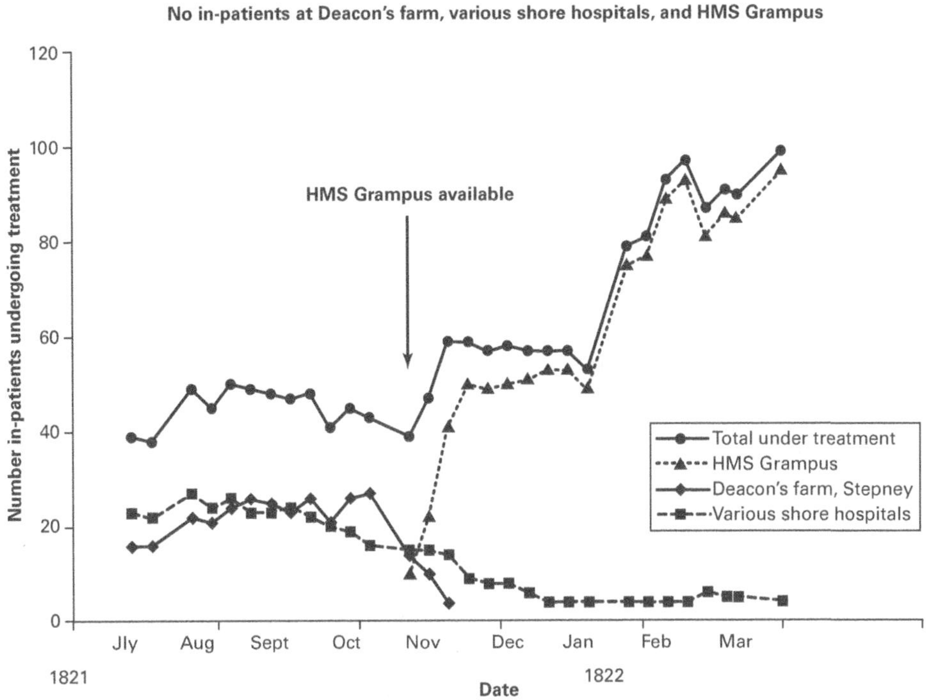

Figure 6.4: Numbers of individuals undergoing in-patient treatment following foundation of the SHS, until several months after HMS *Grampus* became available – on 22 October 1821. The whereabouts of in-patients under the aegis of the SHS during the first year of its existence are indicated.

Honorary Secretary
SIMON COCK, Esq.

Superintendant
Mr DAVID M'CRERY

Resident Surgeon
Mr. D.G. ARNOT.

Secretary and Collector
Mr. RICHARD HARLEY.[33]

Little is known of Harley (the first 'Secretary and Collector') or of the Hon Secretary – Simon Cock – who presumably carried out the day-to-day administration of the Charity and who had played an important part in the transition from CRDS to SHS); at the meeting held on 8 June [1821] it was minuted that Cock should 'be a member of all Committees'.[34]

According to an anonymous document in the SHS archive, the *Grampus* was *officially* opened to patients on 24 October 1821; there was a superintendent, surgeon, three male nurses, and a boatswain and his crew. In addition there was a visiting physician, a surgeon (who gave voluntary service), and a chaplain – who visited every day.

The allowances to the Officers' of the SHS were clearly laid down at a meeting on 11 May:

- The Superintendant £100 per Annum and his Rations
- The Surgeon £150 per Annum & his Rations
- The Steward & Clerk £40 per Annum & his Rations
- The Secretary & Collector. Eighty guineas per Annum & his Rations on the increased Subscription collected by him from and after his appointment.[35]

It is important to understand something of the original medical personnel who staffed the *Grampus*; the success, or otherwise, of the venture was very largely dependent on medical care.

There was mention in the first *Annual Report* of *medical* staffing, and patient care on the *Grampus*:

> the establishment on board the Grampus is placed precisely on the footing of other hospitals; with a Superintendent [Mr David Mc'Crery], Surgeon [Mr D.G. Arnot], Assistant-Surgeons, Visiting Physicians [Sir Andrew Halliday, Dr D Mackinnon, and Dr C.J. Roberts], [and a] Chaplain [The Reverend David Jones], &c, &c.

The first medical member of staff to be appointed was the Resident Surgeon – DG Arnot. At a meeting held on 11 May: '… the consideration of the testimonials for the Candidates for the Office of Surgeon [were] fixed for Friday the 1st of June; and … the Election [was to] be on Friday the 8th of June and that in the interim Advertizements [sic] for a Surgeon be inserted in the daily papers'. At the 8 June meeting: 'The Committee … proceeded to Ballot for a Surgeon. Joseph Dowson Esqr. and Lieut^{t}. J.E. Gordon were appointed [as] scrutineers. At 2 O'clock the Ballot was closed [and] when it appeared that Mr D.G. Arnot had the greatest number of Votes he was declared to be duly Elected. This result was conveyed to him by the Chairman [John Blackburn, Esq.]'.[36] There are references in subsequent minutes to his frequent periods of 'leave of absence'; he was later granted a gratuity (*see* Chapter 12), a salary increase (from £150 to £210), and was later authorised to 'sleep on shore'. He also introduced an Assistant Surgeon (Mr John Irving, a Member of the College of Surgeons of Edinburgh) who was given an allowance of 'one shilling and six pence per day for Rations'; this minute continued: 'in future, Mr Arnot be allowed Rations for himself and one pupil'. Mr Gibson was also nominated as an assistant surgeon.[37]

The first *physician* to be appointed to HMS *Grampus* was Andrew Halliday (1781–1839) (Figure 6.5).[38] A minute of the Committee of Management (of the SHS) for 25 May 1821 states:

> Read a Letter from Dr Halliday, Domestic Physician to H.R.H. the Duke of Clarence [later King William IV – see above], offering his gratuitous Services to the Hospital as an Ordinary or Extraordinary Phisican [sic]. Resolved unanimously: That the Offer of Dr Halliday be accepted, and that a Letter of Thanks be written in reply.[39]

Halliday had been born at Dumfries, Scotland and was initially educated for the Presbyterian ministry; however, he later preferred physic, and graduated MD

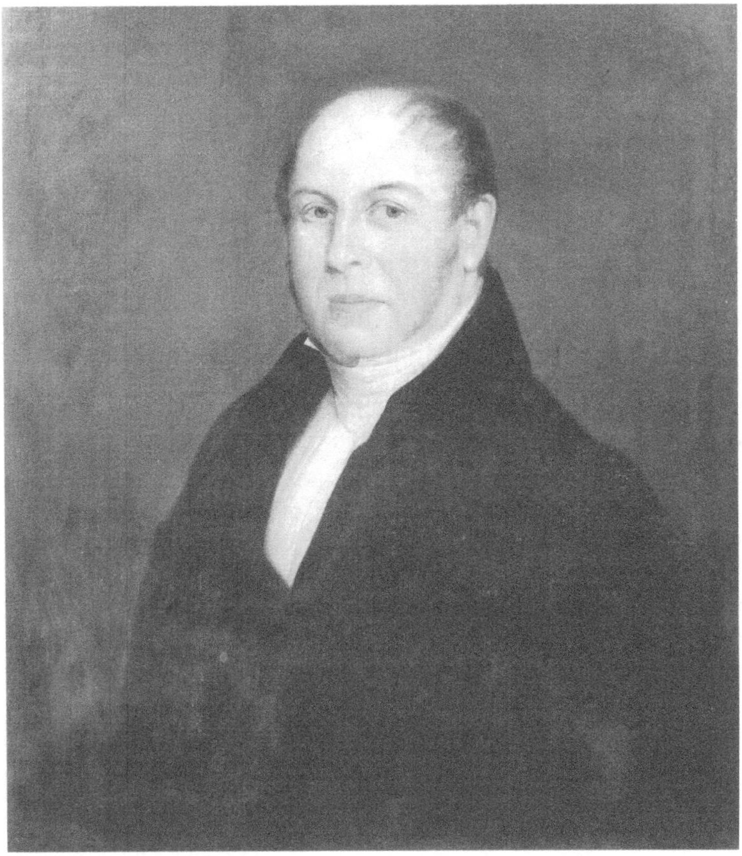

Figure 6.5: Sir Andrew Halliday (1781–1839) – the first visiting physician of the Society. [Reproduced courtesy of the Wellcome Library, London].

(Edinburgh) on 24 June 1806; his thesis (the following year): *De Pneumatosi*, referred to surgical emphysema; this Latin text was enlarged and translated into English: *Observations on Emphysema ...* (which was dedicated to Sir James Pulteney, Bt, Secretary at War).

Halliday was, incidentally, apparently a close friend of a fellow dalesman – Thomas Telford (1757–1834), the eminent engineer. Following travels in Russia and Tartary, he settled at Halesowen, near Birmingham. However, shortly afterwards, he joined the army as a surgeon, serving in the Peninsular Wars with the Portuguese and Spanish armies; returning to Britain he joined the British army, and was present at Waterloo, amongst other battles. Following this, he became domestic physician to the Duke of Clarence, travelling on the continent with him. On 4 November 1817, Halliday was admitted a Licentiate of the (Royal) College of Physicians of Edinburgh; and became a Fellow on 7 August 1827 (despite the fact that on 4 July 1820, he had written to the President requesting that his name be removed from the list of licentiates since the College had until that time refused to make him a fellow). He was also elected to the Royal Society of Edinburgh. On 22 December 1819, Halliday became a licentiate of the (Royal) College of Physicians of London, but was never elected FRCP. Halliday was knighted (through the influence of his Royal patron) by George IV in 1821.

The following letter was, however, received from Halliday later that year:

Hampton Court
27th Sept. 1821

J. Blackburn Esqre.
Sir,

When I took the liberty of offering my services as Physician to the Seamen [sic] Hospital and the Committee were pleased to accept of these Services I did expect that it would have been in my power to give daily nay if necessary hourly attendance at the Hospital. My removal however with His Royal Highness the Duke of Clarence to Hampton Court renders that impossible for the present and although I shall attend as often as I possibly can and at all times when the Committee may think my opinion or advice required – yet as in Winter Season it is both necessary and proper that a Consulting Physician should always be at hand may I be permitted to recommend to the Committee Dr Mackinnon whom I have known for many years as an able physician and to suggest that should the Committee be pleased to appoint Dr Mackinnon jointly with me as physician to the Hospital that there would then be certainty of one of us being always at hand when called upon by the Resident medical officers.

I have the honour to be
&c. &c.
Andrew Halliday[40]

Later (In 1833), Halliday was appointed 'Inspector of Hospitals' in the West Indies; however, his 'health broke down' and in 1837 he retired to Dumfries where he died at Huntingdon Lodge on 7 September 1839.* According to an obituarist in the *Gentleman's Magazine*, Halliday 'was ever ready to do a good deed or speak a kind word; and such was his generous nature, that, though he met with a base return to-day, he was ready to befriend the meritorious tomorrow …'.

---

*Halliday was also a prolific author; amongst his numerous works were: '*Remarks on the Present State of Lunatic Asylums in Ireland …*' (1808) (dedicated to William Wilberforce, MP); '*Observations on the Fifth Report of the Commissioners of Military Enquiry*' (1809); '*Observations on the Present State of the Portuguese Army*' (1811) (which went to two editions); a translation of Professor Franck's '*Exposition of the Causes of Disease*' (1813); '*Letter to Lord Binning … on the State of Lunatic Asylums and on the Insane Poor in Scotland*' (1816); '*A Memoir of the Campaign of 1815*' (1816); '*A History of the House of Brunswick and Lunenburgh …*' (1820); '*A General View of the Present State of Lunatics and Lunatic Asylums in Great Britain and Ireland and in some other Kingdoms*' (1828); '*A letter to Lord R. Seymour with reference to the number of Lunatics and Idiots in England and Wales*' (1829); '*The West Indies: the Nature and Physical History of the Westward and Leeward Colonies*' (1837); and '*A letter to the Right Honble, The Secretary at War, on Sickness and Mortality in the West Indies …*' (1839). He also edited: '*A General History of the House of Guelph*' (1821), and '*Annals of the House of Hanover*' (2 vols) (1826).

At a meeting held on 8 June, letters from Dr C J Roberts (*d* 1851) and Mr T Callaway had been read, tendering their gratuitous services as a Visiting Physician and Visiting Surgeon, respectively to the Hospital. These offers were, however, deferred to a later meeting (see below).[41] Apart from these, the first letter offering his services as a physician came from Dr D Mackinnon (d 1849) following Halliday's recommendation:

No 9 John Street, Adelphi
27th of Sept. 1821

Sir

Sir Andrew Halliday, having, as I am informed, stated his sentiments in the inclosed [sic] letter, it remains for me to offer my services most respectfully to the Committee, and I shall merely beg leave to say, that if these Gentlemen should honor [sic] with their countenance, no exertion on my part shall be wanting, to promote their humane and benevolent objects.

Perhaps it will not be deemed presumptuous in me to state for the information of the Committee, that I took the Degree of M.D. at the University of Edinburgh in 1807, that I am a member of the College of Physicians in London, and that I have been in regular practice as a Physician in the Metropolis for upwards of Twelve years, during which period a considerable portion of my time has been devoted to Charitable Institutions.

I have the honor to be
Sir
Your most obedient servant
D. Mackinnon.[42]

Another testimonial recommending Dr Mackinnon is as follows:

Great Winchester Street
25th September 1821
Jn Blackburn Esqr.

Dear Sir

I beg leave to introduce to you my friend Dr. Mackinnon of the Adelphi who is desirous of being appointed Physician to the new Marine Institution at Deptford. I have known Dr. Mackinnon many years. He succeeded his uncle Dr. Macqueen and for some years past has been Physician at the Westminster Dispensery. The Dr. has attended my family and I have a high opinion of his abilities and character.

I am Dear Sir &c.
Nat. Atchison[43]

The offer of Mackinnon's assistance was unanimously accepted.[44] Donald Mackinnon had graduated MD (Edinburgh) on 12 September 1807; and was admitted a licentiate of the (Royal) College of Physicians on 25 June 1810. Apart from his duties with the SHS (1821–8), he was physician to the Royal Caledonian Asylum and the Westminster Dispensary. Mackinnon died on 10 June 1849.[45]

Shortly after Mackinnon's appointment, a further letter from Dr C J Roberts (see above) was received:

> 20 Earl Street
> October 3rd 1821
> The Committee of the Seamen's Hospital
>
> Gentlemen,
>
> Understanding that you have come to a determination of appointing another Physician to your truly Charitable and highly valuable institution, allow me to renew the tender of my gratuitous services in that capacity.
>
> I am at present Physician to a public Dispensary, and during my residence in Edinburgh (where I obtained my degree) I was actively employed in the Hospital.
>
> I have the honor to remain
> Gentlemen
> C.J. Roberts[46]

This offer was also unanimously accepted by the Committee.[47] Charles Julius Roberts had obtained an MD (Edin) on 1 August 1820, and became a licentiate of the (Royal) College of Physicians on 22 December 1821. In addition to the SHS (1821–8), he served as a physician to many charities: the *Royal South London Dispensary*, the *General Dispensary and Infant Orphan Asylum*, the *Welsh Charity*, and the *Adult Deaf and Dumb Institution*. He became a fellow of the Royal Medico-Chirurgical Society, the Medical Society of London, the Hunterian Society, and the Westminster Medical Society, and wrote on a wide range of topics. Roberts died on 27 September 1851.[48] It must have seemed at this stage that the problems of *medical* cover were thus solved, for the moment at least!

On 2 November, Mackinnon was able to report (to the Committee of Management) that 'the whole of the Patients on board [the Grampus] were in a favorable [sic] way to recovery and [he] stated his perfect satisfaction of Mr Arnot's treatment of them'. At the same meeting it was unanimously resolved 'from the circumstance of the accommodations at Stepney being very inferior to those afforded by the Ship, that such Patients now there, as cannot get admission into Hospitals, be received on board, and thus Mr Arnot be requested to confer with Mr Harkness upon the subject'. Another resolution was 'that Patients having the itch [presumably scabies] be not admitted on board, except in extraordinary cases of Distress, or Accident'.

Medicines for the 'Grampus'

Obviously therapeutic agents were urgently required by the newly formed charity, and at a meeting on 10 August, it was unanimously resolved that 'Mr [J] Blackburn and Mr [J W] Buckle be requested to communicate with the Apothecarys' Company, and ascertain whether they would be disposed to supply the Institution with Medicines … upon advantageous terms'. The reply from Apothecaries Hall stressed that the Society's major objective was *quality* rather than *quanity*, and they would only sell at 'a discount of 10 per cent for money or a running a/c for 12 months. On 31 August, the Committee was given this disappointing news; as a result, the Secretary was requested to write to four 'Druggists': Messrs Allen of Plough Court, Brydon (of Cornhill), Herrings & Burbridge (of Aldersgate Street), and Kirk Herons (of Bishopsgate Street). The outcome of these negotiations remains unclear.[49]

Fund Raising

Of crucial importance to the newly-formed Charity, was of course, fund-raising (see above and Chapter 10). Names of subscribers were published in the first annual reports, and the media of the day (e.g. *The Times*, 12 March 1821, 19 January 1822, and the *Morning Post* 12 April 1821). Large donations were acknowledged in the media, and in fund-raising pamphlets.[50] However, every other effort was utilised, including sermons and even the composition of poems, an example of which is:

> WHILE WE SHED A TEAR OF FEELING, WRITTEN AND PUBLISHED FOR THE BENEFIT OF THE FLOATING HOSPITAL, BY F.W.N. BAYLEY, Esq.
>
> While we shed a tear of feeling
> For the spirits that are fled!
> While we drink a toast in silence
> To the memory of the dead!
> While the First of June recalls us,
> Thousands of the great and free –
> Who, with dying cheers, once shouted
> England! Howe! and Victory!
> Shall it e'er be said that Britons,
> Weeping for the hosts who fell,
> Left forgotten those old sailors
> Who have fought as long and well:
> Those who, maim, and weak, and wounded,
> In their battles on the wave,
> Now are claiming, from their country,
> England's tribute to the brave!
> Veterans, worn in loyal service –
> Friends, when dangers darkly prest –
> Shall we not deserve their blessing,
> Ere the aged sink to rest!
> Go, and gaze in wounds that smarted
> In the toil and tug of war;
> Go, and give them, open-hearted,
> Something for each glorious scar!

This text ended:– 'the words are set to music by J. Addison, Esq., and the song [is] illustrated with a beautiful portrait of Lord Howe.'[51]

By 26 October [1821], the 'State of the Funds' of the fledgling SHS was recorded:

Invested in Exchequer Bills	£1947=15=4
In the Treasurers hands	£628=13=6
	£2576= 9=0

By November, these respective figures stood at: £1900=0=0, £464=18=6, and £2364=18=6.[52]

The first Anniversary Dinner

A year after its foundation, the first *Anniversary Dinner* – which was essentially also a fund-raising occasion, was held on 5 March 1822 and Viscount Melville (the President) presided. Like earlier meetings and dinners, this took place at the City of London Tavern, tickets being priced at £1.[53]

Therefore, the Charity had been firmly established for a full year, and seemed at the time to be financially viable.

References and Notes

1 **George Lyall** M.P. (1778/9–1853) was a politician, who also owned a shipbuilding and merchants business. In 1834, he was to assist in the reform of *'Lloyd's Register'*, and in 1841 was appointed chairman of the East India Company. [*See also*: J A Hamilton, F Harcourt. Lyall, George (1778/9–1853). In: H C G Matthew, B Harrison (eds). *Oxford Dictionary of National Biography*. Oxford: Oxford University Press 2004; 34: 839–40].

2 *Under the Patronage of His Majesty: The first and second reports of the Committee of Management of the Hospital Ship Grampus, for Sick and Diseased Seamen arriving in the Port of London. Supported by donations & voluntary contributions. Established in 1821.* London: W.Gilbert 1823: 2: 51; Anonymous. Seamen's Hospital [Minute Book I]. 1821, undated: 2 [SHS Archive].

3 C Hibbert. George IV (1762–1830). In: H C G Matthew, B Harrison (eds). *Oxford Dictionary of National Biography*. Oxford: Oxford University Press 2004; 21: 856–64.

4 **William Henry Hugh Cholmondeley**, M.P., Earl of Rocksavage (1800–78) was to become the 3rd Marquess of Cholmondeley in 1828. [*See also*: Anonymous. *Burke's genealogical and heraldic history of the Peerage, Baronetage and Knightage*. London: Shaw Publishing Co Ltd. 1938: 573].

5 **Edward Law**, second Baron Ellenborough, and first Earl of Ellenborough (1790–1871) was to become Lord Privy Seal in 1828, and a member of the Board of Control (1828–30). In 1841 he was Governor-General of India; the following year he was responsible for the annexation of Scinde, and in 1844, he subjugated Gwalior. He became first Lord of the Admiralty in Peel's administration (1846) and was President of the Board of Control under Lord Derby in 1858. [*See also*: D Steele. Law, Edward, first earl of Ellenborough (1790–1871). In: H C G Matthew, B Harrison (eds). *Oxford Dictionary of National Biography*. Oxford: Oxford University Press 2004; 32: 747–52].

6 **Admiral Sir Edward Codrington** KCB (1770–1851) commanded the *Orion* at Trafalgar. In 1827, he became Commander-in-Chief in the Mediterranean, and the same year took part in destroying the Turkish fleet at Navarino. Codrington retired from active service in 1842. [*See also*: J K Laughton, R Morriss. Codrington, Sir Edward (1770–1851). In: H C G Matthew, B Harrison (eds). *Oxford Dictionary of National Biography*. Oxford: Oxford University Press 2004; 12: 385–7].

7 **Sir George Grey** Bt, M.P. (1799–1882) was a barrister and statesman. From 1834–9, he was under-secretary for the colonies, and from 1839–41 judge advocate-general. He subsequently became Chancellor of the Duchy of Lancaster (1841 and 1859–61), home-secretary 1846–52, 1855–58 and 1861–6, and colonial secretary (1854–5). He 'carried the convict discipline bill, which abolished transportation'. [*See also*: D F Smith. Grey, Sir George, second baronet (1799–1882). In: H C G Matthew, B Harrison (eds). *Oxford Dictionary of National Biography.* Oxford: Oxford University Press 2004; 23: 839–41].

8 **John Bligh** (1767–1831) had become the fourth Earl of Darnley in 1781. [*See also:* C Mosely (ed). *Burke's Peerage and Baronetage* 106th ed. 1999; 1: 766].

9 **George Granville Waldegrave** CB (1786–1857) had served in the navy from 1798 until 1815. He became a captain in 1807, rear-admiral in 1841 and vice-admiral in 1851. He was the son of William, first Baron Radstock, and became the second Baron in 1825. [*See also*: J K Laughton, A Lambert. Waldegrave, George Granville, second Baron Radstock (1786–1857). In: H C G Matthew, B Harrison (eds). *Oxford Dictionary of National Biography.* Oxford: Oxford University Press 2004; 56: 767].

10 Committee of Management Minutes: 1: 8–12; Anonymous. *Times, Lond.* 1821: 9 March: 2.

11 **George Kenyon** (1776–1855) had become the second Baron Kenyon in 1802, and was a bencher of the Middle Temple. [*See also* J Wolffe. Kenyon, George, second Baron Kenyon (1776–1855). In: H C G Matthew, B Harrison (eds). *Oxford Dictionary of National Biography.* Oxford: Oxford University Press 2004; 31: 343.]

12 **James Gambier**, first Baron Gambier, GCB (1756–1833) was created an admiral of the fleet in 1830. He had had a distinguished naval career, and was Governor of Newfoundland (1802–4). [*See also*: R C Blake. Gambier, James, Baron Gambier (1756–1833). In: H C G Matthew, B Harrison (eds). *Oxford Dictionary of National Biography.* Oxford: Oxford University Press 2004; 21: 353–4].

13 **George Calthorpe** (1787–1851) had become the third Baron Calthorpe in 1807. [*See also*: B Burke. *Burke's Genealogical and Heraldic history of the Peerage, Baronetage and Knightage.* London: Shaw Publishing Co Ltd 1938: 474].

14 **King William IV** (1765–1837) was the third son of King George III, and was created Duke of Clarence and St Andrews in 1789. Often designated the 'sailor king' he rose from being an able seaman to Admiral of the Fleet. He had served with Nelson in the West Indies, and was to succeed King George IV to the throne in 1830. A statue of him is situated at the southern end of King William Walk, Greenwich. [See *also*: M Brock. William IV (1765–1837). In: H C G Matthew, B Harrison (eds). *Oxford Dictionary of National Biography.* Oxford: Oxford University Press 2004; 59: 98–105].

15 **Prince Leopold of Saxe-Coburg-Saalfeld** (1790–1865) became the first King of the Belgians from 1831 until his death. In 1816 he married Charlotte, the only child of the future King George IV of Great Britain. [*See also*: *The New encyclopaedia Britannia* 1995; 7: 283].

16 Anonymous. Seamen's Hospital. *Morning Post* 1821; 12 April: 1. [See also: A E Clark-Kennedy. *The London: a study in the voluntary hospital system.* London: Pitman Medical Publishing 1962, vol 1: 200, 201].

17 H Hobhouse to S Cock: 1821: (24 February); letters received 1821–1837. [SHS Archive].

18 **Admiral Sir Edward Pellew**, first baronet and Viscount Exmouth GCB, M.P. (1757–1833) had a distinguished naval career, and was promoted to Vice-Admiral of the United Kingdom in 1832. [*See also:* Anonymous. Famous naval Vice-Presidents of the Seamen's Hospital Society. *SHS Quart Mag* 1933; 5 (1): 18; C D Hall. Pellew, Edward, first Viscount Exmouth (1757–1833). In: H C G Matthew, B Harrison (eds). *Oxford Dictionary of National Biography.* Oxford: Oxford University Press 2004; 43: 488–92].

19 *Op cit.* See note 10 above (Minutes): J Cotton (5 March); W Money (5 March); G Chester (5 March); T Wilson (7 March); Lord Liverpool (8 March); Lord Hardwick (12 March); W Manning (21 March) to S Cock 1821; *Op cit.* See note 1 above; note 2 above (Minute Book 1): 17–19.
20 *Op cit.* See note 10 above (minutes).
21 J Bold. *Greenwich: an architectural history of the Royal Hospital for Seamen and the Queen's House.* London: Yale University Press, 2000: 207–224.
22 SHS Archive: (?) Peake, (?) Legge, to J.W. Buckle 1820 (6 January) – letters received (1818–1820).
23 *Ibid.* J Barrow to J W Buckle. 1820: 13. (Folio 78)
24 [?] to G Cunliffe Owen. 1820: 1 June. (Folio 79).
25 *Op cit.* See note 1 above (Minute Book 1): 7, 17–19, 20–21, 31–32, 42–44, 62–64, 66; [*See also*: J Barrow to Blackburn 1821; 17 July – letters received 1821–1837].
26 *Ibid*: 5, 19–21, 21–25.
27 *Ibid*: 30–31. [*See also:* N Gould to Committee of the SHS. 1821; 26 May – letters received 1821–1837].
28 *Ibid*: 44–46.
29 Anonymous. Seamen's Hospital. *Times, Lond.* 1821; 12 April: 1.
30 *Op cit.* See note 10 above (Minutes).
31 *Op cit.* See note 2 above (Report 1).
32 *Op cit.* See note 10 above (Minutes): 44–46, 47–48, 67.
33 *Ibid.*
34 *Ibid*: 53, 251, 281.
35 *Ibid.*
36 *Ibid*: 31–32, 58–59.
37 *Ibid.*
38 **Sir Andrew Halliday** (1781–1839) was the first physician to the SHS. Anonymous. Obituary: Sir Andrew Halliday, M.D. *Gentleman's Magazine* 1840: i: 93–94; Anonymous. Sir Andrew Halliday, M.D. *Munk's Roll.* 3: 211–212. [*See also*: N Moore, P Wallis. Halliday, Sir Andrew (1782–1839). In: H C G Matthew, B Harrison (eds). *Oxford Dictionary of National Biography.* Oxford: Oxford University Press 2004; 24: 695–6; G C Cook. Andrew Halliday Kt FRCPE (1781–1839): service in the Napoleonic Wars and West Indies, and first physician to the Seamen's Hospital Society. *J Med Biog* 2004; 12: 136–140].
39 *Op cit.* See note 10 above (Minutes): 27–28; [*See also*: A Halliday to J Blackburn 1821; 23 May – letters received 1821–1837; p 17].
40 *Ibid.* [*See also*: A Halliday to J Blackburn 1821; 27 September – letters received 1821–1837].
41 *Op cit.* See note 2 above (Minutes Book 1): 21–25. [*See also:* C J Roberts to SHS Committee 1821; 4 June; T Calloway to SHS Committee 1821; 8 June – letters received 1821–1837; p 18].
42 D MacKinnon to J Blackburn 1821; 27 September [letters received 1821–1837, p 45–6].
43 *Op cit.* See note 10 above (Minutes). [*See also*: N Atchison to J Blackburn 1821; 25 September – letters received 1821–1837, p 43–4].
44 *Ibid.*
45 *Munk's Roll* 3: 92.
46 *Op cit.* See note 10 above (Minutes): 45–46; [*See also*: C J Roberts to SHS Committee 1821; October 3 – letters received 1821–1837, p 45].
47 *Ibid.*
48 Roberts, C J. *London Medical Directory 1846*: 129; *Munk's Roll* 3: 245.
49 *Op cit.* See note 10 above (Minute Book 1): 47–48. [*See also*: T Morpeth to J Blackburn 1821; 24 August – letters received 1821–1837].

50 *Op cit.* See note 10 above (Minutes); Anonymous. Seamen's Hospital. 1822; 19 January: 2; Anonymous *National Opinion*. 1821; 24 June. [SHS Archive]; Anonymous. *Times, Lond.* 1822; 19 January: 3.
51 Goulding and D'Almaine. Lady Howe's Bazaar [SHS Archive].
52 *Op cit.* See note 10 above (Minutes).
53 Anonymous. Seamen's Hospital Society. *Times, Lond.* 1822: 2 March: 1. [*See also*: J Blackburn to R Harley 1822; 7 February – letters received 1821–1837].

PART II

The days of the Hospital-ships (1821–70)

'Home is the sailor, home from the sea.'

R L Stevenson (1850–94)

Chapter 7

John Lydekker (1778–1832): a benefaction leading to the Act of Incorporation, and other fund-raising initiatives

Eighteen thirty-two was arguably the most important year in the entire history of the Society. The Seamen's Hospital Society (SHS) had been in operation for more than a decade, and had recently taken over HMS *Dreadnought* as its Hospital-ship (Chapter 8), HMS *Grampus* having served this purpose from 1821 to 31. A great deal of goodwill now surrounded the enterprise and numerous benefactors (including HM King George IV – *see* Chapter 6) had made useful financial contributions. However, the charity was still run on a 'shoe-string' and was in dire need of a major 'injection' of capital. This came about, totally unexpectedly, when John Lydekker died suddenly from Asiatic cholera on 23 July 1832.[1] Unfortunately, no known image of Lydekker exists.

John Lydekker (1778–1832)

Lydekker was born in the United States of America (USA) and at five years of age (in 1783) his family moved to, and settled in Britain. In 1804, he began business on his own as a cane and whalebone merchant at 1 Golden Leg Court, Cheapside and, in 1806, moved to 15 Silver Street, Wood Street, where he resided until 1815. In that year, he gave up his wholesale business at Silver Street, and moved to 19 Essex Street, Strand (until 1826); he appears in contemporary directories as: 'merchant, [whale] oil merchant [and] shipowner'. Lydekker's career was based on commerce, and he became increasingly associated with wholesale haberdashery; at that time, whalebone was an important commodity – both for the elaborately shaped ladies' costumes of the period, and also for umbrella frames (steel ones were not to come until many years later). Whale-oil was also at the time a greatly valued commodity in illumination.[2]

Owing to the profitable nature of his business (whaling ships were extremely valuable), he moved from the marketing to the shipping sections of the industry. In 1816 he gave up his wholesale business, moved entirely into shipping, and bought several vessels. At the time of Lydekker's unexpected death he possessed five vessels – all of which traded between London, and the South Seas or Greenland

(Table 7.1). He died suddenly at the house, 4 Brabant Court, Philpot Lane, of his friend and agent, Francis Devereux ('an insurance broker, whalebone and oil and tea merchant') whom he was merely visiting, on Monday 23 July 1832. He was buried in the north vault of St Dionis Backchurch (Figure 7.1) – which stood (until its demolition in 1878) at the corner of Lime and Fenchurch Streets.

Table 7.1: John Lydekker's five ships at the time of his death*

Name	*Captain's name*	*Tonnage (tons)*	*Trading between London and:*
Fanny	Kemp	314	South Seas
Warrens	Rees	324	South Seas
Industry	Bell	289	Greenland
Harriet	Reed[†]	410	South Seas
Fawn	Phillips	445	South Seas

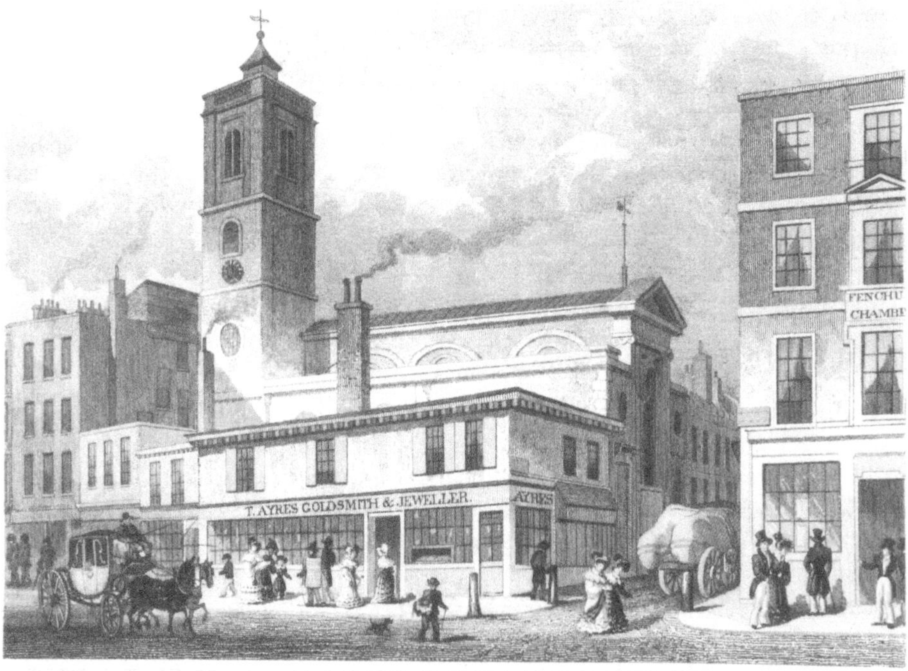

Figure 7.1: St Dionis Backchurch as it was on 20 February 1830 – Lydekker's remains were buried in the north vault. The church was razed to the ground in 1878, and his remains were re-interred in a mass grave in the City of London Cemetery at Ilford. [Engraving by T H Shepherd; reproduced with permission, the Guildhall Library, London].

*Details are recorded in the Royal Exchange *'Register of shipping'* (this became *'Lloyds Register'* in 1834) in 1829; a fire in 1838, destroyed subsequent registers.
[†]A beneficiary of Lydekker's Will.

In addition to the five vessels listed in Table 7.1, Lydekker had also owned the 'Mary' and the 'Adam' (Captain Rozier, 241 tons, which plied between London and the South Seas) until 1826. In the South Seas, the principle target was the Sperm Whale (cachalot); whaling ships usually carried about 25 officers and men, and six boats, and most were equipped for a three-year voyage. After harpooning, the blubber was removed from the whale, reduced to oil and retailed in casks; a large sperm whale yielded up to 80 barrels (three tons) of oil.[3]

Lydekker was a member of Lloyds, then situated at the Royal Exchange building (Figure 7.2).

Lydekker's Will

His Will was short, and drawn up in simple non-legal phraseology. It was written during his dying hours, entirely in his own handwriting, and dated the same day that he died; it was *not* witnessed. The Will was read out (and minuted) at a meeting held on HMS '*Dreadnought*' on 28 July 1832:

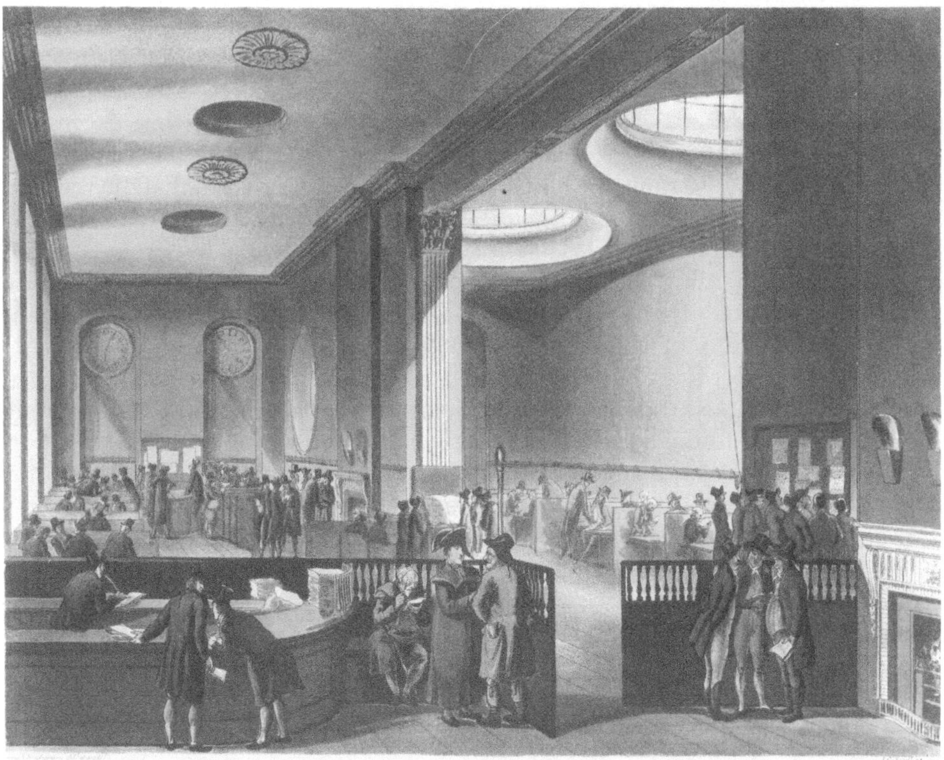

Figure 7.2: Interior of the *Royal Exchange* as it would have appeared in Lydekkers' time – around 1800. [Reproduced with permission, the Guildhall Library, London].

London July 23rd 1832

> This is my last Will and Testament. I direct that all my property consisting of Four Ships and Stores, stock in the 3 percents Consols and 3 per cent reduced and then to be divided as follows. Twenty thousand pounds I give and bequeath to my Brother Richard Lydekker of Henley on Thames, and one Annuity to my Brother William Lydekker of one Hundred per annum. I also give and bequeath to Mr Richard Battersby, High Street Shadwell the sum of Two Thousand pounds, the like sum of Two Thousand pounds to Captain Edward Reed of my ship the Harriet, the sum of one thousand pounds to Mr. Francis Devereux of Brabant Court and five hundred pounds to Mr. Ralph Dunn of Threadneedle Street and all the residue of my property after paying the aforesaid legacies I give and bequeath to *the Trustees of the Seamen's Hospital Ship for Sick and diseased Seamen in the River Thames* [my italics]. I appoint Mr. Ralph Dunn and Mr. Richard Battersby before named my Executors.
>
> John Lydekker[4]

Lydekker clearly had a high opinion of the aims/management of the SHS as '… he was [apparently] so much pleased with the manner in which some of his sailors, principally natives of the islands in the Pacific, were treated on board the [*Grampus*] Hospital Ship that in the month of February 1830, he [had] called at the office of the Society and left a donation of one hundred pounds, at the same time expressing his cordial approbation of the objects, plan, and management of the Institution'.[5] Although Lydekker's family (he had died a bachelor) was advised that the Will was legally invalid because it was not witnessed, they refused to contest it in view of the worthy object to which it was mainly devoted. Later, two of Lydekker's friends testified that the writing was genuine. The Will was proved in London on 27 July, 1832 before the Worshipful John Dauberry, Director of Laws, and surrogated by the oaths of Ralph Dunn of Threadneedle Street in the City of London, and Richard Battersby (the Executors – see above) to whom administration was granted.[6]

The SHS appointed their solicitor, Mr John Young, to deal with the legal matters. He reported to the Society that he had had an interview with the Executors who, owing to the large amount of property left, had 'taken Counsel's opinion upon the Will generally'. Young read the case and opinion, in which the Executors recommended not to pay over the residue of the property except under a 'decree of the Court of Chancery'. The Committee resolved unanimously that Young be instructed 'to take the necessary steps to facilitate the settlement of the buisnefs [sic] and that Mr. Labauchere, the Treasurer, be requested to become the plantiff [sic] in the suite'.[7]

On 31 August, 1832 the termination of the duties of the Executors took place under the direction of the Master of the Rolls. The residue of Lydekker's estate amounted to £45,101.16s.3d. and three per cent stock, the dividends of which were received by the Treasurer of the Society. This was transferred to the Accountant General of the Court of Chancery, in trust for the SHS.

This meant that the SHS, had virtually overnight, become an extremely wealthy charity. With the sale of the ship 'Fawn' in 1835 (which had returned after 38 months absence – carrying 182 tons of whale oil)[8] which raised a further £10,000, the Society was given their much needed financial stability; indeed it gave them not only this but enabled them to obtain *incorporation* by Act of Parliament (see below).

Lydekker's ancestry

The Lydekker family genealogy is of Dutch origin. In the seventeenth century Rich (Richard) Lijdekker settled in the USA, and in December 1654, a grant of land in Long Island, New York was made to him. He became a magistrate and Captain in the local militia, and married Claere Voorniere. His son Gerrit (Gerard) was born in 1650; he was in turn succeeded by his own son Richard (born in 1691), the grant of land being confirmed by an order dated 7 September 1763. He also held the estate of Hackensack, New Jersey, together with land in Jersey.[9]

Gerrit Lydekker graduated BA at Yale College, Connecticut, and was then ordained in Holy Orders; at the outbreak of the War of Independence (1775–83) he 'warmly espoused the Loyalist cause' rendering distinguished service as an active member of that party. As a result, his property was subsequently confiscated and he retired to New York – where he remained until 1783. He and his wife Elizabeth, together with their three sons – Richard, William and John – left the USA, and set out as refugees for England.[10]

The eldest of Gerrit's sons and brother of John, Richard (1772–1844), became governor of Martinique, and was the direct ancestor of the present Lydekkers based at Harpenden Lodge, Hertfordshire. He died aged 72 years, having become a St Albans physician following his return to England, and is buried at St Peter's Church, St Albans.* He had also become a Vice-President of the SHS from 1834 until his death.[11] William (the third son [1775–1840]) remained a bachelor and died in 1840.

A distinguished descendant was Richard Lydekker FRS (1849–1915) eldest son of Gerard Wolfe Lydekker of Harpenden who made major contributions to zoology, palaeontology and geology, and was on the Staff of the Geological Survey of India from 1874–82.[12]

The Lydekker memorial(s)

In order to commemorate his almost unbelievable munificence, a monument was erected (with the sanction of the Gresham Committee) on the north staircase of the second Royal Exchange. In view of his close association with Lloyds, this seemed an entirely appropriate site for the memorial – i.e. at the 'nerve centre of the shipping community'.[13] The formal letter, leading to this proposal was signed by the SHS Secretary, Richard Harley:

---

*A commemorative plaque is situated high on the north wall in the chancel of St Peter's Church, St Albans.

To the Worshipful the Gresham Committee.

The Memorial to the Committee of Governors of this Corporation to Erect a Momument to the memory of John Lydekker Esq a South Sea Ship Owner who died in 1832 bequeathing the residue of his property to this Hospital, after the payment of certain Legacies;– it has ocurred to your Memorialists that the Staircases on the north side of the Royal Exchange would be admirably placed for the Monument to be Erected. Your Memorialists therefore humbly hope that the Gresham Committee will sanction this undertaking which they would have expected at the expense of the Charity and Your Memorialists consider it a tribute due to the benevolent Testator, and it may also be the means of extending the knowledge of a Charity of great importance to the Shipping and Commercial interest of this Country.

Your Memorialists beg to observe that there is a Monument on the South Staircase to the memory of Mr Hicks a Merchant of Hamburg who left considerable property to the Marine Society [Chapter 5].

And your Memorialists are in duty
bound will ever pray.
By order of the Committee
Rd. Harley.
Secretary

19 Bishopsgate St within
1st May, 1834. [14]

Figure 7.3 shows the original monument, which was destroyed in a fire in 1838. The continuing importance, almost a century later, of the Lydekker monument is made clear in a letter in the SHS archive from a later SHS Secretary – P J (later Sir James) Michelli (1858–1935) dated 24 March 1924:

SEAMEN'S HOSPITAL
GREENWICH,
S.E.10
24th March, 1924.

Dear Sir, – I thank you very much for your courteous note saying that you will lay my application before the Committee of Lloyd's. Perhaps you would aid us further by telling the Committee that my Board is very proud of the Lydekker Monument now in the Members' Room at Lloyd's, and I am to express the hope that when Lloyd's is transferred to its new premises [which were opened by King George V (1865–1936) in 1925] this Monument may find a worthy place in their new abode.

The connection between this Society and Lloyd's has existed for such a long period that my Committee would deeply regret the passing of this evidence of the interest that Lloyd's took in the Seamen's Hospital Society in bygone days.

It may be interesting to your Committee to know that there are two descendants of the late Mr. Lydekker mentioned on the Monument still

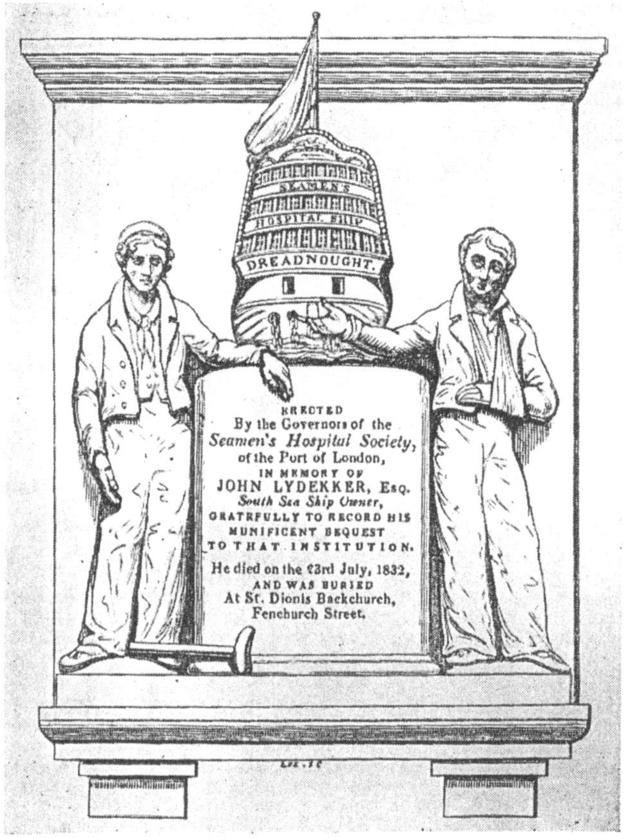
SEAMEN'S
HOSPITAL SHIP
DREADNOUGHT.
ERECTED
By the Governors of the
Seamen's Hospital Society,
of the Port of London,
IN MEMORY OF
JOHN LYDEKKER, Esq.
South Sea Ship Owner,
GRATEFULLY TO RECORD HIS
MUNIFICENT BEQUEST
TO THAT INSTITUTION.
He died on the 23rd July, 1832,
AND WAS BURIED
At St. Dionis Backchurch,
Fenchurch Street.

Figure 7.3: Sketch of the *original* Lydekker memorial at the *Royal Exchange*. This was destroyed when the building was demolished by fire in 1838. Two seamen, in contemporary dress stand in slightly different attitudes; 'the inscription is surmounted with a relief which depicts the stern galleries of the … *Dreadnought* hospital-ship'. [SHS archive].

in association with this Corporation, i.e. Mr. John Lydekker [1851–1934], Barrister at Law, Honorary Counsel, and Mr. Edgar Lydekker [1863–1938], a member of the Board of Management.

Yours very truly,
P.J. Michelli,
Secretary.

W.A.J. Bosford, Esq.,
Lloyd's,
Royal Exchange,
E.C.

It was decided to 'affix another tablet to the memory of that magnificent benefactor'; and it was duly 'placed at the right hand entrance to the Subscription Room at Lloyds' (Figure 7.4). An SHS minute (dated July 1854) refers to this; as far as the sculptor was concerned 'the Monument had been properly taken Care of'. This second memorial has recently been removed to the Museum in Docklands and is on public display immediately inside the entrance.

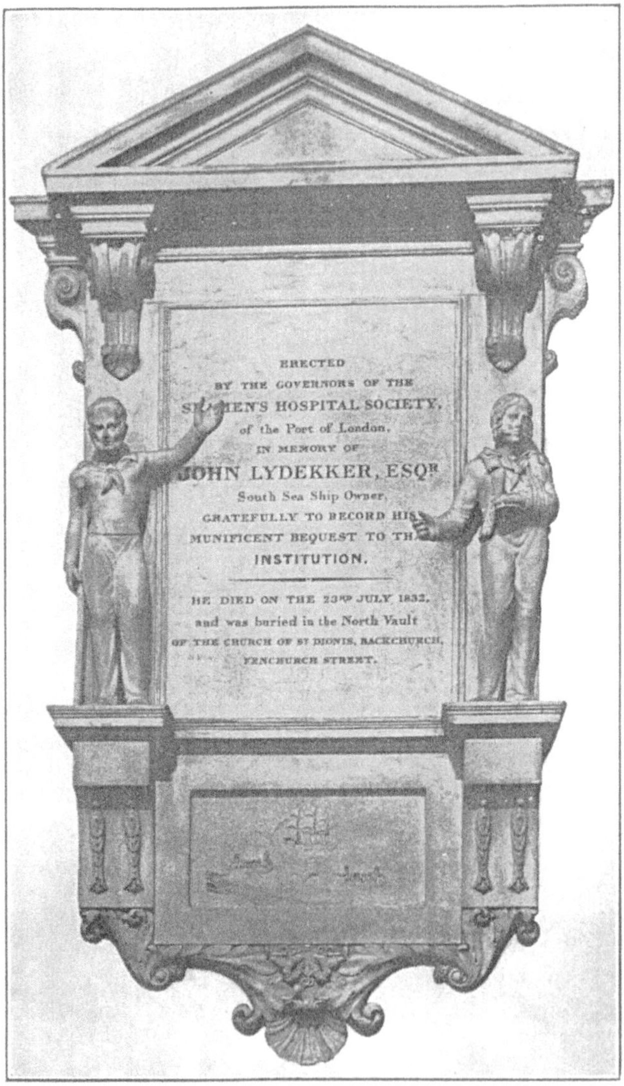

Figure 7.4: The present Lydekker monument (sculpted by a Mr Sanders) – originally erected in the west vestibule of the under-writing room at *Lloyd's*, and recently removed to the *Museum in Docklands*. In the lower part a 'sculptured panel [shows] a spirited whaling scene. In the distance one of Lydekker's ships [which] in full sail stands by, while her crew has manned two of the boats, and are engaged in harpooning a whale [crossing] the foreground'. [SHS archive].

In addition to the Lloyd's memorial, a stained-glass memorial window commemorating John Lydekker was erected in the chapel of the land-based *Dreadnought* hospital at Greenwich (which served as the SHS 'flag-ship' hospital from 1870 until 1986).[15]

The Act of Incorporation

The idea of an 'Act of Incorporation' (i.e. so that the Society should be protected by an Act or by a Royal Charter) had for some years been in the minds of members of the Society.[16] In fact, as early as 2 July 1831, a Committee (which met on board HMS *Grampus*) had been set up to look into this; it consisted of: Captain Bowles RN, Thos Edgar Esq, Charles Francis Esq., Wm Halden (sic), and John Wild Esq. The Committee felt that '… upon the present change of the Hospital Ship [i.e. from HMS '*Grampus*' to HMS '*Dreadnought*' in 1831] it is expedient to adopt such measures as may lead to the speedy attainment of a Royal Charter of Incorporation'.[17]

Little was done, however, until January 1833, when the Committee of Management was specially summoned (on 11 January) to 'obtain an Act of Parliament for the Incorporation of this Charity'. It was resolved unanimously that:

> it appears to the Committee to be expedient to prepare an application to Parliament for an Act of Incorporation, as also the outlines of a Bill for that purpose, in order that the same may be in readiness to enable the Society to apply to Parliament, in the event of the decision in Chancery in the pending question between the Society and the Executors of the late Mr Lydekker being such as to confirm the Society in their present opinion that an Act of Parliament will be desirable and that in the mean while it be ascertained what will be the expense which will thereby be incurred.[18]

The Lydekker bequest therefore made this a clear possibility, and a *special* subcommittee was immediately set up to prepare an application and outline for the Bill; it consisted of: 'Simon Cock, Mr Gray, Mr Grant, and Mr Edgar'. The Act thus gave the SHS permanent legal status. It also enabled it to either continue with their floating establishment, or to build a hospital on shore (Chapter 13).

Joseph Hume, Member of Parliament for Middlesex, presented a petition to the House of Commons, in order for the Society to introduce an Act of Parliament; this petition was dated 19 February 1833, and signed by 21 men, with Wm. Bowles as the first signatory. It began:

> To the Honorable the Commons of the United Kingdom of Great Britain and Ireland, in Parliament assembled The Petition of the Committee of Management of the Society called "The Seamen's Hospital Society".
>
> Humbly Sheweth – That in the winter of 1817–1818 a great number of distressed and destitute seamen were found wandering about the Streets of London, whose wretched condition attracted the attention of several Noblemen and Gentlemen with a view to obtain for the sufferers such relief as the Charity of the Public might be disposed to yield.

The petition continued by describing how the Hospital-ship was set up from *voluntary* funds, and the rules – which included the admission of all seamen without recommendation (Chapter 6):

> ... previous to the establishment of the Seamen's Hospital many Seamen had perished in the Streets and Suburbs of London, through want of friends to procure their reception [into the extant medical institutions].

The Petition continued by describing some of the distressing illnesses found among seamen after long voyages. Figures were given for the number of seamen treated since the foundation of the Charity, and it gave details of some of the donations and legacies given to the Society, mentioning especially that of John Lydekker Esquire which 'will ensure permanency to this Institution'. The Petition then explained why an Act of Incorporation was necessary: 'That your Petitioners are advised that for the [?] of the said Funds so bequeathed to the said Society as well as for providing that the same shall be duly administered for the purpose of the Charity, it is expedient that the Members of the said Society and their Successors should be incorporated by an Act of Parliament'. The Petition ended:

> Your Petitioners therefore humbly solicit that your Honorable [sic] House will be pleased to give leave for the bringing in of a Bill to be entitled "An Act for the Incorporating the Members of a society commonly called the Seamen's Hospital Society and their successors, to be Elected as therein is mentioned and for the better empowering and enabling them to carry on their charitable and useful designs" and that your Honorable [sic] House will be further pleased to pass the said Bill, if after deliberating upon its several provisions, your Honorable [sic] House should in its wisdom deem the same conducive to the purposes of the said charity.
>
> And your petitioners as in duty bound will ever pray.
>
> Wm. Bowles [*et al.*][19]

Passing of the Act

The Bill was duly carried through the House of Commons by Hume (see above). Following that, and assisted by Earl Howe (1796–1870) and Lord Colville (1768–1849) (Vice-President of the SHS), it passed through the House of Lords on 6 May 1833 (see below). The Act gave the Society many rights which it did not formerly possess; for example, the right for perpetual succession, and a Common Seal; it also enabled it to possess property and receive bequests; and it gave power to purchase land to the value of £12,000 per annum. In addition, any person could legitimately sell, give, devise or bequeath property to the Society. The Bill also dealt with the constitution of the Committee and with the Accounts. There were many other privileges also; not least the partial transfer of 'sixpences paid by Merchant Seamen to the Greenwich Hospital, to the society for the relief of aged and 'worn-out' seamen, and for the widows and children. Figure 7.5 shows the first page of the Parliamentary Act (dated 6 May 1833). It is noteworthy that at this early stage in its history '… the said Society [was] desirous of building an Hospital on Shore'. This Act of Incorporation was passed during the reign of the Society's second patron – King William IV (1765–1837).[20]

The SHS (with its new 'Act of Incorporation') felt that it had a right to a portion of the money collected under the Bill to transfer the sixpences paid by Merchant Seamen to the Greenwich Hospital. The SHS Committee therefore sent a Memorandum to the Lords Commissioners of the Admiralty (23 May 1834) 'praying that their Lordships will introduce a clause into Mr [George] Lyall's* Bill … for a portion of the sixpences paid by Merchant Seamen to Greenwich Hospital to be given to this Society'.[21]

However, the Admiralty refused to alter the *status quo* and the Committee had therefore to prepare a further petition (which was taken care of by the Member for Worcester, Mr Robinson) to the House of Commons. This petition, which was sent to Members of Parliament who were also Governors of the SHS, read:

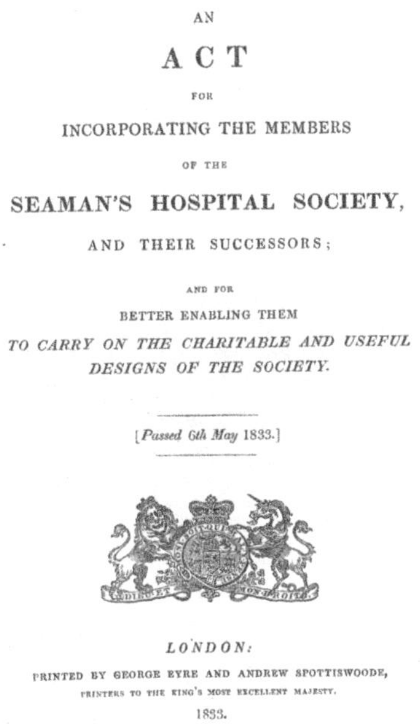

AN

ACT

FOR

INCORPORATING THE MEMBERS

OF THE

SEAMAN'S HOSPITAL SOCIETY,

AND THEIR SUCCESSORS;

AND FOR

BETTER ENABLING THEM

TO CARRY ON THE CHARITABLE AND USEFUL DESIGNS OF THE SOCIETY.

[*Passed 6th May* 1833.]

LONDON:

PRINTED BY GEORGE EYRE AND ANDREW SPOTTISWOODE,

PRINTERS TO THE KING'S MOST EXCELLENT MAJESTY.

1833.

(a)

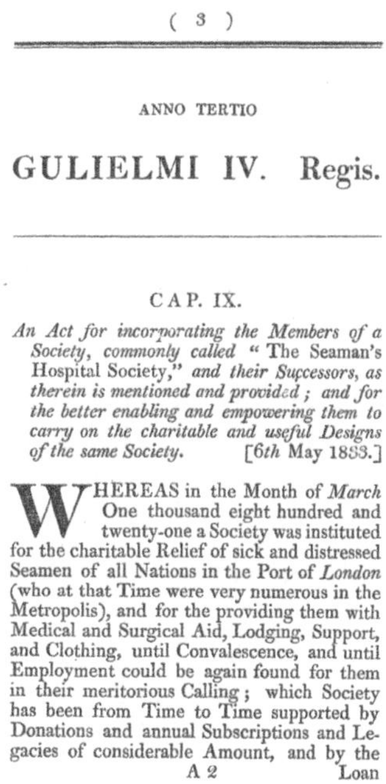

(3)

ANNO TERTIO

GULIELMI IV. Regis.

CAP. IX.

An Act for incorporating the Members of a Society, commonly called " The Seaman's Hospital Society," *and their Successors, as therein is mentioned and provided; and for the better enabling and empowering them to carry on the charitable and useful Designs of the same Society.* [*6th* May 1833.]

WHEREAS in the Month of *March* One thousand eight hundred and twenty-one a Society was instituted for the charitable Relief of sick and distressed Seamen of all Nations in the Port of *London* (who at that Time were very numerous in the Metropolis), and for the providing them with Medical and Surgical Aid, Lodging, Support, and Clothing, until Convalescence, and until Employment could be again found for them in their meritorious Calling; which Society has been from Time to Time supported by Donations and annual Subscriptions and Legacies of considerable Amount, and by the

A 2 Loan

(b)

Figure 7.5 (a & b): Beginning of the Parliamentary Act – which gave the SHS Incorporation of 1833. [SHS archive]. Interestingly there was a mistake in the designation of the Society.

*George Lyall (Chapter 6) was Member of Parliament for the City of London, and a member of the SHS's Committee of Management.

> 9th June, 1834
>
> Sir,
>
> I am desired by the Committee of Management of this Charity (of which you are a Governor) to solicit your attention to Mr. Lyall's Bill now before the House of Commons for transferring the sixpences at present paid to Greenwich Hospital, to the Merchant Seamen's Society Incorporated by 20th Geo 2nd Cap 38 and to state that an application has been made through Mr. Robinson the Member for Worcester to introduce a Clause for a portion to be appropriated to the support of this Hospital.
>
> About 3,000 Seamen are annually relieved by this Hospital, nearly 1,100 of this number belong to vessels of the Out Ports of the United Kingdom trading to London or have travelled up to Town to be cured of their complaints this being the only Hospital for Seamen.
>
> The permanent Income of the Charity is £1,440 and the annual expenses with the utmost economy upwards of £5,000, the deficiency having hitherto been made up by extraordinary exertion and appeals of the Committee to the benevolent public for assistance – now that an opportunity is afforded of enabling Seamen to maintain themselves the Committee hope that you will support their application, Mr. Lyall not objecting to it.
>
> I have &c
>
> R. Harley.[22]

A Petition to Parliament had in fact been submitted (by Harley) a few days previously:

> To the Honorable [sic] the Commons of the United Kingdom of Great Britain and Ireland in Parliament assembled.
>
> The Humble Petition of the Committee of Management of the Corporation commonly Called the "Seamen's Hospital Society."
>
> Humbly Sheweth.-
>
> That your Petitioners having observed that a Bill has been introduced into Your Honorable [sic] House (which has been read a second time) to the effect, that the Sixpences at present paid by Merchant Seamen to Greenwich Hospital under the head of "Hospital Money" should be withdrawn from that Institution and applied to the pruposes of the Merchant Seamen's Society Established by the 20th Geo 2nd Cap 38.
>
> Your Petitioners submit that the [SHS], which was Incorporated by the 3rd of his Present Most Gracious Majesty Cap 9, has for its object the relief of all Sick Seamen, without any recommendation and that since its commencement in 1821 upwards of 21000 have been received, besides 6000 Out-Patients – that the permanent income of this Charity is only £1,443 while the Annual Expenses exceeds £5000, the deficiency having hitherto been raised by the extraordinary exertions of your Petitioners

in annual subscriptions and donations, the amount of which cannot be relied on.

Your Petitioners consider that this Hospital has, by the facilities afforded, been instrumental in restoring many thousand Seamen to their avocation, who would otherwise have become prematurely permanent burdens upon the funds of the Merchant Seamen's Hospital Society – that sick Seamen travel to London from different Out Ports of the United Kingdom confident that the Seamen's Hospital will render them that assistance, which the nature of their Complaints require, and which they consider themselves entitled to in consequence of the deductions from their pay under the head of "Hospital Money".

Your Petitioners humbly hope that as the provisions of the third clause of the Act 20th Geo 2nd Cap 38 almost excludes Seamen from the relief which, when labouring under temporary sickness, they stand in need, and as the Institution which your Petitioners conduct is available for every sick Mariner, that, should the Bill alluded to pass into Law, it is prayed that your Honorable [sic] House will be pleased to introduce a clause when in Committee for such a portion of the said Sixpences as the wisdom of your Honorable [sic] House shall deem to be applied towards the maintenance of the "Seamen's Hospital Society."

And your Petitioners are in duty bound
will ever pray.
By order of the Committee of Management.
R. Harley, Secy.

26th May 1834.[23]

The submission of these petitions had undoubtedly resulted from a discussion at a Committee of Management Meeting on 23 May 1834, during which it was: 'ordered that a Memorial be sent to the Lords Commissioners of the Admiralty praying that their Lordships will introduce a Clause into Mr Lyall's Bill, when in Committee of the House of Commons for a portion of the sixpences paid by Merchant Seamen to Greenwich Hospital to be given to the Society'.[24]

Thanks to Lord Colville [see above], the Bill passed through the House of Lords and as a result, the Society was approximately £500 per annum better off (via the Merchant Seamen's Fund). This move could *not* apparently have been undertaken successfully if the Society had not been incorporated by Act of Parliament!

Permanency at last!

The first General Court of the now *incorporated* SHS was held on 12 July 1833 again at the City of London Tavern. *The Times* for 13 July briefly described the meeting:

> (From a Correspondent) – The First General Court of the [SHS] was held yesterday at the London Tavern, in pursuance of the act of Parliament passed this session, John Labouchere, Esq., treasurer, in the chair: at which a statement of the Society's affairs was laid before the meeting.

> Nearly 1,000 seamen had been relieved during the past three months. The Governors expressed a hope that, from the extensive assistance which the institution affords to sick seamen of all nations, who are received without any recommendation, the charity would meet with support from a benevolent public, corresponding to the great demand upon it.[25]

Other fund-raising initiatives

Clearly the Society could not rest on its laurels, in the light of the Lydekker beneficence. Other fund-raising initiatives were essential and, as with many charities in the early nineteenth century, sermons and dinners were major fund-raising events.

Figures 7.6 and 7.7 show advertisements for Charity Sermons preached by the Reverend John Russell (31 August 1823) and the Lord Bishop of Llandaff (25 March

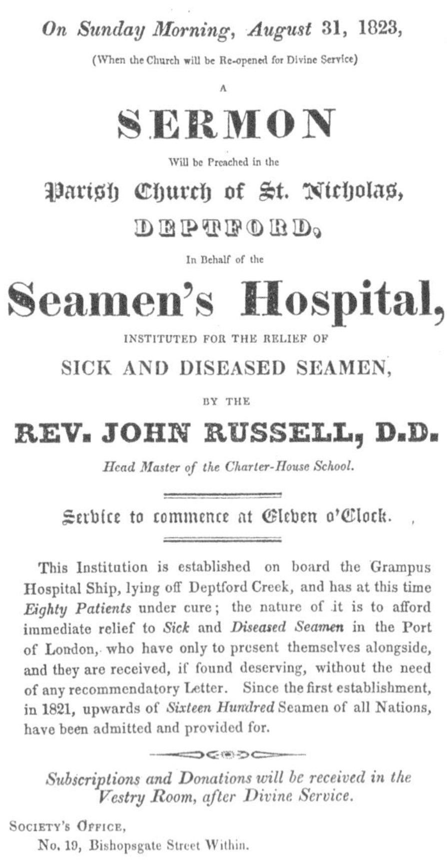

On Sunday Morning, August 31, 1823,

(When the Church will be Re-opened for Divine Service)

A

SERMON

Will be Preached in the

Parish Church of St. Nicholas,

DEPTFORD,

In Behalf of the

Seamen's Hospital,

INSTITUTED FOR THE RELIEF OF

SICK AND DISEASED SEAMEN,

BY THE

REV. JOHN RUSSELL, D.D.

Head Master of the Charter-House School.

Service to commence at Eleven o'Clock.

This Institution is established on board the Grampus Hospital Ship, lying off Deptford Creek, and has at this time *Eighty Patients* under cure; the nature of it is to afford immediate relief to *Sick* and *Diseased Seamen* in the Port of London, who have only to present themselves alongside, and they are received, if found deserving, without the need of any recommendatory Letter. Since the first establishment, in 1821, upwards of *Sixteen Hundred* Seamen of all Nations, have been admitted and provided for.

Subscriptions and Donations will be received in the Vestry Room, after Divine Service.

SOCIETY'S OFFICE,
No. 19, Bishopsgate Street Within.

Figure 7.6: Notice of a Charity Sermon on 31 August 1823 at St Nicholas Church, Deptford. [SHS archive].

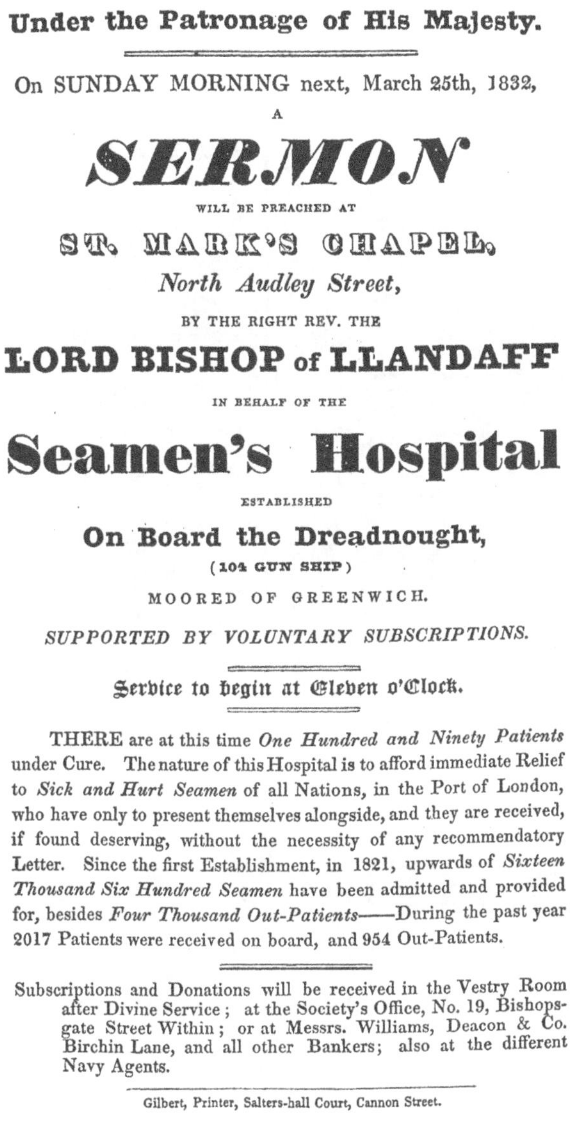

Under the Patronage of His Majesty.

On SUNDAY MORNING next, March 25th, 1832,

A

SERMON

WILL BE PREACHED AT

ST. MARK'S CHAPEL,

North Audley Street,

BY THE RIGHT REV. THE

LORD BISHOP of LLANDAFF

IN BEHALF OF THE

Seamen's Hospital

ESTABLISHED

On Board the Dreadnought,

(104 GUN SHIP)

MOORED OF GREENWICH.

SUPPORTED BY VOLUNTARY SUBSCRIPTIONS.

Service to begin at Eleven o'Clock.

THERE are at this time *One Hundred and Ninety Patients* under Cure. The nature of this Hospital is to afford immediate Relief to *Sick and Hurt Seamen* of all Nations, in the Port of London, who have only to present themselves alongside, and they are received, if found deserving, without the necessity of any recommendatory Letter. Since the first Establishment, in 1821, upwards of *Sixteen Thousand Six Hundred Seamen* have been admitted and provided for, besides *Four Thousand Out-Patients*——During the past year 2017 Patients were received on board, and 954 Out-Patients.

Subscriptions and Donations will be received in the Vestry Room after Divine Service; at the Society's Office, No. 19, Bishopsgate Street Within; or at Messrs. Williams, Deacon & Co. Birchin Lane, and all other Bankers; also at the different Navy Agents.

Gilbert, Printer, Salters-hall Court, Cannon Street.

Figure 7.7: Notice of a Charity Sermon on 25 March 1832 at St Mark's Chapel, North Audley Street. [SHS archive].

1832), respectively.[26] Figures 7.8 and 7.9 show advertisements for the 35th (12 April 1856) and 40th (26 March 1862) Anniversary Dinners at which the chairmen were Sir Charles Wood Bt MP and the Lord Mayor of London, respectively.

In the early days of the Charity, a 'water excursion' on board *The Venus* was also organised on 19 July 1823 to mark the second anniversary of His Majesty (George IV)'s coronation Figure 7.10).

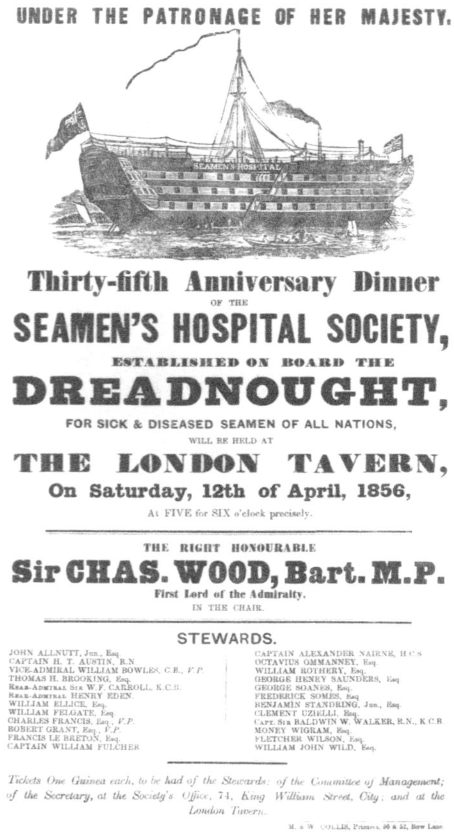
UNDER THE PATRONAGE OF HER MAJESTY.
SEAMEN'S HOSPITAL
Thirty-fifth Anniversary Dinner
OF THE
SEAMEN'S HOSPITAL SOCIETY,
ESTABLISHED ON BOARD THE
DREADNOUGHT,
FOR SICK & DISEASED SEAMEN OF ALL NATIONS,
WILL BE HELD AT
THE LONDON TAVERN,
On Saturday, 12th of April, 1856,
At FIVE for SIX o'clock precisely.
THE RIGHT HONOURABLE
Sir CHAS. WOOD, Bart. M.P.
First Lord of the Admiralty.
IN THE CHAIR.
STEWARDS.
JOHN ALLNUTT, Jun., Esq.
CAPTAIN H. T. AUSTIN, R.N.
VICE-ADMIRAL WILLIAM BOWLES, C.B., V.P.
THOMAS H. BROOKING, Esq.
REAR-ADMIRAL SIR W. F. CARROLL, K.C.B.
REAR-ADMIRAL HENRY EDEN.
WILLIAM ELLICE, Esq.
WILLIAM FELGATE, Esq.
CHARLES FRANCIS, Esq., V.P.
ROBERT GRANT, Esq., V.P.
FRANCIS LE BRETON, Esq.
CAPTAIN WILLIAM FULCHER
CAPTAIN ALEXANDER NAIRNE, H.C.S
OCTAVIUS OMMANNEY, Esq.
WILLIAM ROTHERY, Esq.
GEORGE HENRY SAUNDERS, Esq
GEORGE SOANES, Esq.
FREDERICK SOMES, Esq
BENJAMIN STANDRING, Jun., Esq.
CLEMENT UZIELLI, Esq.
CAPT. SIR BALDWIN W. WALKER, R.N., K.C.B
MONEY WIGRAM, Esq.
FLETCHER WILSON, Esq.
WILLIAM JOHN WILD, Esq.
Tickets One Guinea each, to be had of the Stewards; of the Committee of Management; of the Secretary, at the Society's Office, 74, King William Street, City; and at the London Tavern.
M. & W. COLLIS, Printers, 50 & 52, Bow Lane.

Figure 7.8: Advertisement for the 35th Anniversary Dinner at the *London Tavern* on 12 April 1856. [SHS archive].

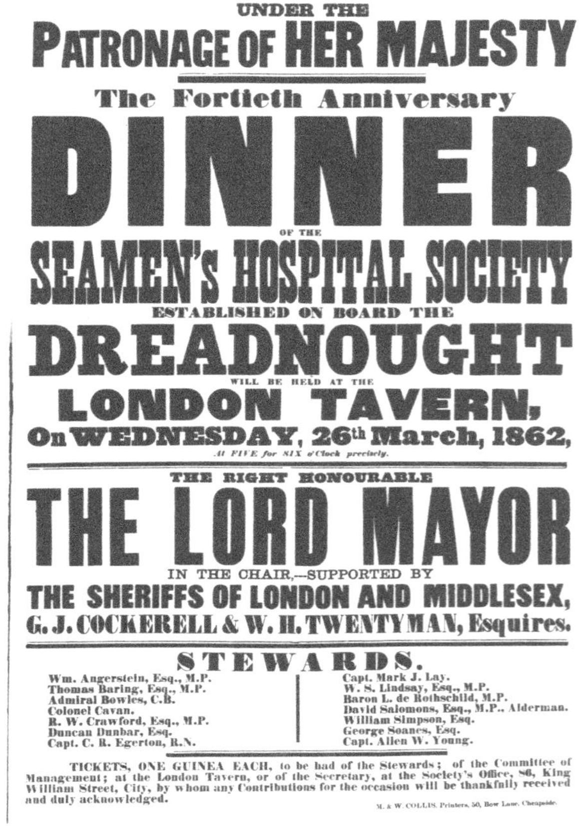
UNDER THE
PATRONAGE OF HER MAJESTY
The Fortieth Anniversary
DINNER
OF THE
SEAMEN'S HOSPITAL SOCIETY
ESTABLISHED ON BOARD THE
DREADNOUGHT
WILL BE HELD AT THE
LONDON TAVERN,
On WEDNESDAY, 26th March, 1862,
At FIVE for SIX o'Clock precisely.
THE RIGHT HONOURABLE
THE LORD MAYOR
IN THE CHAIR,—SUPPORTED BY
THE SHERIFFS OF LONDON AND MIDDLESEX,
G. J. COCKERELL & W. H. TWENTYMAN, Esquires.
STEWARDS.
Wm. Angerstein, Esq., M.P.
Thomas Baring, Esq., M.P.
Admiral Bowles, C.B.
Colonel Cavan.
R. W. Crawford, Esq., M.P.
Duncan Dunbar, Esq.
Capt. C. R. Egerton, R.N.
Capt. Mark J. Lay.
W. S. Lindsay, Esq., M.P.
Baron L. de Rothschild, M.P.
David Salomons, Esq., M.P., Alderman.
William Simpson, Esq.
George Soanes, Esq.
Capt. Allen W. Young.
TICKETS, ONE GUINEA EACH, to be had of the Stewards; of the Committee of Management; at the London Tavern, or of the Secretary, at the Society's Office, 86, King William Street, City, by whom any Contributions for the occasion will be thankfully received and duly acknowledged.
M. & W. COLLIS, Printers, 50, Bow Lane, Cheapside.

Figure 7.9: Advertisement for the 40th Anniversary Dinner at the *London Tavern* on 26 March 1862. [SHS archive].

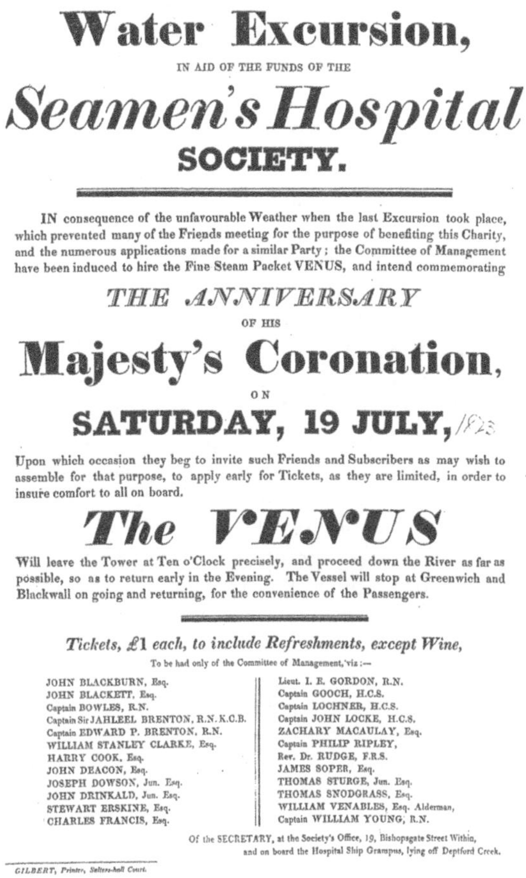
Water Excursion,
IN AID OF THE FUNDS OF THE
Seamen's Hospital
SOCIETY.
IN consequence of the unfavourable Weather when the last Excursion took place, which prevented many of the Friends meeting for the purpose of benefiting this Charity, and the numerous applications made for a similar Party; the Committee of Management have been induced to hire the Fine Steam Packet VENUS, and intend commemorating
THE ANNIVERSARY
OF HIS
Majesty's Coronation,
ON
SATURDAY, 19 JULY,
Upon which occasion they beg to invite such Friends and Subscribers as may wish to assemble for that purpose, to apply early for Tickets, as they are limited, in order to insure comfort to all on board.
The VENUS
Will leave the Tower at Ten o'Clock precisely, and proceed down the River as far as possible, so as to return early in the Evening. The Vessel will stop at Greenwich and Blackwall on going and returning, for the convenience of the Passengers.
Tickets, £1 each, to include Refreshments, except Wine,
To be had only of the Committee of Management, viz:—
JOHN BLACKBURN, Esq.
JOHN BLACKETT, Esq.
Captain BOWLES, R.N.
Captain Sir JAHLEEL BRENTON, R.N. K.C.B.
Captain EDWARD P. BRENTON, R.N.
WILLIAM STANLEY CLARKE, Esq.
HARRY COOK, Esq.
JOHN DEACON, Esq.
JOSEPH DOWSON, Jun. Esq.
JOHN DRINKALD, Jun. Esq.
STEWART ERSKINE, Esq.
CHARLES FRANCIS, Esq.
Lieut. I. E. GORDON, R.N.
Captain GOOCH, H.C.S.
Captain LOCHNER, H.C.S.
Captain JOHN LOCKE, H.C.S.
ZACHARY MACAULAY, Esq.
Captain PHILIP RIPLEY,
Rev. Dr. RUDGE, F.R.S.
JAMES SOPER, Esq.
THOMAS STURGE, Jun. Esq.
THOMAS SNODGRASS, Esq.
WILLIAM VENABLES, Esq. Alderman,
Captain WILLIAM YOUNG, R.N.
Of the SECRETARY, at the Society's Office, 19, Bishopsgate Street Within, and on board the Hospital Ship Grampus, lying off Deptford Creek.
GILBERT, Printer, Salters-hall Court.

Figure 7.10: Advertisement for a 'water excursion' on board *The Venus* to mark the second anniversary of the coronation of the Society's Patron, King George IV, on 19 July 1823. [SHS archive].

References and notes

1 12th Annual Report. In: *Origin and progress of the Hospital for Sick and Diseased Seamen in the Port of London, on board the Dreadnought, 104 Gun Ship, moored off Greenwich. Supported by Donations and Voluntary Contributions. Established in 1821.* London: W Gilbert 1833: 20– 3; *Ibid.* 13th Report 1834: 18– 21; *Ibid.* 14: 17– 21; *Ibid.* 15: 19– 22; *Ibid.* 16: 19– 22; W R Dawson. John Lydekker: the Memorial at Lloyd's. Supplement to *Lloyds List and Shipping Gazette* (reissued by the Seamen's Hospital Society in pamphlet form). London: E G Berryman & Sons Ltd. 1927: 11 March: 20; Anonymous. John Lydekker, South Seas Shipowner and benefactor of the Seamen's Hospital Society. *SHS Quart Mag.* 1932; 4 (3): 12; SHS Committee of Management Minutes 3: 260– 3.

2 *Ibid* (Dawson); Anonymous. John Lydekker: the memorial at Lloyd's. *SHS Quart Mag* 1930; 2 (1): 3-7; R Hopkins. From coffee house to palace: the romantic rise of Lloyds. *SHS Quart Mag* 1935; 7 (1): 10– 11, 21.

3 *Ibid.* (Anonymous).

4 *Op cit.* See note 1 above (Minutes): 3.

5 *Op cit.* See note 1 above (Reports): 12.

6 *Op cit.* See note 1 above (Minutes): 3: 263–5; V Corstophine. *Some aspects of the history and development of the Seamen's Hospital Society between 1821 and 1870.* 1968: 19–22. [SHS Archive].

7 *Op cit.* See note 1 above (Dawson, Anonymous).

8 *Op cit.* See note 1 above (Reports): 14, 15, 16.

9 *Op cit.* See note 1 (Dawson, Minutes: 2 and 3.

10 *Op cit.* See note 1 above (Dawson).

11 *Op cit.* See notes 1 above (Dawson) and 2 (Anonymous).

12 **Richard Lydekker** (1849–1915) was a distinguished zoologist and Fellow of the Royal Society. [*See* also: *Proc R Soc Lond B* 1917; 89: iii–vi; Anonymous. Lydekker, Richard. In: *Who Was Who: a companion to 'Who's Who' containing the biographies of those who died during the period 1897–1915 with addenda and corrigenda.* London: A & C Black 1935: 443].

13 *Op cit.* See note 1 (Reports, Dawson); W A Flere. Lloyd's: early marine insurance: Lloyd's coffee-house and "Lloyd's News": granting of charters: development and changes of quarters: *La Lutine:* The Corporation of Lloyd's and the new Head Office. *PLA Monthly* 1928: 175–82; *Op cit.* See note 2 above (Hopkins).

14 R Harley to Gresham Committee. Letters received 1821–1837; 1834 1 May: 224. [SHS Archive].

15 W R Dawson. *The Treasures of Lloyds: a descriptive catalogue of the monuments, drawings, plate, medals, manuscripts, and other objects of historic interest preserved at Lloyd's, London.* 2nd ed. London: Lloyd's 1930: 1–2. [*See also*: Anonymous. John Lydekker, South Sea Shipowner and benefactor of the Seamen's Hospital Society. *SHS Quart Mag* 1932; 4 (3): 12; Anonymous. James Michelli. *Who Was Who 1929–1940* London: A&C Black 1947: 937].

16 *Op cit.* See note 1 above (Dawson).

17 *Op cit.* See note 1 above (Reports): 12: 22 ; 13: 19–20; 42: 18 ; 44: 2; (Minutes): 3: 148–51, 332, 334, 338.

18 *Op cit.* See note 1 above (Minutes) 3: 295–300.

19 W Bowles *et al.,* to Parliament. Letters Received 1821–1837. 1833: 19 February: 184–8 [SHS Archive].

20 Anno Tertio Gulielmi IV Regis. The 3rd Act of His Most Gracious Majesty William IV. Cap IX. *An act for incorporating the Members of a Society, commonly called "The Seaman's [sic] Hospital Society", and their Successors, as therein is mentioned and provided; and for the better enabling and empowering them to carry on the Charitable and useful Designs of the same Society [6th May 1833].* London: George Eyre and Andrew Spottiswoode 1833: 125–136; [MFT]. Centenary of the Incorporation of the Seamen's Hospital Society. *SHS Quart Mag* 1933; 5 (2): 7; Anonymous. The sailor king's new home. *SHS Quart Mag* 1936; 8 (4): 6; Anonymous. The Lord High Admiral: William IV, a sailor king. *SHS Quart Mag* 1938; 10 (1): 15–16; P Newell. *Greenwich Hospital: a Royal Foundation 1692–1983.* London: Trustees of Greenwich Hospital 1984: 145–6; [*See also:* **9th Lord Colville of Culross, Richard William Penn,** 1st Earl Howe. In: B Burke, A P Burke. *A genealogical and Heraldic History of the Peerage and Baronetage and Knightage* 77th ed. London: Harrison and Sons 1915: 498, 1074].

21 *Op cit.* See note 1 above (Minutes): 3.

22 R Harley to Governors of SHS who were also MPs. Letters received 1821–1837. 1834: 9 June: 228–9. [SHS Archive].
23 R Harley to Parliament. Letters received 1821–1837. 1834: 26 May: 226–7. [SHS Archive].
24 *Op cit.* See note 1 above (Minutes). 3: 431–3.
25 Anonymous. *Times, Lond.* 1833; 13 July: 5 [*See also* notes 1 (Dawson) and 13].
26 G C Cook. Parish Church of St Nicholas, Deptford. *Mariner's Mirror* 2002; 88: 350–1.

Chapter 8

The Hospital-ships

Many of the medical problems (Chapter 11) which seafarers contracted in the early to mid-nineteenth century would now be considered *infective* in origin, but it was not until the late nineteenth century that this was seriously considered to be the case. In the early days of the hospital-ships, the sole illness considered to be *contagious* and a danger to immediate contacts, was smallpox; the remainder, it was felt, were caused by 'miasmas'. Although John Snow (1813–58) had demonstrated, on epidemiological grounds, that cholera was water-borne (in the 1853–4 outbreak in London), this was not widely accepted until very late in the century. Tuberculosis (*see* Chapter 23) (which was of major importance in seafarers) was also not considered an infectious disease until at least, the mid-nineteenth century. Smallpox (variola) was of course readily identifiable on *clinical* grounds. [1]

Little was known in the early nineteenth century about disease *prevention* (Chapter 1); Southwood Smith (1788–1861)[2] formed strong views on *sanitation* and *ventilation* to combat 'miasmas' – themes which were later taken up by Edwin Chadwick (1800–1890) and Florence Nightingale (1820–1910) (*see* Chapter 1).

The three hospital-ships

Why did the SHS, for almost 50 years, house its hospital on three successive ships?[3] The accepted *raison d'être* was that most sailors would *not* have considered attending (or be admitted to) a land-based establishment. But there were other reasons also (*see* Chapter 6), not least that of expense. Equally important was the fact that communities surrounding the Port of London were seriously concerned about the risk of contracting one or more of the 'exotic' diseases imported from tropical countries. There was at the time a great deal of local antagonism, and even positive hostility, to smallpox and 'fever' hospitals being established in heavily populated areas, and this continued until at least the late nineteenth and early twentieth centuries. For that reason, such cases were transferred to one of the Thames hulks which were moored at Dartford – HMS *Dreadnought* (after it had completed its period with the SHS) (see below), and later HMS *Atlas*, HMS *Endymion*, and HMS *Castalia*.[4] Table 8.1 summarises details of the three hospital-ships successively loaned, between 1821 and 1870, to the SHS by the 'Lords Commissioners of the Admiralty'.

Table 8.1: Details of three warships – the hulks of which were subsequently used by the SHS as *permanent* Hospital-ships – lent by the Admiralty.

Name and date of launch (HMS)	*Site of mooring (and date of loan)*	*Description*	*Guns (no)*	*Complement (men)*	*Length/width* Gun Deck	*Length/width* Keel	*Length/width* Beam	*Depth of hold*	*Tonnage*
GRAMPUS (originally TIGER) (1802)	Deptford (1821)	4th rate 2-decker	50	343	151′ 0″	124′ 7″	41′ 0″	17′ 3″	1,114
DREADNOUGHT (1801)	Greenwich Reach (1831)	2nd rate 3-decker	104	738	184′ 11″	152′ 3″	51′ 2″	21′ 6″	2,123
CALEDONIA (renamed DREADNOUGHT on 21 June 1856) (1808)	Greenwich Reach (1857)	1st rate 3-decker	120	875	205′ 0″	170′ 9.5″	53′ 8″	23′ 2″	2,616

HMS Grampus

Figure 8.1 shows a painting of the *Grampus* – which was in use as the SHS's hospital-ship between 1821 and 1831. Events preceding the loan of this hulk by the Admiralty, are recorded in Chapter 6.

HMS *Grampus* was lent to the SHS in 1820, and served as the first hospital-ship moored off Deptford from 1821. She had seen service in the East Indies (1803–5, 1811, 1814–15), Cape of Good Hope (1806–9), South America (where she was the flagship of Sir George Cockburn (1810–12), and Leeward Islands (the flagship of Sir Francis Laforey)[5] (1813). HMS *Grampus* had also been used as a troopship in 1817 and subsequently a store-ship at Chatham. When taken over by the SHS, the ship was in urgent need of caulking. Following 10 years' service with the SHS (1821–1831), she was sold by the Admiralty (in 1832).[6]

In September 1822, a minute of the Committee of Management states:

> Mr Snodgrass reported, that, finding by a late Act of Parliament, that no Ship or Vessel except those of His Majesty's Navy were allowed to wear a Union Jack or Pendant, and apprehending that information might be laid against the Grampus for hoisting those colours, he had instructed the Secretary to desire the Superintendent to discontinue hoisting them, until the Sanction of the Lords of the Admiralty should be obtained for that purpose; to which end the Secretary had … written to John Wilson Croker, Esq. [Secretary of the Admiralty] but has not yet received an answer.

Later that month a letter to Harley from the Admiralty Office dated 27 September gave the desired information:

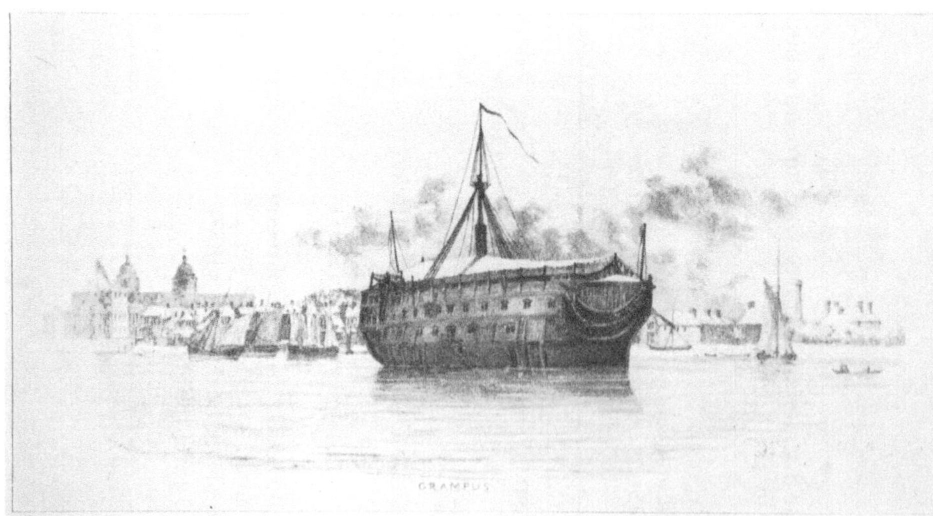

Figure 8.1: Painting of HMS *Grampus* – artist unknown. [SHS Archive].

Sir,

Having laid before my Lords Commissioners of the Admiralty your letter of the 20th instant … I have it in command to send you herewith their Lordships warrant authorising the said ship to wear the said colours until further orders.

I am

Sir,

John Barrow [Second Secretary of the Admiralty]

The following letter, under the Admiralty Seal and signed by J Osborn and G[eorge] Cockburn, was enclosed:

> … whereas we think fit that the 'Grampus' used as a Seamen's Hospital in the River Thames shall be allowed to wear an Union Jack and Pendant whilst she is so employed, or until further orders. We do hereby authorize you to hoist an Union Jack and Pendant on board the 'Grampus' and to wear the same whilst she is so employed as abovementioned or until further orders, accordingly and for you wearing the said Jack and Pendant this shall be your warrant.

Merchantmen were at that time fined £500 for wearing these flags, which were usually restricted to the Sovereign's Ships (i.e. those of the RN). The *Dreadnought's* pendant (see below) was the subject of an article in the *SHS Quarterly Magazine* for 1934.[7]

A suitable pendant was therefore requested for the *Dreadnought* (see below); a minute in April 1833 states that the SHS Committee 'Ordered that a New Ensign lettered 'Seamen's Hospital' and a Union Jack be procured of larger dimensions than the present'. A new figure-head was also ordered in 1854 from the Deptford and Woolwich Dockyards at a cost of £15=00 to replace the present one which was beyond repair; however, at the following meeting, the carver considered that he could repair (and paint red) the original at a cost of £1=10=00. This and wire-rope (for the awnings of the ship) were subjects for discussion at Council of Management meetings.

HMS Dreadnought

By 1830 the hulked *Grampus* was considered too small to house the increasing number of patients undergoing treatment by the SHS (*see* Chapter 9) – the 'crowded state of the Wards … excluded a great number of Patients'. The 'Committee [the 10th annual report – written like all the previous ones by Richard Harley – recorded] flatter themselves that ere long [the *Dreadnought*] will occupy the place of the Grampus'. The following report confirmed the Admiralty's loan: 'the Society is indebted [to His Majesty's Government] for being now in possession of an Hospital Ship worthy of the Port of London, and of the British Nation'. HMS *Dreadnought* (Figures 8.2–8.3) was to serve as the SHS Hospital-ship at Greenwich from 1831 until 1857.

The 10th report also gave details of the 'fitting-out' process – the cost of which was borne by the SHS, although various Thames shipbuilders gratuitously supervised

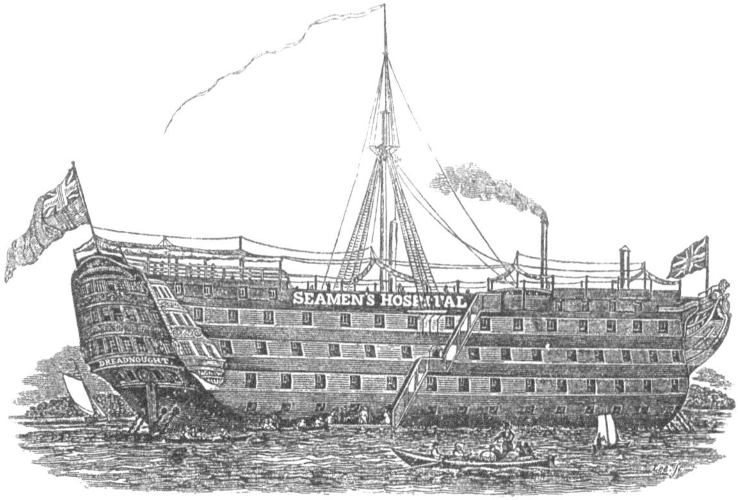

Figure 8.2: Engraving of HMS *Dreadnought:* artist unknown. [SHS Archive].

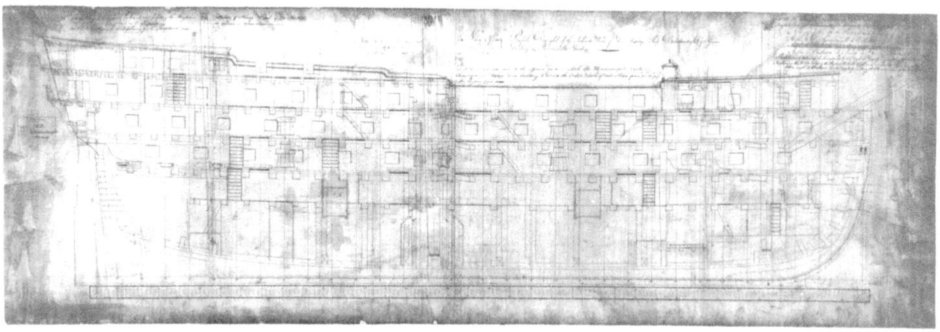

Figure 8.3: Profile of HMS *Dreadnought* [reproduced with permission, the National Maritime Museum Archive].

these alterations and obtained 'all materials on the lowest terms, for ready money'. Despite this, the overall cost to the Society was £2893=18^{s}=7^{d}, which included addition of 'Bedsteads, Bedding, Clothing, and other necessities, in readiness for the maximum number of 250 Patients, over and above 150 Convalescent and men fit for duty – and likewise the cost of the *Hot-Water Apparatus*, by which the Wards are warmed'. It was hoped that the latter expenditure would soon be justified by a reduction in fuel-consumption and 'an improved atmosphere for the Sick'.[8]

The *Dreadnought* (draft of about 18 feet) had been used as a Lazaretto at Milford between 1827 and 30. She was the sixth of that name – launched at Plymouth on

13 June 1801, having been 13 years on the stocks; the ship was coppered and eventually sent to sea in six hours, joining the fleet in the middle of the Napoleonic wars. On 17 May 1803 she had sailed from Cawsand Bay, flying the flag of Admiral William Cornwallis,[9] at the head of ten ships of the line, and several frigates; she also took part in the blockade of Brest. From 1804–5, the *Dreadnought* flew the flag of Vice-Admiral Cuthbert Collingwood[10] – when she was again engaged in the blockade of French ports. Ten days before the battle of Trafalgar (21 October 1805), Collingwood (who had apparently trained his crew with 'efficiency and gunnery skill') was ordered to move his flag to the '*Royal Sovereign*'.[11]

ACTIVE SERVICE

At the Battle of Trafalgar, the *Dreadnought* (under the command of Captain John Conn) was one of 27 ships of the line, together with four frigates and two small craft, under the direction of Vice-Admiral Viscount Nelson – whose flag was on HMS *Victory*. The *Dreadnought* was the eighth ship of the lee line and engaged the Spanish vessel *San Juan Nepomuceno*, which she captured in a quarter of an hour. She then engaged the *Principe de Asturias*, which managed to escape, despite the fact that the Spanish Commander-in-Chief, Admiral Gravina was killed in the fight. Overall, the *Dreadnought*'s casualties at Trafalgar were: seven killed and 26 wounded. On 9 September 1810, (commanded by Captain Valentine Collard), and flying the flag of Rear-Admiral Thomas Sotheby, she took part in an unsuccessful attack on a French vessel lying behind the west side of Ushant. Her last experience of active service was in the Baltic in a fleet commanded by Admiral Sir James Saumarez with his flag on HMS *Victory*.[12]

SERVICE WITH THE SHS

The Admiralty were to keep the hulk of HMS *Dreadnought* in good repair during the 16-year period on loan to the SHS, this fact being acknowledged in several Annual Reports.[13] Unfortunately, however, in 1840, the ship 'sprung a leak' and was towed to Sheerness (at the Admiralty's expense), where the repairs were carried out in dry dock in a mere four days. During this brief period, it was obviously necessary to evacuate the patients from the vessel and they were temporarily transferred to Guy's and King's College Hospitals. The 'Marine Society' also supplied 'valuable assistance, in the hour of need'.

In 1847 the ship sprung another leak (albeit a minor one) and the Master Shipwright of Woolwich Dock Yard (directed by the Lords Commissioners of the Admiralty) considered that the ship would need to be docked the following spring. Fortunately, this was unnecessary – as the leak had by then 'diminished considerably'; however, docking was felt advisable later that year, and extensive alterations – which improved the 'ventilation of the several Wards' (at the Admiralty's expense) were made. Other modifications included the introduction of 'Large and lofty skylights' on the upper deck, [and] other decks were 'widely opened', while the 'ports or windows' were greatly enlarged. The whole of the ship was also 'thoroughly cleansed' – the 'spaces between the timbers having been injected with Sir

W. Burnett's Fluid'.[14] The 1850 SHS report concluded that the 'Sanitary conditions of the Hospital [had] been improved to a remarkable extent', this having a beneficial effect on 'cases of Erysipelas' and also the management of wounds, sores, and severe injuries. These alterations took three months to complete, during which time their Lordships granted a loan to the SHS of HMS '*Devonshire*' (*see* Table 8.2) (*see* Chapter 11); the patients were therefore transferred to this vessel and 'no injury [was] sustained by any [of them]'.[15]

DICKENS' VISIT

Charles Dickens (1812–70) alluded to the Seamen's Hospital (ship) in chapter 23 of his novel *Dombey and Son* (1848). He also included an article entitled 'The Dreadnought' in the weekly journal *Household Words* which he edited (*see* Chapter 9), which was published on 23 August 1851; whether Dickens wrote this descriptive piece himself remains open to question; however, the medical officer who showed the author round the ship (probably Dickens himself) was identified by Kemball Cook (the SHS Secretary) as Dr A H Churchill (*see* Chapter 12).[16] Figure 8.4 shows interior views of wards in the *Dreadnought* and its successor, the *Caledonia*. The 'convalescents' slept (he wrote) in hammocks on the main-deck; the middle deck was *surgical*, and the lower *medical*, while the orlop deck was reserved for 'minor cases of illness'. This article also dwelt on the part the ship had played at Trafalgar (see above), and the history of the two SHS hospital-ships. The total number of patients *received* at that time amounted (wrote the author) to 'sixty-three thousand three hundred and forty-five'. The Museum seems to have been of particular interest to Dickens: 'Here we behold [he wrote] a collection of skulls of all nations; a geographical Golgotha which is, to the ethnographer, of illimitable interest. Each skull is wrapped up in paper, and duly labelled'. The collection had presumably been assembled by George Busk FRS (Chapter 12), who was at that time one of the two surgeons on board. The author ended with a comment about 'the bluff fat nurse [a] remarkable old woman [who] tucks up [a handsome Prussian]'.[17]

The *Dreadnought* was broken up in 1857 – the task being completed on 31 March of that year – i.e. shortly after her term as Hospital-ship with the Society (1831–1857) had ended.

A *Lancet* reporter wrote rather romantically that the old *Dreadnought* which had 'braved a thousand storms, the battle [of Trafalgar], and the breeze' would be 'shortly towed away to some nautical knacker's yard, and there broken up'. He then quoted Sir Walter Scott (1771–1832):[18]

> "Oh! Caledonia, stern and wild,
> Meet nurse for a poetic child …"

However, 'the patients now to be nursed are of somewhat tougher sort and courser grain'. A subsequent *Lancet* report recorded the end of the *Dreadnought's* life: 'On Tuesday last [10 March 1857] commenced the sale of this old vessel, which has been used for so many years as a floating hospital off Greenwich. Eighty-five lots of timber, &c., fetched £370. It is computed that her copper will fetch £2000'.[19]

Table 8.2: Details (where known) of six hulks loaned temporarily – most as cholera ships (*see* Chapter 11) – to the SHS by the Admiralty.

Name	*Date lent to SHS*	*Description (and date launched)*	*Guns (no)*	*Complement (men)*	*Length/width*				*Tonnage*	*Site of mooring (and date of loan)*
					Gun deck	*Keel*	*Beam*	*Depth of hold*		
DOVER	1832	5th rate (1806)	–	–	131′ 6″	110′ 4″	34′ 4″	8′ 11″	692	Deptford (1832)
ECHO	1835	Paddle-vessel (1827)	2–6	–	111′ 9″	92′ 4″	24′ 10″	13′ 6″	295	Sheerness (1835)
IPHIGENIA	1849	5th rate (1808)	30	274	137′ 0″	113′ 1″	38′ 2″	13′ 5″	896	Deptford (1849)
DEVONSHIRE	1853	– (1808)	–	–	–	–	–	–	–	Deptford (1854)
BACCHANTE	1854	5th rate (1811)	46	–	154′ 0″	–	–	–	1,077	Deptford (1854)
BELLE-ISLE	1867	3rd rate (1819)	74	–	–	–	–	–	–	Sheerness (1867)

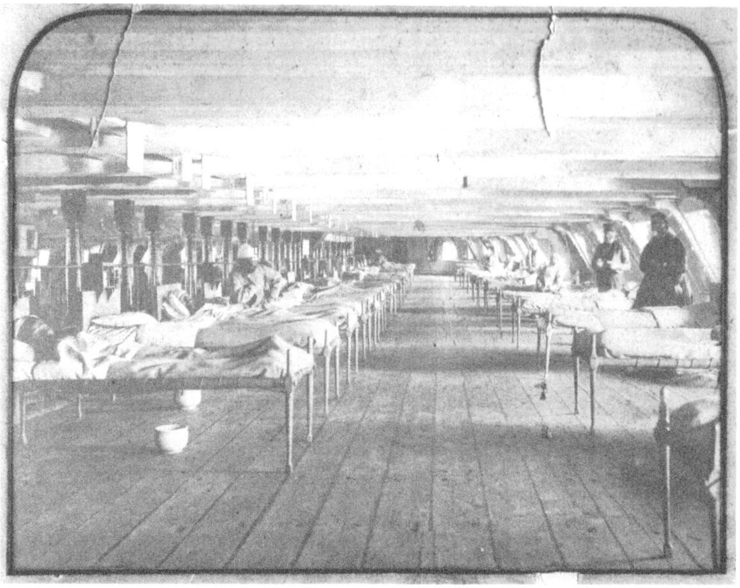

(a)

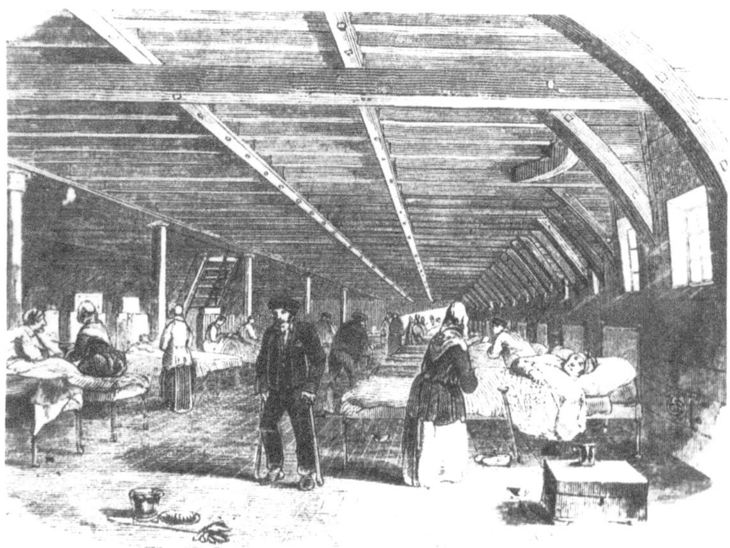

(b)

Figure 8.4 (a, b & c): Illustrations (undated) showing the interiors of wards on HMS *Dreadnought* and HMS *Caledonia*. [SHS Archive].

HMS Caledonia *(renamed* Dreadnought*)*

In June 1856, the Lords Commissioners of the Admiralty granted the SHS use of the hulk of HMS *Caledonia* (Figures 8.5–8.7), a 'large, and more commodious vessel' which was to serve as the SHS Hospital-ship from 1857–1870. Furthermore,

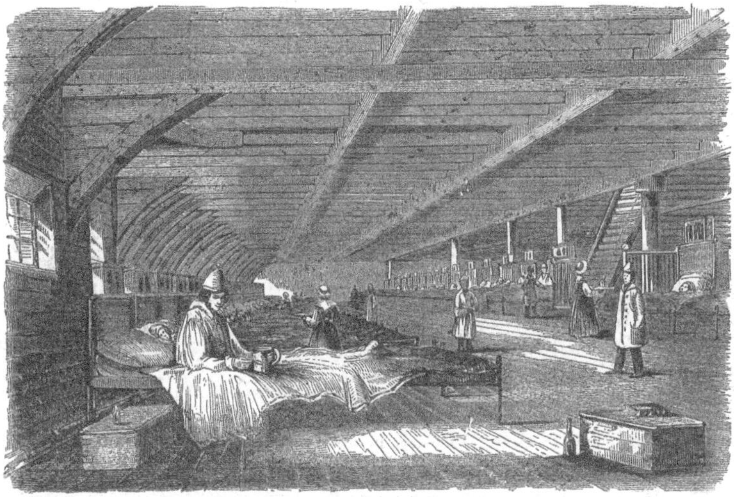

INTERIOR OF THE DREADNOUGHT.

Figure 8.4c

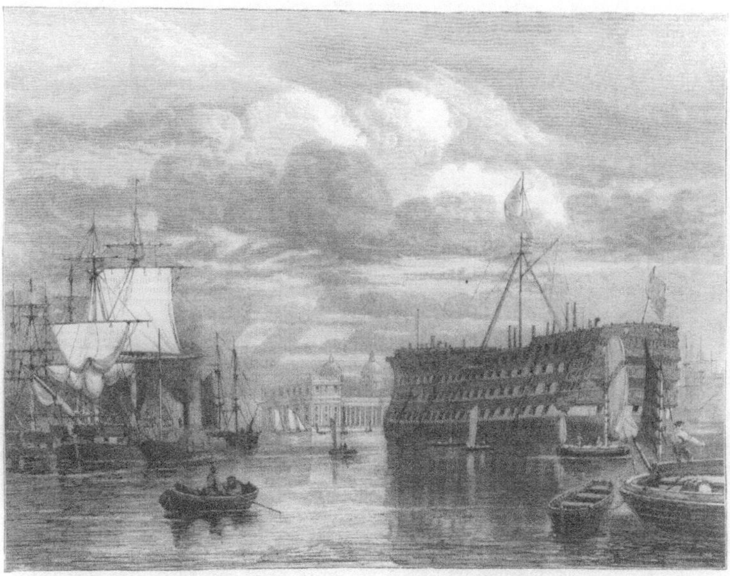

THE SEAMEN'S HOSPITAL SHIP DREADNOUGHT, OFF GREENWICH

Figure 8.5: Engraving of HMS *Caledonia* (renamed *Dreadnought*). [*The Graphic* 1870: 28 May].

in accordance with the wishes of the Committee, they had altered her name to '*Dreadnought*' on 21 June 1856.[20] The 36th Annual Report also summarised the 'fitting-out' of this third vessel at the Woolwich Dock Yard. The cost of alterations, with the exception of 'removal of some bulky and superfluous iron and timber', and 'cutting the ports on the Orlop deck', was borne by the Society, which was

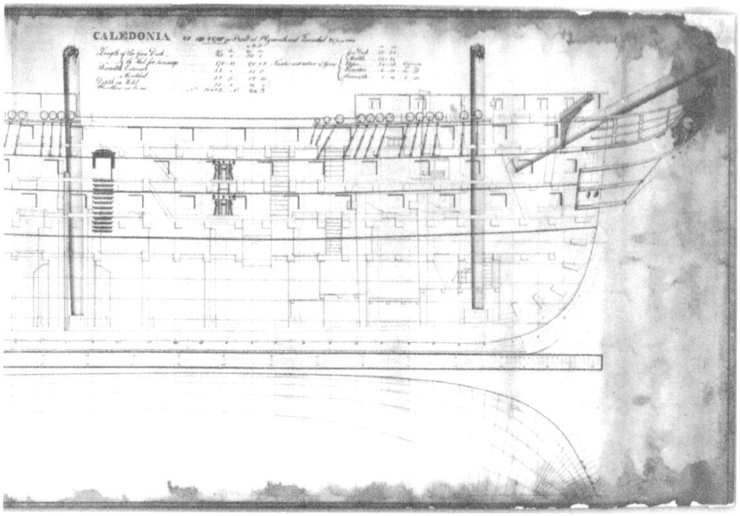

(a)

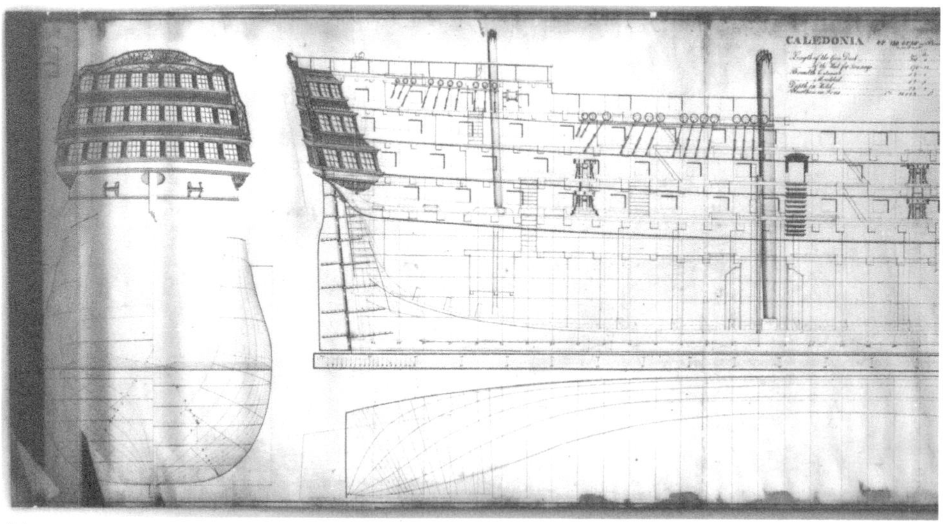

(b)

Figure 8.6 (a & b): Profile of HMS *Caledonia* (renamed *Dreadnought*): (a) fore and (b) aft views. [Reproduced with permission, the National Maritime Museum Archive].

represented throughout the re-fit ('almost every day … for six months') by Captain W E Farrer, HCS an Elder Brother of Trinity Corporation. This report continued: 'The warming and ventilation of the Ship are subjects to which the Committee have devoted much attention'. The alterations cost the Society £11,000 (which ultimately escalated to £15,038=18^{s}=2^{d}). The 36th report concluded: '… as the Ship is now brought to her moorings, she will in the course of a few days supersede the present

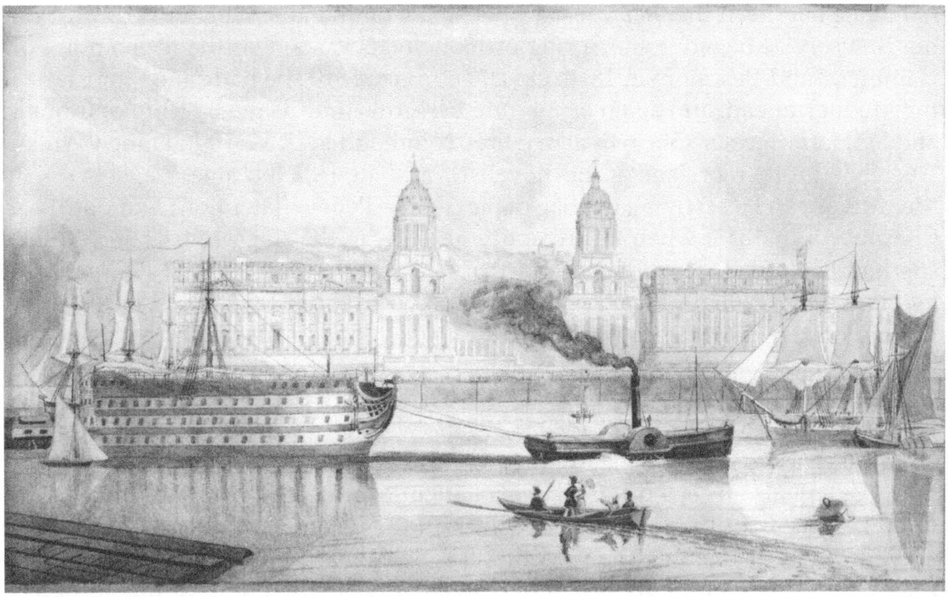

Figure 8.7: HMS *Caledonia* (renamed *Dreadnought*) being towed away from Greenwich in 1872. She served as a small-pox ship following her use by the SHS. [SHS archive].

Dreadnought'.[21] The saga of 'fitting-up' was the subject of an article in *The Lancet*; unfortunately there were several inaccuracies in the account which were corrected in a follow-up letter by Kemball Cook – the SHS Secretary: *'Every deck is devoted to the use of the patients'* [he stressed], there being 'no accommodation exclusively [used by the Committee]'; the weather deck was to be used by the convalescents, the main deck both as a 'chapel for Divine worship' and as sleeping accommodation for the convalescents, the middle deck for 70 surgical patients, the lower deck for 80 medical patients, and the orlop deck for 65 venereal cases. In the hold are [he wrote] 'the furnaces, boiler, &c, for warming the decks, and for hot-water baths, space for 100 tons of coals, besides coke and various store-rooms'. [Kemball Cook ended his letter]: 'The officers' and attendants' cabins, the various offices, provision and store rooms, surgery, dispensary, operating-room, lavatories, &c. &c. are placed at the fore and after part of the various decks, as most convenient for the purposes of the hospital'.[22]

HMS *Caledonia*, had been designed by Sir W Rule, and took part in the French wars; but she became notable chiefly because she was the favourite ship of Vice-Admiral Sir Edward Pellow (later Lord Exmouth – *see* Chapter 6). The *'Caledonia'* was probably ordered in 1794, and modelled on the 'Commerce of Marseilles' which had been captured from the French at Toulon in 1793. Her keel was probably laid in 1796 in King's Yard, Plymouth dock, Devonport; subsequent work was carried out until 1805, and she was completed on 25 June 1808; the 'biggest ship [to be] launched from an English Yard' she possessed 120 guns. Her original name had been the '*Impregnable*'; her first Commander William Bedford,[23] and her first service began in the Spring of 1809. In 1809, she was the flagship of Lord Gambier,[24] and Pickmore in 1810. On 20 February 1810 she had sailed for Cadiz in the Mediterranean, and again on 14 June 1811, this time as the flagship of Gambier and Sir Harry Neale.[25] She was at one time commanded by Captain Francis William Austen[26] (brother of Jane – the novelist), and in 1811 became Flagship of the Mediterranean Fleet (flying the flag of Sir George Pellew [later Lord Exmouth] – *see* Chapter 6). In 1843, when at Plymouth and flying the flag of Sir David Milne,[27] she had been visited by Queen Victoria. She flew the flag of Sir J Louis in 1846 and that of Sir William Parker[28] the following year. From 1851– 6 she was based at Devonport. HMS *Caledonia* (renamed *Dreadnought)* had thus had an eventful life – which probably lasted a total of 75 years.[29]

The 37th Annual Report summarised the transfer of patients to the new venue – which took place on 17 February 1857 – 'the weather being most propitious'. The emphasis was on ventilation, lighting, while heating and the 'sanitary condition of the Hospital' also received a great deal of attention; 'the Committee [Kemball Cook wrote] derive considerable gratification from the testimony borne by the medical and surgical officers, that the present "Dreadnought" in a sanitary point of view is second to none of the Metropolitan Hospitals'. The high cost of the 're-fit' (see above) was largely attributed to the 'high rate of wages at the time', and the fact that the contribution of the Lords Commissioners of the Admiralty was 'comparatively trifling'.[30]

Eighteen fifty-eight was of course the year of 'the Great Stink' – when Parliament had to be dissolved due to the unacceptable (noxious) state of the River Thames at Westminster, which was heavily contaminated with sewage.[31] The medical and surgical officers of the *Dreadnought* had given their assurance that 'no pernicious effects [of the Thames contamination] were produced on board'; however, as a contingency measure if things were to worsen, they recommended that at an hour's notice the ship be removed from her moorings (off Greenwich Reach) and transferred to new ones off Greenhithe; although this strategy met with the approval of their Lordships 'no occasion was found to call for the anticipated removal'.[32]

The following year (1859), it became clear that the *Dreadnought* required an entire re-caulking; although sympathetic, the Lords Commissioners of the Admiralty were unable 'to give orders for the execution of this work' due to the pressure of work in Her Majesty's Dock Yards. Caulking was not in fact undertaken until 1868; during this process (which was carried out at the expense of the Lords Commissioners of the Admiralty), the Society was loaned HMS *Belle-isle* (see Table 8.2).[33]Also in 1859, the Committee decided to attend to the water-supply of the *Dreadnought*. At a cost of £120=00=00, a 'larger and more regular supply of filtered water [was obtained] at a considerable reduction of expense'; this was achieved by 'having pipes laid from the filtered basins of the Kent Water Works Company'.[34]

Appendix IV gives extracts from the Ship's *Log* between 1865 and 68; every detail of day-to-day activities was recorded.

Subsequently the *Caledonia* was broken up (in 1875), i.e. some five years after her 13 years of service with the SHS had expired (see below).

The decision to move to land (*see also* Chapter 13)

Concern arose in the early 1860s about the position of the mooring site of the *Dreadnought*, as the 44th Annual Report makes clear:

> Of late years [Kemball Cook wrote] the position of the Dreadnought has been injuriously affected by the gradually increasing occupation of the banks of the river on both sides of it, as Iron Ship-building Yards; the incessant noise from which (often by night as well as day) is stated by the Physicians to interfere with the proper treatment of their patients, and to impede their recovery.

However, all efforts to find a more congenial site had so far failed due to the following factors: 'the fear of impeding the navigation of the river – the want of depth of water – the necessity of remaining near the bulk of the Shipping and the Docks – and the means of convenient communication with the shore'.[35] By 1864, a decision to move to dry-land (preferably at Greenwich) had been made; this had been first aired in the 44th Annual Report; (see above): 'A great change … has taken place in the mind of the Sailor [when compared with the time the SHS was founded – in 1821] as he now undoubtedly prefers a Hospital *ashore*'. Kemball Cook continued: 'The general establishment of Sailor's Homes, and the Seamen's Savings Banks, have doubtless greatly contributed to elevate the tone and improve the habits of seafaring men'. The major factors which underlay this radical move were: poor ventilation and light, excessive noise, and limited access to the ship. The events leading up to, and the actual move to dry land are related in Chapter 13.

The removal of the *Dreadnought* from her moorings at Greenwich and the subsequent 'breaking-up' at Chatham Dockyard are pictured in two engravings in the *Illustrated London News* for 1872 and 1875 respectively (*see* Chapter 13).[36]

Table 8.2 gives details of other ships loaned by the Admiralty, for various reasons, between 1821 and 1870 (*see also* Chapter 11).

Although the SHS was therefore to abandon the use of Hospital-ships in 1870, similar 'floating hospitals' had an important future elsewhere. They have in fact served an important rôle in military operations over the last century.[37]

References and Notes

1 H. Richardson (ed.). *English Hospitals 1660–1948: a survey of their architecture and design.* Swindon: Royal Commission on the Historical Monuments of England 1998; S J Snow. Snow, John (1813–1858). In: H C G Matthew, B Harrison (eds). *Oxford Dictionary of National Biography.* Oxford: Oxford University Press 2004; 51: 495–8.

2 **Thomas Southwood Smith** (1788–1861) was a leading pioneer of sanitary reform. He wrote important works on epidemics and sanitary improvements – especially sewage disposal and ventilation. He was a founder of the 'Westminster Review', The Health of Towns and other bodies. [*See also*: G C Cook. Thomas Southwood Smith (1788–1861): leading exponent of diseases of poverty and pioneer of sanitary reform in the mid-nineteenth century. *J Med Biog* 2002; 10: 194–205].

3 Anonymous. His Majesty's Ships: Grampus – Dreadnought – Caledonia. *SHS Quart Mag* 1929; 1: 59–61.
4 J Burne. *Dartford's capital river: paddle steamers, personalities and smallpox boats.* Buckingham: Barracuda Books Ltd. 1989: 44–58.
5 **Admiral Sir Francis Laforey** KCB Bt (1767–1835) commanded HMS *Spartate* at the Battle of Trafalgar in 1805. He later became Commander-in-Chief at the Leewood islands from 1811 until 1814. [*See also:* J K Laughton, A G Jamieson. Sir Francis Laforey (1767–1835). In: H C G Matthew, B Harrison (eds). *Oxford Dictionary of National Biography.* Oxford: Oxford University Press 2004: 32: 210].
6 *Op cit.* See note 3 above.
7 Council of Management Minutes. [See Appendix 1 for minute-book dates] 1: 150, 153; 3: 329; 7: 189, 198, 477; B. Cable. The Dreadnought's pendant. *SHS Quart Mag* 1934; 6(1): 11, 14. [*See also*: C H Gaye-Hexham. Masthead pendants. *The Nautical Magazine* 1948; September; C H Gaye-Hexham. The Dreadnought's Jack and Pendant. *The Trident* 1949; 2: 171–2].
8 10th Annual Report (1830): 21; 11th Annual Report (1831): 21–2.
9 **Admiral Sir William Cornwallis** GCB (1744–1819) took part in several naval actions, and became Commander-in-Chief in East India waters from 1789 until 1793. In 1801 and 1803–6 he commanded the Channel fleet. [*See also*: A Lambert. Cornwallis, Sir William (1744–1819) In: H C G Matthew, B Harrison (eds). *Oxford Dictionary of National Biography.* Oxford: Oxford University Press 2004; 13: 489–92].
10 **Admiral Lord (Cuthbert) Collingwood** (1748–1810) took part in numerous naval actions before Nelson's death at Trafalgar. He commanded the *Royal Sovereign* and was Nelson's second in command at the battle of Trafalgar, taking charge on Nelson's death. [*See also:* C H H Owen. Collingwood, Cuthbert, Baron Collingwood (1748–1810). In: H C G Matthew, B Harrison (eds). *Oxford Dictionary of National Biography.* Oxford: Oxford University Press 2004; 12: 670–5].
11 *Op cit.* See note 3 above.
12 R Harding (ed). Bicentenary of Trafalgar. *Mariner's Mirror* 2005; 91: 133–383; A B Sainsbury. Saumarez, James, first Baron de Saumarez (1757–1836). In: H C G Matthew, B Harrison (eds). *Oxford Dictionary of National Biography.* Oxford: Oxford University Press 2004; 49: 21–5].
13 *Op cit.* See note 8 above. 15: 21; 17: 21.
14 C Penn. Sir William Burnett (1779–1861), professional head of the Royal Navy Medical Department and entrepreneur. *J Med Biog* 2004; 12: 141–6.
15 *Op cit.* See note 8 above. 20: 18; 27: 20; 28: 18; 29: 19–20; 30: 18.
16 **Augustus Henry Churchill** qualified with the MRCS Eng (1836) and LSA (1837) diplomas, from St Bartholomew's Hospital. Before he joined the SHS as an assistant surgeon on the *Dreadnought*, he had been surgeon to the Carnarvon and Anglesea Infirmary. He subsequently became Resident Medical Officer to the Westminster Hospital and the Chelsea, Brompton and Belgrade Dispensary. His final appointment was as Medical Officer of Health for Walton-on-the-Hill. He died in either 1896 or 97. [*See also*: Anonymous. *Medical Directory*: London: J & A Churchill; 1896: 615].
17 C. Dickens. *Dombey and Son.* London: Penguin Books 1970; 411; C. Dickens (ed). 'The Dreadnought'. In: *Household Words: a weekly journal.* London: Ward, Lock and Tyler 1851; 3: 516–9. [*See also*: Anonymous. When Charles Dickens visited the old 'Dreadnought' Hospital Ship: her early career as a man-of-war. *SHS Quart Mag* 1932; 4(4): 13–14 & 26; When Charles Dickens visited the old 'Dreadnought' Hospital Ship in 1851 (continued). *SHS Quart Mag* 1933; 5(1): 15–16].
18 Anonymous. *Lancet* 1857; i: 152; D Hewitt. Scott, Sir Walter (1771–1832). In: H C G

Matthew, B Harrison (eds). *Oxford Dictionary of National Biography.* Oxford: Oxford University Press 2004; 49: 490–510.
19 Anonymous. *Lancet* 1857; i: 281.
20 *Op cit.* See note 8 above. 36: 18–19.
21 *Ibid.*
22 Anonymous. *Lancet* 1857; i; 152; S. Kemball Cook. Seamen's Hospital Society. *Lancet* 1857; i; 208.
23 J K Laughton, A Lambert. Bedford, William (1764?–1827). In: H C G Matthew, B Harrison (eds). *Oxford Dictionary of National Biography.* Oxford: Oxford University Press 2004; 4: 777–8.
24 **Admiral James Gambier, first Baron Gambier** GCB (1756–1833) had a most distinguished naval career. He was a Lord of the Admiralty from 1795–1801 and 1804–06, and from 1802–04 Governor of Newfoundland. From 1808 until 1811, he commanded the Channel fleet, and in 1814, was a commissioner for the treaty with the United States of America. [*See also* Chapter 6].
25 **Admiral Sir Harry Burrard Neale** Bt GCB GCMG MP (1765–1840) was a Lord of the Admiralty in 1804. He became Commander-in-Chief in the Mediterranean from 1823–6. [*See also*: J K Laughton, A Lambert. Neale, Sir Harry Burrard, second baronet (1765–1840). In: H C G Matthew, B Harrison (eds). *Oxford Dictionary of National Biography.* Oxford: Oxford University Press 2004; 40: 296–7].
26 J K Laughton, A Lambert. Austen, Sir Francis William (1774–1865). In: H C G Matthew, B Harrison (eds). *Oxford Dictionary of National Biography.* Oxford: Oxford University Press 2004; 2: 957–8.
27 **Admiral Sir David Milne** GCB MP (1763–1845) served initially with the East India service. He became Commander-in-Chief in North American waters, and ultimately Commander-in-Chief at Plymouth. [*See also*: J K Laughton, A Lambert. Milne, Sir David (1763–1845) In: H C G Matthew, B Harrison (eds). *Oxford Dictionary of National Biography.* Oxford: Oxford University Press 2004; 38: 292–3].
28 **Admiral Sir William Parker** Bt GCB (1781–1866) saw naval service in many parts of the world. In 1841, he was Commander in China and captured Amoy, Ningpo, Woosung and Shanghai; he also captured Chin-kiang-foo. In 1846 he was nominated to command the Channel fleet, and from 1854 until 57 he was Commander-in-Chief at Devonport. [*See also*: J K Laughton, A Lambert. Parker, Sir William, first baronet (1781–1866). In: H C G Matthew, B Harrison (eds). *Oxford Dictionary of National Biography.* Oxford: Oxford University Press 2004; 42: 756–8].
29 C N Parkinson. The story of a ship. *SHS Quart Mag* 1933; 5 (4): 15–16 & 1934; 6 (1): 15–16. [*See also*: B Cable. Clippers and cut-throats. *SHS Quart Mag* 1933; 5 (1): 13–14; Anonymous. Lord Exmouth. *SHS Quart Mag* 1933; 5 (1): 18; *Op cit.* See note 3 above].
30 *Op cit.* See note 8 above. 37: 18–19.
31 S. Halliday. *The Great Stink of London: Sir Joseph Bazalgette and the cleansing of the Victorian Metropolis.* Stroud: Sutton Publishing 1999. [*See also*: G C Cook. Joseph Willam Bazalgette (1819–1891): a major figure in the health improvements of Victorian London. *J Med Biog* 1999; 7: 17–24; G C Cook. Construction of London's Victorian sewers: the vital role of Joseph Bazalgette. *Postgrad Med J* 2001; 77: 802–4].
32 *Op cit.* See note 8 above. 38: 18–19.
33 *Ibid.* 39: 18; 48: 18.
34 *Ibid.*
35 *Op cit.* See note 8 above. 44: 19.
36 Anonymous. *Illustrated London News.* 1872; 61: 505, 1875; 66: 69.

37 J H Plumridge. *Hospital ships and ambulance trains.* London: Seeley, Service & Co 1975; G Clark. *'Doc': 100 year history of the sick berth branch.* London: H M Stationery Office 1984; R M Bruce-Chwatt. The Wartime use of merchant vessels as hospital ships. *Sea Breezes.* 1994; vol 68, no 577.

Chapter 9

Service on the Hospital-ships

The *permanent* Society had got off to a good start in 1821 (*see* Chapter 6); however, it began on a small scale, and admissions to HMS *Grampus* were at first on a modest scale, being of the order of 400 per year. Numbers of in-patients soon escalated, however, until they amounted to around 2,000 admissions annually, and after five years the Society also attended to out-patients (*see* Figure 9.1), but its existence was still *not* widely known!

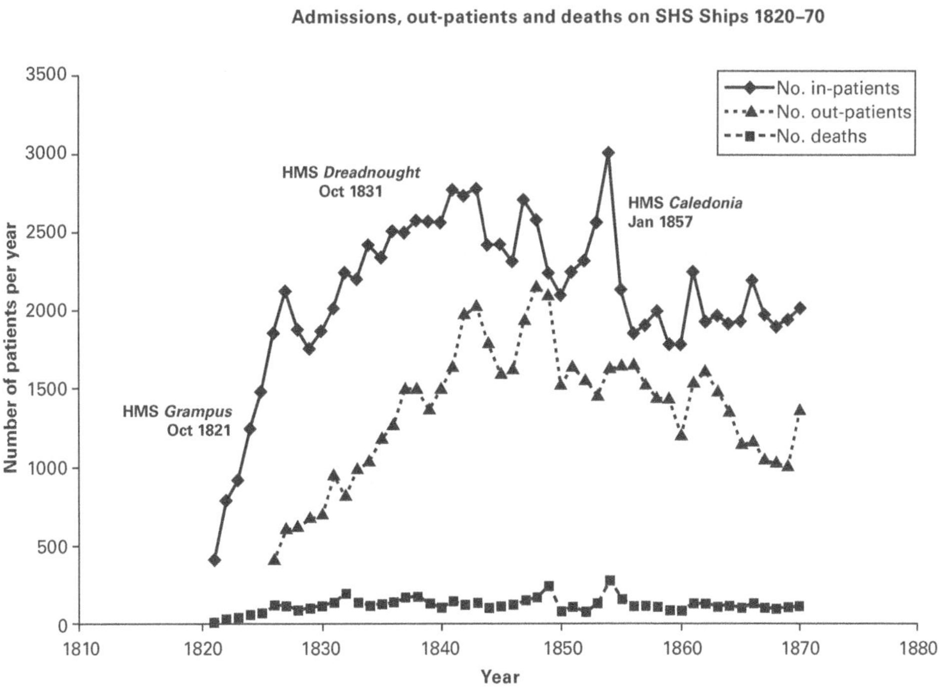

Figure 9.1: Admissions, numbers of out-patients, and deaths on the three hospital-ships between 1821 (i.e. when alterations to the *Grampus* were completed – *see* Chapter 6) and 1870 (i.e. when the hospital-ships were abandoned).

The Society's *raison d'être*

The Society had been founded to care for the overall well-being of merchant sailors; emphasis had been, from the outset, not solely on medical aspects, but also on improving 'their habits, by the daily religious services and regular discipline they are called upon to witness on board'. This aim was reflected in the *first* report of the SHS, which had succintly spelt out the function(s) of the Charity (*see* Chapter 6):

> ... seamen, when they return home in ill health, frequently fall into the hands of ignorant wretches, who fill them with pernicious drugs as long as their money lasts, and then turn them out half naked, and in a worse condition than when they received them, to perish with cold and hunger in the streets. During the period of their remaining under the care and protection of this charity, every effort is used, to impress upon their minds the great importance of religion; to which end they are amply furnished with such religious tracts as are suited to their several capacities, and are properly exhorted and instructed by the Chaplain.

The Report then focused on the prevalence of ship-wrecks around England, and the severe injuries resulting there from, and also emphasised that typhus was a real health hazard facing the seafarer.

The 35th Annual report (written by Kemball Cook – the Society's Secretary) also contains a somewhat verbose statement, which again emphasised the *religious* objective(s) of the Charity:

> Great indeed are the benefits of a *temporal* character conferred by the Society upon the invalided Sailor. He arrives at the Hospital racked with pain or enfeebled by fever and disease. *Here* he receives all the relief and attention which medical science and surgical skill can apply to his particular case. Neither is he again cast adrift on the first symptoms of returning health and renewed vigour. He rises from the bed of sickness and of languor, and the Hospital Ship becomes for a time his home, – a home in which he is well fed, and, if need be, clothed. This, however, is not all. It may be that, amid the active and bustling pursuits of a seafaring life, his thoughts have been but little directed to that Being who has yet been guiding all his course, and who has in His mercy at length laid him low for a season to bring him nearer to Himself. *Now*, indeed, he has time for reflection; – neither in this respect is he left to grope his way to light and to life unassisted and uncared for. He enjoys the daily ministrations of a faithful Minister of religion, the appointed Chaplain of the Institution, – and though, in the Providence of God, the bed of sickness may prove to him the bed of death, yet are his last days and hours cheered by the sacred consolations of religion, and in his dying moments he is enabled to look with a living faith to that Saviour in whom he has learnt at length to place all his confidence and all his hope.

Some years later (i.e. 10 years before the Hospital-ships were abandoned) Kemball Cook again wrote on the virtues of the Charity:

> The ready access ensured to Seamen on board the Dreadnought would [now] appear to be known in every maritime port in the world. Here he finds a comfortable abode, well warmed and ventilated – shipmates at hand who can cheer and sympathize – nurses accustomed to his peculiarities – well-skilled medical and surgical relief – food and nourishment adapted to his particular case – a home during convalescence – clothing or a passage home, if required – and, above all, the kindly ministrations of a Messenger of GOD's Word to him.
>
> Thankful we may well be that our Sailors, – both in peace and war so valuable to our country, – are no longer left in their sickness and disease, to wander uncared for in our streets; or to be the victims of base harpies* as soon as they receive the wages which should comfort their families and make a provision for their future wants.
>
> The friends of the Seaman may well rejoice in the review of the past Forty years – not only from a consideration of the amount of good effected by this Society, but in the formation of those Institutions, where, though not afflicted with any bodily ailment, he may comfortably shelter himself when in port, from the haunts of vice and infamy so abundantly prepared for him, and learn to live a useful, honourable, and happy life. To the successful establishment of this Hospital may probably be traced in a great degree the commencement, some fourteen years later, of Sailors' Homes, of which those whose thoughts and labours from year to year are especially directed towards Seamen, can never speak too highly.[1]

An SHS minute of 1854 refers to the fact that the *Holy Scriptures* should be read to 'Lascars or Asiatic Seamen' in their own language. The following SHS minute written in 1840 also emphasises the value of the SHS to the seafarers of the world:

> The Superintendent and Surgeon reported the destitute condition of 22 Lascars sent from the Repulse, lately arrived from Calcutta, and stated that they found it necessary to destroy the Rags which partly covered some of them, their complaints Scurvy, one since dead'. It was ordered that the Secretary write to the owners of the Repulse requesting them to send 'a sufficient supply of warm clothing' as soon as possible.[2]

Limitations of care

Early reports contain reference to the fact that when first seen (on HMS *Grampus*) illness was frequently so far advanced that the physicians and surgeons had no chance of saving men who were 'almost beyond the reach of medical skill'. As the Charity became better known, however, patients were seen in a much earlier stage of sickness.

---

*A rapacious, plundering, or grasping person; one that preys on others. J A Simpson, ESC Wiener (eds). *The Oxford English Dictionary* 2nd ed. Oxford: Clarendon Press 1989; 6: 1129.

The Report for 1825 (i.e. before Lydekker's beneficience) contained gloomy news that owing to the 'declining state of their funds', the Society could only accept 'such Seamen as had been on shore the six months preceding their application'. In other words, they could no longer take *all* seafarers. The 21st Report directed the reader's attention to Lascars '[many of whom were] afflicted with scurvy in its most aggravated form'. Other Lascars also suffered from the effects of the cold, wet British climate. Also, 'upon their arrival in this country they frequently cease to be under the control of their European officers, and they persue ... a course which entails severe suffering, and even produces death'.[3]

A second *special* group consisted of '*incurable* [my italics] seamen'. It was unanimously resolved in late November 1824 that 'whenever a patient [especially one suffering from 'Rheumatic and Pulmonary complaints'] shall be declared to be incurable that immediate steps be taken for his removal'.

A disturbing incident, involving a patient at a very advanced state of illness (in fact 'in extremis') is recorded in a minute for 1864. This man had been visited repeatedly by two women, and ultimately 'contrary to advice' they conveyed him to the Shipping Office in the Minories in order to obtain his wages. The Shipping Master, believing that the man was *in extremis* refused to pay them and he died that same evening. It was Ordered (by the Society's Committee) 'that a discretionary power be given to the Medical Officers to prevent a patient leaving the Ship when they believe that death is imminent, or that his removal would endanger his life'. Furthermore, it was also ordered that 'the Superintendent shall remove from the ship persons of questionable character whose visits to a patient are considered injurious to his recovery or made with a view to obtain his property or wages'.

Several reports also addressed the issue of *urgent* cases. A minute in 1857 for example, states: 'Read a letter [from] Mr. Tudor and Mr. Busk stating that the admission of urgent cases had always been left to the discretion of the Surgeon', a sentiment reiterated in a later minute.[4]

The sailor in the Port of London

Repeated attention was given to the appalling conditions under which seamen then lived while in London:

> It may be remarked, that amongst the Seamen admitted, great numbers contract complaints *after* [my italics] their arrival in London, or labour under diseases incurred at other ports: This is attributed chiefly to their sudden removal from a good atmosphere and regular diet, into the wretched and filthy hovels in which Seamen are immured when on shore, and the irregular mode of living consequent upon the great change they experience. The conduct of many publicans and lodging-house keepers increases this evil, for possessing themselves of the Seamen's money and clothes, they keep them in their power until the whole of their means are exhausted, and they are then left pennyless and without friends.

> The effect of this system is very clearly defined by the fact, that very few of the men boarded at the 'Sailor's Home', have occasion to apply to this Hospital for relief; which is a proof of the steady management at that excellent establishment – of wholesome food, regularity of living, comfort and good example. This statement the Committee recommend to the notice of owners and ship masters; and suggest that they use their influence to produce a diminution of the injurious practices complained of, and exert their best energies to improve the moral as well as physical condition of Seamen.

Another insight into the life of the newly-arrived seaman in the Port of London is provided in the 1843 Report:

> It is a custom generally practiced by the crimps and the low house-keepers, who derive a living by their traffic with Sailors, to visit ships immediately upon their arrival, in order to persuade the Seamen to resort to their houses for board and lodging, where so little care is devoted to the wants of the inmates, that Seamen, seriously ill, when they land, are, through neglect or improper treatment, reduced to a worse – even to a hopeless – condition and, in such state – their money being spent, and their effects disposed of – they are inhumanly 'turned out to perish in the streets', as asserted in the First Report of this Hospital [see above]… On some of these occasions the Boarding-house keepers have been known to hold large balances belonging to their deceased lodgers, which, of course, never fell into the hands of their relatives; so that fraud – which is of minor importance – would seem to be the inducement which leads to the more weighty injury …
>
> Fully informed of the character of such houses, and of the habits of their proprietors, the Thames Police Magistrates have directed that their surveillance shall have the especial attention of the Police force of the district; but, it has been truly observed, that the offending parties are too wary to be detected in their iniquitous dealings, and have too perfect a knowledge of the law to place themselves directly within its reach.
>
> The Press also has animadverted upon the misdeeds of these men, but without its usual effect; their proceedings are not to be stayed by mere censure: and upon a consideration of these facts, the Committee hope that they shall stand excused for soliciting from the Shipping interest the exercise of its influence, through the Commanders of vessels, in favour of the 'SAILOR'S HOME' which is a large building, well constructed, and eligibly situated [at Well Street, London Docks] and furnished, as an abode for Mariners. From that excellent establishment the Committee must in justice remark, that the 'SEAMEN'S HOSPITAL' receives but few cases, and of those few, none have presented the dreadful features which have characterized the cases of patients admitted from lodging-houses kept by crimps.

The 1845 Report admirably outlined legislation which had recently been introduced protecting seamen in London, and other cities of Britain against the *crimps* (*see* Chapter 3):

> In the view of bettering the condition of the sailor during his temporary sojourn on shore, the Committee has noticed with singular satisfaction during the past year, the wise provision of the legislature, on the suggestion of Sir George Cockburn, to restrict the procuring of Seamen for Merchantmen to persons duly approved of and licensed by the Board of Trade, with the intention to suppress the evils of crimping, which has so long existed, with all its nefarious concomitants of crimps' lodging houses, their demoralization, plunder, and ruin of the sailor; the Dreadnought has been the too frequent receptacle of the wretched victims of these dens of infamy, for the Committee and the officers of the Hospital not to feel deeply the importance of pointing out such places of destruction to the sailor's health, morals, and social worth.
>
> In the establishment of sailors' homes in every great port, ... the nation would reap a gratifying reward in the physical, moral and general improvement of the entire class of sailors; who would thence become a credit to the country whose greatness and defence they so largely contribute to support. From sailors' homes a seaman's hospital would never receive those pitiable cases of neglected or ignorantly treated diseases, which are frequently brought into the wards in hopeless exhaustion, from the squalid haunts of infamy and vice, called Sailors' Lodging Houses. A sailor's health would be properly attended to, and medical relief, when needed, sought in time; and what is not the case in crimp's keeping, his property would be secured to him on his restoration to health.[5]

CHARLES DICKENS' VISIT IN 1851

It is difficult today to visualise life on the Hospital-ships, but the following account is of value in this context. In 1851 (i.e. some 20 years after the *Dreadnought* had replaced *Grampus)*, Charles Dickens (1812–70) or one of his journalist colleagues, recorded impressions of the Hospital-ship (*see* Chapter 8). The author seems overall to have viewed this experience with satisfaction:

> As we sighted Blackwall, the chequered sides of the old craft [the '*Dreadnought*'] dawned on our vision, and a steamer that was passing her looked like a pigmy. We landed at the pier, took a boat, and bobbed quietly alongside. 'That's the way up,' said the waterman, pointing to what, in the service, we call the 'accommodation ladder.' ... We mounted the ladder with a firm step (to borrow a well-known newspaper phrase); the great, high black-and-white sides seemed so familiar once more. The ports were open; but we missed the grim black gun-muzzles which protrude so calmly from your active-service vessels, and which usually,

with their brilliant polish, and their ornate 'tompions' corking them neatly, look as if they were meant only for ornament . . .

One's first sensation on reaching the deck was of a white bareness – it seemed so odd to be in a ship without rigging; but glancing round, we observed what a clear, broad promenade it made – how clean and orderly everything was. The first hospital feature presented itself, in two or three 'convalescents'; white caps covering them, and the inevitable pipe soothing their returning vigour. We moved first aft, and visited the office where the ship's books are kept. There a curiosity of historical interest was shown to us – a piece of glass from a cabin skylight of the 'Dreadnought' of old days, scrawled over with the names of those officers who were in her at Trafalgar . . .

The total number of patients received has been [63,345]. Of these, the British make up about [50,000]. The Norwegians and Swedes are the next in point of number; after these, come Prussians, East and West Indians, and Americans; then Germans, Russians, Danes, Italians, and Portuguese; then Dutchmen, Spaniards, and Africans. The list, too, comprises [182] South Sea Islanders, [16] Turks, and [38] Chinese, besides [181] 'born at sea'; – anomalous citizens of this planet, whom we defy any overseer going to keep to their proper parish. From all parts of the globe, you see, these poor fellows come to the 'Dreadnought': mankind has a family resemblance in disease, which in spite of their fightings, makes them brothers in pain. There, within the bulwarks originally built for the purpose of smashing mankind at large, they get tenderly doctored and nursed, and flannelled and gruelled, and almost petted, till they become once more able-bodied . . .

I observe fore-and-aft ten rows of little beds, each tenanted by its patient and covered by its little brown coverlet. Above each hangs a little board, whereon is marked his diet, his name, times of admission, and so forth. Some are dozing languidly; some are reading papers; some are curiously inspecting tracts; some are simply peering out from their night-caps with the clear sad eyes of illness – the clear look that seems to go so far, and fare so ill. A black man leans up with his queer comic negro expression. Presently, we come to a bed, and see a young fellow with a cheerful enough face. 'Amputation', says our guide, quietly, 'at the ankle', and the patient cocks up a gutta percha contrivance at the end of the severed limb; grinning as if it was rather a joke than otherwise ... One youth, with something between a grin and a blush, hints that milk diet is scarcely substantial enough for the existing state of his constitution, and receives an accession accordingly. Then we come to a brown fellow, who looks quite like an Englishman, but who is a Norwegian, and whose language is unintelligible. However, surgical tact joined to experience soon understands his case. The next patient is very, very far gone with consumption – he, poor fellow, asks for lime-juice; one is glad to think that there is still anything which can promise him pleasure here.

> One feels the emotion or relief at parting from this scene of pain and weariness – and feels it to be a somewhat ungrateful emotion – thinks how anxious everybody ought to be to aid an institution so valuable and so peculiar – an institution which appeals to what is best in the heart, and by so much that is attractive to the imagination.[6]

Two other reports concentrated on the future of the sailor, *after discharge* from the '*Dreadnought*'. The 1862 Report told how clothes, together with 'sufficient money to [enable him to] reach his home, if he be fortunate enough to possess one, would be provided from SHS funds'; others were found ships, or sent to their respective Consuls for assistance. The 1864 Report, on a slightly different tack, stressed that the sailor is 'generally alone in the world – but once within this Hospital, he finds a home until he is able to resume work on board ship'.[7]

Staffing of the Hospital-ships

It is important at this juncture to focus on some of the problems faced by the *staff* (Figure 9.2 and Appendix III) (*see also* Chapter 12).

Nursing staff

In the very early days, only male staff were employed on the Hospital-ships. On 21 November 1825, two female nurses joined, and an SHS meeting on 3 December 1831 heard that a female Matron had been appointed to the *Dreadnought* at a salary of £2=8=0 per month in order to 'take the general charge of the Hospital Clothing and Linen'. Hours of duty came under review, and it was decided in 1835 that in summer time they should start at 6.00am and in winter at 7.00am. Rules for nurses were strict; a Committee of Management minute dated June 1836 states: '... that the Superintendent should have power over the Nurses in seeing that wards are kept in proper order, and that they should not leave the ship without the superintendent's permission as well as that of the surgeon or his assistant'.

Another problem was *accommodation* for the female nursing staff, this was discussed by the Committee in November/December 1854. A later minute (in 1858) indicated that Mr Corner had advised that a female, rather than a male nurse should 'superintend the Medical deck'; but after obtaining the opinion of Mr George Busk [*see* Chapter 12) this suggestion was abandoned. The nursing staff was sometimes the subject of criticism: '... George Belt ... was discharged yesterday having been repeatedly intoxicated' and 'Nurse Vallance had been supplying [a patient] with articles of food without the surgeon's permission, charging the man for them and keeping back part of the money'.[8]

Allegations against the medical and other staff

Mr Chrystie, a *Lancet* reporter wrote a piece (published on 11 October 1828) alleging defects in the surgical practice of the *Grampus* (*see also* Chapters 11 and 12). The

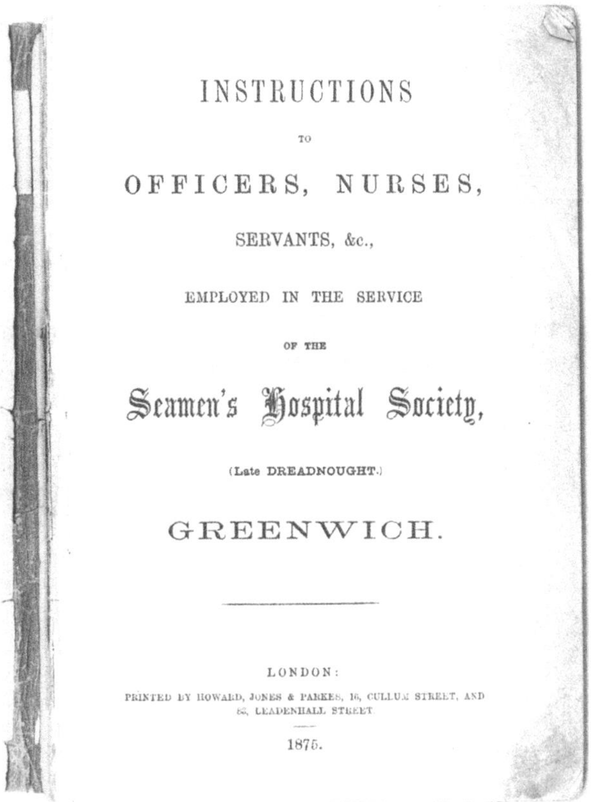

INSTRUCTIONS

TO

OFFICERS, NURSES,

SERVANTS, &c.,

EMPLOYED IN THE SERVICE

OF THE

Seamen's Hospital Society,

(Late DREADNOUGHT.)

GREENWICH.

LONDON:

PRINTED BY HOWARD, JONES & PARKES, 16, CULLUM STREET, AND 83, LEADENHALL STREET.

1875.

Figure 9.2: Instructions given to patients and staff [SHS archive]. This document is slightly later, but rules were of necessity very precise.

reporter assured the Committee of Management that he had obtained the information from Dr Roberts (a Visiting Physician – *see* Chapters 6 and 12). Some years later, in 1833 a complaint was received 'that a man sent by [a firm of subscribers] to the Hospital-Ship … with a serious injury of the hand and had not been properly treated'. Another (in 1858) from Guy's Hospital alleged (erroneously, as it transpired) that a patient 'had died there & that his death was hastened if not caused by removal from the Dreadnought'.

A complaint was received from the Honourable Company alleging that one of their Petty Officers 'had declared that he was neglected when on board the *Grampus*, as a Patient, that he saw no surgeon for several days, and was discharged not cured'; this complaint had had an adverse effect on the subscription(s) received by that ship. A later communication (from the Well Street Sailors' Home) complained (apparently justifiably) about the way in which applicants from the Destitute Sailors' Asylum (DSA) had been received by Mr Croft and Mr Corner. Mr Rooke (*see* Chapter 12) was involved in a complaint from the DSA; it was alleged that two men had been discharged from the *Dreadnought* before they were fit. Rooke (when questioned) told the SHS Committee that one of them had never been admitted to the *Dreadnought*, and the other was discharged cured! Staff discipline on board-ship was also a matter of intense interest. Mr Arnot (the Resident Surgeon) had, for example, at one stage been 'absent from his duty for two days'.

The chaplain was not above criticism: the SHS Committee were 'Unanimously of opinion that Mr Jones had acted improperly throughout [he had used 'intemperate language to the Carpenter before the congregation'] and requested the Chairman to admonish him accordingly'.[9]

On a more sensitive note, several discussions took place regarding delays in conducting inquests – with emphasis that a body should be inspected *on board* the *Dreadnought*, and also the place and cost of the burials of those unfortunate enough to die on the hospital-ship. A letter dated 11 October 1827 from the Revd Mr. Jones of St Nicholas Church, Deptford recorded that 'the Churchwardens should demand from henceforth *double dues* for all bodies taken there for interment from [the Society's Ship *Grampus*]'. It was ordered by the SHS Council of Management that the 'Secretary do wait upon the Revd. M^{r}. Mathew Vicar of Greenwich [in which parish the *Grampus* lay] and solicit that his parish will remit the fees usually demanded as the funds of this charity are very low'.[10]

Other matters during the days of the Hospital-ships

In July 1831, it is clear from the SHS minutes, that there was a growing feeling of impatience regarding the date upon which HMS *Dreadnought* would be ready to receive patients. And in 1857, the *Dreadnought* was replaced by HMS *Caledonia* (renamed *Dreadnought*) after a good deal of modification (*see* Chapter 8). A minute dated 1857 states that:

> ... the patients were all transferred safely and comfortably on Tuesday last, the weather being most propitious [*see* Chapter 8].

Ventilation, sanitation, water-supply (six tons of filtered water was used weekly) and heating (an ongoing problem without a simple solution) were all matters of crucial importance. Improvement in ventilation was given high priority as indicated by the following minute (June 1838):

> ... that Dr [George] Budd and Mr [George] Busk recommended that on the middle and Lower Decks the port tackle pennant holes which have been closed with Free nails should again be opened in every other Port on each side of the ship, the outside to be protected from the rain by a small hood the inside to be covered with a copper mouth piece, perforated with many holes to permit the foul air to escape. That on each Deck the present night lanterns be altered in shape and placed at

> the mouth of the air funnels to increase the Draft. On the spur Deck the present wooden covers of the air funnels be removed and Zinc cowls be substituted which can be turned with the wind.[11]

At a later date (February 1848), two Visiting Physicians – Black and Blackall (*see* Chapter 12) – again wrote to the SHS Committee with regard to inadequate ventilation, which they believed was exerting a significant influence on disease (especially diarrhoea and erysipelas) prevalence, and therefore delaying convalescence.

There is also frequent reference to the state of the Water Closets on board; in 1833, a minute states that they were to be 'lined with lead and ... a 12 Gallon Tank with Ball Cock be fitted on the larboard side of each deck ...'. In 1837, a careful examination of the WCs concluded that no change was required, but that 'six night stools be made'. A subsequent meeting however agreed with another recommendation that 'the Bath Rooms and Water Closets be removed forward on each of three decks, which alteration the Committee think will improve the atmosphere and prove a considerable saving of experience'.

The hospital lending library, for in-patients, was mentioned in several annual reports; gifts from the Society for Promoting Christian Knowledge, the Religions Tract Society and the British and Foreign Bible Society had significantly boosted numbers of books. These were by no means restricted to religious and moral works, but included: 'Accounts of voyages and travels, and works on several scientific subjects'. 'The Committee are much gratified [wrote Kemball Cook] by finding [the books] in constant use'. An inventory of specimens in the museum was requested by the SHS Committee in 1852.[12]

Another matter was control of vermin; in early 1832, the *Dreadnought* was 'much infested with rats' and to deal with this 'ten gallons of sperm oil and three Dozen Birch Brooms' were procured.[13] There must also have been a problem with security. Figure 9.3 for example, shows a notice announcing that a patient had been convicted of theft on board the third of the hospital-ships.

Maintenance of the ships themselves was of course important – painting, scraping, whitewashing and caulking.[14]

Owing to accommodation problems (see below) and overcrowding at the London Hospital (*see* Chapters 5 and 6), the SHS Committee was asked if it would consider co-operating with the establishment of another hospital on the Isle of Dogs; this offer was however declined![15] Another issue involved medicines and drugs for use on the Hospital-ships; for example leeches were supplied to the *Dreadnought* at 6/6 per 100 from a Mr. Potter.

Recognition of 'clinical material' by the University of Edinburgh

A minute in December 1837 stated that: 'The Surgeon reported that Certificates of attendance on the practice of this Hospital were received by the Examiners of the Royal College of Surgeons at Edinburgh'. The 1837 Annual Report enlarged upon this and recorded the fact that the University of Edinburgh had recognised the Hospital for *practical* training of medical students in surgical and anatomical studies; it was hoped, the report continued, that 'other Medical Bodies [would]

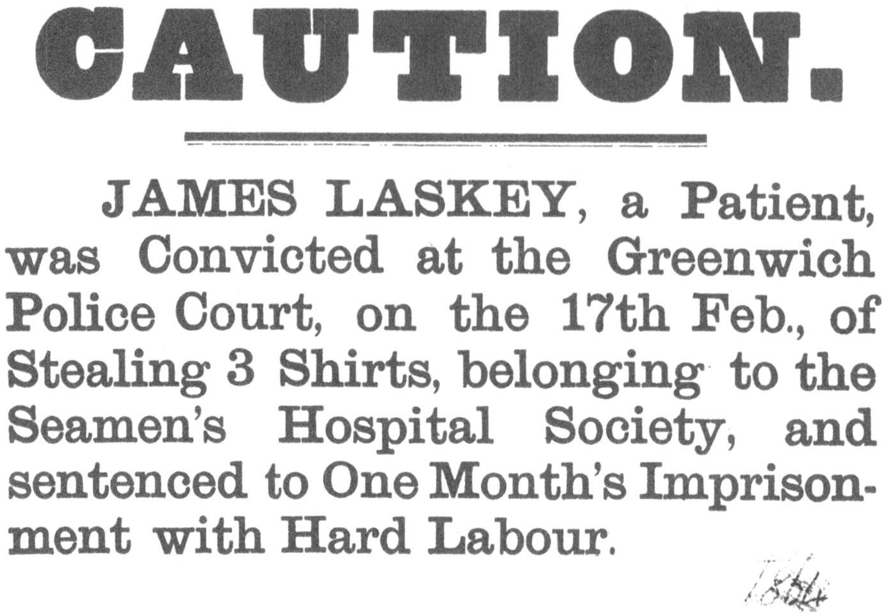

CAUTION.

JAMES LASKEY, a Patient, was Convicted at the Greenwich Police Court, on the 17th Feb., of Stealing 3 Shirts, belonging to the Seamen's Hospital Society, and sentenced to One Month's Imprisonment with Hard Labour.

Figure 9.3: Notice (dated 1864) indicating that a patient undergoing treatment on the third of the hospital-ships had been convicted of theft. [SHS archive].

discover, and admit the propriety of granting similar privileges to students in the profession'.[16]

The SHS log-book

During the years of the Hospital-ships, the SHS kept meticulous log-books. In 1831, for example, they were kept 'just as if the [Grampus] was still in commission'. Day-to-day activities including the state of the weather, the times of arrival and departure of medical and surgical staff and the chaplain, times of morning and evening prayers, patients' diet, etc, were all recorded. Of interest, activities on Christmas Day 1831 were precisely the same as on any other day. Appendix IV records extracts from the log-book for 1865–8 preserved in the SHS Archive. Subscriptions, it is recorded, were received at 'the bar of Lloyds, Jerusalem, Jamaica and the principal coffee houses and taverns in the Metropolis'.[17]

Extraneous factors affecting the hulks

The temperature of the River Thames water was the subject of considerable interest, the precise reason remaining unclear. A minute written in 1857, for example, states: 'Read a letter from the Registrar General requesting that he might be furnished ... with the daily temperature of the Thames water taken by the apparatus provided by the Astronomer Royal'. Pollution from Deptford Creek was a further matter of concern. The Phoenix Gas Co. was discharging 'gas water' into the Creek, a practice that the Lord Mayor ordered to be discontinued.

The major extraneous factor was, however, the intense pollution of the river in the mid-nineteenth century – culminating in the 'Great Stink' of 1858. A minute for June, 1858 records:

> Read a letter from the Physician stating that though there appeared to have no injury to the patients at present from the polluted state of the River they deemed it advisable to consider the Expediency of mooring the Dreadnought lower down the River.

As a result of this it was Ordered that the Admiralty be asked, if the 'state of the river' proved injurious to the patients, the ship could be moved to Greenhithe (*see also* Chapter 8). This was agreed, but as the Secretary of the SHS pointed out that this was as yet a precautionary arrangement.[18]

Patient accommodation

Owing to escalating numbers of in-patients (*see* Figure 9.1), accommodation on the *Grampus* had by the late 1820s become hopelessly inadequate; therefore a larger hulk (*see* Chapter 8) was sought, and obtained – again on loan from the Lords Commissioners of the Admiralty.

References and Notes

1 SHS Annual Reports. 1*:* 17–18; 29*:* 19; 40*:* 18–19.
2 *Ibid*. 21*:* 20; Committee of Management Minutes 5*:* 38; 7*:* 499. [See Appendix I for dates].
3 *Op cit*. See note 1 above. 2*:* 21; 5*:* 20; 6*:* 21–2; 12*:* 18–29.
4 *Op cit*. See note 2 above (Minutes): 2*:* 10; 388; 5*:* 143–4; 7*:* 476; 504; 8*:* 411.
5 *Op cit*. See note 1 above. 18*:* 21; 23*:* 18–19; 25*:* 19.
6 C. Dickens (ed). The "Dreadnought". *Household Words: a Weekly Journal*. 1851; 3: 516–9.
7 *Op cit*. See note 1 above. 24*:* 21; 26*:* 20. *Op cit*. See note 2 above (Minutes) 7*:* 202.
8 *Op cit*. See note 2 above (Minutes): 2: 80; 3*:* 42, 187; 4*:* 70; 7*:* 238, 246, 464, 520, 523; 9*:* 255. (*See* note 6 above).
9 *Ibid*. 2*:* 70, 108, 109, 116, 140, 178, 217, 253; 3*:* 216, 245–6, 337, 434; 5*:* 216; 7*:* 496, 499, 508.
10 *Ibid*. 2*:* 22, 261, 313; 4: 46–7; 5*:* 85–7; 7*:* 507, 546, 549, 551; 9*:* 61, 78.
11 *Ibid*. 3*:* 161, 170, 331–4; 4*:* 122, 178, 214, 233, 356–7; 5*:* 48; 6*:* 197–8; 7*:* 291, 379–80, 385, 404, 435, 520.
12 *Ibid*. 7*:* 60, 110, 114, 184.
13 *Ibid*. 3*:* 207.
14 *Ibid*. 2*:* 182; 3*:* 244–5, 329, 334; 4*:* 440, 552; 6*:* 415, 499, 7*:* 39, 181, 283, 549, 552–3.
15 *Op cit*. See note 1 above. 25*:* 18–19; 38*:* 19; 39*:* 20; *Op cit*. See note 2 above (Minutes) 7*:* 90, 97–8, 99.

16 *Op cit.* See note 1 above. 17: 20; *Op cit.* See note 2 above (Minutes): 4: 306.
17 Anonymous. A hundred years ago. *SHS Quart Mag* 1931; 3 (4): 9–10.
18 *Op cit.* See note 2 above (Minutes): 7: 448; 8: 8, 15, 18–19. [*See also*: G. C. Cook. Joseph William Bazalgette (1819–1891): a major figure in the health improvements of Victorian London. *J Med Biog* 1999; 7: 17–24; G.C. Cook. Construction of London's Victorian sewers: the vital role of Joseph Bazalgette. *Postgrad Med J* 2001; 77: 802–4; S. Halliday. *The Great Stink of London: Sir Joseph Bazalgette and the cleansing of the Victorian metropolis.* Stroud: Sutton Publishing. 1999: 210].

Chapter 10

Fund-raising in the days of the ships

The crucial subject of fund-raising has been addressed in Chapter 7. Raising the profile of the Charity, as well as increasing the 'index of awareness' to a far wider circle of individuals was under constant review. This was again emphasised in the 1861 Report:

> The Seaman who enters the Port of London, being in many cases ignorant of the English tongue and in almost every instance unable, from his mode of life as well as his state of health, to seek on shore a Governor of some Hospital, to give an order for admission – is admitted to the Dreadnought, by virtue of his calling. On presenting himself alongside [the ship], he receives the best Medical or Surgical advice, with careful Nursing, and whatever diet is considered best adapted to his particular case.

The following Report concluded:

> The only charitable Institution existing in England for the exclusive benefit of sick Sailors [i.e., the SHS], will never be suffered to languish while this Nation assumes the proud position she has so long maintained as a Maritime Power.

And the 1863 Report again highlighted the excellence of this under-recognised Institution:

> Among the many public institutions that proclaim individual exertions in the cause of charity, few, if any, stand so prominently forward in a national character, as the SEAMEN'S HOSPITAL. Situated close to the bulk of our Mercantile Marine, and gazed at daily by hundreds to whom the Thames is a highway for business or pleasure [*see* Chapter 2], it is, nevertheless believed that this Hospital is far better known abroad than at home. Its unique character; its high estimation in the mind of that amphibious creature, the Sailor, to whatever nation he may belong, should of itself create public interest.[1]

Finance and fund-raising

The 1829 and 1830 reports had highlighted also, presumably for fund-raising purposes, the fact that 'numerous accidents' (amounting to 80 in 1830) occurred on the River and the victims were 'immediately taken on board the Grampus'. A further line taken by Harley was to point out that before the SHS had been founded, many seamen used 'to conceal [disease] from their officers'; on long voyages this produced a 'danger [both] to the invalid himself and also the ship [which] must be too apparent to those acquainted with the restricted number of the crew of a merchant vessel'. Yet another tack to raise income was used by Harley in his 1837 Annual Report; by 'checking sickness, disease and misery, in the Port of London [in the absence of an Asylum, the SHS offered] protection to the *general health of the community* [my italics]'.

Anniversary Dinners were, as was the case with numerous charitable institutions in the nineteenth century, the highlight of the year's activities (*see* Chapter 7). Amongst others, the Duke of Wellington[2] and W E Gladstone[3] presided at two of these occasions; the 1838 Report recorded that that year the Chairman of the 17th Anniversary Dinner was 'Field Marshall His Grace the Duke of Wellington'.

In 1859, the SHS attempted to raise funds by other methods, there being so many Anniversary Dinners which were designed to boost the funds of various Charities; however, the 'amount of donations [was] so much lessened' by abandoning them that it was deemed 'advisable to resume the plan which had prevailed for 38 years'.[4] The 1843 Annual Report also stressed that the Society had an important rôle in *preventive* as well as in *curative* medicine.

The Merchant Seamen's Fund

In 1844, a Bill was brought before Parliament to amend the law relating to the Merchant Seamen's Fund (MSF). A clause had been inserted in the Merchant Seamen's Fund Act, allowing the SHS 5 per cent on any money collected from ships belonging to the Port of London. The draft new Bill provided for a financial grant to seamen from this fund. Unfortunately it omitted the former provision of 'appropriating five per cent. on the collections from ships belonging to the Port of London to the funds of the [SHS]'. This meant therefore that the sick sailor could receive his grant directly from the MSF, and then seek (free) treatment from the SHS! In any event this Bill was abandoned, and 'the legislature … recognised the service rendered to sailors by the [SHS], but assigning all fines, forfeitures, and penalties under the Act to its funds'. This was clearly laid out in the Act for the Registration of Seamen (7 & 8 Vic. c. 112) which came into operation on 1 January 1845. In this context, problems arose with payments from the Corporation of Liverpool – outlined in the Society's Annual Reports of 1847–9 and 1851.

However, the question of the rights of the SHS to penalties and forfeitures imposed by the 'General Merchant Seamen's Act' were materially affected by the 'Mercantile Marine Act' of 1849 – which came into effect on 1 January 1850. Under this Act, all dues made payable to the SHS were to be paid to the Board of Trade. There was naturally considerable apprehension regarding the MSF Winding-up Act of 1851, and this seems to have had serious financial repercussions for the [SHS]; however, the Board of Trade paid first an annual, then a lump sum to the SHS in lieu of their 5 per cent per annum on money collected by the Merchant Seamen's Society; nevertheless 'the receipts [were] considerably diminished'. The sum total was that (after some 20 years) due to this piece of legislation, the SHS would lose 'about one-fifth of the sum requisite to meet the yearly expenditure', amounting in monetary terms to £1150 per annum.[5]

Other funding initiatives

The Chatham Chest had come into being in 1588, i.e. following defeat of the Spanish Armada. Sir Francis Drake (1540–96)[6] and Sir John Hawkins (1532–95)[7] inaugurated a fund for the 'relief of naval seamen. Out of the wages of 'every mariner, seaman, and shipwright, receiving ten shillings per month or more, sixpence [was deducted] per month; out of the wages of every grommet [servant or valet], receiving seven shillings and sixpence per month, fourpence per month; and out of the wages of every boy receiving five shillings per month, threepence per month'. In 1803, administration of the Chatham Chest had been transferred to Greenwich Hospital for the payment of Out-pensions, and in 1814, these funds had been merged with those of the Greenwich Hospital (*see* Chapter 7).[8]

In order to attempt to boost the Society's funds, a Bill had been introduced into Parliament by George Lyall, Esq, MP for the City of London (*see* Chapter 7) to transfer part of the wealth accumulated by the 'Greenwich sixpences' to the Society. Unfortunately this had failed on two occasions, the matter being eventually raised successfully in the House of Lords by Lord Auckland.[9]

Assistance from HM Government?

The tenuous financial position of the Society in the early days of the Charity was summarised in the 1861 Annual Report:

> The constant aim of the successive Committees of this Institution has been to invest (in Government Funds), all the Legacies that may be received during their term in office, in order to create therewith a fund for the permanent endowment of the Hospital. In this endeavour they have so far been successful, that nearly half the ordinary expenses can now be met by the dividends on Stock purchased by money bequeathed to the Society from the time of its formation. But, during the last eight years, it has been found impossible to invest the whole amount annually received from bequests, a portion of such money having been repeatedly required for the service of the year.
>
> This necessity has arisen from the withdrawal of all the accustomed receipts of the Society, under two separate Acts of Parliament, known as "Merchant Seamen's Acts", whereby a diminution of income to the extent of about £1,700 per annum has been occasioned.
>
> As it appears by the accounts presented annually to Parliament, by the Mercantile Marine Department of the Board of Trade, to whom the payment of the monies withdrawn from this Society was transferred, – that a very large amount of money, gathered from Seamen in vari-

> ous ways is accruing, the Committee in the early part of last year drew up a memorial upon this subject, and a deputation from their number, headed by their Chairman ... had an interview with the President of the Board of Trade to present the same, and urge its consideration – they were told, however, that inasmuch as the destination of all this money was the National Exchequer, their object could only be accomplished by an appeal to Parliament, which in the present financial condition of the country the members of the Government could not advise.
>
> The Committee have, therefore, taken no further step, but they still feel that at least some portion of the loss sustained by the withdrawal of money which Parliament directed to be paid to them for the support of the Hospital, should be made up by a grant from the large sum received annually by Her Majesty's Government, as the unclaimed wages and effects of deceased Seamen.

The 43rd (1863) Report (also written by Kemball Cook) maintained that:

> The proposal by the Chancellor of the Exchequer ... to levy Income Tax on the receipts of Charitable Institutions, led the [SHS] Committee (in common with other similar Societies) to petition the House of Commons on the subject by way of remonstrance. For the information of the public generally, the Committee think it well to quote a passage from that petition, as explanatory of the financial condition of this Institution. "The Society was in the habit of receiving, for many years, a considerable income, amounting to nearly £1,200 per annum, arising from various fines imposed on Seamen, under the provisions of the Mercantile Marine Acts, and by those Acts directed to be paid over to this Society.
>
> At the instance of the Board of Trade, the Committee were induced to forego their right to such fines, and to accept in lieu thereof certain specified sums of nearly equivalent amount, received by the Board in each year as fines on the loss of register tickets, and which were accordingly directed by the Merchant Seamen's Amendment Act to be paid over to the Society. But on the very day on which such Amendment Act came into operation, the Board of Trade issued orders for discontinuing the system of registering Seamen by means of tickets; whereby the Society was at once, and without notice, deprived of nearly one-sixth part of its entire income".[10]

Donations from ships crews?

Fund-raising continued, however, to be a matter of monumental importance, but improvement was only possible if the profile of the Charity was raised (see above): Kemball Cook considered in his 1857 Report that, for example:

> When it is considered that in each year about 28,749 vessels (including repeated voyages) enter the River Thames and that the 58,307 men employed therein find there a Hospital into which, free of all expense,

> the sick among them can be at once sent to be provided with experienced Medical and Surgical skill, careful Nursing, and everything that can contribute to their comfort and restoration to health and strength, the Committee feel it but just to remind Captains, Officers and Crews, that the payment of a very small sum on each return voyage, would provide the Hospital from this source alone, with sufficient to meet its necessities.[11]

The 1836 report – which was written some five years after transfer to HMS *Dreadnought* – was again written with funding (see above) in mind:

> The appearance of the noble Ship Dreadnought must draw every reflecting mind to consider to what defence, when at war, this Country is chiefly indebted; – how much England has to thank her undaunted Seamen for her present position; – to whose exertions, in time of peace, she is equally indebted for her commercial wealth and prosperity. A contemplation of these facts cannot but lead to a just and favourable opinion of the value of the Seamen's Hospital.[12]

References and notes

1 Annual Reports 41: 20; 42: 18; 43: 19–20.

2 **Arthur Wellesley, first Duke of Wellington** MP, KB, GCB (1769–1852) had a distinguished military career, culminating in his defeat of Napoleon at Waterloo (1815). He subsequently became Prime-minister of Great Britain. [*See also*: Chapter 1].

3 **William Ewart Gladstone**, MP (1809–1898) was an eminent British statesman and Prime Minister on four occasions. [*See also:* H C G Matthew. Gladstone, William Ewart (1809–1898). In: H C G Matthew, B Harrison (eds). *Oxford Dictionary of National Biography.* Oxford: Oxford University Press 2004; 22: 383–409; R Jenkins. *Gladstone.* London: MacMillan 1995: 698].

4 Committee of Management Minutes. 4: 319, 340, 421; 5: 255; *Op cit.* See note 1 above (reports). 18: 18; 40: 21.

5 *Op cit.* See note 1 above. 24: 21; 25: 20; 27: 19-20; 28: 21; 29: 19; 31: 19; 30: 18-19; 31: 18–19; 34: 18.

6 H Kelsey. Drake, Sir Francis (1540–1596). In: H C G Matthew, B Harrison (eds). *Oxford Dictionary of National Biography.* Oxford: Oxford University Press 2004; 16: 858–70.

7 B Morgan. Hawkins, Sir John (1532–1595). In: H C G Matthew, B Harrison (eds). *Oxford Dictionary of National Biography.* Oxford: Oxford University Press 2004; 25: 919–27.

8 Anonymous. The chest at Chatham. *SHS Quart Mag* 1934; 6 (1): 20.

9 *Op cit.* See note 1 above. 14: 18–19; '*Sixpences paid by Merchant Seamen to Greenwich Hospital, to the Society for the relief of aged and worn-out Seamen, their Widows and Children'.* [SHS Archive].

10 *Op cit.* See note 1 above. 41: 20–21; 43: 19–20.

11 *Ibid.* 9: 21–2; 10: 22; 15: 20; 17: 20, 32: 21; 22: 18; 37: 20.

12 *Op cit.* See note 1 above. 16: 20. *Op cit.* See note 4 above (Minutes): 3: 149; 7: 435–7; 439–40, 446–7.

Chapter 11

Disease(s) on the Hospital-ships

In the first half of the nineteenth-century, i.e. when the Society was founded, disease was in the main still classified according to symptoms/signs, without any understanding of a causative agent being responsible; this had to await the advent of the 'germ-theory' of disease in the latter days of the century. Therefore, diseases were classified in much the same way as during the Hippocratic era. 'Fevers' were considered to be generalised forms of non-specific disease which (with the exception of smallpox – which was readily identifiable) were generated by 'foul air and putrefying matter'. It was not until 1837 that typhus was separated (in the USA) from typhoid fever; first recognition of this distinction in Britain in 1850 was due to (Sir) William Jenner FRS (Figure 11.1) – physician to the London Fever Hospital. It was not until 1843 that relapsing fever was recognised as a separate entity.[1,2]

In 1804, Parliament produced a report on the '*Infectious fever*'; most cases were probably examples of epidemic typhus, which had existed in London for many years, and had presented a major problem at the London Fever Hospital established at Gray's Inn Lane in May 1801; 29 out of 325 'Fever Patients' admitted there had died. This hospital had been followed by a 'House of Recovery' opened in the same Lane, in February 1802; it was 'open to all applicants, at all days and hours' and patients were conveyed there 'in a litter belonging to the establishment, thereby [obviating] the use of coaches or sedan chairs'. This disease, which was prevalent 'among the poorer Parts in confined Situations', was estimated to have produced a total of 3,000 deaths annually in the previous few years. The report pointed out that the present hospitals were too small to exert a significant impact on the incidence of disease generally, and that more funds would be required to expand this facility.

A larger enquiry carried out by a 'Select Committee' (again followed by a *Parliamentary Report*) was held 14 years later – in 1818. Evidence was taken from many eminent physicians both from the House of Recovery, and from all major London Hospitals, and it was concluded that the 'contagious fever in London' had assumed epidemic proportions in 1817, especially amongst the *poorer classes*. The disease was in fact so common, that London's hospitals could *not* cope with all cases requiring admission. Also, infection was sometimes contracted *within* the hospitals; however, 'As long as fever cases can be diluted through a large ward, with proper attention to ventilation [there was, it was concluded], scarcely any danger of contagion ...'. This report ended by regretting that '[no] hospital in the Metropolis [possessed] a register of diseases':

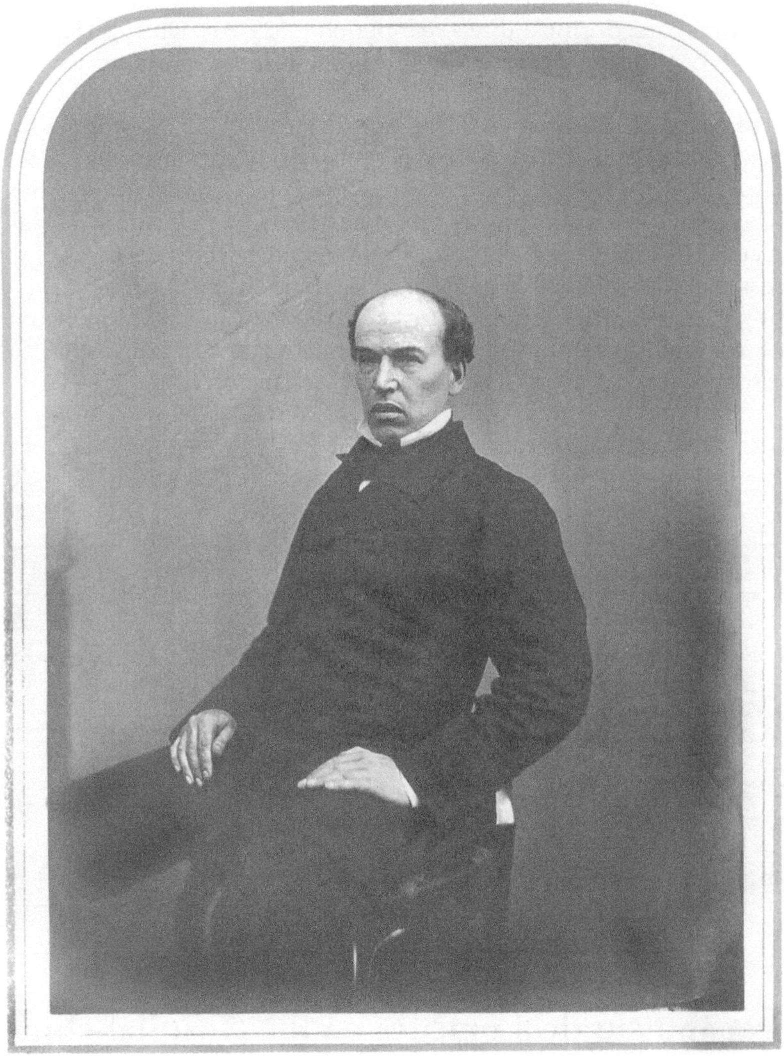

Figure 11.1: Sir William Jenner Bt GCB FRCP FRS (1815–98). Courtesy, the Wellcome Library, London.

> … in their opinion [it] would be advisable to register, not only the diseases, but also the name and profession of the patient. It must at all times be a matter of useful knowledge to be able to learn the quality and extent of the different diseases that prevail at different periods; and Your Committee have felt the want of that information, arising out of this strange irregularity, in not being able to ascertain the average fever cases that have occurred for some years past in the Metropolis.[3]

With this background, it is not surprising therefore that 'Fevers' heads the list of *acute* cases admitted to the '*Grampus*' in the early days of the SHS. One of the SHS physicians, George Roupell (*see* Chapter 12) provided a detailed 'breakdown' of cases under his care, during a three-year period (1829–31). During 1829 there were 181 cases of 'continued', and 112 of 'intermittent' *fever*; mortality was, however, limited to seven cases. On the list of diagnoses were also: 'Inflammation of the lungs' (118 cases), 'Inflammation of the bowels' (62), 'Affections of the brain' (28) and 'Rheumatism' (91); deaths were recorded as ten, ten, three and zero in these four groups respectively. The *chronic* admissions were dominated by 'Phthisis' (presumably in most cases, tuberculosis, and many cases were in South Sea Islanders); no less than 25 out of 30 sufferers died. The remainder were: 'Diseases of the heart' (8), 'Diseases of the stomach' (29), 'Dropsy' (11), and Scurvy (19); mortality in these four groups was two, zero, three and zero respectively. In the following two years, the same Visiting Physician also recorded the diagnoses of admissions under his care; the diagnoses and mortality rates in 1830 are shown in Table 11.1.[4]

Table 11.1: Roupell's classification of medical cases admitted to HMS *Grampus* (the first SHS Hospital-ship) under his care during 1830 (i.e. 22 January 1830–23 January 1831).

	No. admitted	*Deaths*
Fevers	273	6
Inflammation in the chest	126	15
Diseases in the Abdomen	69	5
Affections of the Brain	24	7
Rheumatism	141	2
Phthisis	22	12
Scurvy	11	–
Dropsy & Diseases of the Heart	25	13
Diseases of the General Health	10	1
TOTAL	701	61

Medical and surgical practice on the Hospital-ships

Mortality-rate on HMS *Dreadnought* was the subject of much public interest. Following a statement in the *Morning Post* for 10 February 1837, and some years later an anonymous letter to the *Times* (in August 1845) speculated that the mortality rate on the *Dreadnought* was excessive (both statements were subsequently corrected), there was a good deal of discussion, and George Budd (Visiting Physician) (*see* Chapter 12) produced evidence from 400 cases under his care over a four-month period, that most morbidity in the seafaring community arose from disease contracted *while the sailors were in fact in the Port of London*.[5] It was left to Richard Goolden (also a Visiting Physician) (*see* Chapter 12) however, to produce a breakdown of comparative mortality-rates at St Thomas's and St Bartholomew's Hospitals in the years 1843–44 (Table 11.2). It transpired that in 1844, only one in 25.46 died on the *Dreadnought*, compared with one in 15.23, and one in 15.71 at

Table 11.2: Goolden's summary of (overall) death-rates at St Thomas's and St Bartholomew's Hospitals over a 12-year period (1833–1844).

Year	*St Thomas's*		*St Bartholomew's*	
	Admitted	*Died*	*Admitted*	*Died*
1833	2866	284	5164	392
1834	2904	237	5267	346
1835	2974	283	5644	366
1836	3025	298	5548	424
1837	2971	303	5452	572
1838	3033	300	5135	480
1839	3086	244	5038	364
1840	2897	317	5015	419
1841	3143	341	4724	320
1842	3284	220	4839	339
1843	3609	249	5372	377
1844	3731	245	5673	361
Average death-rate (%)		8.6		7.6

St Thomas's and St Bartholomew's, respectively. The Registrar General's report on the overall average death-rate in London gave a ratio of one in 44.[6]

Controversy also arose regarding *surgical* competence on board the *Grampus*. A correspondent to *The Lancet* suggested in 1828, for example, that the late [resident] surgeon (D G Arnot) transferred his 'lithotomy cases' either to the London or another metropolitan hospital. This allegation brought forth a rapid response from the SHS secretary – Richard Harley – who pointed out that only a single case of bladder stone had been received on the *Grampus*, and due to the 'express desire of the parents of the patient, this man was transferred to St Thomas' Hospital where, owing to consent not being granted, the operation was *not* performed'.[7]

Although five 'specific' diseases (see below) are highlighted in the SHS Committee of Management Minutes and Annual Reports, the sole detailed 'breakdown' of medical admissions on the Hospital-ships (apart from those of Roupell) is due to Stephen Ward (Chapter 12) – writing in 1860; Table 11.3 summarises his diagnoses/symptoms in 1,000 *consecutive* admissions under his care. It was the author's intention to dissuade '… many medical men, that the *Dreadnought* is little better than a refuge for patients suffering under scurvy and chronic dysentery'. As well as a source for study of 'organic and blood diseases contracted in tropical climates', together with a comparison of the 'disease of different races', many of the cases [he wrote] were similar to 'acute and chronic diseases … met with in other metropolitan hospitals'.[8]

Several of the individual medical cases, excluding the major entities covered in the Minutes and Annual Reports, were recorded in contemporary medical journals. Thus, two sailors suffering from diphtheria, both of whom recovered, were documented in 1859.[9] A case of 'idiopathic tetanus' was described by Harry Leach (see

Table 11.3: Diagnoses/symptoms in 1000 consecutive admissions under a single physician (Dr Stephen Ward) to the third of the Hospital-ships, in 1860.

Brain and Nervous System		
Cerebral congestion	5	
Delirium tremens	19	
Epilepsy	10	
Insanity	2	
Neuralgia	2	
Paralysis	24	
Spinal debility	1	
Sciatica	11	
Tetanus	1	
	75	
Thoracic Viscera		
Heart and large vessels	23	
Asthma	3	
Bronchitis – acute, 24; chronic and slight, 42	66	
Emphysema	3	
Haemoptysis	6	
Laryngitis (subacute and chronic)	5	
Pleuritis	5	
Pleurodynia	1	
Pneumonia and pleuro-pneumonia	41	
Phthisis	77	
	230	
Abdominal Viscera		
Oesophagus, schirrus of	1	
Constipation	1	
Colic	5	
Diarrhoea	47	
Dysentery	56	
Dyspepsia	5	
Epiploitis	1	
Peritonitis	6	
Stomach, derangement and disease of	7	
Tonsillitis	15	
Worms	4	
Spleen, disease of	7	
Liver, disease of, including cirrhosis and abscess	23	
Kidneys, disease of	17	
	197	
General Diseases		
Fever – typhoid, 60; typhus, 1; relapsing, 2; febricula, 46	109	
Ague, 94; hemicrania, 1; ague cachexia, 7	102	
Anaemia and debility	40	
Rheumatism – acute, 53; chronic and slight, 44	97	
Exanthemata – measles, 5; scarlatina, 11	16	
Erysipelas	11	
Skin diseases	14	
Periostitis	3	
Anasarca	8	
Cholera	1	
Opium-eating, effects of	1	
Scurvy	96	
	498	
		1000

below) in 1870;[10] the patient was managed (unsuccessfully) with chloral hydrate and chloroform – when tetanic spasms occurred. A further communication concerned the use of zinc phosphate in the management of a woman who was under the care of Robert Barnes suffering from epilepsy (*see* Chapter 12). [11]

Surgical disease seems to have been dominated by venereal disease – syphilis and gonorrhoea – and its complications [see below]. Regrettably, however, no 'breakdown' of surgical cases (comparable to that for medical ones) seems to have survived, although John Tudor, Visiting Surgeon provided his impressions of hygienic standards, together with the outcome of several major surgical operations. Only one out of 14 operations had been followed by death: ten of these consisted of amputations, and the others: excision of an elbow, removal of a 'large tumour of the left temporal region', trephining of the skull, and removal of three large tumours from the legs, respectively.[12] Several case-reports of operative intervention were subsequently recorded in the medical literature. A case of advanced disease (possibly tuberculosis) involving the hip-joint[13] under Henry Rooke (Resident Surgeon) (*see* Chapter 12), and presumed malignant disease of the testicle – with liver metastases[14] (also under Rooke) were, for example, documented. Mr Croft, a house-surgeon recorded four cases 'of interest' (all under George Busk) from the 'return for the month of March': cases of urethral stricture, amputation, necrosed bone, and 'removal of tumours'.[15] This was an era when chloroform anaesthesia was first given, sometimes with serious complications.[16]

The surgical benefits of acceptance of the 'germ-theory' which had to await Joseph Lister (1827–1912)'s observations; the emphasis on medical care, therefore continued to be on cleanliness and ventilation, together with the prevention of contagion – conveyed in the main by unwashed hands, etc.

Surviving documents concentrate on five diseases which were prevalent on the Hospital-ships: typhus fever, venereal disease, cholera, scurvy and smallpox. In addition tuberculosis must have been a major problem – but was *not* recognised as a single affliction in the years 1821–70.

Typhus Fever

There seems little doubt that early descriptions of 'fever' on the *Grampus* usually represented epidemic typhus (a louse-borne rickettsial infection). Roupell had written a 20-page pamphlet on 75 cases (12 of whom died) of a febrile illness encountered amongst the sailors on the SHS Hospital-ships – which he had personally seen between 1 January and 18 April 1831. Most cases had originated at an 'asylum' (i.e. a place of shelter) situated at Globe Street, Wapping, established 'to relieve by food and Shelter the misery in which numbers of the lower class of maritime people are involved during the spring'. Roupell considered that these cases (at Wapping) were 'produced by the crowded and ill ventilated state of that place'.[17]

At a meeting of the SHS Committee on 11 February 1831 it was 'ordered that a letter be written to the Committee of that Asylum requesting them not to forward any more cases of Fever to the Grampus as they cannot be taken on board'. A week later a minute refers to a letter signed by Roupell and Edward Seymour (*see* Chapter 12) stating that: 'The nature of the disease [a 'Fever of an unusual character'] may induce a fear that the Disease may spread in the present crowded state of the Hospital, [and they strongly recommend] that the admissions should be restricted to such a number as can be beneficially accommodated'. On 2 April the Committee ruled that: 'following admission of three cases of fever from the 'Sailors Rest' ... letters be written to the Asylums for Seamen informing them that no other cases of Fever will be admitted on board'.[18]

George Busk (*see* Chapter 12) reported to the Committee on 18 November 1842 that most cases of this epidemic febrile illness occurred in men 'received from Colliers'; it was thus 'ordered [by the SHS Committee] that ... this subject [be brought to] the notice of ship owners in the North'. In an attempt to eradicate typhus (by that time theoretically separable from typhoid fever), the 1842 Annual Report stated: 'The Committee have reason to expect that by impressing upon the Owners and Masters [of colliers] in which this disease is found mostly to exist, the very great value of attention to cleanliness and ventilation [which] may contribute materially to reduce the frequency of Typhus Fever'. This theme was vented again in the 1847 annual report: '... in the present days of sanitary precautions, their benefits may be made to reach the floating habitations of the useful and laborious class of men engaged in the coasting trade of this country'.[19]

There seems little doubt therefore, that most cases of 'fever' on board the hospital-ships were associated with the poorer stratum of society [see Chapter 1] and/or overcrowding, and resulted from epidemic typhus, or 'Jail Fever'. In 1863, the Committee received a report that the Boatswain's wife had typhus fever; she had lived with her husband and three children in the same cabin [on the third hospital-ship] in which the former boatswain had died of typhus'.[20]

Venereal Disease

No surviving SHS document records the true prevalence of venereal disease (which was considered *surgical*) during the years 1821–70. This disease was however a colossal problem in the nineteenth century merchant navy. During the latter days (1864–65) of the Hospital-ships, the Admiralty appointed a committee to investigate the problem(s) associated with VD in the British Army and Navy; many leading physicians and surgeons including: Arthur Farre FRS (1811–87), William Jenner FRS (1815–98) (see above), Erasmus Wilson FRS (1809–84), Jonathan Hutchinson FRS (1828–1913), James Paget FRS (1814–99) and James Syme (1799–1870) were invited to give evidence; the Society's representative was Busk (*see* Chapter 12), the most experienced surgeon on the *Dreadnought's* staff.

Busk gave his evidence to the *Committee on Venereal Disease in the Army and Navy* (at the Admiralty) on 2 May 1865. In a pre-amble, he estimated that the average number of patients on the *Dreadnought* ('in my time') had been 170 or 180, and that the annual admission rate was 1,500–2,000. The patients, he maintained, were 'Entirely sailors in active employment, with the exception of a few cases of accidents from manufactories on shore'. 'The Hospital [he continued was] intended entirely for sailors who have been at sea within six months'. They were from 'Wapping, Poplar, Limehouse,

Gravel-lane, and those places [from up the river],' and their general class, habits, ages and constitutions were similar to 'those at Portsmouth, Devonport, and Chatham'. Management on board the *Dreadnought* was aimed at getting 'the men well as fast as [possible], and to get rid of them; we cannot [he continued] keep men under treatment for six months [as was done in the Peninsular War 1808–14]'.

Was there anything in the 'constitution' which predisposed to the development of *syphilis,* Thomas Balfour FRS (1813–91) asked? Busk's reply was in the negative; 'men who have been drinking hard, or, as sailors call it, "knocking about", very often come in with greatly inflamed sloughing sores [on their genitalia], which I attributed to their neglect'. He was also asked by Spencer Smith, Secretary of the Committee whether he felt that:

> 'the cases … on board the "Dreadnought" do as well as in [land-based] hospitals, or that the locality of the ship, or a miasma from the river, might exercise any effect [on venereal disease in the sailors]?'

His reply was that he did not consider that 'cases [of VD] are affected in that way'. Although he had seen 'A great many' cases of gonorrhoea, he recognized 'gonorrhoeal rheumatism, the major (venereal) problem was undoubtedly syphilis. He had seen numerous sores on the genitalia (usually 'about the frenum, or the lining of the prepuce [foreskin]) … and less often the rectum and 'about the verge of the anus [a not infrequent site of primary sores]'. Busk also claimed to have seen sores 'on the hands of the nurses', which did not possess a venereal connection.

He firmly believed (correctly in the light of later evidence) that having once had a sore, an individual was never 'safe from the secondary symptoms'; 'tertiary syphilis [he claimed] rarely [occurred] within three years after a primary sore'. Asked about the high prevalence of *phagedenic* (or *sloughing*) *sores* (which are probably more common on the *Dreadnought* than elsewhere and had to be differentiated from 'simple primary sores' (ordinary abrasions) – which were not often seen – and 'indurated sores', he considered that the sole cause was 'the bad habits of the men'; 'Generally [he continued] when they come ashore they set out to drink, and they perhaps eat very little, and drink a great deal, and they are incessantly going about with women with all kinds of diseases upon them; and in that way they get very foul sores'.

Another line of questioning related to whether or not this disease (VD) was related to (or worsened by) climatic factors. Busk again answered in the negative, but in reply to a question from Benjamin Babington FRS (1756–1833), he considered that the worst disease was in men 'coming from China and the East'. Some of these men who had come from these parts, he maintained (when questioned by Frederic Skey FRS [1798–1872]) had sores which were 'as intractable as a cancer, destroying the whole penis, and sometimes the scrotum, and eating under the arch of the pubis'… 'that is [Busk continued] a peculiar form of syphilitic disease, if it be such, that I am not acquainted with as occurring in this country [England]'.[21] In reply to Balfour, Busk said he did *not* consider that the disease 'resulted from the scorbutic condition … after a long voyage', although he *had* often seen syphilis in a scorbutic patient.

Regarding treatment, the most dramatic form according to Richard Quain FRS

(1816–98) was: 'very extensive amputations [sic] of the prepuce [which was most frequently performed] by the Assistant-Surgeon on board the Dreadnought'. Busk however, felt that 'except in the case of a long narrow prepuce [that procedure] should be avoided'. A great many less invasive ('medical') measures were also used to manage syphilis; there are for example, numerous references to the use of mercury (usually administered as a 'blue pill' – one grain three times daily – but also 'rubbed in' locally); in fact all 'indurated sores' were so managed. This was not, however, the treatment recommended for phagedenic sores. Mercury was usually given in conjunction with a 'good diet', and continued for 'at least six weeks'. Alternative regimens involved 'sarsaparilla [which was *not* very effective] and iodide of potassium [especially for periostitis]'. For small, recent soft sores 'nitric acid or caustic' (or escharotics) were used – but that did not necessarily protect against 'secondary symptoms'. For large soft sores, Busk apparently used 'black-wash'. The correct treatment for *gonorrhoea*, Busk claimed in a reply to James Donnet (1816–1905), was an 'injection of a solution of acetate of zinc, or by cubebs and copaiba'.[22]

Cholera

The *Asiatic cholera* was undoubtedly the most alarming disease encountered on the Society's Hospital-ships, for the disease progresses so rapidly. Major outbreaks (with peak prevalence rates) in London occurred in: 1831–2, 1848–9, and 1853–4. Drinking water in the ships was derived from the mainland supply and delivered via a pipe; it is likely therefore that most, if not all, cases had their origin in London. However it is not impossible that a minority of cases were 'imported', but owing to the short incubation-period (two or three days) of *Vibrio cholerae* infection, this seems unlikely. Some sailors had consumed drinking water from ports up and down the country, e.g. Sunderland and Guernsey; while others seem to have been infected in Hamburg.

The first London outbreak

First indications that this 'pestilence' had reached England were recorded in late 1831, and first evidence of the *'visitation'* onboard the *Dreadnought* did not occur until May 1832. However, at a Committee of Management meeting in November 1831, Roupell (see above) requested clear guidelines regarding the course of action, if the disease appeared on the ship; it was decided 'after mature consideration' to *refuse* admission, and to instruct Mr Lawson (Resident Surgeon) to report to the Parochial Authorities at Greenwich and Deptford (the Central Board of Health [CBH] having been apprised), and for the Superintendent to 'exercise all necessary precautions against the risk of the ship being placed under quarantine'. There was obviously concern that this serious malady might spread throughout the Port of London, and it was felt that the Steam Washing Company's premises on the Isle of Dogs might be designated a site for the reception of cholera patients.[23]

On the morning of 4 May 1832, the SHS encountered its first case. The affected patient was 'brought alongside the Dreadnought', and since the *Dover** (*see* Chapter 8) moored off Limehouse had already been 'paid off' there was apparently nowhere to send him. The Committee ordered that Mr Lawson (surgeon in charge) contact the Thames Police Magistrates to seek suitable accommodation. The *Dover* (*see* Chapter 8) at that time moored off Deptford (and under the orders of the CBH) was immediately allocated by the Admiralty as a lazaretto or cholera-ship. Details of other hulks loaned by the Admiralty as cholera-ships, are given in Chapter 8.

In August, the Committee was furnished with an update of *cholera* cases on board the *Dreadnought* over the previous week: 'admitted 13, discharged cured 3, died 7, remaining 9'. The CBH was kept in the picture throughout; both Roupell and Lawson continued with their conviction that 'cholera cases [should not be] received on board the Dreadnought'. In January of the following year, Lawson reported that 'the cholera ship is now clear of patients'. However, that was not the end of the epidemic, for in 1833 he was to inform the Committee that: 'two cases were received yesterday: one 'a suspicious and the other a decided case of cholera ...' the Committee ordered that Busk and Harley contact the London Hospital to ask them to receive the cases.[24]

The overall SHS experience during 1832 was summarised in the Annual Report for 1832: Lawson had volunteered to take charge of the Lazaretto (i.e. HMS *Dover*) on condition that the CBH provide nurses, medicines, etc. – which they declined to do! Instead the CBH offered '... thirty shillings per diem to meet all charges, including burials'; as the Committee had had direction of the Lazaretto for 166 days (i.e. until 31 October 1832), they received £249 (including the cost of 90 burials). In the entire outbreak there had been 161 cases, of whom 93 had died. However, this outbreak smouldered on and the 14th Annual Report (1834) informed its readership that under the Lords of the Admiralty, the Society 'had taken charge of the *Echo*† hulk (*see* Chapter 8), stationed off Deptford ...' where 35 cases had been received, of whom 11 had died.[25]

But the disease lingered on! On 19 October 1837 an emergency meeting of the Committee of Management was told that cholera had broken out on the Orlop Deck of the *Dreadnought*; there had been 11 cases with three deaths; 'two others had recovered from that complaint, but had died of other diseases'. It was resolved that these cases be reported to Sir John Russell, Secretary of State for the Home Department, and that Busk and Harley should attend the Home Office in order to provide further information.[26]

*HMS *Dover* (formerly *Bellona*) had been built at Venice in 1806 (see Chapter 8); she was a 692 ton 5th Rate with a gun deck length of 131′ 6″. In 1819 she had served as the flagship of A B Bingham, and the following year Sir J P Beresford. The hulk was sold on 21 January 1836.

†HMS *Echo* had been built at Woolwich in 1827; she was a 295 ton Paddle Vessel, possessing 2–6 powder guns. Most of her existence was devoted to surveying the River Thames, but later, she was a tug at Portsmouth.

The second major outbreak

The second major London epidemic took place during 1848 and 1849. In August 1848, the Society gave their assurance to the Lords Commissioners of the Admiralty that they were ready, if the need arose, to take 'medical charge of any Floating Cholera Hospital for Seamen in the Port of London'. It was not long before Busk was to report two cases of cholera on board – one in a man who had been on the *Dreadnought* for six months, and the other who had been admitted with that ailment. At this point there seems to have been a reversal of the former policy, in reply to a letter from Sir J Hall, Secretary of St Katherine's Docks: 'isolated cases would be received on board [the *Dreadnought*] for the present'. The disease was to re-emerge however, but the '*Iphigenia*' (*see* Chapter 8),* which became a hospital-ship, had been moved to Woolwich. An assurance was given by the Admiralty that 'the *Iphigenia* would be placed close to the Dreadnought on Monday 23rd ult. clean and ready for use'. It is clear that this 'visitation' reached its peak in early 1849; 250 cases were admitted to the *Iphigenia* up to 28 June of that year, and 'Cholera medicines, prepared by the Society's Medical Officers' seemed to prove beneficial. On 21 December 1849 the Committee was read a letter from the Chaplain of the Thames Church Ship (the '*Swan*') thanking the SHS for a 'liberal supply of Cholera Medicine which has proved highly beneficial'. In the autumn of 1852, further cases were admitted to the *Dreadnought*, but these were limited to about 40.

In August 1849 it was 'Resolved unanimously that the Surgeons be allowed to give such Wine or Porter as they may deem proper to the nurses on board the Cholera Hospital Ship'. A later minute refers to the allocation to the nurses of such 'wine, brandy or Porter they [the medical officers] may deem desirable'.[27]

The last of London's outbreaks

The third (and last) of London's major cholera epidemics raged during 1853 and 1854. In 1853, HMS *Devonshire*† (Figure 11.2) was loaned by the Admiralty as a 'Cholera-ship' (*see* Chapter 8) and a minute in October of that year records: 'Ordered that the Secretary draw up a Bill exhorting Captains of ships to send Sailors on board the Cholera Hospital Ship on the first symptoms of Diarrhoea appearing [Figure 11.3]; the same to be printed and circulated'. The Principal Harbour Master was helpful in distributing 2,000 copies of this pamphlet. When the *Devonshire* was suddenly removed to Sheerness in mid-1854 for the reception of prisoners of war (from the Crimea), the Admiralty replaced her with HMS *Bacchante*.‡ In 1853, '182 patients

*HMS *Iphigenia* was built at Chatham in 1808; she was an 896 ton 5th Rate with a gun-deck length of 137′ 0″. After service in the Mediterranean, Jamaica and Africa she was lent to the Marine Society between 1833 and 1850. This ship was subsequently broken up at Deptford in May 1851.

†HMS *Devonshire* was built at Deptford in 1808, and was ultimately hulked in 1849.

‡HMS *Bachante* was built at Deptford in 1811. She was a 1,077 ton 5th Rate with 46 guns and a gun-deck length of 154′ 0″. She had taken part in many naval actions. Between 1837 and 46 she was in quarantine service at Stangate. After serving as a cholera-ship for the SHS, she was broken up at Deptford in 1858; the process being completed on 20 February.

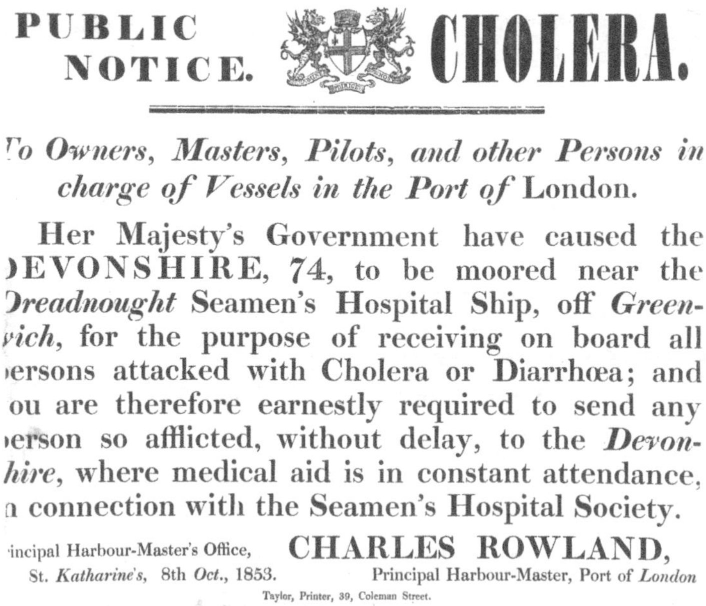

PUBLIC NOTICE. CHOLERA.

To Owners, Masters, Pilots, and other Persons in charge of Vessels in the Port of London.

Her Majesty's Government have caused the)EVONSHIRE, 74, to be moored near the *)readnought* Seamen's Hospital Ship, off *Green-vich*, for the purpose of receiving on board all ›ersons attacked with Cholera or Diarrhœa; and ou are therefore earnestly required to send any ›erson so afflicted, without delay, to the *Devon-hire*, where medical aid is in constant attendance, n connection with the Seamen's Hospital Society.

'incipal Harbour-Master's Office, St. *Katharine's*, 8th *Oct.*, 1853.

CHARLES ROWLAND,
Principal Harbour-Master, Port of *London*

Taylor, Printer, 39, Coleman Street.

Figure 11.2: Announcement that HMS *Devonshire* had been loaned by the Admiralty as a cholera-ship. [SHS archive].

suffering from this fearful Epidemic' were received on board HMS *Bacchante* and 80 were 'restored to health'. The occurrence and prevalence of cholera between 1848 and 54 is succinctly summarised in Annual Reports of the SHS.[28]

A minute of 29 September 1854, however, makes sombre reading: 'Ordered that the Society do bear the Funeral Expenses of Nurse Mary Scott who died of cholera this Morning on board the Dreadnought after 36 hours' illness'. It was soon after this that Roupell (one of the Visiting Physician) also died of cholera; he did *not* however, contract the disease during the course of his work, but whilst visiting a friend at Boulogne.[29]

Lingering fears

London, as well as most parts of England, was thus (not at that time knowingly) over the worst. However, as late as 1865–6, cholera remained a matter of concern for the Society; at a meeting on 1 September 1865, the Physician's Assistant and Apothecary, Harry Leach (*see* Chapter 12), requested (and was granted) two months leave of absence in order to study the disease in 'the neighbourhood of the Black Sea' – he subsequently wrote a book on cholera in Turkey.[30]

The Committee heard in May 1866, that Rooke had requested the 'grant of a ship for reception of Cholera [cases] to be moored near the Dreadnought'; this request

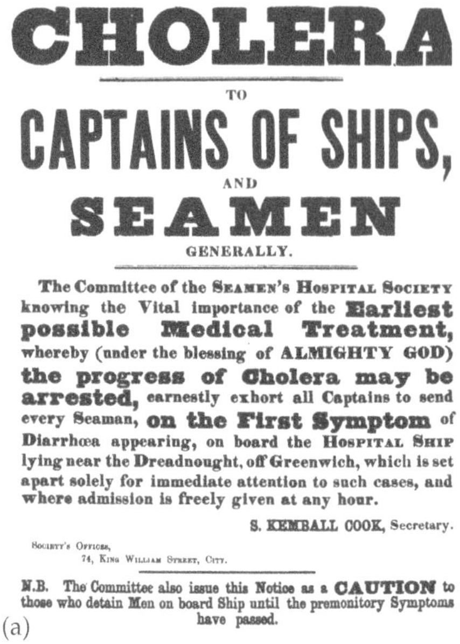

CHOLERA

TO

CAPTAINS OF SHIPS,

AND

SEAMEN

GENERALLY.

The Committee of the SEAMEN'S HOSPITAL SOCIETY knowing the Vital importance of the **Earliest possible Medical Treatment,** whereby (under the blessing of ALMIGHTY GOD) **the progress of Cholera may be arrested,** earnestly exhort all Captains to send every Seaman, **on the First Symptom** of Diarrhœa appearing, on board the HOSPITAL SHIP lying near the Dreadnought, off Greenwich, which is set apart solely for immediate attention to such cases, and where admission is freely given at any hour.

S. KEMBALL COOK, Secretary.

SOCIETY'S OFFICES,
74, KING WILLIAM STREET, CITY.

N.B. The Committee also issue this Notice as a **CAUTION** to those who detain Men on board Ship until the premonitory Symptoms have passed.

(a)

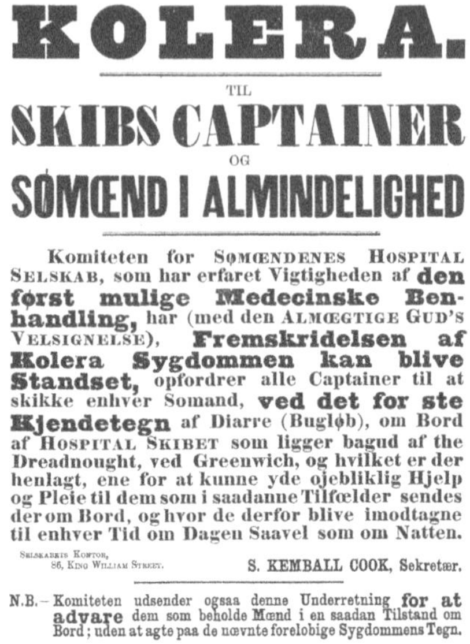

KOLERA.

TIL

SKIBS CAPTAINER

OG

SØMŒND I ALMINDELIGHED

Komiteten for SØMŒNDENES HOSPITAL SELSKAB, som har erfaret Vigtigheden af **den først mulige Medecinske Benhandling,** har (med den ALMŒGTIGE GUD'S VELSIGNELSE), **Fremskridelsen af Kolera Sygdommen kan blive Standset,** opfordrer alle Captainer til at skikke enhver Somand, **ved det for ste Kjendetegn** af Diarre (Bugløb), om Bord af HOSPITAL SKIBET som ligger bagud af the Dreadnought, ved Greenwich, og hvilket er der henlagt, ene for at kunne yde ojebliklig Hjelp og Pleie til dem som i saadanne Tilfœlder sendes der om Bord, og hvor de derfor blive imodtagne til enhver Tid om Dagen Saavel som om Natten.

SELSKABETS KONTOR,
86, KING WILLIAM STREET.

S. KEMBALL COOK, Sekretær.

N.B.– Komiteten udsender ogsaa denne Underretning **for at advare** dem som beholde Mœnd i en saadan Tilstand om Bord; uden at agte paa de nœvnte forelobige Sygdommens Tegn.

(b)

Figure 11.3 (a, b): Notice to captains of ships (in English and Swedish) that cases of cholera and diarrhoea) should be *immediately* sent to HMS *Devonshire*. [SHS archive].

resulted in the loan of the *'Belle-isle'** (then moored at Chatham) provided that the SHS pay 'all Expenses connected with her removal and maintenance'; after a protest by the SHS Committee, financial aspects were dropped. However, minor alterations were deemed necessary in order to convert her into a Cholera-ship, and the SHS was told to pay £100 for these to be carried out; this too was, however, contested successfully by the SHS! The promise of the loan of the ship was subsequently negated by the Admiralty on the grounds that 'there appeared to be no immediate necessity for a cholera hospital and she might [in any case] be required before long for service elsewhere'.[31]

On 18 July 1866, a case of cholera was in fact received on the *'Belle-isle'* and this was reported to the Admiralty. Details of the SHS and its previous role in dealing with cholera patients were demanded by Sir Mordaunt Wells, Chairman of the Mansion House Cholera Relief Fund; the SHS was granted £250 and a deputation was told that more money might be forthcoming if they were to re-apply.[32]

The events of the 1860s were recorded in full in the 46th SHS Annual Report; in all, 85 cases of cholera had been admitted to the *Belle-isle*, and regular cholera inspections (from 11 August to 10 November 1866) aimed to detect *early* cases. The

*HMS *'Belle-isle'* was built at Pembroke in 1819, and was a 74 gun 3rd Rate which amongst other activities had served as a troopship. In 1854 she became a Hospital-ship – serving in the Baltic, East Indies and China. Her break-up was completed at Chatham on 12 October 1872.

River Thames from London Bridge to Woolwich – including the Regent's and City Canals – was divided into four districts, each being visited by a Medical Visitor who was provided with a man and a boy in a boat who hoisted a white flag marked SH (Seamen's Hospital). This scheme was supervised by Leach and Rooke, and the total number of ship visits was no less than 31,346! Fourteen out of 37 cholera cases had previously died, but *after* it was instituted, the corresponding figure was eight out of 48.[33]

Little more was done until 1871, when correspondence with the Privy Council and the Lords of the Admiralty addressed the mode of dealing with cholera cases, should the situation again arise; the *Dreadnought* was *not* available as it had been lent by the Metropolitan Asylums Board for smallpox cases (*see* Chapter 8). A case of cholera infected at Caen (in northern France) which was admitted to the land-based *Dreadnought* Hospital (*see* Chapter 13) on 8 October 1873, and reported in the *Times* the following day brought the cholera era in London to a close. Details of later *sporadic* cases of the disease admitted to the Society's Hospital-ship were recorded in the *Lancet*: five cases of 'choleroid diarrhoea' admitted under Barnes, and two cases (both of whom recovered) under Ward.[34]

Scurvy

Although far less dramatic than cholera, and with a far lower mortality-rate, scurvy was numerically a major problem on the Hospital-ships. Scurvy had, in the light of Lind's work (Chapter 4) and others, almost disappeared from the RN by the early nineteenth century. However, many Annual Reports refer to the frequent occurrence of this disease on the hospital-ships amongst seafarers in the Mercantile Marine.[35]

The Reports for 1839 and 1841 allude to an investigation carried out and followed by a recommendation by George Budd (*see* Chapter 12); both stressed that 'a plentiful supply of vegetables, limejuice and fruit' is vital in prevention. Budd's obvious concern about the relatively high incidence of the disease in the Mercantile Marine is clear from entries in 1838–9. Budd was asked therefore to 'trace the causes which … have led to its appearance after a lapse of many years'. The 1846 and 1847 reports referred to the Merchant Seamen's Registration Act (7 & 8 Vic cap 112) which 'enjoins ship-owners to supply [daily] lime juice and sugar'. But as pointed out in the latter report, that Act 'does not apply to vessels registered and belonging to any British colony having a legislative assembly', and even in British registered vessels, implementation of the Act is often 'shamefully evaded'. This report also pointed out that 'unwholesome compounds are not unfrequently substituted for lime or lemon-juice', a fact which was highlighted in the 1851 report as 'ill-judged parsimony'. The 1861 report referred to 'a brief statement drawn up by the Medical Officers, showing the various means whereby Scurvy may be prevented' (*see* Figure 11.4).[36]

A great deal of attention was given to circulation of Budd's notes on *prevention*, copies of which were sent to East India House and the Trinity Corporation for free distribution to ship owners and Ship Masters – especially those trading with the East Indies, Australia, and the Southern Fisheries.

SCURVY.

CAUSE. Privation for a considerable length of time of Fresh Vegetables.

MEANS FOR PREVENTION.

WHEN AT SEA.

1. A proper quantity of *Lime Juice* should be supplied to every ship on a long voyage. Each man should have at least two ounces (4 tablespoonsful) twice a week, to be increased to an ounce daily, if any symptoms of scurvy manifest themselves. The giving out of Lime Juice should not be delayed longer than a fortnight after the vessel has put to sea.

2. *Preserved Vegetables;* of these Potatoes and Onions are the best; next Greens, Carrots, Turnips, &c.

3. A *good* supply of *fresh water*.

4. Attention to *cleanliness* and *ventilation*, more particularly of the quarters of the crew.

5. If the Lime Juice should fail or become bad, an excellent substitute is the Salts of Potash. It is strongly recommended that every Ship's Medicine Chest should be supplied with some preparation of this salt; the bicarbonate is perhaps the cheapest and best. Five grains twice a day may be given.

WHEN IN PORT, a full supply of such Vegetables as may be most easily procured, such as Potatoes, Greens, Radishes, *Watercresses;* the latter vegetable is a powerful antiscorbutic and easily procurable. Fruits, as Oranges, Lemons, Shaddocks.

Seamen's Hospital Office,
86, King William Street, London, E.C.

Figure 11.4: Advice for prevention of scurvy – provided by the Seamen's Hospital Society. Undated, but probably 1840s. [SHS archive].

In order to learn more about the disease, 'names of the ships … and the ports they arrived from' were carefully recorded. Numbers of cases 'admitted into the Seamen's Hospital from 1822 to 1842' were given to the Inspector General of the Navy, at Somerset House. Later, in 1843, Busk was also asked by the Committee to draw up notes on *prevention* of the disease; these were circulated, a number being 'sent to the Sailors Home for distribution'.[37]

Owing to the gravity of the situation, Lydekker (a descendent of John [*see* Chapter 7], and Hon. Consul to the SHS was consulted about the legal aspects with respect to enforcement of the prevailing Act. He found it 'full of difficulties owing to the loose and careless way in which the act [had been] drawn up'. The Naval Department of the Board of Trade, and subsequently, the Secretary of Lloyd's were duly involved, but although a great deal of correspondence was generated, little seems to have been accomplished.[38]

The 43rd Report gave a summary of cases encountered on the Hospital-ships between 1851 and 63 (*see* Figure 11.5); very few had originated, it was stated, on ships 'belonging to the Port of London', and it seemed to be a disease of 'small vessels, whose forecastle accommodation is ill suited for tropical voyages'. The fact, the Report continued, 'that such cases are never received from certain lines of vessels trading to China and the East Indies, is positive evidence that this malady may be prevented in the Mercantile Marine'.

Despite this much needed publicity, the disease continued to occur in the Merchant Navy, and the *Dreadnought* authorities reported many new cases to the Marine Department of the Board of Trade. The 1864 Report made a recommendation that lime-juice should be 'carried in small jars, instead of in bulk as is mostly done'. A year later, the Annual Report recorded an actual *increase* in admissions from scurvy (*see* Figure 11.5); of the 102 cases received during a 12-month period, 99 were from *British* (38 of these in ships belonging to the Port of London, 31 Liverpool, and 10 Glasgow and Greenock), while only three had served on *foreign* vessels. This unsatisfactory state of affairs was reiterated in the 1866 Report, although by then the number of 'London cases' had fallen.[39]

The following Report (for 1865) continued by quoting a Parliamentary Paper (no: 404, Sess. 1865) on the subject, and both this and the report for 1866 gave advice on the origin, inspection and storage of lime-juice. This disease, the 46th Report rightly claimed, 'is now practically unknown in Her Majesty's Navy [RN], and in the first-class ships of our Merchant Service'.[40]

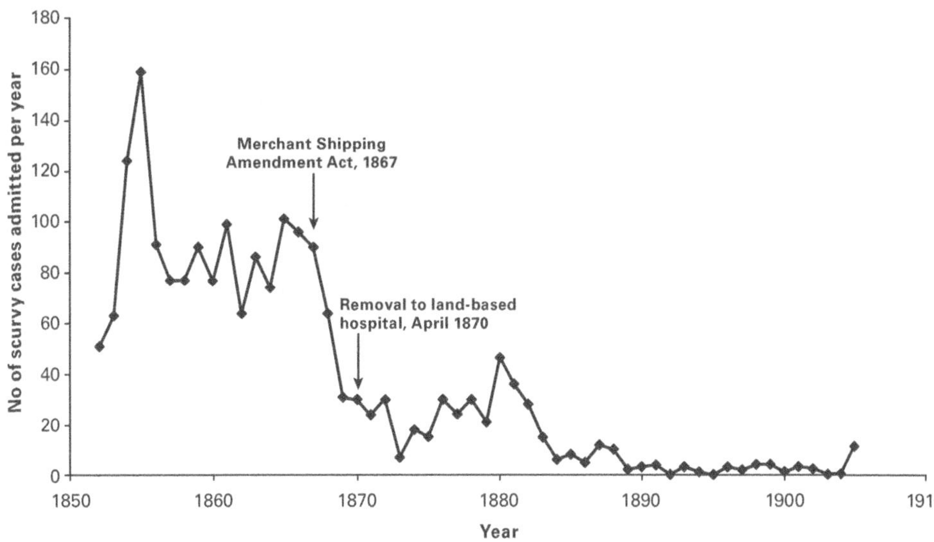

Figure 11.5: Numbers of cases of scurvy admitted to the second and third Hospital-ships between 1850 and 1870. [Cases admitted between 1870 and 1905 are also shown]. The Merchant Shipping Amendment Act (1867) came into effect on 1 January 1868; this was followed by a dramatic decline in numbers of cases on HMS *Dreadnought* and in the land-based hospital (see text).

The fact that scurvy continued to be a major problem on the *Dreadnought* is clear from numerous entries in the SHS minutes for 1865–66, and correspondence with the Marine Department of the Board of Trade; there are numerous references to scurvy occurring on specific ships. An entry at a meeting held on 12 May 1865 is particularly revealing:

> Read a letter from the Board of Trade in Reference to the cases of Scurvy received into the Dreadnought from the "French Empire" stating that the provisions of the Merchant Shipping Act had not been Complied with – first, by there being no Entries in the Official log book of several cases of illness, in Contravention of Sec. 282 – Secondly, that no lime or lemon juice was issued to the Crew as required by Sec. 284 and that the Master of the Vessel was to blame for not procuring at St. Helena or Ascension those supplies of which his Crew stood so much in need.[41]

Solution of the scurvy problem

1867 proved to be a significant year in the history of this, by then, well-established Charity, thanks largely to the initiative of Harry Leach (Resident Medical Officer on the *Dreadnought*),[42] for scurvy was shortly to become a rarity in the Mercantile Marine. The 47th Report addressed his major contribution to the health of the seafarer in the merchant service: '... although a large proportion of the Patients in the Dreadnought are from *Foreign* Ships, the cases of Scurvy are almost exclusively confined to *British* Vessels'. In a series of letters to the editor of *The Times*, Leach stressed the importance of pure lime-juice in the prevention of this disease; he recommended 'certain modifications in the supply and storage ... and inspection of lime-juice by an authorised officer' and 'insisted ... on the necessity of a strict and full inquiry in every case of scurvy occurring on board ship'. A leading article in *The Times* for 10 January 1866 had concentrated on the Board of Trade's recently published memorandum (1863) on the subject – which was almost certainly instigated by Leach himself. Leach was certain that scurvy could be prevented/cured by good quality lime-juice, when properly stored; he also brought the true prevalence of the disease, from his extensive experience with the SHS, to public attention.

Leach's initiative resulted in an amendment (ratified in 1867) to the *Merchant Shipping Act* of 1854 to 'provide effectually for inspection of antiscorbutics and for such other precautions as had been suggested'. This Bill (which received the Royal Assent on 20 August 1867) had been 'laid before Parliament' by His Grace the Duke of Richmond,[43] President of the Board of Trade, to improve legislation with regard to the prevention of scurvy; it became mandatory, amongst other things, for all lime-juice to undergo a Medical Inspection 'before the Ship goes to Sea'. The following minute of a meeting of the Committee of Management held on 18 October 1867 summarised this new legislation:

> Read a letter from the Board of Trade transmitting a copy of the 30th & 31st Victoria Cap 124 the principal object of which is to make better provision for securing the health of seamen with especial reference to Sea-scurvy and conveying to the Committee of the Seamen's Hospital Society, and

> personally to the Secretary & Mr Leach the acknowledgements of the Board for the very valuable and ready assistance at all times rendered to the Board whilst Endeavouring to deal with this important subject.[44]

An analysis of admission data to the *Dreadnought* Hospital following implementation of this Act confirms a steep decline in *new* cases of scurvy.[45] Three years later the number of scorbutic patients on the *Dreadnought* had been reduced by 84%.

During his long period of service on the *Dreadnought* Hospital-ship, Leach had of course had constant 'opportunities of witnessing the terrible sufferings and … deaths among the crews of trading ships from scurvy, due to defective provisions and want of pure and good lime-juice'. The 1869 Report alluded to the fact that, thanks to the new legislation – which took effect on 1 January 1868 (see above) – the number of cases of scurvy 'admitted [the previous] year was forty, whilst in 1865 and 1866 they had exceeded one hundred per annum'. The 1870 Report (the year of removal to the land-based hospital – Chapter 13) recorded that 'Since the 20th October last, no case of Scurvy has come to the Hospital'.

On 25 October a letter from the Board of Trade was read to the Committee: Harry Leach had, under the 1867 Act, been designated *Inspector of Lime-juice*; this appointment, the Committee agreed, was consistent with his continuing his post at the SHS. From then onwards the prevalence of scurvy in the merchant navy declined steeply and ultimately disappeared – thanks to the Society, and particularly to Leach (*see* Figure 11.5).[46]

Smallpox

It had been a 'golden rule' of the Society since its foundation in 1821, that smallpox cases should *not* be admitted, but referred to one of the smallpox hospitals on shore. During the early days of the Hospital-ships, this system functioned well, as there seems to have been a great deal of goodwill between the Society and the Surgeon to the St. Pancras Smallpox Hospital – James Marson.[47] According to the Minutes of the Committee of Management, the Society regularly gave a donation (usually £10 or ten guineas) to the Smallpox Hospital for services rendered. There are also several friendly reports (from Marson) involving deaths in patients referred for his care; funeral expenses had to be paid on all deaths in patients referred by the Hospital, but *not* for direct admissions in which the Society was *not* involved. It was therefore 'Resolved unanimously that the funeral expenses of all seamen, sent by, or from, this Hospital be paid'.[48]

Eighteen forty-eight seems to have been a 'bad year' as far as smallpox was concerned. The Secretary to the Smallpox Hospital (Mr Clift) requested: '… an increased subscription in consequence of the great number of Patients admitted [the previous] year, 45 of whom were sent from this Hospital, and their funds having [proved] inadequate to meet the increased expenditure – [it was] Resolved [by the SHS Board of Management] that under the special circumstances of the case a further donation of £20 be given to the Small Pox Hospital'.[49]

Some five years later (in 1854), Marson seems to have become very difficult to deal with, for in a letter addressed to the SHS Secretary he:

> … called upon him to remove immediately a man sent from the Dreadnought, complaining of reluctance in several cases to do so, & threatening that if this request were not complied with no man recommended by this Society should obtain admission to the Small Pox Hospital. The Secretary was instructed to write to [Clift] on the subject & in the meantime, as the man in question was a South Sea Islander, ignorant of the English language, to make arrangements for his removal.

The result of this altercation was that the SHS Committee of Management resolved to discontinue donations to the Smallpox Hospital; instead, they decided to pay one guinea for each patient sent to the Hospital, but *not* for seafarers with smallpox who were not referred by the Society! The *Daily News* and the *Morning Herald* of 31 May 1855 contained the following statement (apparently written by Mr Thwaites, Receiving Officer of the City of London Union, St. Mary Axe):

> If the authorities at the Dreadnought do not admit cases of Small Pox, they surely ought to have the power of … admissions to the Small Pox Hospital.

In order to attempt to reach an amicable arrangement it was decided that a deputation from the Society should meet one from the Smallpox Hospital. This meeting, however, proved extremely difficult to arrange; the best that the Smallpox Hospital could suggest was that a deputation from the SHS should attend one of their meetings at 'The Freemason's Tavern'! However, in the meantime, a Quartermaster from the *Dreadnought*, who had been sent by the SHS Superintendent, travelled with a patient to the Smallpox Hospital but without one guinea in his pocket (see above); he received 'rough treatment' from Marson 'who [gave] the cabman money to bring the man back to the Society's Office and leave him there'.[50]

The joint meeting eventually took place, and the Smallpox Hospital authorities issued an ultimatum which stipulated:

(i) a demand for an annual subscription of ten guineas;
(ii) a letter of introduction and one guinea [must] be sent with each patient;
(iii) a demand for an undertaking to remove any patients when requested to do so;
(iv) a demand for an undertaking to bury patients if required!
(v) payment of arrears [which amounted to] – £37=16=00, or the 'lapsed Anl. Sub$^{\underline{n}}$ of Ten guineas for 1855-6-&7'.

The Committee readily agreed to iii & iv, but considered that 'No. 5 [v] Cannot be Entertained'. Regarding i and ii, they recommended an annual subscription of fifteen guineas, on condition that all patients referred from the *Dreadnought* was received into the Smallpox Hospital. The Smallpox Hospital Committee however responded that they could *not* accept an Annual Subscription of *less* than twenty guineas; this was 'subject to a proportionate increase should the average number of patients sent from the Dreadnought exceed that cost …'. The proposal was in any case subject to the arrears account being settled! This was the unsatisfactory state of negotiations at the time of removal to the land-based *Dreadnought* in April 1870 (*see* Chapter 13).

There is little mention of smallpox in the Annual Reports. This had always been a highly contentious area, and these acrimonious discussions with the senior staff of the St Pancras Smallpox Hospital, which obviously reached the 'media', must surely have been a disinterrant to potential benefactors of the Society![51]

The 'Ship Captains Medical Guide'

In 1868, Harry Leach (see above and Chapter 12) published his most important work *The Ship Captain's Medical Guide* (*see* Figure 11.6), which in a modified form continues to this day. In it, he classified medical and surgical diseases in seafarers of the Mercantile Marine (i.e. the group of individuals for which the SHS had been set up to care for). Table 11.4 summarises Leach's 1868 classification.[52]

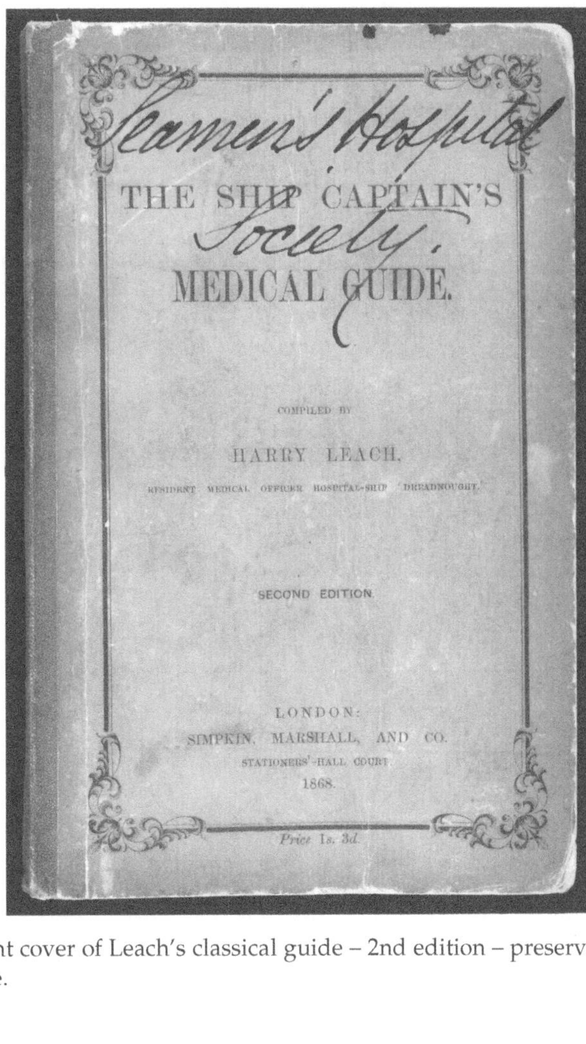

Figure 11.6: Front cover of Leach's classical guide – 2nd edition – preserved in the Society's archive.

Table 11.4: Leach's classification of medical and surgical diseases in his monograph '*The Ship Captain's Medical Guide*' first published in 1868 (i.e. two years before the *clinical* facilities were transferred to the land-based hospital).

Medical:	Fever
	Ague, or Intermittent Fever
	Scarlet Fever, Small-pox, Measles and Erysipelas
	Yellow Fever
	Cough, Bronchitis, Inflammation of the Lungs, and Consumption
	Quinsy
	Heart Diseases
	Jaundice, and Liver Diseases
	Constipation
	Indigestion
	Diarrhoea
	Cholera
	Dysentery
	Colic
	Kidney Diseases
	Fits
	Sunstroke
	Palsy
	Delirium Tremens
	Scurvy
	Rheumatism
	Itch
Surgical:	Venereal (Pox, Clap, &c.)
	Rupture
	Retention of Urine
	Dribbling of ditto
	Boils
	Ulcers
	Piles
	Gum-Boil
	Bleeding from the Nose

References and Notes

1 T Baker (ed.) *The common nature of epidemics, and their relation to climate and civilization. From writings and official reports by Southwood Smith, M.D.* London: N Trübner & Co. 1866: 130; W F Bynum, V Nutton (eds.). *Theories of fever from antiquity to the enlightenment.* London: Wellcome Institute for the History of Medicine. 1981: 154; H Richardson (ed.). *English Hospitals 1660–1948: a survey of their architecture and design.* London: Royal Commission of the Historical Monuments of England. 1998: 1–15. [*See also*: G C Cook. Robert Robertson,

FRS (1742-1829): physician to the Royal Hospital Greenwich, 18th century authority on 'fever', and early practitioner in care of the elderly. *J Med Biog*. 2006; 14: 42–54].

2 **Sir William Jenner** Bt GCB FRCP FRS (1815–98) qualified in medicine at University College London in 1837, where he subsequently became a physician and Professor of Medicine. He subsequently became President of the Royal College of Physicians, and was physician to both Queen Victoria and the Prince of Wales. He is best known as the first Englishman to clearly distinguish typhus from typhoid fever. [*See* also: W I McDonald. Jenner, Sir William, first baronet (1815–1898). In: H C G Matthew, B Harrison (eds). *Oxford Dictionary of National Biography*. Oxford: Oxford University Press 2004; 30: 10–12; Anonymous. Jenner, Sir William, Bart., GCB. *Munk's Roll* 4: 67–69].

3 *Parliamentary papers*. Report on the Petition respecting the Fever Institution 1804; 5 July: 4; *Parliamentary papers*. Report from the Select Committee on Contagious Fever in London. 1818; 20 May: 52.

4 G L Roupell. Committee of Management Minutes, 3: 17–19; G L Roupell. *Ibid*. 3: 121; [*See also*: G C Cook. Disease in the merchant navies of the world in the days of sail.The Seamen's Hospital Society's experience. *Mariner's Mirror* 2005; 91: 46–51)].

5 Anonymous. *Morning Post*. 1837; 10 February; Anonymous. *Times, Lond*. 1845; August. [*See also*: *Op cit*. See note 4 above (Minutes) 4: 222; G Budd. 1839; 23 February: 425; 5 1845: 8 August: 491].

6 R H Goolden. *Op cit*. See note 4 above (Minutes): 491–2.

7 Anonymous. *Lancet*. 1828; i: 64; R. Harley. Seamen's Hospital Society. *Lancet*. 1828; i: 113.

8 S Ward. Analysis of 1000 consecutive cases admitted into the Seamen's Hospital, "Dreadnought". *Lancet*. 1860; ii: pp 78–9.

9 Anonymous. Dreadnought Hospital. Two cases of diphtheria, followed by recovery. (Under the care of Dr Barnes). *Lancet*. 1859; i: 629.

10 H Leach. The Dreadnought Seamen's Hospital. A case of idiopathic tetanus. *Lancet*. 1870: ii: 435.

11 Anonymous. The 'Dreadnought' and metropolitan free hospitals. Phosphate of zinc in epilepsy. *Lancet*. 1858; i: 119.

12 J Tudor. The hygienic condition of the "Dreadnought" hospital ship in the year 1857–8, as exemplified by the result of surgical operations. *Lancet*. 1859; i: pp 361–2.

13 Anonymous. 'Dreadnought' Hospital Ship. Excision of head of femur with great trochanter for hip-joint disease; subsequent perforation of the floor of the acetebulum from extensive caries; death. (Under the care of Mr Rooke). *Lancet*. 1869; ii: 507–8.

14 Anonymous. 'Dreadnought Hospital'. Fungous disease of the testicle associated with deposits of encephaloid cancer in the liver; sudden death. (Under the care of Mr Rooke). *Lancet*. 1870; ii: 154–5.

15 Anonymous. Seamen's Hospital ship, 'Dreadnought'. *Lancet*. 1856; i: 457.

16 Anonymous. 'Dreadnought' Hospital Ship. Death during the inhalation of chloroform. *Lancet*. 1859; ii: 412.

17 G L Roupell. *Some account of a fever prevalent in the year 1831*. London: William Nichol 1837: 20; H Sandwith. *A history of the epidemic fever, which prevailed in Bridlington and the neighbourhood, in the years 1818 and 1819*. London: Burchess and Hill. 1821: 173; G C Cook. George Leith Roupell FRS (1797–1854): significant contributions to the early nineteenth-century understanding of cholera and typhus. *J Med Biog* 2000; 8: 1–7.

18 *Op cit*. See note 4 above (Minutes). 3: 111; E Seymour, G L Roupell. *Ibid*. 113, 127.

19 *Ibid*. G. Busk. 1842; 18 November: 232; SHS Annual Reports 22, 27.

20 *Op cit*. See note 4 above (Minutes). 8: 321.

21 This is certainly *not* a description of any form of syphilis as seen today. The condition

described by Busk is probably *granuloma inguinale* – a sexually-transmitted infection caused by *Calymmatobacterium granulomatis* (formerly named *Donovania granulomatis*). [*See also*: J Richens. Granuloma inguinale. In: G T Strickland (ed). *Hunter's tropical medicine and emerging infectious diseases.* 8th ed. London: W.B. Saunders Co. 2000: 369-372].

22 Minutes of evidence taken at the Admiralty before a Committee on Venereal Diseases in the Army and Navy 1864-5 [G C Cook: personal archive]; [*See also*: G C Cook. Disease in the nineteenth-century merchant navy: the Seamen's Hospital Society's experience. *Mariners' Mirror*. 2001; 87: 460–471].

23 *Op cit.* See note 3 above (Minutes). 3:179–180. [*See also*: G L Roupell. *The Croonian lectures, delivered at the Royal College of Physicians in MDCCCXXXIII, on cholera.* London: G & W Nicol. 1833: 91; J Fayrer. *The natural history and epidemiology of cholera: being the annual oration of the Medical Society of London, May 7, 1888.* London: J & A Churchill. 1888: 71].

24 *Op cit.* See note 4 above (Minutes) 3: 235, 269, 257, 299, 349. [*See also*: Anonymous. Dark days a hundred years ago: the Seamen's Hospital Society lend a hand. *SHS Quart Mag* 1935; 7(3): 10–11].

25 *Op cit.* See note 19 above (Reports): 12, 14. [*See also*: *Op cit.* See note 3 above (Minutes) 4: 4].

26 *Op cit.* See note 4 above (Minutes) 4: 291–2.

27 *Ibid.* 6: 243, 256–7, 259, 261, 353; 7: 137.

28 *Ibid.* 7: 142, 225. *Op cit.* See note 17 above (Cook).

29 *Op cit.* See note 19 above (Reports): 28, 29, 30, 34.

30 *Op cit.* See note 4 above (Minutes) 8: 464. [*See also:* G C Cook. Harry Leach MRCP (1836–1879): control of scurvy in the British Mercantile Marine, and first Port Medical Officer for the City of London. *J Med Biog* 2000; 8: 133–139].

31 *Op cit.* See note 4 above (Minutes). 9: 504–5, 508–9: 511, 512–3.

32 *Op cit.* See note 4 above (Minutes). 9: 519; 527–8.

33 *Op cit.* See note 19 above: 46; *Op cit.* See note 4 above (Minutes) 9: 284–6.

34 Anonymous. Cholera. *Times, Lond.* 1873; 9 October: 7; Anonymous. "Dreadnought" hospital ship. Cholera and choleroid diarrhoea. (Under the care of Dr Barnes). *Lancet.* 1859; ii: 137–8; Anonymous. Dreadnought Hospital Ship. Two cases of cholera; recovery. (Under the care of Dr S. Ward). *Lancet.* 1868; ii: 77.

35 G C Cook. Scurvy in the British Mercantile Marine in the 19th century, and the contribution of the Seamen's Hospital Society. *Postgrad Med J* 2004 ; 80: 224–9.

36 *Op cit.* See note 19 above (Reports): 18, 19, 21, 22, 26, 27, 31, 41, 43. *Merchant Shipping Act* 1854; 17° & 18° Victoriae c 104; A.G. Course. *The merchant navy: a social history*: 208–9, 214–215; G C Cook. George Budd FRS (1808–1882): pioneer gastroenterologist and hepatologist. *J Med Biog* 1998; 6: 152–159.

37 *Op cit.* See note 4 above (Minutes) 4: 358–9, 497, 502; 5: 69, 190–1, 279.

38 *Op cit.* See note 4 above (Minutes) 6: 70, 483–5, 489; 7: 12–15; 8: 209, 332.

39 *Op cit.* See note 35 above.

40 *Op cit.* See note 19 above: 44, 45, 46.

41 *Op cit.* See note 4 above (Minutes) 8: 1863: 341, 372–3, 409–10, 442, 446, 450, 452, 456, 475, 479, 483, 489–90, 495, 500, 532, 554.

42 *See also* Chapters 12 and 15; G C Cook. Harry Leach MRCP (1836–1879): control of scurvy in the British Mercantile Marine, and first Medical Officer for the City of London. *J Med Biog* 2000; 8: 133–9; G C Cook. Leach, Henry (1836–1879). In: H C G Matthew, B Harrison (eds). *Oxford Dictionary of National Biography.* Oxford: Oxford University Press 2004: 32: 950–1.

43 **Charles Henry Gordon-Lennox, sixth Duke of Richmond** (1818–1903) ultimately became Lord President of the Council in Disraeli's government. He had served as President of

the Board of Trade from 1867–8. The Prince of Wales (later King Edward VII) referred to him as 'the farmers' friend'. [*See also:* F M L Thompson. Lennox, Charles Henry Gordon – sixth Duke of Richmond, sixth Duke of Lennox, and first Duke of Gordon (1818–1903). In: H C G Matthew, B Harrison (eds). *Oxford Dictionary of National Biography.* Oxford: Oxford University Press 2004; 33: 369–71].

44 *Op cit.* See note 4 above (Minutes); 9: 38; *Op cit.* See note 19 above: 47, 49, 50. [*See also*: *Merchant Shipping Act*, 1854; 30° & 31° Victoriae, Cap 124; 1867: 1296–1302]

45 *Op cit.* See note 35 above.

46 *Op cit.* See note 4 above (Minutes). 9: 39–40.

47 **James Furness Marson** FRCS (?–1877) was Surgeon to the Small-pox and Vaccination Hospital for 40 years; he was also the Principal Vaccinator of the National Vaccination Establishment. His practical knowledge of Smallpox and vaccination was unparalleled in his time, and he wrote extensively on this subject and was also a member of the Epidemiological Society of which on at least one occasion. He declined the Presidency on the grounds of ill health. Marson subsequently lived, in retirement, at Worthing and following a 'painful malady' died there on 15 November 1877. His greatest literary achievement was: '*An Analytical Examination of all the cases admitted, during sixteen years, at the Small-pox and Vaccination Hospital, London, with a view to illustrate the Pathology of small-pox and the protective Influence of Vaccination, in degrees varying according as the Vaccination has been perfectly or imperfectly performed.*' (*Medico-Chir Trans* 1847; 30: 121–9). [*See also*: Anonymous. *BMJ* 1877; ii: 773; Anonymous. James Furness Marson, FRCS *Trans Epid Soc.* 4: 128; Marson, James Furness. In: *Plarr's Lives.* 1930; 2: 32].

48 *Op cit.* See note 4 above (Minutes) 4: 349–50.

49 *Ibid.* 6: 295.

50 *Ibid.* 8: 241, 254, 281, 473.

51 *Ibid.* 9: 485, 512–3, 522.

52 *Op cit.* See note 30 above (Cook).

Chapter 12

Administrators, physicians and surgeons who served during the ship era

Before describing those individuals who served the Society in the days of the Hospital-ships, this chapter records the site(s) of the SHS office, and gives details of meetings of the Committee of Management.

The Society's Office (1821-70)

As with many Victorian charities, the SHS, in the days of the Hospital-ships, had its office – not at Deptford or Greenwich – but in the *City* of London. The situation of the office was, however, somewhat peripatetic. In the initial Annual Report, the address was stated as: 'No. 2, Hatton Court, Threadneedle Street'. The first report to be written (by Richard Harley) from a new address was that of 1826: '19, Bishopsgate Street Within'. However, the Society was soon to move its office once again, and the 1836 report contained the following notice:

> The Office of this Society has been removed from Bishopsgate Street, and is now situated in King William Street, two doors West of Clement's Lane.

The precise address was – '74 King William Street'. Later, the 1857 Annual Report (written by the Secretary, Silas Kemball Cook) informed its readership: 'The Office of the Society has been removed from No. 74 to No. 86, King William Street'. This removal had probably taken place in 1856, and that is where it remained during the remainder of the Hospital-ship days.[1]

Meetings of the Committee of Management (1821–70)

In early years, meetings of the Committee were held at the Society's city office – either on Fridays (three or four times monthly), and once a month on Saturdays (usually the first or last in the month) 'on board [the *Grampus* Ship'; all meetings took place at 'two o'Clock'. However, from 1835 the Saturday meetings started at 'Three o'Clock' between 1 April and 30 September, and at the 'old time' from 1 October until 31 March. During those years, a General Meeting of Subscribers was held annually (in early February). From 1841, in addition to the weekly meetings of the Committee of Management, an Annual Court was held on the first Wednesday in February, and Quarterly Courts on the second Friday in January, April, July and October. This arrangement remained unchanged until removal to land (*see* Chapter 13).[2]

This chapter is concerned (for the most part) with the physicians, surgeons and apothecaries who served the SHS during the Hospital-ship days. It is pertinent however, to first mention some of the non-medical personnel.

Administrators

Table 12.1 summarises those individuals who held key positions in the Society between 1821 and 1870. The death of the first President – the second Viscount Melville[3] – who had served from the foundation of the Society, was announced at the SHS Committee of Management Meeting on 13 June 1851. In 1865, the second President of the Society – His Grace the 4th Duke of Northumberland,[4] a prominent politician and former First Lord of the Admiralty – also died; this was recorded at a meeting on 17 February of that year.[5]

Little is known about the first Chairman of the Management Committee – John Blackburn – but his distinguished successor has been well documented – Admiral Sir William Bowles.[6]

The death of the original Secretary and Collector – Richard Harley (?–1849) – who had held this office for 'nearly 28 years' took place on 18 February 1849, and was minuted at a special SHS meeting held on 23 February at the Society's office. Unfortunately little is known about him, although he was obviously held in very high regard by the Society. Although Silas Kemball Cook (1818–74)'s career as the second Secretary with the SHS was to extend into the era following the Hospital ships (Chapter 15), the bulk of his input had been prior to this. He joined the Society as Secretary in 1849 (i.e. following the death of Harley). His father, a schoolmaster, was also named Silas and his mother was (formerly) Emily Archer; Cook was baptised at St Mary's Church, Rotherhithe on 21 January 1818, but the family moved at some stage to Montpellier Crescent, Brighton. One of his sons, Sir Edward Cook, KBE (1857–1919) became a well-known author and editor, and wrote a two-volume biography of Florence Nightingale. When the Society removed to the Infirmary of the Royal Hospital (*see* Chapter 13), he was given the title of House Governor (in addition to that of Secretary) with a residence in the Infirmary itself, and received a salary of £600 per annum. He died at the 'land-based' *Dreadnought* hospital on 25 June 1874, having previously been granted sick leave for at least six months; he had become ill in late 1873. His death, the precise cause of which is unknown, was recorded in the *Times*, and the following notice appeared in the *Shipping Gazette* for 27 June 1874:

> THE LATE MR KEMBALL COOK – Our impression of yesterday contained the announcement of the death on Thursday last of this lamented gentleman. Mr Cook was in his 56th year, and for the last 25 years had

Table 12.1: Non-medical personnel who served the SHS in the years of the Hospital-ships (1821–70).

Patron:	1821–30:	King George IV (1762–1830)
	1830–37:	King William IV (1765–1837)
	1837–[70]:	Queen Victoria (1819–1901)
President:	1821–51:	The Rt. Hon. the 2nd Viscount Melville KT (1771–1851)
	1852–65:	His Grace the 4th Duke of Northumberland KG FRS (1792–1865)
	1865–[70]:	Position vacant
Chairman, Committee of Management:*	1821–24:	John Blackburn, Esq. (?–1824)
	1825–69:	Capt (Later Admiral) Sir William Bowles RN[4†] (1780–1869)
	1869–[70]:	Francis Le Breton, Esq. (?–1880) (*see* Chapter 15)
Hon. Secretary:	1821–33:	Simon Cock (?–?)
Secretary & Collector:	1821–49:	Richard Harley (?–1849)
	1849–[70]:	Silas Kemball Cook (1818–74)
Clerk & Collector:	1849–53:	Henry Swift
Superintendant:	1821–30:	Lieut. David McCery RN
	1831–37:	Lieut. William Bowers RN
	1837–56:	John Sanders RN
	1856–69:	Commander Crang RN
	1869–[70]:	Position vacant
	1821–54:	Rev. David Jones
Chaplain:	1854–70:[5‡]	Rev. J J W Harris
	1870–[70]	Rev. W F Mothersole

been closely connected with the Dreadnought Seamen's Hospital. He was appointed Secretary in 1848, and to this office was added that of House Governor in 1870, when the Hospital was, mainly owing to Mr Cook's exertions, established on shore in a portion of Greenwich Hospital rendered vacant by the removal of Pensioners. We have frequently had occasion, when advocating the claims of this excellent Institution, to

*The members of the Committee of Management were very numerous; for details, *see* the SHS Annual Reports between 1821 and 1870.

†Bowles received a KCB on 10 November 1862.

‡[Between 1854 and 1866, the Rev von Bulow served as Chaplain to 'Foreign' Patients.]

speak in terms of deserved commendation of the services rendered to it by the late Mr. Cook, and we cannot doubt that by his death the Society have sustained a very serious loss.[7]

The records relating to the medical staff are better documented, and are summarized in Tables 12.2–12.4. Details of the founding Physicians and Surgeon have been recorded in Chapter 6.

Physicians

Table 12.2 lists the physicians during the Hospital-ship years. For information on Sir Andrew Halliday, and Doctors Mackinnon and Roberts (the founding physicians) the reader is referred to Chapter 6.

Roupell

George Leith Roupell FRCP FRS (1797–1854) (Figure 12.1) served the SHS as a Visiting Physician from 1828, becoming a Consulting Physician in 1832. He had graduated MB (1820) and MD (1825) from St Bartholomew's Hospital, London,

Table 12.2: Physicians on the Hospital-ships (1821–70) with dates.

Name	*Physician*	*Visiting Physician*	*Consulting Physician*	*Physician's Assistant/ Resident Physician*
Sir Andrew Halliday*	1821–28	–	–	–
D Mackinnon	1821–28	–	–	–
C J Roberts	1821–28	–	–	–
G L Roupell FRS	–	1828–32	1832–54	–
E J Seymour FRS	–	–	1828–66	–
A Mower	–	1832–37	–	–
G Budd FRS	–	1837–40	1841–[70]	–
P Black	–	1840–51	–	–
R H Goolden	–	1840–46	–	–
T Blackall	–	1846–55	–	–
J W Hue	–	1851–56	–	–
R Barnes	–	1855–[70]	1882–1904	–
S H Ward	–	1856–[70]	–	–
H Leach	–	–	–	1869–[70]
J H Jackson FRS	–	1870–[70]	–	–

*Also personal physician to the Duke of Clarence (later King William IV); knighted 26 January 1821.

Table 12.3: Surgeons on the Hospital-ships (1821–70) with dates.

Name	*Resident Surgeon*	*Assistant Surgeon*	*Consulting Surgeon*	*Surgeon*	*First Surgeon*	*Second Surgeon*	*Visiting Surgeon*
D G Arnot	1821–28	–	–	–	–	–	–
J Y Thorburn	1828–30	–	–	–	–	–	–
J T Blenkin	–	1828–30	–	–	–	–	–
(Sir) Richard Dobson FRS[7]*	–	–	1829–47	–	–	–	–
T Lawson[8†]	1830–34	–	1834–7	–	–	–	–
F D Bennett	–	1830–1	–	–	–	–	–
G Busk FRS	1834–37	1831–4	1855–86	1837–40	1840–53	–	1853–65
F Tuckett	–	1834–40	–	–	–	1840–43	–
W Clapp	–	–	–	–	–	1844	–
C L Norton	–	–	–	–	–	1848–49	–
J Tudor	–	1853–55	–	1855–[70]	–	–	–
H T L Rooke	–	–	–	1853–55 & 1860–70	–	1849–53	–
J Croft	–	1855–60	–	–	–	–	–
R J Beaford	–	1860–68	–	–	–	–	–
W J Smith	–	1863–[70]	–	1870– [70]	–	–	–

*Also surgeon of the Royal Hospital, Greenwich; knighted 17 August 1831.
†Resided on the *Dover* cholera-ship during 1832.

Table 12.4: Apothecaries on the Hospital-ships (1821–70) with dates.*

	Apothecary	*Assistant Surgeon & Apothecary*	*Physicians Assistant & Apothecary*
W Baker	1828–29	–	–
F D Bennett	1829–30	–	–
G Busk FRS	1830–31	–	–
T Hays	1831–37	–	–
R F Salter	1837–40	1840–41	–
W Clapp	–	1841–44	–
J Hudson	–	1844–47	–
C L Norton	–	1847–48	–
H T L Rooke	–	1848–49	–
J H Lakin	–	1849–51	–
A H Churchill	–	1851–[70]	–
E J Complin	–	–	1853–54
J Vaux	–	–	1854–55
W T Plowman	–	–	1855–56
F M Corner	–	–	1856–58
R J Bedford	–	–	1858–60
J Cooke	–	–	1860–62
H Leach	–	–	1862–69

and following continental travels, was appointed to HMS *Grampus* in 1828; whilst there he assembled much information leading to his major publications – on *cholera* and *typhus* – as well as recording the diagnoses of patients admitted under his care during 1829–31 (Chapter 11). With the SHS, he also acquired information on several other infectious diseases – which formed a major source for several subsequent books. On 19 June 1834, Roupell was appointed physician to St Bartholomew's; he then held the appointment of Consulting Physician to the SHS from 1832 until his death on 29 September 1854 from Asiatic cholera, which had been contracted in Boulogne whilst visiting a relative stricken with this disease.[8]

EXPERIENCE WITH CHOLERA

Roupell's three Croonian lectures for 1833 on *cholera* (those for 1832 had addressed 'General pathology') were subsequently published in book format: '*The Croonian Lectures delivered at The Royal College of Physicians in MDCCCXXXIII*'. The Asiatic cholera had begun its first 'visitation' to England (via Sunderland) in October 1831 and was the subject of much nation-wide anxiety; the disease dominated the medical (and lay) press of the day. Much of Roupell's experience with the infection was

*In early 1870, the following *junior* appointments were made: House Physician: H C Martin, M.B.; House Surgeon: W M Campbell, M.B.

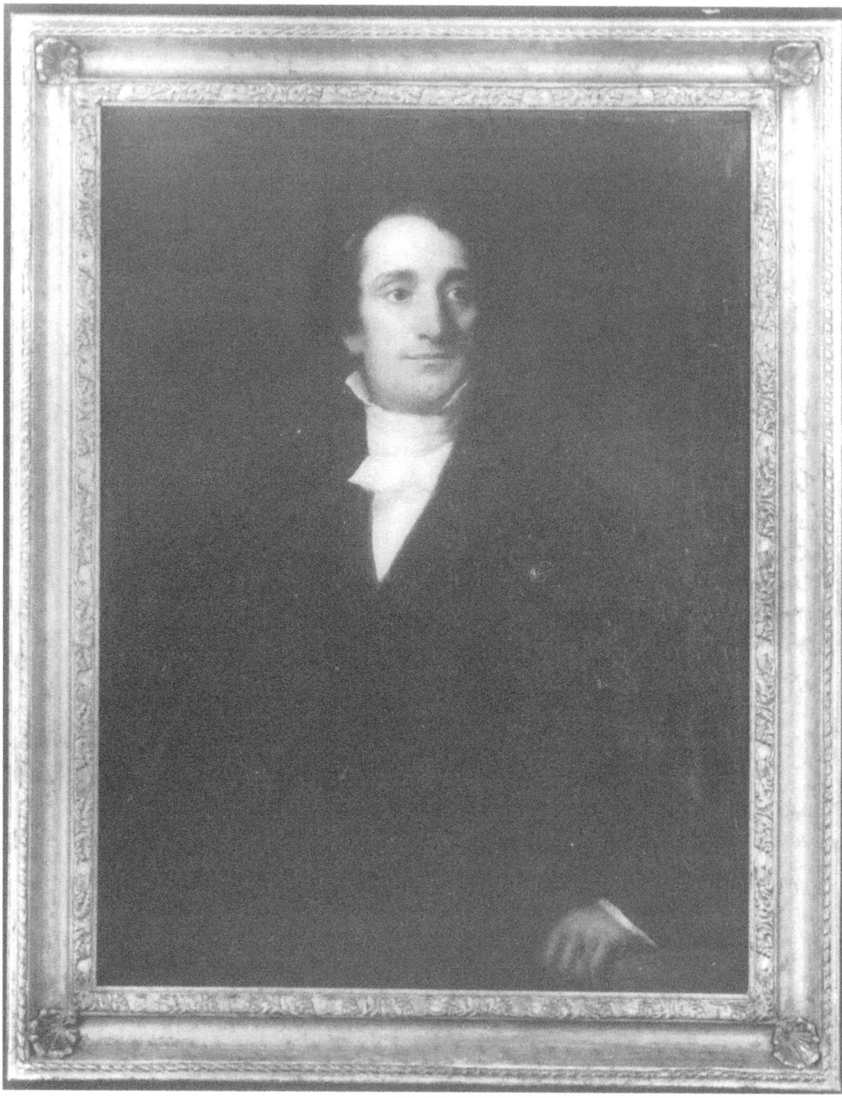

Figure 12.1: George Leith Roupell FRCP FRS (1795–1854). [Courtesy, the Archivist, St Bartholomew's Hospital, London].

acquired during this outbreak. He was also 'one of the medical officers attached to the City of London Board of Health (CBD), as the physician entrusted with the charge of … Cholera patients at St Bartholomew's Hospital during the months of June, July and August [1832] …'.

He attempted a distinction between malignant (Asiatic) cholera (or 'Cholera morbus') and the common cholera of England – a disease of the summer months. His historical and clinical descriptions (based largely on those of Mr Curtis – a ship's surgeon who recorded cases [in the *Madras Reports* for 1782] acquired at an infected port in Ceylon) of this disease remain excellent today. The third Croonian lecture addressed *pathogenesis* (which was *not* at that time understood). He stressed the *normality* of the mucous membranes in cholera; was the disease therefore due to 'an increased vitiated secretion from mere distention of vessels?' He mentioned 'suppression of urine' in a severe case.[9]

He also summarised many theories concerning the cause of cholera, and considered that poor sanitary regulations in the 'native towns of India' were aetiologically important. Roupell also advocated 'under-ground sewers' and removal of 'cemeteries beyond the confines of the city …' which was in line with the writing of Southwood Smith.[10] The (wet) state of the atmosphere was considered relevant, which was apparently the case when the disease first appeared in London in February 1832. Roupell also stressed that there was a great deal of 'under-reporting'.

MANAGEMENT OF CHOLERA

Whilst medical treatment was of value in 'common' (or sporadic) cholera, nothing seemed effective in the Asiatic variety. He was *not* an enthusiast for venesection, but gave detailed accounts of two patients (suffering from presumed *cholera*, although 'ordinary purging' was not excluded) whom he attended on board the *Dreadnought* in 1831 – James Ward and Robert Blair, men of 56 and 32 years, respectively, and both of whom had recovered after venesection. Roupell also gave details of a patient later treated at St Bartholomew's who had 20 ounces of blood venesected – and who, like the *Dreadnought* cases, duly recovered.

He advocated emetics (ipecacuanha or salt emetics) in management but usually in conjunction with venesection. 'Stimulants (including alcohol, mercury, [and] nitric acid), cold, purgatives (e.g. rhubarb given early in the disease after a 'large does of calomel'), and narcotics were discussed at length. Roupell was one of the first physicians to use 'saline injections', which became widespread in subsequent years:

> If the simple supply of those principles which are usually found in the blood, and which we know to be deficient in the advanced stage of Cholera, be all that is required for its cure, we cannot have a more direct or more certain method of supplying them, than by the easy and simple process of *injecting into the veins* [my italics] … this plan I have tried, and it was eminently successful in one of the cases …, yet in many others it proved quite unavailing …

Roupell continued:

> … for I have seen the indisputable improvement by saline injection quickly subside from the increased discharges by the bowels, which have come on soon after the injection, and in a short time reduced the patient to his former state.

Regarding the *limitations* of intravenous therapy, an important complication of which was 'phlebitis', Roupell wrote:

> I imagine that the saline injection does good, if the lost constituents of the blood be supplied in those cases in which exhaustion has been rapid, and the disease is disposed to cease, but it is a remedy far from innocent in its nature, and it is to be borne in mind, that it can do harm as well as good …

Roupell was therefore one of the first physicians to attempt correction of the underlying biochemical defect by the *intravenous* route (a technique which was not in general use until very much later).[11]

TYPHUS FEVER

In 1839 Roupell produced *'A Short Treatise of Typhus Fever'*, which contains an historical account, with some later impressions of the disease gained while at St Bartholomew's. This work had been preceded, however, by an account of a febrile illness – presumably epidemic (louse-borne) typhus (which occurred 'especially during the Spring of the two last years') on board HMS *Grampus* in 1831 (Chapter 11); 12 out of 75 cases had died of this entity which he termed: *'febris typhodes rubeoloida'*. He wrote in this report:

> this institution to which I was physician [i.e. HMS *Grampus*] furnished ample scope for studying acute diseases of all kinds, and especially fevers, for to them, as might be supposed, the sailor would be particularly obnoxious – his thoughtless character and reckless career on shore soon leaving him destitute of money, and exposing him to wants and privations of every sort. Hence fevers of the intermittent and remittent character during spring and autumn, and of the continued type during the summer, presented themselves almost daily; and offered nothing remarkable, except that during the preceding summer, the continued fever chiefly affected the head and was relieved by active depletion.

Some of the cases contained in his *magnum opus* were probably suffering from enteric (typhoid) fever; it was not until 1850 that a clear distinction was made (in Britain) between typhus and typhoid – by Sir William Jenner (1815–98) (*see* Chapter 11). Differentiation between the two diseases had already been made in 1837 in the USA by W W Gerhard (1809–72) working at Philadelphia. The *Grampus* 'epidemic' at a 'refuge … on the north side of the River Thames' seems to have convinced him that typhus was in fact a *communicable* disease.[12]

ROUPELL'S LEGACY

Munk has summarised Roupell's life by quoting extensively from an obituary notice in the *Medical Times & Gazette*: his 'public life was that of an upright and honourable man, and in private he was courteous, kind, and generous, almost to a fault. Habits of close industry, together with deep interest in the subjects of his study, stood him in the place of brilliancy of intellect, and furnished him with a rare extent of professional knowledge'. But the same journal also considered: 'As a lecturer (Figure 12.2), he could not be considered eloquent, his compositions being

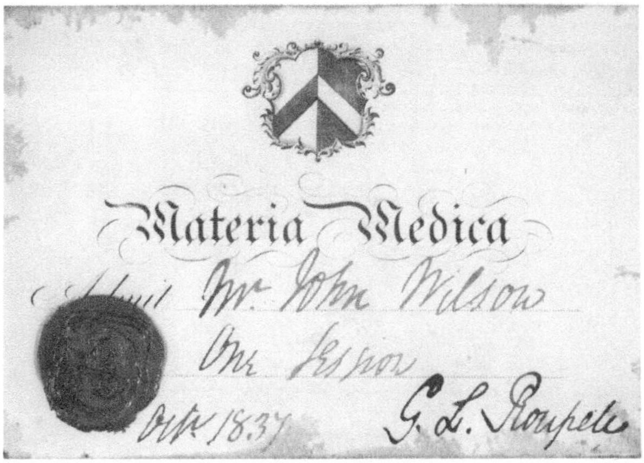

Figure 12.2: Ticket (dated October 1837) for admission to one of Roupell's *Materia Medica* lectures at St Bartholomew's Hospital. [Courtesy the Archivist, St Bartholomew's Hospital, London].

rather distinguished by the soundness of their subject-matter than any more attractive qualities'. The *Lancet's* obituarist considered: 'Although not of robust constitution, Dr Roupell could endure a considerable amount of mental and bodily labour. His great activity, his simple and temperate habits, and his constant cheerfulness of disposition, gave promise of a lengthened honourable career …'. He ended: '… the medical profession has [in his death] sustained a most severe loss, such indeed as can be ill afforded from its ranks'.[13]

Seymour

Edward James Seymour FRCP FRS (1796–1866) (Figure 12.3) was also appointed to the Society in 1828, as a Consulting Physician; he continued in that capacity until his death. Seymour was the son of a Brighton solicitor, and after attending a school in Richmond, Surrey, he entered Jesus College, Cambridge, from which he matriculated – proceeding to BA (1816) and MA (1819) degree. In 1822 he was granted a *licence ad practicandum* and proceeded to the MD degree in 1826. Before settling in London, he spent 'some years' in Italy (mainly Florence); in London, he had an upper class practice as a physician, and as well as joining the SHS, he was elected Physician to the Asylum for Recovery of Health (1825) and Physician to St George's Hospital (8 November 1828) ultimately becoming Senior Physician – which he served until 1846. On 1 September 1836, Seymour was appointed a metropolitan commissioner in lunacy; he was apparently a pioneer in the use of opium in the management of 'insanity'. He was also physician to the Duke of Sussex. His latter days were obscured by 'Broken health and … fortunes' and he died as a result of 'organic disease of the stomach and liver' on 16 April 1866.

At the College of Physicians, Seymour was admitted as an Inceptor-Candidate on 22 December 1823, a Candidate on 30 September 1826, and a fellow on 1 October 1827. He was successively Gulstonian lecturer (1829), Censor (1830), Croonian lec-

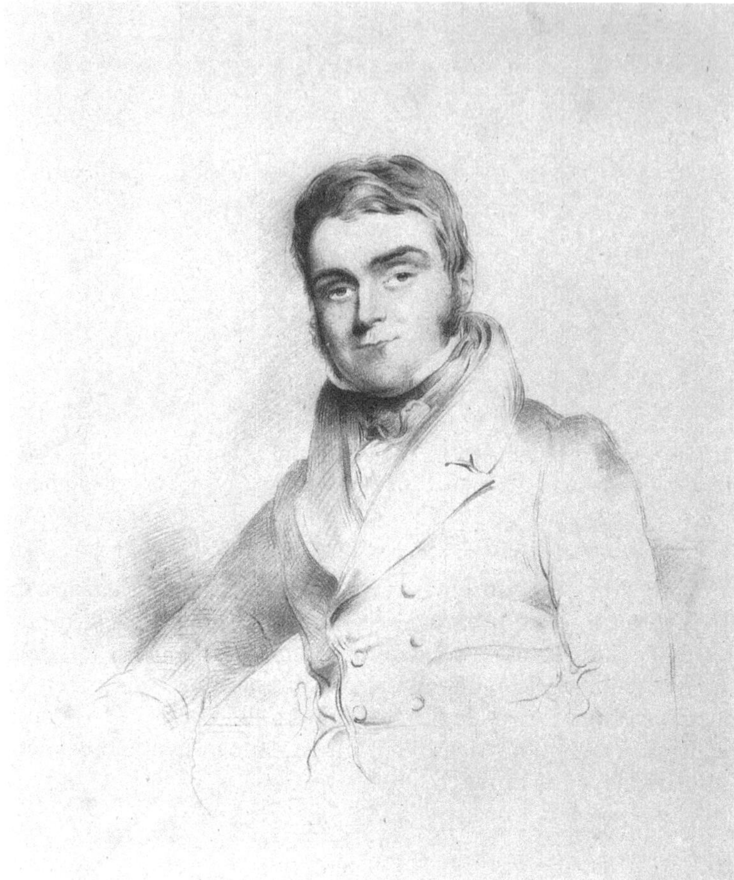

Figure 12.3: Edward James Seymour FRCP FRS (1796–1866). [Courtesy, Wellcome Library, London].

turer (1831) and Consilarius (1836). He was 'considered one of the most distinguished of the staff [of St George's Hospital], an able physician, a good teacher at the bedside, and a friend to the students'.[14]*

Mower

Arthur Mower FRCP (?–1837) was a graduate of Edinburgh University and served as Visiting Physician to the *Dreadnought* hospital (at Deptford) from 1832 until his death. During the years 1832–34 and 1836, he was also a curator of the Royal College of Physicians' Museum, and in 1835 he served as a Censor of that College.[15]

*Seymour's publications included: '*Illustrations of Diseases of the Ovaria, with Observations on their Structure and Functions*' (1830), '*Observations on the Medical Treatment of Insanity*' (1832), '*On the Nature and Treatment of Dropsy*' (1837) and '*Thoughts on the Nature and Treatment of Several Severe Diseases of the Human Body*' (1847).

Budd

George Budd FRS (1808–1882) (Figure 12.4) was born on 23 February 1808 at North Tawton, Devon. Early education was 'at home', but in 1827 he entered St John's (later moving to Caius) College, Cambridge. His clinical studies were carried out in Paris and at the Middlesex Hospital, London. At the age of 29 Budd was appointed Visiting Physician to the SHS.

RESEARCH ON SCURVY

The year after his appointment, an SHS minute records:

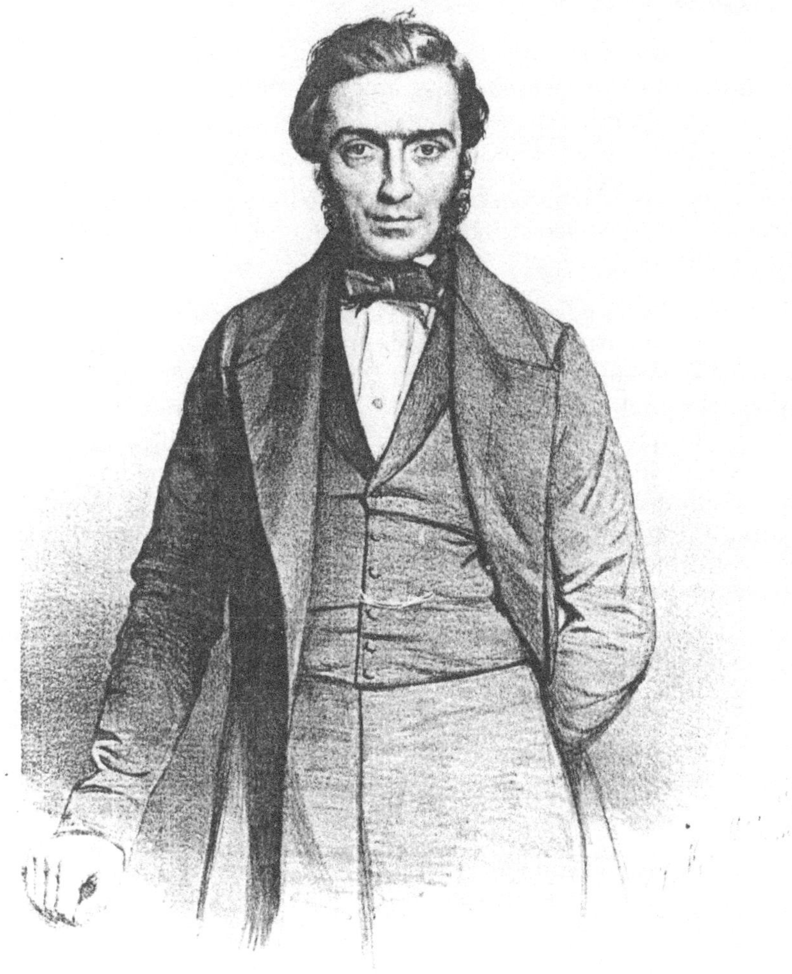

Figure 12.4: George Budd FRCP FRS (1808–82). [Courtesy, Royal College of Physicians, London].

> Read a letter from Dr. Budd Visiting Physician of the 12th inst stating that since he has been attached to the Hospital 31 cases of Scurvy have been admitted. Ordered [the minute continued] that Dr. Budd be requested to give a more detailed account of these cases and attend the Committee next Friday.

Later at that meeting:

> … Dr. Budd was requested to favour this Committee, in writing, with his opinion of the *causes* [my italics] of the Disease and the remedies he recommends that this Society may print it for circulation among Merchant Vessels.

Writing on *scurvy* in 1840, Budd considered:

> … its real cause is prolonged abstinence from fresh succulent vegetables or fruits, or their preserved juices; and that cold, defective ventilation, and the various other causes assigned for it, have no influence in bringing it on, except in so far as they waste the body or impair nutrition.

Budd's observations with proposed solution(s) to the scurvy problem (see Chapter 11 and below) were deemed sufficiently important to obtain mention in the SHS *Annual Report* for 1840:

> The Committee, in their last report [1839], felt it their duty to allude to the frequent occurrence of Cases of Scurvy among Seamen; since which time the Committee have requested DR. BUDD, the Visiting Physician to this Hospital, to trace the causes which in his opinion have led to its re-appearance after a lapse of many years. In obedience to which request, DR. BUDD investigated every case admitted, and has given to the Committee the result of his research, and the means by which so fearful a disease may be prevented in Merchant Ships. This valuable document, adding as it does to the essential services already rendered by DR. BUDD, has been printed by direction of the Committee, and is now in course of circulation among ship-owners and captains, with whom in a great measure rests the future application of the remedy.

OTHER SERVICE WITH THE SHS

Budd's medical interest(s) was, however, by no means limited to scurvy, for in February 1839, a minute stated:

> Read a letter from Dr. Budd Visiting Physician giving an account of 400 medical cases which have come under his treatment in four months, tracing the origin of the complaint in most cases to causes *while in port* [my italics]. Ordered that the thanks of the Committee be given to Dr. Budd and that his letter be printed for circulation.

Budd's three to four years service with the Seamen's Hospital Society gave him a wealth of experience – upon which he drew for numerous subsequent lectures and publications (see below). He was, for example, to set out his opinion(s) on amoebic liver 'abscess' in his book on Liver Disorders (see below). He clearly had a profound knowledge of Sir James Annesley [1780–1847]'s work in India, which he combined with his own experience at Greenwich.

Budd's tenure as Visiting Physician was, however, to be short-lived owing to escalating duties at King's College Hospital. In July 1840, a minute recorded:

> Read a letter from Dr. Budd Visiting Physician stating that his Duties at King's College demanding a great deal of his attention and that he finds he cannot devote so much time, as he has hitherto done, to the Patients under the charge of this Hospital and requesting this Committee will appoint him a Colleague with the understanding that no additional expense is to be incurred. Ordered [the minute continued] that the Committee be specially summoned for this day fortnight to consider the same.

The Committee duly met in late July, when his request was upheld. A fortnight later, Budd again wrote to the SHS Committee:

> 9 Bedford Place
> August 12 1840
>
> Gentlemen …
>
> I have engaged my Brother Dr. Wm. Budd [1811–80 – well known for his work on typhoid fever] to assist me in the performance of my duties at the Dreadnought. In making this choice I have in some measure consulted my own wishes, but I can assure you that I should not have done so, had I not been fully assured that I was at the same time promoting the real interests of the Institution … He has [since obtaining the Edinburgh MD with gold medal] had extensive opportunities of practice and I have no doubt that he will perform the duties that may devolve on him to the satisfaction of myself and of the Committee.
>
> I have the honour to be
> George Budd

Shortly afterwards, Budd resigned from the Society, and at the same time his brother was 'laid up' with Typhus fever. In November 1840, the following letter – received by the SHS Committee from Budd – was read:

> 2nd. Novr. 1840
>
> I have been considering your proposal to appoint two Physicians to the Dreadnought instead of one and I have no doubt that it would be for the advantage of the Institution to do so. The number of patients – 60 – that fall under the Physicians charge is exactly double the number I have at King's College Hospital. To make my visit well and to keep good registers of my cases takes at least an hour and half for each visit – for a man to do the same at the Dreadnought would require three hours at each visit, which together with the time consumed in coming and going is more than most men can afford to give. It may be done at first,

but it cannot be done when a man gets any private practice. With two Physicians the work would be easier and therefore in the long run better done. Another advantage that would result from the appointment of two is that in case of absence or illness, one might replace the other.

I am

George Budd

FUTURE CAREER

The Annual Report for 1841 recorded Budd's resignation, and added: '... the Committee, at DR. BUDD's suggestion, took into consideration the increased demand upon the time and attention of whoever might fill the responsible office; they therefore took the opportunity offered by the resignation of DR. BUDD, to appoint two Visiting Physicians, and after due enquiry they selected, from many candidates, DRs [Patrick] BLACK and [Richard] GOOLDEN [see below], who have been appointed accordingly'. Budd was then made a Consulting Physician.

At the Royal College of Physicians he was to become Gulstonian (1843) and Croonian (1847) lecturer. His principal literary works were: *On diseases of the Liver* (1845) and *Diseases of the Stomach* (1855).

Few contemporary descriptions of Budd as an individual have survived; however, one obituarist gave a brief insight; he referred to '[his] tall and spare frame, his academic style, his keen glance, and intellectual physiognomony'. Budd was also, he continued: '... eloquent and learned [as a lecturer]' and ' ... earnest, emphatic and practical [as a bedside teacher]'. Budd died at his home at Ashleigh, near Barnstable (to which he had retired due to ill-health), on 14 March 1882.[16]

Black

Patrick Black FRCP (1813–79) was born in Aberdeen, and educated at Eton and Christ Church, Oxford. His medical training was at St. Bartholomew's Hospital, where he became assistant physician in 1842, and warden of the college; he became a full physician in 1860. Between 1840 and 51, Black was a Visiting Physician to the *Dreadnought* Hospital, and a physician to Christ's Hospital. His publications were on chloroform (which he regularly administered), respiration, scurvy and diseases of the spleen. Black was a Censor and Croonian Lecturer (1855) at the Royal College of Physicians, and in 1867 revised the Latin part of their *Nomenclature of Diseases*. One of Black's house-physicians at Bart's was the future poet-laureate Robert Bridges OM, FRCP (1844–1930). Black married the daughter of William Mark (HM Consul at Malaga) in 1843 and they had several children. He died on 12 October 1879.[17]

Goolden

Richard Henry Goolden FRCP (1810–80) was a Visiting Physician to the SHS from 1840–6. Educated at the Merchant Taylors' School, Queen's College Oxford, and King's College, London, he graduated BA (1832), BM (1836), and DM (1838).

From 1844 until 70, he was either Assistant Physician, or Physician to St. Thomas' Hospital, London. Goolden also lectured at the Grosvenor Place School of Anatomy and Medicine. In 1861, he delivered the Harveian Oration to the Royal College of Physicians. He died on 10 March 1880.[18]

Blackall

Thomas Blackall FRCP (1814–99) was educated at Exeter Grammar and Westminster Schools, and at Caius College, Cambridge, graduating BA in 1837. His medical training was at St. George's Hospital; following qualification, he served as a Visiting Physician on the *Dreadnought* Hospital-ship, as well as developing a practice in Mayfair. On the death of his father, in 1860, he inherited (at the age of 46) a fortune which enabled him to retire to Devon, where he became a 'cultured member of local society' and a benefactor to local charities. He died on 11 May 1899.[19]

Hue

John William Hue FRCP (1820–1903) was persuaded to enter medicine by his father – a physician at St. Bartholomew's Hospital. After graduating BA at Pembroke College, Cambridge he entered St Bartholomew's Hospital in 1843. Between 1851 and 56 he was a Visiting Physician to the *Dreadnought* Hospital, but in 1858 (at the age of 38) he retired from active medical practice; this followed an unsuccessful application for a post as Assistant Physician at St Bartholomew's. From thence he lived on the Isle of Wight and spent a great deal of time abroad; he was apparently very fond of music! Hue died on 24 December 1903.[20]

Barnes

Robert Barnes FRCP (1817–1907) (Figure 12.5) was educated at Bruges, and (privately) at his father's home in Norwich. At the age of 15 years, he was apprenticed to a local surgeon; in 1842, he qualified in medicine following studies at University College and St. George's Hospital, London. In 1848 he obtained the MD (Lond) and was elected FRCP in 1859. He then spent a year in Paris – apparently maintaining himself by giving English lessons. On his return to London, after short spells at University College and the Bethlem Royal Hospitals, he entered General Practice at Notting Hill, but in 1859 was appointed Assistant Obstetric Physician, and in 1863, Obstetric Physician to the London Hospital. He also lectured to St Thomas's and St George's Hospitals. In 1865 he transferred to St. Thomas's Hospital in the same discipline.

Ten years later he moved back to St. George's. Barnes was a Visiting Physician to the *Dreadnought* Hospital (1855–70), Consulting Physician (1882–1904) and a Vice-President (1900); he also held appointments at the *East London Hospital for Children* and the *Royal Maternity Hospital*. In 1858 he gave the Lettsomian lectures to the *Medical Society of London*, and in 1873 the Lumleian Lectures of the *Royal College of Physicians* – where he was also a Censor. Around 1887, he moved to Eastbourne,

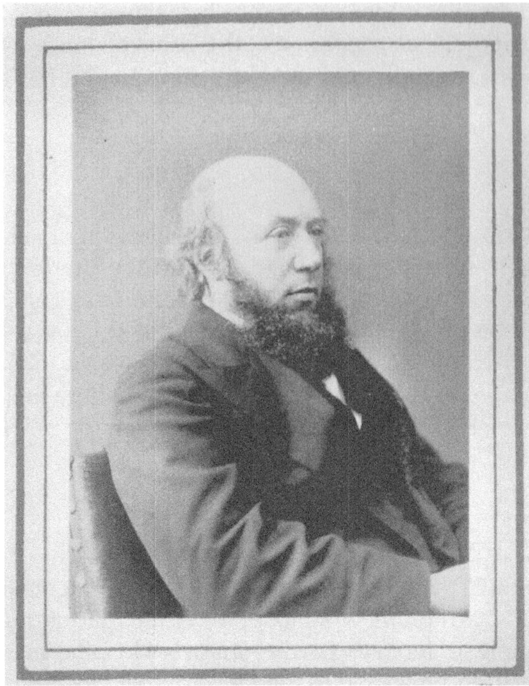

Figure 12.5: Robert Barnes FRCP (1817–1907). [Courtesy, Wellcome Library, London].

having retired from active practice. Barnes married Eliza Fawkener (daughter of a London solicitor) by whom he had a son and two daughters, and secondly (in 1880) Alice Maria (daughter of Captain WG Hughes J P) who bore him a son and a daughter.* He died on 12 May 1907 from a 'thrombotic episode'.[21]

Ward

Stephen Henry Ward FRCP (1819–80) was a Visiting Physician at the *Dreadnought* Hospital from 1856 until his death; he thus served on the latter two hospital-ships, and the land-based hospital, also. Ward was the son of a distinguished botanist/ microscopist – Nathaniel Bagshawe Ward FRS, and was educated at Hackney and the London Hospital. In addition to his appointment to the SHS, he had been appointed in 1864 as a physician to the London Hospital for Diseases of the Chest. He became Treasurer, and later President of the Hunterian Society, and was an examiner for the Worshipful Society of Apothecaries of London. Ward contributed an important paper to *The Lancet* in 1860, entitled 'Analysis of 1000 consecutive cases admitted into the Seamen's Hospital, "Dreadnought"'. [*Lancet*, 1860; ii: 78–9]. His publications also included a book on diseases of the liver – on which he became

*Barnes wrote a great deal; his best-known works were: *Lectures on Obstetric Operations* (1870), and *Medical and Surgical Diseases of Women* (1877).

an authority. He married a sister of E W Cooke RA FRS – the distinguished maritime engraver – and had one daughter. Ward died on 10 July 1880.[22]

Leach

Harry Leach MRCP (1836-79) died early in his fifth decade from pulmonary tuberculosis, he had a distinguished career with the SHS, and devoted a great deal of time and energy to the improvement of the health of sailors in the Mercantile Marine. He was initially appointed to the SHS as an apothecary, and served in that capacity on the third of the hospital-ships from 1862–9. In 1869–70 his title was 'Physicians Assistant'; his subsequent career took place on the land-based *Dreadnought* Hospital until his premature death.

Leach was born at Wisbech, Cambridgeshire into 'a family long known and esteemed in that borough'. Educated at St. Albans School, he subsequently became a pupil of a Peterborough practitioner Dr. Thomas Walker. Leach entered St. Bartholomew's Hospital in 1853, and qualified with the MRCS and LSA diplomas in 1858. Following a brief spell as House-Surgeon at Peterborough Infirmary, and after several voyages to India and back, he was appointed (in 1862) Physicians Assistant and Apothecary to the SHS – serving for most of his professional life on the *Dreadnought* hospital-ship, and from 1870 onwards at the land-based *Dreadnought* Hospital at Greenwich (see above). A close colleague at the SHS was H T L Rooke (see below); when Rooke died in September 1870 (i.e. soon after removal to land), Leach was appointed Principle Medical Officer (PMO) at the *Dreadnought* Hospital. He was also a medical inspector on the Turkish Railways.

HEALTH OF THE MERCHANT NAVY

In 1867, he published (anonymously) a series of five articles in the *British Medical Journal* entitled: '*Report on the Hygienic Condition of the Mercantile Marine, and on the Preventable Diseases of Merchant Seamen*'. This excellent series of articles (based on his experience with the SHS) dealt with general matters, and health problems associated with ocean-going ships, coasters, barges and training ships, and scurvy; he concentrated on the necessity for inspection of all shipping arriving in the Thames, as well as the sanitary control of the Port – with a view to improving the health and comfort of the vast community of seamen and their families passing to and from the Port of London. The series was subsequently reprinted in book format, and under his *General Remarks*, Leach considered: 'Fever exists to a great extent in our coasting, scurvy in our ocean-going ships, and venereal diseases in both'! The timing of Leach's publication was admirable for the appalling conditions in the Mercantile Marine, especially from a health viewpoint, had by 1867 become the subject of much public – including parliamentary – concern. Amongst several other topics, mercantile marine reform became a dominant theme in Queen Victoria's speech at the opening of parliament that year.

RESEARCH ON SCURVY AND CHOLERA

Leach contributed an important series of letters on *scurvy* to The Editor of *The Times* (which began with a reply to a leading article in that newspaper [Chapter 11]). He was not, of course, the first medical officer serving with the SHS to take an interest in scurvy; Budd (see above) had, many years before, written two treatises on the cause and prevention of this disease, and had composed notes which were widely circulated to captains of ships.

During an anticipated *cholera* epidemic in 1866, Leach took charge of the hospital-ship *Belle-isle* – which, like the *Dreadnought*, had previously served at Trafalgar (*see* Chapter 8). He organised (with his colleague, Rooke – see above) an 'extensive programme of ship-to-ship visitation on the river Thames'. This work was undertaken by the SHS at their own expense after an application to the Privy Council had proved unsuccessful; for three months, 'every vessel between London-bridge and Woolwich was visited daily'; in all a total of 31,346 ship-visits were made!

OTHER CONTRIBUTIONS

Leach formed the opinion during his term of residence on the last of the Hospital-ships 'the utter unfitness of the old wooden hulk for hospital purposes'. Together with his colleagues (Rooke included) he whole-heartedly supported a campaign for removal to dry land – which, after much administrative as well as parliamentary intervention, eventually came to fruition on 13 April 1870 (Chapter 13).

Leach either wrote or compiled several books.* An Official Notice in his most important book recommended: (at the price of 'One shilling and Threepence') 'The Ship Captain's Medical Guide' compiled by 'Harry Leach, resident Medical Officer of the 'Dreadnought' Hospital Ship, and Inspector of lime and lemon juice appointed by the Board of Trade for the Port of London'. In 1873, Leach resigned from the SHS, and became the first Port Medical Officer of the City of London, but two years later he was appointed Visiting Physician to the SHS (*see* Chapter 15).

Socially, Leach was described as 'the most genial of companions, hospitable, kindly, considerate, and possessed of the happy faculty of adapting himself in personal intercourse to every variety of social and mental demand'. He was also 'well read in men, and had added much to his abundant store of knowledge by extensive travel abroad'.[23]

Jackson

John Hughlings Jackson FRCP FRS (1835–1911) (Figure 12.6) was appointed Visiting Physician to the *Dreadnought* Hospital in early 1870 – immediately prior to the removal to dry-land – on 13 April. Born at Green Hammerton, Yorkshire and educated at Tadcaster and Nailsworth, Gloucestershire, he became apprenticed to a York practitioner and attended the York Medical and Surgical School. After qualification at St Bartholomew's Hospital in 1856, he served as house-physician at the York Dispensary. Returning to London, Jackson was appointed to the staff of the *Metropolitan Free Hospital* in 1859, and to a Lecturership in Pathology at the London

*Amongst Leach's publications were: *Brief Notes on the last epidemic of Cholera in Turkey* (1866) (based on an epidemic of 1865), *Hygienic Condition of the Mercantile Marine* (1867) (previously published anonymously in the *British Medical Journal*), *The Ship's Captain's Medical Guide* (1868), *Pocket Doctor for the Traveller and Colonist* (1875) and *A Bit of Bulgaria* (1877).

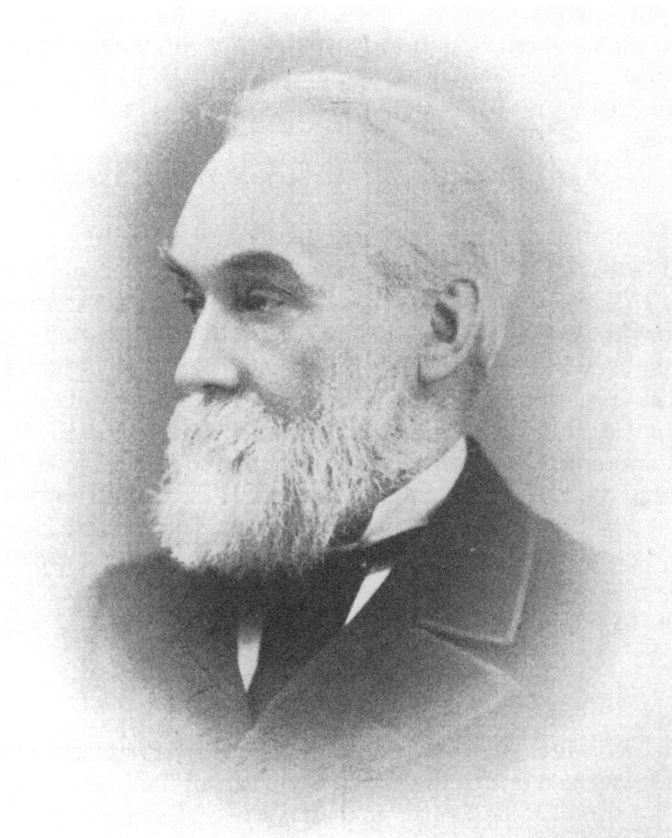

Figure 12.6: John Hughlings Jackson FRCP FRS (1835–1911). [Courtesy, Wellcome Library, London].

Hospital; he was also appointed to the Islington and Moorfields Eye Hospitals. However, his distinguished career in neurology (he was to become the 'father of English neurology') began with his election as assistant physician to the *National Hospital for the Paralysed and Epileptic* in 1862. In 1869 he became a full physician there, and in 1874 a physician to the (Royal) London Hospital.

Hughlings Jackson subsequently became a Censor of the Royal College of Physicians, and delivered the Goulstonian Lectures in 1869; he also gave the Croonian in 1884 and the Lumleian Lecture in 1890. He married a cousin in 1865. Hughlings Jackson died on 7 October 1911.[24]

Surgeons

Table 12.3 lists the surgeons serving the SHS during the years of the Hospital-ships. Unfortunately their lives have not been as meticulously recorded for posterity as those of the physicians who served the SHS between the years 1821–70. Full biographies are available in only a minority of cases. As with the founding physicians, those who served the Society at its origin are mentioned in Chapter 6. Without doubt, the most distinguished of the surgeons during this period was George Busk FRS (see below).

Dobson

(Sir) **Richard Dobson** FRS (1773–1847) was a Consulting Surgeon to the SHS from 1829 until 1847. He had joined the Royal Navy in May 1795, served at Haslar Hospital, and was made a full surgeon on 17 February 1797. He had served on various ships in the West Indies and on the 'home station'. In 1794, he had been Surgeon of the *Lively* at the capture of the Spanish treasure ships at Cadiz. Following this, he was appointed Surgeon to the *Trusty* Hospital-ship in the Medway. In 1814, Dobson was appointed Surgeon to the Royal Marine Infirmary at Chatham and 10 years later to the Royal Hospital, Greenwich. He was therefore well placed in relation to the SHS. Dobson was knighted in 1831, and elected FRS in 1835. He subsequently became Medical Inspector of Hospitals and Fleets. He seems to have been instrumental in 'abolishing … the office of physician', and placing all patients at Greenwich Hospital under a surgeon.[25]

Busk

George Busk FRCS FRS (1807–86) (Figure 12.7). As well as being an outstanding surgeon, Busk was also one of the great polymaths of the nineteenth century. He was the second son of Robert Busk a merchant of St. Petersburgh, and was born in that city on 12 August 1807. Busk was the grandson of Sir Wadsworth Busk – Attorney-General of the Isle of Man – and nephew of Hans Busk (1772–1862), a scholar-poet; his cousin, also Hans Busk (1816–62), was the principal founder of the Volunteer Movement in England. His mother was the daughter of John Westly, Custom House clerk at St Petersburgh.

He was initially educated at Dr Hartley's School, Bingley, Yorkshire, and studied medicine at St Thomas's Hospital; he also attended (for one session) St Bartholomew's Hospital – from October 1828. For six years he was an articled student with George Beaman under the aegis of the Royal College of Surgeons of England (RCS), and was elected FRCS on 11 December 1843. Busk married a first cousin, Ellen – youngest daughter of Jacob Hans Busk of Theobalds, Hertfordshire. He subsequently occupied many influential positions, not only in the surgical world (he served as President of the Royal College of Surgeons of England in 1871), but also in many learned scientific societies (see below).

Busk was appointed to the SHS in 1831 – having served (in 1830) as Apothecary on HMS *Grampus*; the following year he was appointed Assistant Surgeon on HMS *Dreadnought*. By 1834, he was designated Resident Surgeon; in 1840 as 'First Surgeon', in 1853 as 'Visiting Surgeon' and in 1866 as 'Consulting Surgeon'; the SHS Reports describe him in this latter capacity until his death. In addition to his day-to-day activities on board *Dreadnought*, he 'worked out the pathology of cholera, and

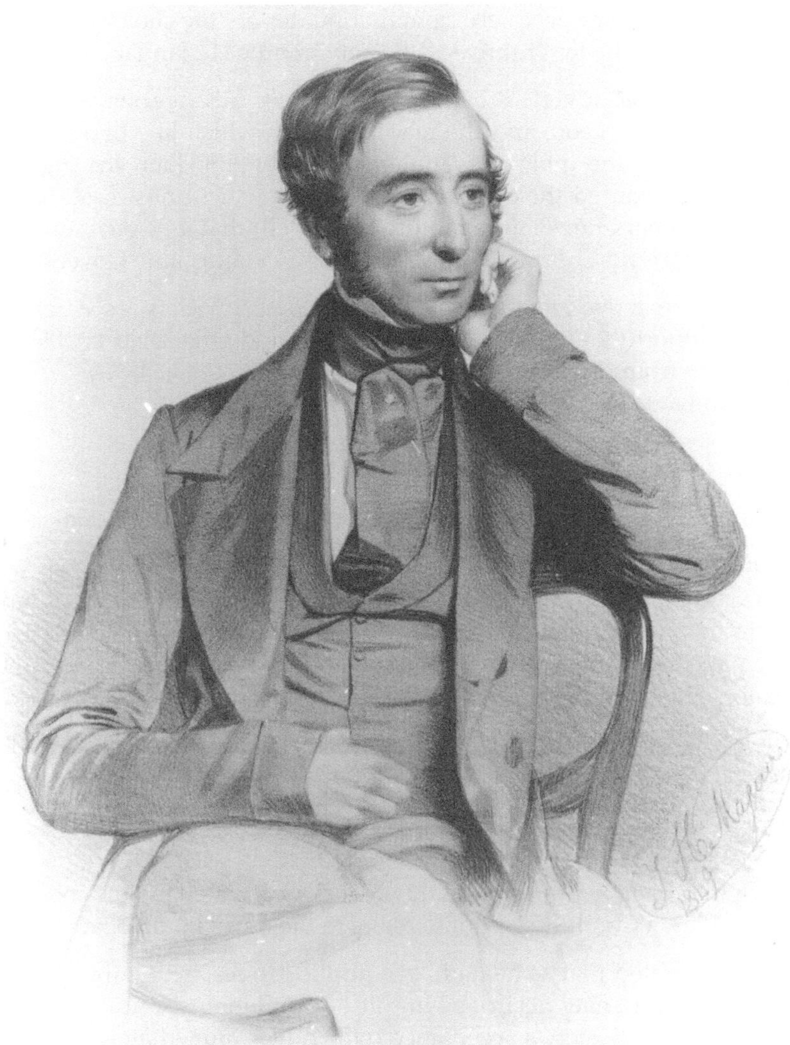

Figure 12.7: George Busk FRCS FRS (1807–86). [SHS Archive].

made important observations on scurvy'. He thus served as surgeon to the SHS for 24 or 25 years – until 1855 (a period which '[had] embraced the strictly professional [years] of his life') after which he retired from surgical practice.

CHOLERA RESEARCH

Busk's work on cholera was dominated by a joint report with Budd (see above); together they documented clinical details of 20 cases of cholera on the *Dreadnought* between 8 and 28 October 1837 (see Chapter 11). The 28th and 29th *Annual Reports* (dated 1849 and 1850 respectively) contain updates on 'the cholera' on the Thames in London's second major outbreak. A Society minute (12 January 1849) records:

> The Committee adverted to the unabated zeal and attention of Mr Busk their Senior Surgeon, and the readiness with which he volunteered to the charge of the Iphigenia Cholera Hospital Ship [and in August of that year recorded the sites on the River at which most cases arose]. Resolved unanimously [the minute continued] that it be recommended to the Quarterly Court to elect Mr Busk an Honorary Life Governor.

Busk (already an active member of the Microscopical Society – see below) was 'a recognised authority on multicellular organisms and other objects'. He examined faecal-samples from cholera patients (on board HMS *Dreadnought*) – with, according to Edwin Lankester, *negative* (erroneous) results.

RESEARCH ON OTHER DISEASES

Busk also carried out work on scurvy (jointly with Budd – who wrote a report for the SHS – see above). On Friday 12 May 1843, an SHS minute stated:

> Ordered a paper drawn up by Mr Busk the Surgeon "Hints to Seamen as to the prevention and cure of scurvy" be printed and circulated to the patients on their being discharged and that a number be sent to the Sailors Home for distribution.

A further disease which proved troublesome during Busk's period on the *Dreadnought* was 'Typhus Fever' (see Chapter 11).

BUSK'S MUSEUM

Beginning in his active professional days, Busk was a meticulous 'collector'! On 3 November 1843, a Committee minute refers to the museum on board *Dreadnought*:

> Mr Busk stated that as he had been applied to respecting the Museum on board and being desirous himself of promoting surgical science he requested the Society's acceptance [which was immediately forthcoming] of his anatomical preparations, which he hoped to see increased as opportunity offers.

After the *Dreadnought* ship had given way to the land-based *Dreadnought* Hospital in 1870 (*see* Chapter 13) the *new* School of *Clinical Medicine* (Chapter 19) also contained a Museum, the content(s) of which: '...include a collection of skulls [see below], interesting from an ethnological point of view, made by Mr Busk who was at one time surgeon to the *Dreadnought*'.

OTHER DISCIPLINES

Busk also made important contributions to several other disciplines: in helminthology he was the first individual to visualise *Distoma* (later *Fasciolopsis*) *buski* – a fluke infecting the upper gastrointestinal tract of man); he also advanced knowledge in zoology and palaeontology (his significant contributions to understanding of 'Neanderthal man' culminated in the demonstration of the 'Gibraltar skull' at the British Association's meeting at Bath in September 1864 (at which Dr David Livingstone [1813–73] was present). Busk also contributed to, and held office in, many learned societies – including the Zoological Society, the Linnean Society (Busk was the Zoological Secretary when the Darwin/Wallace papers were presented to the 'special meeting' on 1 July 1858), and the Geological Society.

LATER LIFE

Following 25 years at Greenwich, where he both lived and worked, he moved to London – at number 15 and subsequently 32 Harley Street, where he died after a protracted illness associated with 'long-continued neuralgic suffering, consequent on an attack of herpes' on 10 August 1886; it is probable that ill-health in latter years prevented him accepting the Presidency of the Linnean Society of London. The *Annual Report* for 1886, contained the following notice:

> The Committee desire to place on record that death has ... deprived them of the valued services of Mr. George Busk, F.R.S, who was first associated with the Society in 1830, and became the Consulting Surgeon in 1866. For 56 years Mr. Busk was connected with the Hospital, and when Consulting Surgeon he was always ready to place his skilled experience at the disposal of his Colleagues ...

Of Busk's overall personality the anonymous writer in *Plarr's Lives* considered: 'He was a man of unaffected simplicity and gentleness of character, without a trace of vanity, a devoted friend, and an upright, honest gentleman'. Busk's two daughters later endowed a bed at the *Dreadnought* Hospital (the plaque remains extant) in memory of their distinguished father.[26]

Clapp

William Clapp FRCS (1814–88) received his medical education at Guy's and St Thomas's Hospitals, London. He obtained the MRCS (1839) and LSA (1840) diplomas, and became FRCS on 16 December 1847. In 1844 he served as Second Surgeon on HMS *Dreadnought*. Following service with the SHS he practiced at Exeter – where he was the first Surgeon-Apothecary (House Surgeon) to the Devon and Exeter Hospital. He seems to have 'hived off' administrative duties in order to devote more 'time to profession work in the wards'. He died at his residence – Southernhay Place, Exeter on 27 May 1888.[27]

Tudor

John Tudor (?–1908) qualified at King's College, London – with the MRCS diploma in 1847, and LSA in 1853. He published a paper in *The Lancet* for 1859 on 'The Hygienic Condition of the "Dreadnought" Hospital-ship in 1857–8 ...' [*Lancet* 1859; i: 361–2]. Tudor later became Senior Surgeon to the Dorset County Hospital.[28]

Rooke

Henry Turner Lane Rooke (1824–70) qualified MRCS and LSA at King's College, London and Edinburgh Universities in 1846. He served in the Crimean War (1854–7) as a surgeon on the civil list. Rooke was appointed junior medical officer of the *Dreadnought* in September 1848. From 1848–54 he served under Busk on the *Dreadnought* hospital-ship. In 1857, Rooke obtained the LM from the Rotunda Hospital, Dublin and then entered general practice at Wisbech, Cambridgeshire. He rejoined the SHS as Principal Medical Officer. When the post of Surgeon on the *Dreadnought* became vacant (following the resignation of Tudor), Rooke was appointed. He died of complications from an epithelioma of the tongue.[29]

Croft

John Croft FRCS (1833–1905) (see Figure 12.8) was born at Pettinghoe, near Newhaven, Sussex. Educated at the Hackney Church of England School, and following a short apprenticeship with Thomas Evans of Burwash, Sussex, he entered

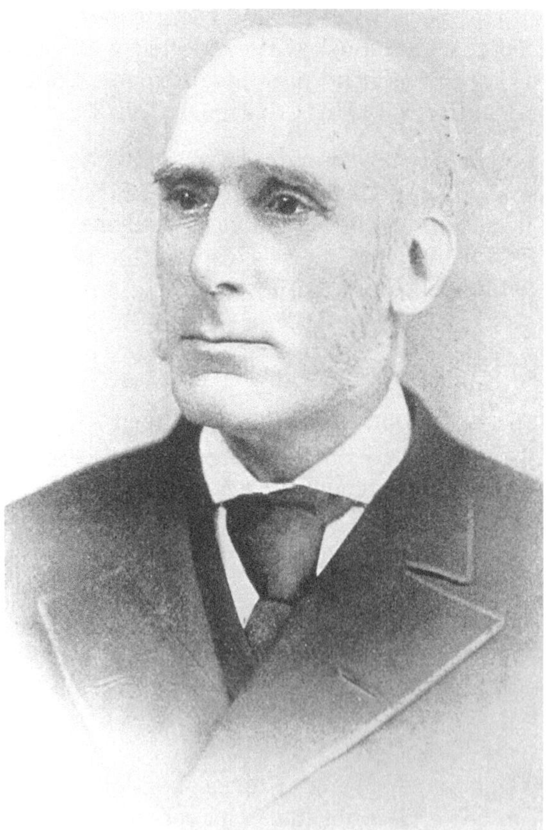

Figure 12.8: John Croft FRCS (1833–1905). [Courtesy, Wellcome Library, London].

St Thomas's Hospital in 1850, where he subsequently served as a House Surgeon. From 1855 until 1860, he was Resident Surgeon on the SHS Hospital-ships. He then returned to St Thomas's as Surgical Registrar and Demonstrator of Anatomy. When St Thomas's Hospital's *new* building opened, he became successively Resident Assistant Surgeon (1863), Assistant Surgeon (1871), and Surgeon (1871); in the Medical School, he was also Demonstrator of Anatomy, Lecturer on Practical Surgery, and Lecturer on Clinical Surgery. In 1891 he was elected Consulting Surgeon to the SHS. He was also Surgeon to the Surrey Dispensary, the National Truss Society, the Magdalen Hospital Streatham, and the National Provident Assurance Society. At the RCS, he was elected to Council in 1882 but resigned in 1890; he served as Vice-President in 1889, and was a member of the Court of Examiners from 1881 until 1886.

Croft was apparently one of the first surgeons in London to adopt 'Listerian methods'. He also introduced 'Croft's splints' (plaster of Paris cases made with scrubbing flannel and shaped to the limb it was desired to immobilize), which were superseded by 'celluloid splints'. He married Annie, daughter of Alexander Douglas. Croft died on 21 November 1905, and was buried at Kensal Green Cemetery.[30]

Smith

William Johnson Smith FRCS (1840–1912) (see Figure 12.9) studied medicine at King's College Hospital – qualifying with the MRCS (1862) and LSA (1863) diplomas; he obtained the FRCS on 14 December 1865. Smith was appointed Assistant Surgeon to the SHS – at Greenwich in 1863, and later to the Albert Dock Hospital.

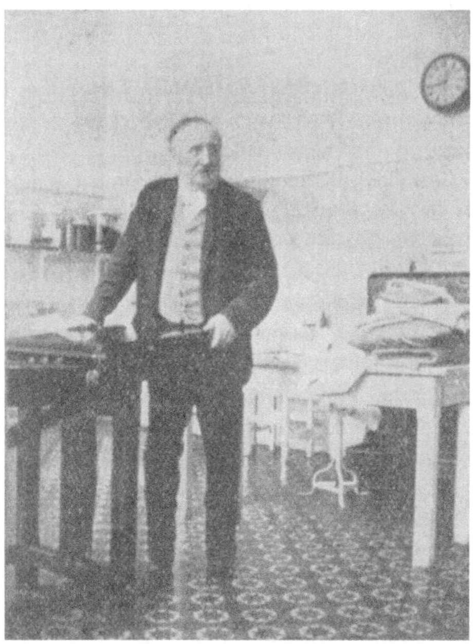

Figure 12.9: William Johnson Smith FRCS (1840–1912). [SHS Archive].

He was also surgeon to the Cottage Hospital at Eltham, Kent. In 1867 he gained the Jacksonian Prize at the RCS with an essay: 'The various deformities resulting from severe burns, etc'. For many years he '... had a monopoly on the teaching of operative surgery on the dead body, owing to the number of unclaimed bodies at the Seamen's Hospital'.

Johnson Smith was one of the few surgeons to span the hospital-ship days and those of the land-based *Dreadnought*. His subsequent career (after 1870) is related in Chapter 15.[31]

Apothecaries

Table 12.4 lists the apothecaries, 'assistant surgeons and apothecaries', and 'physician's assistant and apothecaries' from 1821 to 70. Some of these proceeded to become members of the SHS's *senior* staff (e.g. Busk, Clapp, Rooke and Leach), but the majority left after one or two year's service on the Hospital-ships.

References and notes

1 SHS Annual Reports. 21, 22, 23.
2 *Ibid.* 1824: 4; 1831: 8; 1833: 8; 1835: 7; 1841: 7; 1851: 7; 1861: 7.
3 M Fry. Dundas, Robert Saunders, second Viscount Melville (1771–1851). In: H C G Matthew, B Harrison (eds). *Oxford Dictionary of National Biography.* Oxford: Oxford University Press 2004; 17: 292–4.
4 F M L Thompson. Percy, Algernon, fourth Duke of Northumberland (1792–1865). In: H C G Matthew, B Harrison (eds). *Oxford Dictionary of National Biography.* Oxford: Oxford University Press 2004; 43: 684–6.
5 Committee of Management Minutes. 6: 292–294; 510; 8: 430.
6 A Lambert. Bowles, Sir William (1780–1869). In: H C G Matthew, B Harrison (eds). *Oxford Dictionary of National Biography.* Oxford: Oxford University Press 2004; 6: 967–9.
7 *Op cit.* See note 5 above. 6: 1849; 23 February; Anonymous. *Times Lond* 1874; 27 June: 1; 'The late Mr Kemball Cook'. *Shipping Gazette* 1874; 27 June: 5. [*See also*: SHS Annual Report 1874; B H Kemball-Cook. *A memoir – ancestors.* Hitchin – Calliope Press 2001: 19; A J A Morris. Cook, Sir Edward Tyas (1857–1919) In: H C G Matthew, B Harrison (eds). *Oxford Dictionary of National Biography.* Oxford: Oxford University Press 2004; 13: 92–4].
8 Anonymous. *Times, Lond.* 1854; 30 September: 10; *Lancet* 1854; ii: 303–4; *Medical Times and Gazette* 1854; 9: 374; *Munks Roll*: 3: 293–4; *Gentleman's Magazine* 1854; ii: 520–21; N Moore, K Bagshaw. Roupell, George Leith (1797–1854) In: H C G Matthew, B Harrison (eds). *Oxford Dictionary of National Biography.* Oxford: Oxford University Press 2004; 47: 947. [*See also*: G.C. Cook: George Leith Roupell (1797–1854): significant contributions to the early nineteenth-century understanding of cholera and typhus. *J Med Biog* 2000; 8: 1–7; G C Cook. Medical disease in the Merchant Navies of the world in the days of sail: the Seamen's Hospital Society's experience. *Mariner's Mirror* 2005; 91: 46–51].
9 *Op cit.* See note 11 below (Roupell); G C Cook. Management of cholera: the vital role of rehydration. In: B S Drasar, B D Forrest (eds). *Cholera and the Ecology of* Vibro cholerae. London: Chapman and Hall, 1996: 54–94. [*See also: Op cit.* See note 8 above (Cook 2000)].

10 G C Cook. Thomas Southwood Smith FRCP (1788–1861): leading exponent of diseases of poverty, and pioneer of sanitary reform in the mid-nineteenth century. *J Med Biog* 2002; 10: 194–205.

11 G L Roupell. *The Croonian lectures delivered at the Royal College of Physicians in MDCCCXXXIII*. London: G & W Nicol 1833: 96; G C Cook. The Asiatic cholera: an historical determinant of human genomic and social structure. In: B S Drasar, B D Forrest (eds). *Cholera and the Ecology of* Vibro cholerae. London: Chapman and Hall, 1996: 18–53.

12 G L Roupell. *A short treatise on typhus fever*. London: W Wright, S Highley, J Churchill. 1839: 301; G L Roupell. *Some account of a Fever Prevalent in the year 1831*. London: William Nichol: 1837: 20; *Op cit*. See note 8 above (Cook 2000).

13 *Op cit*. See note 8 above (Cook 2000).

14 Anonymous. *Lancet* 1866; i: 473–4; *Munk's Roll* 3: 277–8: 142; *London Medical Directory* 1866; W W Webb, M Bevan. Seymour, Edward James (1796–1866) In: H C G Matthew, B Harrison (eds). *Oxford Dictionary of National Biography*. Oxford: Oxford University Press 2004; 49: 877–8.

15 Anonymous. *London Medical Gazette* 1837; 20: 56; *Munk's Roll* 4: 5.

16 Anonymous. *Lancet* 1882; i: 49; *Proc R Soc Lond* 1882: 34: i–iii; *Medico-Chirurg Trans* 1883; 66: 8-10; *Munk's Roll* 4, 27; S J A Salter, M E Gibson. Budd, George (1808–1882) In: H C G Matthew, B Harrison (eds). *Oxford Dictionary of National Biography*. Oxford: Oxford University Press 2004; 8: 550; [*See also:* Minute Book 1: 219; G Budd. *On diseases of the liver*. London: John Churchill. 1845; G. Budd. *On the organic diseases and functional disorders of the stomach*. London: John Churchill. 1855; G C Cook. Scurvy in the British Mercantile Marine in the 19th century, and the contribution of the Seamen's Hospital Society. *Postgrad Med J*; 2004; 80: 24–9; Anonymous. William Budd M.D. *SHS Quart Mag* 1936; 8(3): 13; G C Cook. George Budd FRS (1808–1882): pioneer gastroenterologist and hepatologist. *J Med Biog* 1998; 6: 152–9; William Budd and typhoid fever *J Roy Soc Med* 2003 ; 96: 54].

17 Anonymous. *Lancet* 1879; ii: 595–6; *St Bartholomew's Hospital Reports* 1879; 15: 29; *Munk's Roll* 4: 39–40; S J Snow. Black, Patrick (1813–1879) In: H C G Matthew, B Harrison (eds). *Oxford Dictionary of National Biography*. Oxford: Oxford University Press 2004; 5: 911–2. [*See also:* G C Cook. The medical career of Robert Seymour Bridges FRCP (1844–1930): physician and Poet Laureate. *Postgrad Med J* 2002; 549–554].

18 Anonymous. *Munk's Roll* 4: 22.

19 Anonymous. *Munk's Roll* 4: 48. [*See also*: Presidential Address to the Royal College of Physicians 1900: 20].

20 Anonymous. *Munk's Roll* 4: 85–6. [*See also*: Presidential Address to the Royal College of Physicians 1904: 36].

21 Anonymous. *Times, Lond* 1907: May 12; Anonymous. *Lancet* 1907; i; 1465–9; *Br Med J* 1907; i: 1221–2; Annual Report 1906; *Munk's Roll* 4, 99; O Moscucci. Barnes, Robert (1817–1907) In: H C G Matthew, B Harrison (eds). *Oxford Dictionary of National Biography*. Oxford: Oxford University Press 2004; 3: 1009–10.

22 S H Ward. Analysis of 1000 consecutive cases admitted into the Seamen's Hospital, "Dreadnought". *Lancet* 1860; i: 78–9; Anonymous. *Lancet* 1880: ii: 154; Anonymous. *BMJ* 1880; ii; 155; S H Ward. *On some affections of the liver and intestinal canal with some remarks on ague and its sequelae, scurvy, purpura, etc.* London: J & A Churchill 1872: 260; *Medical Times Gazette* 1880; SHS Annual Report 1880; ii: 196; *Munk's Roll* 4: 189–190.

23 Anonymous. *Lancet* 1879; ii: 842 and 855–6; *BMJ* 1879; ii: 870; *Medical Press & Circular* 1879: 10 December: 506; *Morning Advertiser* 1879: 29 November: 3; *Ill London News* 1879; 75: 539; *Modern English Biog* 1851–1900, 6 (suppl to vol 3): 23; *Suppl to Allibone's critical dictionary of English Literature* 2: 982; SHS Annual Reports 1873 and 1879; G C Cook.

Harry Leach MRCP (1836–1879): control of scurvy in the British Mercantile Marine, and first Port Medical Officer for the City of London. *J Med Biog* 2000; 8: 133–9; G C Cook. Leach, Henry (1836–1979) In: In: H C G Matthew, B Harrison (eds). *Oxford Dictionary of National Biography*. Oxford: Oxford University Press 2004; 32: 950–1; [*See also:* [H Leach] Anonymous. Report on the hygienic condition of the Mercantile Marine, and on the preventable diseases of Merchant seamen. *BMJ* 1867; i: 36–7, 64–6, 89–91, 120–2, 147–8; H. Leach. *The Ship Captain's Medical Guide*. London: Simpkin, Marshall, and Co. 1868: 93; *Op cit*. See note 8 above (Cook, 2005)].

24 Anonymous. *Lancet* 1911; ii: 1103–7; Anonymous. *BMJ* 1911; ii: 950–4: 161–3; *Arch Ophthalmol* 1937; 17: 241–89; *Munk's Roll* 4; J Taylor, Walton of Detchant. Jackson, John Hughlings (1835–1911). In: H C G Matthew, B Harrison (eds). *Oxford Dictionary of National Biography*. Oxford: Oxford University Press 2004; 29: 504–6.

25 *Naval Intelligence. Times, Lond* 1847; 3 September: 7; Anonymous. Sir Richard Dobson, M.D., F.R.S. *Medical Directory* 1848: 336–7. G C Cook. Richard Dobson Kt, MRCS, FRS (1773–1847) and the inferior status of naval medicine in the early nineteenth century: end of the Fleet physicians. *Notes Rec R Soc* 2005 ; 59: 35–43.

26 Anonymous. *Times, Lond*. 1886: 11 August. *Proc. Linnean Soc* 1886–7: 36–8. *Plarr's Lives* 1930; 1: 174–6; G C Cook. George Busk FRS (1807–1886), nineteenth-century polymath: surgeon, parasitologist, zoologist, and palaeontologist. *J Med Biog* 1997; 5: 88–101; Woodward BB, Y Foote. Busk, George (1807–1886). In: H C G Matthew, B Harrison (eds). *Oxford Dictionary of National Biography*. Oxford: Oxford University Press 2004; 9: 100–1; [*See also:* G Budd, G Busk. Report of twenty cases of malignant cholera that occurred in the Seamen's Hospital-ship, Dreadnought, between the 8th and 28th of October, 1837. *Medico-Chirurgical Transactions* 1838; 21: 152–86].

27 Anonymous. *Plarr's Lives* 1930; i: 227.

28 Anonymous. John Tudor. *Times, Lond* 1808; 12 November.

29 Anonymous. Henry Turner Lane Rooke, M.D. *Lancet* 1870; ii: 453.

30 Anonymous. *Lancet* 1905; ii: 1656; *St Thomas's Hospital Rep* 1905; 34: 505; *Plarr's Lives* 1930; i: 297; D'A Power, J S Reznick. Croft, John (1833–1905) In: H C G Matthew, B Harrison (eds). *Oxford Dictionary of National Biography*. Oxford: Oxford University Press 2004; 14: 247–8.

31 Anonymous. *Plarr's Lives* 1930; i: 325–6; *See also* Chapter 15.

PART III

The SHS in 'full swing' (1870–1914)

'When we build, let us think that we build for ever.'

John Ruskin (1819–1900)

Chapter 13

Transfer of facilities to the Infirmary of the Royal Hospital, Greenwich in 1870

The decision to transfer *clinical* facilities from Hospital-ship to a land-based establishment was one of the most important events in the history of the Society. In August 1869 a leading article in the *Times* referred to: 'An Order in Council just published [which] completes a great reform in the administration of an important national institution [namely The Royal Hospital, Greenwich]'. It indicated that a decade ago a mere 500 out of 1900 inmates of that Institution were 'genuine seamen'; the remainder were the 'dregs of society'. When an offer was made to the prisoners 'nearly 1,000 out of 1,400 in-pensioners [the writer recorded] at once accepted out-pensions (amounting to 36=1=10s each) while many others would have availed themselves of the offer if it had been applicable to their case'. 'It is [he continued] intended at once to reduce the inmates to such a number as can be accommodated in the Infirmary [of the Royal Hospital], which is a distinct building from the Hospital'. It was the *long-term* intention to empty the Infirmary entirely and to place it 'at the disposal of the [SHS which was at the time] established in the Dreadnought [Hospital-ship]'. By so doing the 'merchant seamen will [he considered] reap a tangible benefit from the contributions [i.e., the Greenwich sixpences – see below] they have so long made from their wages to the income of the Hospital'. 'Admission to the Hospital [had until then] been subject to restrictions which have excluded from its benefits many whose relief was doubtless designed in its original institution' for it was 'notorious that our workhouses [he concluded] contain numerous disabled sailors who have hitherto had no hope of public aid'.

Removal from HMS *Dreadnought*

On 13 April 1870 (i.e. after six years of negotiation) the occupants of the last of the Hospital-ships (the *Caledonia* renamed *Dreadnought* – see Chapter 8) were removed to the now virtually empty Infirmary (and adjoining Somerset Ward) of the Royal Hospital (see Figure 13.1) which had been formally 'closed for pensioners of the Royal Navy [RN] on 1 October 1869'. These events were well described by Kemball Cook (see Chapter 12).[1] This venue for the *clinical* facility of the SHS (in fact, its *clinical* flagship) continued until 1986, and in 1999 became the *Dreadnought* library of the University of Greenwich.

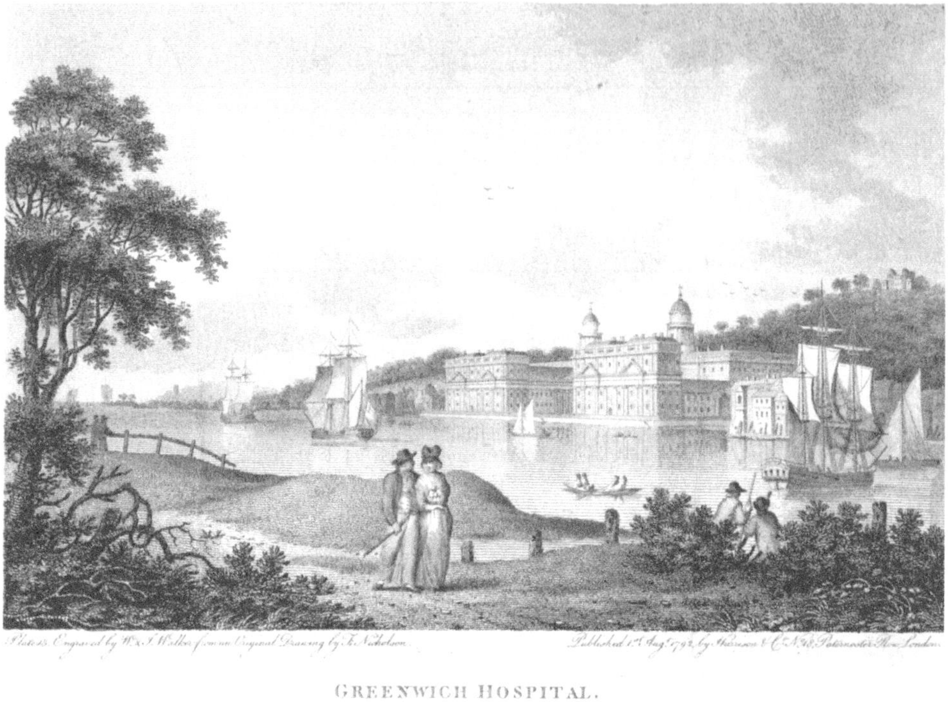

Figure 13.1: The Royal Hospital, Greenwich – engraving published in 1792 (artist unknown). [SHS Archive].

Removal of patients from the last of the Hospital-ships to the Infirmary (and Somerset Ward) of the Royal Hospital is described in an SHS minute for April 1870; it was:

> effected between the hours of Eleven & One (when the tide was favourable & the weather also) … The [patients] numbered 120. That 107 of them were removed in a Steam ferry hired for the purpose (at the reduced charge of One penny each). They were landed at Greenwich pier and Entered the Grounds of the Hospital almost immediately, by means of a private gate – the use of which was granted by Mr Arthur Jones the Steward of Greenwich Hospital – and by the good arrangements & personal attendance of all the Medical Officers [of the SHS], they were speedily settled in the beds allotted for them. The remaining thirteen, who could only be removed in a recumbent position, were brought in their beds to the Shore in a pinnace (lent for the occasion by the Dock Yard), and thence in an omnibus and a large & broad waggon provided with trays, stretchers and bedding. That the Patients Expressed themselves very much pleased with the Wards – Especially of not sleeping with an open Port close to their heads. That there had been three deaths but these were in no way attributed to the removal.[2]

Figure 13.2 shows a contemporary notice (signed by Kemball Cook) announcing the removal from the last of the Hospital-ships to the Royal Hospital's *infirmary*.

Initiation of the move to dry-land

Moves to transfer clinical facilities from ship to dry-land began in 1864 with an initiative from the SHS's medical staff;[3] an SHS minute records:

> Read a letter from Mr George Busk[4] [the Visiting Surgeon to the SHS] on the question of removing the Hospital from a ship to a building ashore. Ordered that this letter together with the report of Mr Henry Rooke[5] [the senior surgeon on the *Dreadnought* Hospital-ship] on the same subject be taken into consideration specially when the attendance of a larger number of the committee can be secured.

SEAMEN'S HOSPITAL SOCIETY,

LATE

DREADNOUGHT HOSPITAL SHIP.

NOTICE IS HEREBY GIVEN, that this Hospital is **REMOVED FROM THE "DREADNOUGHT"** to that part of Greenwich Hospital formerly known as the Infirmary, where **SEAMEN OF ALL NATIONS,** requiring Medical or Surgical treatment, will be received in the same manner as heretofore.

This Building is situate a few minutes' walk from the River, and near the Greenwich Steam Boat Pier and the Stairs adjoining.

Those who come by land will find it a few minutes' walk from the Greenwich Railway Station, Trains to which run every 20 minutes from London Bridge, Cannon Street and Charing Cross Stations.

Hours for Admission of Patients, 9 to 3 daily, (Sundays excepted.)

Accidents and urgent cases at all hours.

KEMBALL COOK,
House Governor and Secretary.

SEAMEN'S HOSPITAL, GREENWICH, S.E.
April 1870.

Figure 13.2: Notice issued by the Society in April 1870 announcing the removal of *clinical* facilities from the last of the Hospital-ships to land. [SHS Archive].

In a paper printed for the SHS late in 1864 (see Figure 13.3), the 'Visiting Physicians' (Robert Barnes[6] and Stephen Ward[7] – writing on 1 July 1864), the 'Surgeon on Board' (Henry Rooke – 11 August 1864) and the 'Visiting Surgeon' (George Busk –18 August 1864) expressed in writing their serious disquiet at conditions on the *Dreadnought* [hospital-ship].

The medical staff saw 'no advantages attendant upon a floating hospital' and referred to: lack of ventilation, 'want of light' – especially during the winter months, constant noises (both internally and externally) – which had increased during the previous two years, the impossibility of 'secluding refractory and delirious patients' (e.g. those suffering from delirium tremens), lack of facilities for convalescent patients, and the 'Deficient remedial arrangements, as to baths, &c'. Rooke (whose report occupied seven out of the ten pages of this publication) was

SEAMEN'S HOSPITAL SOCIETY.

COPY OF THREE LETTERS RECEIVED BY THE COMMITTEE.

No. 1.—From the Visiting Physicians.

LONDON, *July 1st*, 1864.

GENTLEMEN,

We have long entertained a conviction that there are many and serious objections to a floating Hospital such as the "Dreadnought." Some of these objections have of late become so seriously aggravated, that we should not be acting in accordance with the larger view of our functions as your Visiting Physicians, did we longer refrain from communicating with you upon the subject.

We will not occupy your time with any needless preamble, but at once ask your attention to the following, as among the more serious, objections to the present Hospital Ship :—

1. The impossibility of procuring effective ventilation, in consequence of the want of height between the decks. To effect any ventilation, it is necessary to open the ports, whereby patients are exposed to draughts. In foggy weather, the ports must either be kept closed, or, if opened, to the serious detriment of patients suffering from rheumatic and chest affections.

2. The want of light, especially during the winter months. The influence of light as a remedial agent has long been recognised by medical men.

3. Constant noises: (A.) *Externally*, from the iron-ship building yards, not only affecting the patients, but rendering a proper physical examination of chest affections almost impracticable. We would lay the greatest stress upon this annoyance, as one of comparatively late growth, increasing aggravation, and not likely to terminate. (B.) *Internally*, from walking over-head, and the traffic incidental to the Hospital. Under this head must be noticed, the noise arising from the necessary repairs of the ship, especially from caulking, and the shocks from collisions, which usually occur at night.

4. Impossibility of secluding refractory and delirious patients; the other patients being thereby deprived of rest. It is necessary only to mention cases of delirium tremens and fever, both of which are common on board, in illustration of this point.

5. No opportunity for convalescent patients to take air and exercise; the deck and forecastle being too exposed for most cases, especially in the colder seasons.

6. Deficient remedial arrangements, as to baths, &c.

We are not aware of any advantages attendant upon a floating hospital which can counterbalance the disadvantages. We leave the subject, however, in your hands, feeling assured that it will receive your earnest consideration.

We have the honour to remain,
Gentlemen,
Yours faithfully,
ROBERT BARNES, M.D.
STEPHEN H. WARD, M.D.

Figure 13.3: First of three letters – addressed to the Committee of the Seamen's Hospital Society, which initiated the move from the last of the Hospital-ships to a land-based institution. [SHS Archive].

particularly concerned with the inadequate *ventilation* on board the *Dreadnought* and in his report he compared it to the 'Black Hole of Calcutta' – which he felt encouraged erysipelas, pyaemia and hospital gangrene. Rooke cited Florence Nightingale's *Notes on Hospitals*.[8]

He was then, of the opinion that a 'Deficiency of Light' on board ship encouraged hospital gangrene. He also alluded to the unreliable water supply ('The ship is supplied by a pipe from the shore [which is] frequently broken by accident [and] takes some hours to repair') and that the 'dead-house [was too] close to the orlop-deck'. He produced data indicating that 391 sailors had, during the course of a single year, been admitted to nine London shore-based hospitals (rather than the *Dreadnought)*; there were of course many more outpatients (who had suffered 'slight accidents' or venereal disease). From this, Rooke concluded that 'sailors whose cases [are] interesting, or who require operation, are willingly admitted into the Metropolitan Hospitals ...'.

Another serious disadvantage was

> 'want of accommodation for [the] staff of Nurses. [Although the men nurses' have each a small cabin at the extremity of the wards [he wrote] the women have only two sleeping cabins common to six nurses; the best nurses [he concluded] will not accept an engagement on board the *Dreadnought* [despite the fact that the rate of pay is] better than at the London Hospitals.'

In his report, Busk (see above) agreed with most of Rooke's conclusions (the ship had 'become more and more saturated with a septic poison'), but he pointed out that since the *Dreadnought* was 'surrounded by a wide and open space' it certainly had some advantages over a *land-based* hospital, which must inevitably be situated in a heavily built-up area. In conclusion, Busk considered: 'The only real and effective remedy for most of these evils is the erection of a Hospital on shore, in as open and airy a situation [a suitable site 'seems to exist opposite to Greenwich Hospital'] as can be found in immediate reach of the river'.

In fairness, it should be stated that the Committee of the SHS 'aided by the co-operation of the Conservators of the Thames [had endeavoured], to find a less objectionable site [on the River Thames] for the *Dreadnought*'.[9] Their efforts were rendered fruitless by one or other of the following considerations: 'The fear of impeding the navigation of the river – the want of depth of water – the necessity of remaining near the bulk of the Shipping and the Docks – and the means of convenient communication with the shore'. This ten-page report continued by reminding its readership that whereas in 1821 (when the SHS was founded) the sailor demanded medical attention afloat, by 1865 a great change had taken place in that 'he now undoubtedly prefers a Hospital *ashore*'. 'Private bounty and public legislation [Kemball Cook continued] have been exerted very energetically on behalf of this most useful, and formerly most neglected, class of men. The [widespread] establishment of Sailors' Homes and the Seamen's Savings Banks, have doubtless greatly contributed to elevate the tone and improve the habits of seafaring men'. The 'Act of Incorporation [of 1833] had given the [SHS] Committee power to build a Hospital ashore' the report emphasised.[10]

The Society immediately formed a Sub-Committee to consider the practicalities and cost of removal; this consisted of: 'Admiral Warden, C.B; Captn E Littlehales R.N., Captn A Henning R.N., Captn Farrer & Captn V Budd together with Captn Hon. F Maude R.N. and (if his consent can be obtained) Mr Brooking, a Vice-President of the Society.' The Sub-Committee was also 'Empowered to obtain the services of Mr E L Bracebridge, Architect & Surveyor, to assist them'.[11] But, as this chapter will show, an enormous amount of negotiating was necessary before the removal was actually to take place.

Purchase of land in (East) Greenwich

In January 1865, the Quarterly General Court of Governors 'unanimously agreed ... that the Hospital should be moved ashore, provided a suitable site [could] be secured on the banks of the river [in Greenwich] with a frontage thereto and access by boat'. It was hoped therefore that the public (both at home and abroad) would support 'the erection of a Hospital of a permanent character contiguous to the Thames, for the relief at all times without introduction or recommendation, of every Seaman who is afflicted with sickness or disease'. Following the granting of permission of the Admiralty, an offer for the freehold of land valued at £5,500 owned by the Commissioners of Greenwich Hospital, and formerly the property of Crowley-Millington of East Greenwich (see Figure 13.4) was accepted. The purchase of this land from the Greenwich Hospital Commissioners was not completed until May.[12] This indenture (see Figure 13.5) gives details of the land purchased by the Society:

> All that plot/piece or parcel of ground situate lying and being at Greenwich in the County of Kent containing by recent admeasurement a 2..r 0..p17 or thereabouts abutting Northward upon the River Thames Southward upon Hog Lane otherwise the Old Woolwich Road Westward upon Norfolk College [now Trinity Hospital] and Eastward upon Land and premises belonging to Morden College on which plot or parcel of ground recently stood or within it were comprised the Ancient Mansion House called Crowley House and the Offices and Gardens belonging thereto and sundry large warehouses some of which warehouses were erected or projected over and supported upon the Quay wharf or passage running in front of Crowley House and the adjoining premises.[13]

Kemball Cook was in correspondence with the Secretary of Greenwich Hospital (J W Nickols). The cost of the plot of land was confirmed by the Commissioners of Greenwich Hospital as £5,500; 'They [i.e. the Commissioners, it was stated] must decline to entertain any offer less than £5,500'. A fourth letter stated that 'the Lords Commissioners of the Admiralty have given their consent to the Sale of the Plot of Ground in East Greenwich the Property of the Hospital consisting of 2 acres and 17 Perches to your Committee for the sum of £5,500'.[14]

MORDEN COLLEGE LAND

Shortly afterwards, negotiations also proceeded for the acquisition of an adjoining plot; an offer of £150.00 per annum was made to the tenants of Morden College[15] for

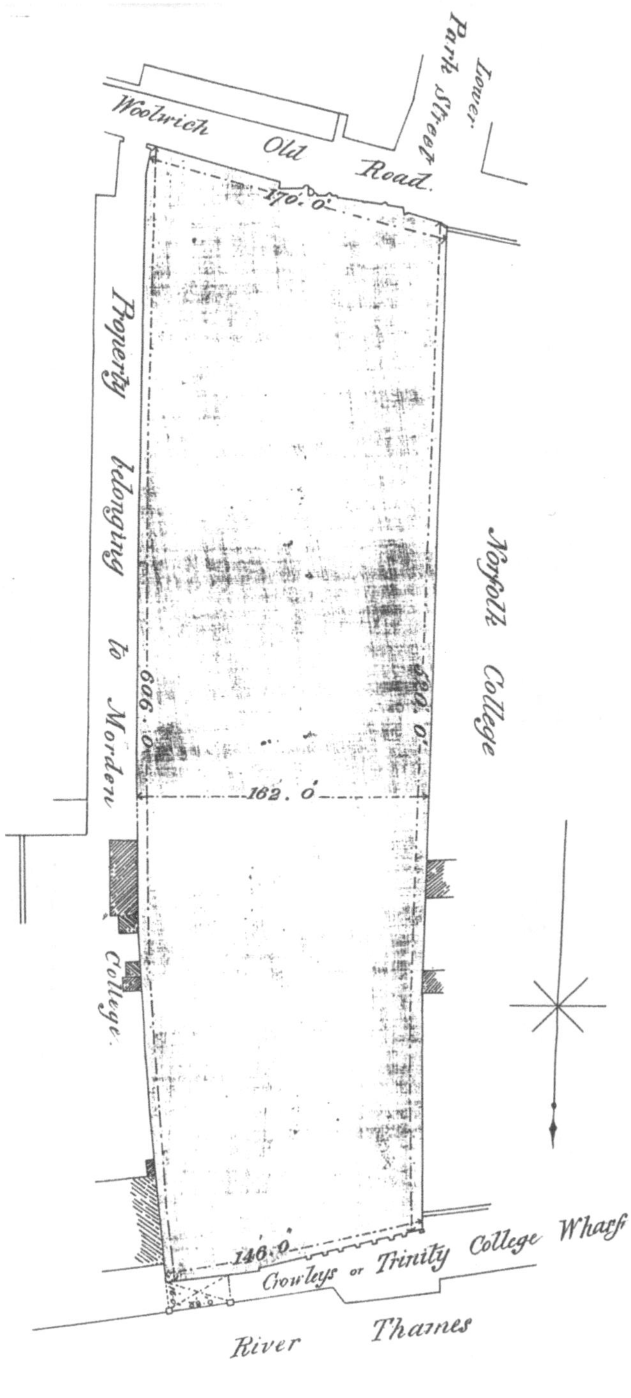

Figure 13.4: Map showing the plot of ground purchased by the SHS from the Commissioners of Greenwich Hospital for £5,500. [SHS Archive].

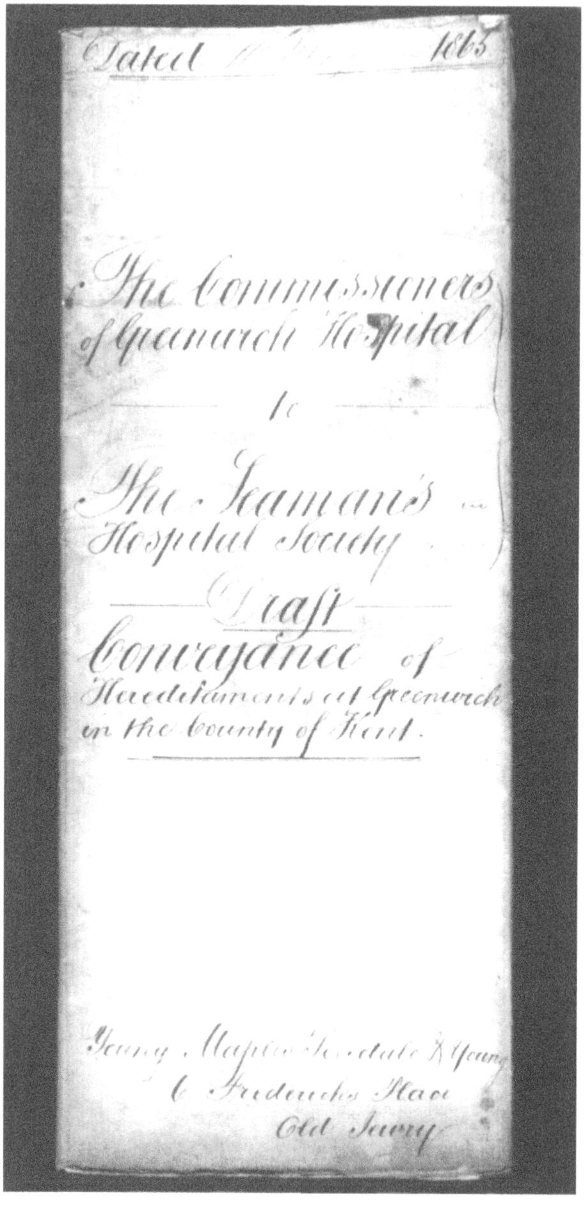

Figure 13.5: Draft of 'conveyance' document referring to the purchase of land by the SHS from the Commissioners of Greenwich Hospital – dated 11 May 1865. [SHS Archive].

the transfer of a lease (to the SHS) for this site – which was presently in their hands; meanwhile the SHS Solicitor (Mr Young) was instructed to explore the possibility of purchasing this land *freehold*. A later Committee of Management minute indicates that a Mr Hardwick had 'surveyed the land & buildings adjoining the [site which was now owned by the SHS] the property of the Trustees of Morden College and that he Estimated the present value of the freehold to be £3,300'.[16]

A Morden College minute dated July 1865 reads:

> The Surveyors reported that in conformity with the Trustees' instructions, they had communicated with the Solicitors, Secretary, & Surveyor to the [SHS] with a view to agree if possible upon a sum as it might be advisable for the Trustees to accept for the property on lease to Mess[rs] J. Taylor & Co & also that agreed to be let to Mess[rs] Seymour & others, and Mess[rs] Walker & Neale [sic] as well as some vacant Ground adjoining in Bennett [now Hoskins] Street, the whole situate South of the Anchor Wharf, Greenwich, at rents amounting altogether, with the exception of the piece of vacant ground, to £141 per Annum. The said Surveyors now beg to submit an offer from the Secretary of the Society of the sum of £3,300 which sum they would advise be accepted, subject to the existing Leases and Agreements, & subject also to the Society taking upon themselves the repairs & liabilities of the River Wall & inclosures, & to their paying up the Arrears of Rent, as well as, in the rebuilding of the passage at the East side of the property, to the not building over again of the said passage. The Surveyors likewise advise that, if the above terms be entertained, they shall be subject to the legal Arrangements & to the consent of the Charities' Commissioners to the Sale, & also to all costs and expenses attendant thereon being paid by the Society. Resolved, that the offer from the [SHS] be referred to the consideration of the Charities' Commissioners, and that it be accepted, if it receive their sanction, provided the acceptance have the concurrence [sic] of one or more of the absent Trustees likewise.[17]

The matter was again referred to in a further Morden College minute dated March 1866:

> The Surveyors reported, that the [SHS] have agreed to the terms fixed by the Trustees on the 12th July last for the purchase of certain Houses and Ground near the Ballast Quay.[18]

The 'conveyance' document (dated 31 December 1866) (see Figure 13.6) gives details of the land purchased by the SHS:

> All those 3 messes or tenem[ts] sit[e] at or near The Ballast Quay & Anchor Wharf in the Parish of St Alphege Greenwich in the Cty of Kent consisting of a Public House called the Golden Anchor … Secondly all those 3 messes or tenem[ts] … with the gardens to the same running down to the Old Woolwich Road … Thirdly all that piece or parcel of ground … now used as a Cooperage lying at the rear of the heredits … fronting Bennett Street … And Fourthly all that piece or parcel of vacant ground … also fronting Bennet St[t] .[19]

The Society now had a large plot of land, i.e. that bought from the Royal Hospital plus the smaller piece purchased from Morden College, in its possession (see Figure 13.7). In order to attempt to cover the cost of these transactions, and also to build a new hospital, the SHS Chairman, Admiral Sir William Bowles, delivered a Memorial

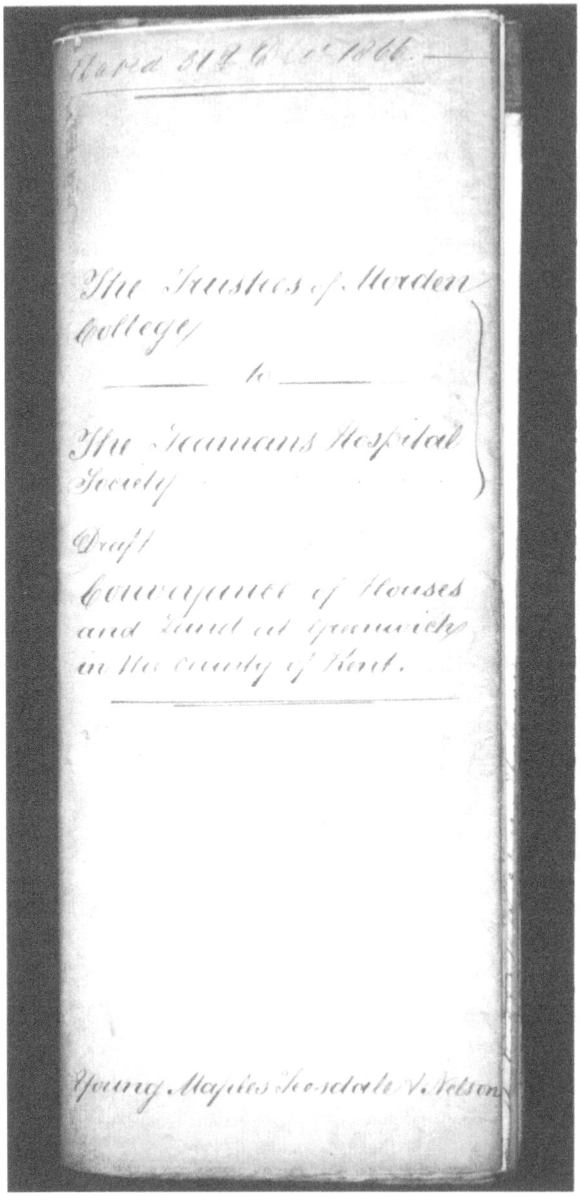
Dated 31st Dec. 1866.

The Trustees of Morden College

to

The Seamans Hospital Society

Draft

Conveyance of Houses and Land at Greenwich in the County of Kent.

Young, Maples, Teesdale & Nelson

Figure 13.6: Draft of 'conveyance' document referring to the purchase of land by the SHS from the Trustees of Morden College, Blackheath – dated 31 December 1866. [SHS Archive].

to the Lords of Her Majesty's Treasury (dated March 1865) requesting a grant of at least £20,000 'from the wages and effects of deceased Seamen [collected from the 'Greenwich sixpences'] as set out in Act 14 and 15 Victoria, Cap. 102. Sec 36; such an

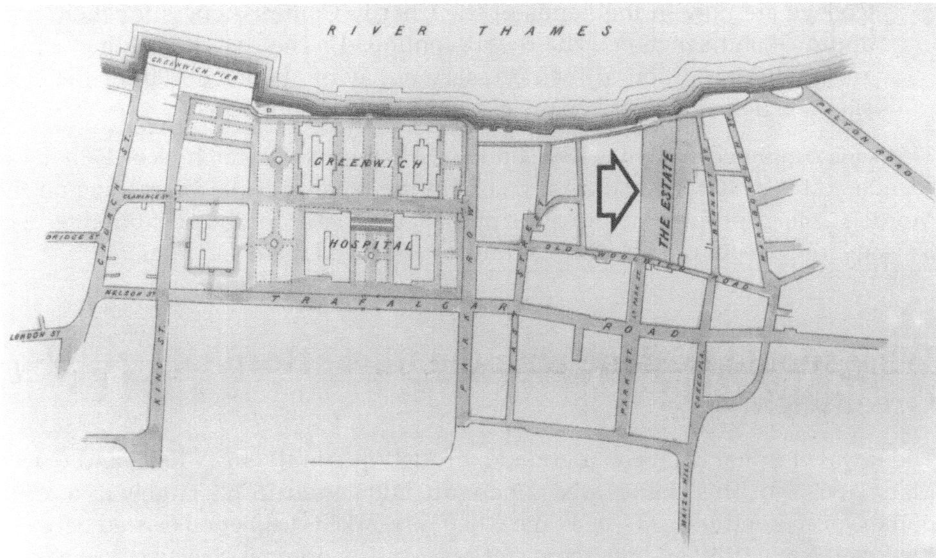

Figure 13.7: Map, undated, showing the plot of ground purchased from the Royal Hospital and Morden Colleges upon which it was envisaged a land-based hospital would be erected. [SHS Archive]. This land was bordered by the Old Woolwich Road (south), the River Thames (north), Trinity Hospital (formerly Norfolk College) (west) and Bennet Street (east).

award would [he pointed out] have to be made by Parliament on the recommendation of their Lordships'. This request, which was set out in the Memorial, was however declined. This led to a further communication from Kemball Cook on behalf of the SHS Committee to HM Treasury in which the claims of the Society were succinctly laid out; this was arranged under three major headings: (1) Merchant Seamen's Fund, (2) Unclaimed wages and effects of deceased Seamen, and (3) Fines and Forfeitures levied on Seamen. In the reply it was emphasised that none of the points made in this Memorial (see above) had been challenged. In support of clause 1, Kemball Cook cited Acts 4 & 5 William IV. Cap 52, 2 Parliamentary paper, No 23, of 1852, and clause 3, Acts 7 & 8 Victoria cap 112, and 8 & 9 Victoria cap 116.[20]

The overall position in early 1865 summarised

The 45th annual report succinctly summarised the position regarding the future venue for *clinical* facilities; the society:

> ... have purchased (from the Commissioners of Greenwich Hospital) the freehold of a plot of ground ... within sight of the present anchorage of the Dreadnought – having a good river frontage (with landing place) and extending to the old Woolwich Road. The committee have also become tenants of an adjoining strip of ground of the same length, and the terms for sale of the freehold thereof by the Trustees of Morden

> College are now in the hands of the Charity Commissioners for their approval and sanction. [The report continued]: The cost of building a Hospital (in addition to the necessary outlay of about £10,000 for the site) will demand a very heavy expenditure of money ...[21]

This saga continued well into 1866, and an SHS minute of March records that: the Secretary stated that 'he had arranged with the tenants of the Cooperage on the Morden College property to purchase of them their lease for the unexpired term of 35 years for the sum of £150. The committee approved thereof'.[22]

What should be done with the Royal Hospital, Greenwich?

The Royal Hospital had been founded by King William III (1650–1702) and Queen Mary (1662–94). This charity was apparently initiated in 1696 – largely as a result of the Queen's enthusiasm – at a time when no marked distinction existed between the Royal Navy [RN] and the merchant service. The original objective was to provide 'an asylum for those who had served in the fleet, to afford additional encouragement to Seamen to enter the [RN]', and to offer maintenance to widows and education of children of 'those killed or disabled in the Royal Service'.

Some years after the establishment of the Hospital, it was found that the subscriptions of the Seamen of the fleet, unless largely supplemented from the coffers of the State, would be insufficient for the maintenance of the foundation and, in 1745, an Act was passed authorising the Government to enforce subscriptions of 6d per man every month from *Merchant* Seamen. During 138 years (from 1696 to 1834) in which they were taxed, the merchant seamen had therefore subscribed an estimated (approximately) two million pounds sterling. In 1711, a further Act stipulated that only those who had served in the RN were eligible for admission to the Royal Hospital, despite the fact that 'great sums had been constantly paid towards the support of the Hospital from the wages of seamen employed in the merchant service'. In 1746, a later Act (the 'Merchant Seamen's Fund Act') (*see* Chapter 9) was passed following a recommendation by a House of Commons Committee, on the 'stoppage of another monthly sixpence from the wages of ... merchant seamen in order to provide them with similar relief in a separate hospital [from that in the RN]'. There was no doubt, therefore, that the mercantile marine had 'donated' vast sums of money to Greenwich Hospital, and in return had received *no* benefits; this was therefore a serious bone of contention.[23]

Future rôle of Greenwich Hospital

In March 1865, Hugh Childers FRS (1827–96) (then Junior Lord of the Admiralty) had initiated a Parliamentary discussion on the future of Greenwich Hospital; details of his plans were outlined the following month in an introduction of a Bill to provide 'better government of Greenwich Hospital'. In the eyes of a *Times* leader-writer, 'The original conception of Greenwich Hospital [see above] was a mistake.

It was a pretty thought to collect together in those magnificent halls on the banks of the Thames those battered hulks of humanity, to spend their time alternatively in dreaming over the past and holding up their withered hands in prayer'. The writer was firmly of the opinion that the pensioners would be far better off integrated with their families.

It was proposed [Childers claimed] to 'limit the admission to infirm and *helpless* [my italics] seamen, and seamen who required medical assistance of a temporary character, making the Hospital for Seamen what Haslar [the Royal Naval hospital at Portsmouth] was, and the harbour to which seamen, when helpless, might continue to retire. The number estimated to be provided for would be reduced [from 1,600 to 2,300 at present] to 600 seamen and marines'. The 'income [of Greenwich Hospital] was now about 154,000/ (£) a year and it arose from the interest on money invested, 20,000/ from the Consolidated Fund in lieu of what were called Seamen's sixpences (which was 'little better', the *Times* claimed 'than robbery'), and from rents of estates in the north and in the neighbourhood of Greenwich amounting to 40,000/ a year. Childers outlined the means for streamlining management of the institution; Government proposed (he continued) 'that an officer should be appointed by law to be called 'The Controller of the Greenwich Hospital Estate' and that the estates themselves should be vested in the Board of Admiralty. He recommended giving 'Greenwich out-pensions' to all out-pensioners exceeding a certain age. The pensioners at that time varied in age 'from about 40 to about 80 years of age. The Government proposed to take 55 as the age at which the pensioner should be entitled to some additional boon, and to provide that, at that age, an additional pension of 5d a day should be granted to him …'; for 70 year olds who had been pensioners for 10 years or more, 9d a day should be paid.

In subsequent discussion following Childers' speech, Frederick Lygon (1830–91) (MP for Worcestershire West) asked what was to be done with the remainder of Greenwich Hospital, i.e. after reduction of the number of pensioners to 600, he suggested that 'the surplace accommodation [be used] to provide naval barracks, which were much wanted'. Henry Liddell (1797–1878) (MP for Northumberland) suggested that in the event of 'a future naval war … extra accommodation for wounded seamen would arise; therefore it would be prudent to maintain all the wards in a state of preparedness'.[24]

A leading article in *The Times* referred to the Parliamentary discussion on the '*Greenwich Hospital Bill*': 'From first to last scarcely a glimpse of intelligence [has] irradiated the discussion'... 'To assume, as was done in the House of Commons … that the income of the Derwentwater Estates [which had contributed a major sum to Greenwich Hospital] must always be applied to the relief of disabled seamen of the [RN] because an Act of the eighth year of George II directed such an application, is about as irrational as it would be to argue that certain apartments in Somerset House and at Whitehall must always be used as Admiralty offices because they were so occupied in the time of George III'. This leader-writer received the unconditional support of a writer in the *Shipping and Maritime Gazette.*[25] In any event, the second reading of the Bill took place late in May; and Acton Ayrton (1816–86) (MP for Tower Hamlets) suggested that 'some consideration should be paid to the commercial marine of the country. The Hospital [had been] established for the benefit of seamen of *every kind* [my italics]'. Childers responded: 'with respect to the mercantile navy, [he cited authorities, including an Act of Parliament passed in 1747, which excluded merchant seamen from the ordinary benefits of the hospital] unless wounded in [naval] actions'.[26]

An alternative view was directed to the 'evasive reply of Childers, when asked by Sir J[ohn] Pakington Bt (1799–1880) and Mr J P Hennessy (1834–91) why surgeons were not included in the Greenwich Hospital pensions'. These doctors, subsequently argued a Naval Surgeon, were employed on short-term contracts (unlike other officers of the establishment) and if they were excluded from 'any share in the pensions' it would cause a great deal of dissatisfaction.[27]

Following Childers' speech and the following discussion (see above), the Government decided to close the Royal Hospital (with the exception of the Infirmary); the sole exceptions were to be the wounded and very infirm – who required medical care and treatment. The 'old … and worn out mariners' who did not require medical attention would be transferred to Belvedere [at Erith].[28]

Challenge to the SHS's proposed strategy

A parliamentary debate devoted to this issue was immediately followed by two letters (to *The Times)* from a correspondent who signed himself 'Justitia' (and who was an outspoken supporter of the merchant navy's claims to Greenwich Hospital). In his first letter 'Justitia' was critical of the reasoning of the SHS on the grounds that a hospital *on shore* would suffer from all of the defects which had been exposed at Greenwich Hospital: 'has it not now been established [he asked] that such an institution is quite unsuited to present days, demoralising to its inmates, injurious to their wives and children and little attractive to the better class of seamen?' … 'An out-pension [he claimed] of 10/ a year, which an old seamen can spend among his family or his friends, is better for him than any in-door provision which will cost the charity from 50/ to 100/'. The Greenwich Hospital, he argued, had accrued millions of pounds from the Greenwich sixpences – which should now be available to *merchant* seamen, who should be cared for in the Royal Hospital, four-fifths of which would in the future be empty.

In his second letter, 'Justitia' alluded to the urgency of the situation as he had only just heard of the SHS's intention to move to a site adjacent to Greenwich Hospital, which would be exceedingly costly. They are about to spend (which 'cannot be allowed'), he continued, the 'greater part of 44 years' savings and benefactions, at least 60,000/ in erecting, within a stonethrow ('at the very doors') of the ancient and now half-vacant Greenwich Hospital, a new hospital to hold 300 beds'. The claims of the mercantile marine for space in Greenwich Hospital was reiterated by an anonymous writer to the *Lancet*. 'Justitia' reminded his readers that in the eighteenth century (when the Royal Hospital had been founded), 'The old monastic feeling for collecting and sheltering under one large roof all whose wants and needs and habits were akin, lingered still in the minds, and coloured the action, of the Legislature'. Views had changed and therefore, he argued, now was the time for 'reviving the claims to Greenwich Hospital of the merchant service'.

'To the Duke of Somerset ['Justitia' wrote], whose statesmanlike memorandum of April 1864 has established the principles which must henceforth rule the administration of our great national charities, I would earnestly and respectfully appear at the present time on behalf of the merchant seaman's claim to share in the Infirmary of Greenwich Hospital'. 'Justitia' suggested further 'that a great medical school [could be started] for the practice and employment of the surgeons of the [RN]'. The SHS (which had a modern hospital established in 1821 to care for sick and injured seafarers – including the relief of 3,511 sailors of the RN during its 44 years of its existence) should be installed in the Royal Hospital; the alternative was to build a new hospital in close proximity to the Royal Hospital – which would be very costly to the SHS. It should be remembered that in 1853 the Board of Trade, with the sanction of Parliament, repealed a former decision to pay the SHS 550/ annually in lieu of unclaimed wages and the effects of deceased merchant seamen which had been unclaimed for seven years. Since 1854 the SHS had received *no* assistance from Parliament. Therefore, 'Why should not the eastern moiety of the Hospital, composed of Queen Anne's and Queen Mary's quarters, be assigned at once to the use of the [SHS], for the benefit of the mercantile marine?'[29]

A leader-writer in *The Times* largely concurred with 'Justitia's' views; 'Greenwich Hospital [he wrote] is not a Hospital in the modern sense of the word, and because, in the present state of things, the use is made for it, and not it for the use?' He continued, '... a Hospital is wanted for our Merchant Seamen. ['It is the Merchant Service that feeds the Navy' and] leading merchants, shipowners, and shipping companies have bought Belvedere, the picturesque pile commanding the Thames near Erith, and are adapting it for this purpose'. He therefore strongly supported the use of Greenwich Hospital (or part of it) by the SHS.

But not all (the Admiralty included) were in agreement; one correspondent to *The Times* for example outlined the merits of Belvedere (which was to become 'the last retreat of aged men worn out in their country's service who have no prospect at a workhouse, no natural ties to sooth [sic] the evening of their days, and to whom a pension compared to the comfort of such a home would be valueless') where there was 'ample room for extension, but it is not proposed to receive more than 500, as it is hoped that similar retreats for our old tars will be established at Liverpool and other places on the coasts, so that they may be as near as possible to their own localities'.[30]

Uncertainty continues

In early June 1865, T*he Times* published a letter from a correspondent who signed himself 'Vigil'. He was concerned that the 'Admiralty Bill for improving Greenwich Hospital [would] saddle the country with an unjust tax of at least 20,000/'. In 1834, Mr [G] Lyall (1784–1853), had brought forth his Bill for discontinuing the payment to the Hospital of the merchant seamen's sixpences (a move opposed by the First Lord, Sir James Graham [1792–1861]); this meant that to be financially viable the Hospital had to 'apply for 20,000/ from the consolidated Fund'. In 1848, a naval Lord of the Admiralty, Sir Alexander Milne (1806–96) had instituted 'a great change in the mode of granting the out-pensions'; since at that time, the proportion of out-pensioners had increased, whereas the number of in-pensioners had diminished – leaving vacancies (which in 1865 totalled 1,300) in the Hospital. The result was that between 1834 and 1865, the number of in-pensioners had diminished from 2,710 to 1,400 and of these 1,000 were now to become out-pensioners. This would leave 400 in-pensioners and the Treasury would have to pay 'not 1,000 but 2,310 additional out-pensions, not 15,000/ *l* but 35,000/ a year in excess of the annual sum which if the Hospital were full we should have to vote for naval out-pensions'. This correspondent was therefore unhappy with the *financial* aspects of the Bill.

The *British Medical Journal* summarised, what its anonymous reporter considered, important aspects of the debate concerning the Bill; salaries and pensions (which dominated the discussion) for officers did not (Hennessy claimed) include medical officers or chaplains (the latter however were dealt with by a subsequent clause); however Childers considered that the term officers should *include* medical officers! In a Parliamentary debate, (Sir) Stephen Cave (1820–80) considered that part of the vacant hospital should be given over to the SHS, while Ayrton felt that a clause should be inserted to make entirely clear that 'the Greenwich Hospital was for the benefit of the merchant marine as well as of the [RN]'. Childers conceded that there was nothing in the Bill to 'prevent the Admiralty letting a portion of the building for the purposes of a hospital in lieu of the Dreadnought'. Another hotly debated matter was the recommended abolition of the title 'Master and Governor of Greenwich Hospital.'[31]

Childers made it clear that a definitive plan for the future of Greenwich Hospital had yet to be formulated (see below). *The Times* for 30 June stated that the 'Greenwich Hospital Bill had passed through [a House of Lords] committee', and a subsequent leading article in that paper (which welcomed the reforms) began: 'One of the most valuable of the many good measures passed [the Bill was enacted on 5 July that year] during the last session of Parliament is now being most successfully carried into execution. Within the next few days Greenwich Hospital will be cleared of two-thirds of its inmates'. The article continued: 'In place of hundreds of elderly but still hale and athletic veterans wandering listlessly about the terraces and colonnades of Greenwich, ('half a century of naval peace' had changed things immeasurably since the battles of the Nile and Trafalgar) and, if the truth must be said, sometimes overstepping the bounds of sobriety in the numerous public houses of the neighbourhood, there will be but a limited number of indoor pensioners'.[32]

The Royal Hospital in late 1865 – a summary

The day before publication of the above article, the *Times* summarised the current situation at Greenwich Hospital; 200 out of 900 pensioners who had elected [the previous day] to become out-pensioners left the Hospital for 'various parts of the country [fares and cost of transportation of their 'chest of clothes' were being paid by the Admiralty] they have selected for their future home'. The writer considered that by the end of that week all 900 would have left, leaving a mere 450 in-patients (mostly 'cripples, or persons otherwise infirm') at Greenwich Hospital. Details of out-patient pensions was given; in all they would be entitled to '316 1 10s a year'. Pensioners could be readmitted to the Hospital 'at any time hereafter on becoming infirm and helpless'. At this point, the editor of *The Times* reproduced an account of Greenwich Hospital and its Pensioners – written by Charles Dickens in '*All the year round*'; he emphasised perceptively that the best parts ('almost exactly one-half') of the Royal Hospital (i.e. King Charles's and Queen Anne's quarters) had been taken over by officials (largely for residential purposes) – leaving the principal beneficiaries, i.e. the seafarer, *in the less distinguished parts*.

This sudden decline in the number(s) of in-pensioners inevitably meant that the caring staff also had to be reduced, and in December the *British Medical Journal* recorded: 'Fifty of the female nurses, who have been for years engaged in this establishment have been discharged by order of the Admiralty upon pensions varying according to length of servitude'.[33]

Chance of SHS removing to the Royal Hospital becomes a realistic possibility

A leader-writer in *The Times* readdressed the subject of a *future role* for Greenwich Hospital; in it, he considered '... if the increasing trade of the Port of London requires more hospital accommodation for seamen, there can be no valid objection to giving relief to the sick or wounded merchant seaman within the Hospital walls'. An SHS minute for July described an interview between Kemball Cook and J H Farrar (Secretary of the Marine Department of the Board of Trade); the first realistic possibility – provision of accommodation in Greenwich Hospital – was raised. Farrer felt that 'the Board had advised the Treasury that, although it could not recommend the grant of public money to the Society ashore in lieu of the *Dreadnought* might well be granted in the Greenwich Hospital building.'

The Treasury had viewed this proposal so favourably that they had made an application accordingly to the Lords of the Admiralty who had 'promised to give due consideration to any application from the Society'. A week later, a formal application for use of part of the Hospital was made (by the SHS). In late October 1865, *The Times* considered: 'We believe that nothing has yet been decided [regarding the empty quarters of Greenwich Hospital], but it is said not to be improbable that they may eventually substitute the Dreadnought floating hospital, in the reception of invalid *merchant* [my italics] seamen'.[34] However, in December, an SHS Minute recorded: 'Read a letter from the Admiralty dated the 12th instant stating that their Lordships are *not* [my italics] able at present to entertain the question of giving over a part of Greenwich Hospital to the [SHS]'. This negative attitude was echoed in the SHS Annual Report for 1866; however, it remained the view that either the Charity should 'be received into a portion of the empty Greenwich Hospital, to which the Mercantile Marine had for so long paid forced contributions although deriving no advantage from it – or, to receive a grant from Parliament, on giving up Her Majesty's Ship Dreadnought, and thereby putting an end to the annual charge upon the National Exchequer for keeping the Ship in good repair, and for providing ship's stores'.[35]

'The uses and abuses of Greenwich Hospital': the future remains in the balance

The year 1866 passed without much headway being made – a situation which was admirably summed up in the 46th Annual Report: 'The Committee regret ... that little progress has been made with reference to the plan for removal of the Hospital from the Dreadnought'. This report made clear that they still wanted either: (i) part of the vacant Greenwich Hospital; or (ii) 'a money grant [from HM Government] in aid of the cost of Erecting a Building in lieu of the Dreadnought'.[36]

The year had, of course, begun optimistically enough; the *Lancet* had recorded (in early February): '... the future of this great mass of buildings is a matter for grave consideration. It is important that its occupation should be speedy, for it would be a reproach to the nation that these walls should be tenantless a month longer than is absolutely necessary'. This anonymous writer strongly supported the SHS's case: 'An annual income of upwards of £1000 was granted by Parliament (through the Board of Trade) towards the support of the *Dreadnought*, which sum was entirely taken away in the year 1853 by the passing of the Mercantile Marine Amendment Act. By this means the *Dreadnought* had at once been deprived of nearly one-sixth of its income, at a time when, from the annually increasing commerce of the port of London, it was (as it still is) ill able to bear such a loss'. He ended: 'In the absence of regular Government occupation, the House of Commons can hardly resist this request of the [SHS] ...'

This viewpoint was rapidly endorsed by the *Shipping and Mercantile Gazette*:

> 'We have always felt that the position of the *Dreadnought* Hospital Ship, more especially during the summer months, moored as that ship is in about the foulest part of the polluted waters of the Thames, is most unfortunate, and must seriously interfere with the successful treatment of disease ...' [The anonymous leader-writer continued:] 'At present there is no provision for the infirm, the worn-out, or disabled Sailor, who has spent his days and his strength in the service on which the prosecution of England's Maritime Commerce depends. We are happy to say that an effort has been made to remedy this glaring neglect of a national duty, but it is an effort on the part of private individuals, and entirely independent of the State and of the Government.[37]

Shortly after this, the SHS forwarded a further Memorial to the Lords Commissioners of the Admiralty; this was again signed by Kemball Cook and contained an outline of the history of the SHS, together with a renewed plea for the use of part of the vacant Greenwich Hospital premises – preferably Queen Anne's Quarter - which 'would be sufficient for all the purposes of this Society'.[38] However this approach was again rejected by the Admiralty: '... their Lordships cannot consent to appropriate a portion of Greenwich Hospital for the purposes of this Society [and they] anticipate that it will be required for the use of the Seamen of the Fleet under arrangements now being considered'. The matter was reported by the *Shipping and Mercantile Gazette* in March; the leader-writer indicated that the sole option left to the SHS was an 'appeal to Parliament'. He continued: '... to appropriate the whole of the Institution to the [Sailor of the Fleet], ignoring utterly the claims of the [Merchant Service], is an act of gross injustice, which we do not believe the Legislature will sanction'.[39]

Meanwhile, towards the end of 1866, the *Lancet* continued with its campaign on behalf of the SHS and the mercantile marine: '... the now closing year still finds one of our noblest charitable institutions [Greenwich Hospital] in a state of disgraceful emptiness and desolation ... we cannot believe that the present Government will allow another year to pass without some legislation on this question'. 'It will be well [the writer concluded] if, at the commencement of the [Parliamentary] Session, the future uses of Greenwich Hospital are determined without further delay'. In an article in the *British Medical Journal,* the writer drew attention to the (unnecessarily) large administrative staff still at Greenwich Hospital, which meant that the cost of maintaining each pensioner had risen from £60 to over £100 annually. A later issue of the *Lancet* put the latter figure at £114 per annum, and this writer urged the Admiralty to 'make the hospital and the staff both useful, by drafting in patients of the Dreadnought and employing this hospital as a training school [Netley and its role in training doctors for the Army was cited] for young naval medical men'.[40]

An SHS delegation meets the Prime Minister

1867 proved to be the major year for negotiation both regarding the way forward for the Royal Hospital, Greenwich and also the future of the SHS. An SHS minute in early March read: 'The secretary [Kemball Cook] reported that he had obtained an appointment for the reception by the Earl of Derby,[41] the Prime Minister, of a delegation of Members of the House of Commons on behalf of this Society – with a view to obtain the loan of part of Greenwich Hospital for the use of the Society – or, a grant of money to aid in the Cost of Erecting a Hospital – in lieu of the Dreadnought'.[42]

This delegation initially proved successful, as reported in an SHS minute for 8 March (Founder's Day):

> '... the Deputation to the First Lord of the Treasury at No 10 Downing Street ... consisted of the following members of the House of Commons, viz. – Messrs Ayrton – Sir C. Bright – R. Brooks – Rt Hon. G J Goschen – J Hartley – R. Ingham – Hon. Arthur Kinnaird – J Laird – Alderman Lawrence – Alderman Lusk – Hon. C. Waldegrave Leslie - & Coll [sic] Norwood by Admiral Sir W[illiam] Bowles KCB Chairman & the following Members of the Committee, viz. Hon. Capt F. Maude RN – Admiral Buckle, CB – Captn C R Egerton R.N. – Messrs. Le Breton – Mr Grouther – Captains Sleight & Toller and the Secretary of the Society. That Lord Derby was accompanied by Sir John Pakington Bart. [see above], First Lord of the Admiralty and by Sir Stafford Northcote, Bart. C.B. [1818–87] President of the Board of Trade because, as his Lordship stated, the Society had been in frequent Communication with these departments of Her Majesty's Government. That the Chairman having addressed Lord Derby as to the Nature of the Society's operations, the

> support granted to it by the Nation, and the need of removal from a Ship stated that the immediate object of the Deputation was to request that Her Majesty's Government would grant the loan of so much of Greenwich Hospital fronting the river (he thought one-third) as would be necessary for the purposes of the Society in lieu of the Ship Dreadnought. That Lord Derby then stated that he was glad to find that no portion of the revenues of Greenwich Hospital was asked for, and that the deputation did not apply for the *gift* of any portion of that building, to both of which Her Majesty's Government would have been unable to agree. With regard however to the loan of so much of the building as the Society needed *he was happy to say that the Government were quite prepared to grant that to the Society* [my italics]'. The outcome of the meeting was recorded in the *Times* and the *Shipping and Mercantile Gazette* the following day. The latter emphasised that the deputation had obtained what it wanted i.e. a loan, because 'there is little chance of the patients being disturbed, except in the event of a war, which might necessitate the re-appropriation of the Hospital to the Seamen of the Fleet'.[42]

From the beginning of 1867 both national and medical press recorded developments at Greenwich in detail; *The Times* correspondent who signed himself 'Beta' (an ardent supporter of the SHS) dominated those contributions. In January, he wrote: 'that [the SHS] ought to have some public aid at the present time, the Board of Trade, the Treasury, and the Admiralty alike agree; but here their harmony ends'. He again emphasised that to build a *new* hospital would be exceedingly costly and that the capital of the SHS was being seriously depleted by the 'stoppage of Government aid'; between 1835 and 1854, Parliament had contributed 'about 450/ per annum'. In addition, the 'wages and effects of deceased seamen [amounting to 'more than 8,000/'] used to be paid to the Dreadnought, and are now paid to the Board of Trade'.

The surplus of the contributions which form the Merchant Seamen's Fund and the Mercantile Marine Fund ought [he wrote] in all justice to be spent as far as possible in the several ports whence they have proceeded'. He referred to the fact that the SHS had purchased land in east Greenwich (which had cost Greenwich Hospital 4,000/, for 5,500/), and in addition had brought adjoining land from Morden College at 4,000/; to build a new hospital would cost a further 80,000/. This letter was accompanied by a highly supportive leading article in the same issue; the writer emphasised that there was so much vacant accommodation in Greenwich Hospital, that the Admiralty could easily accommodate the SHS and [also] keep sufficient for any contingency demanded by the RN. He continued: '... the interests of the [RN] and the mercantile marine should not be thus sharply distinguished or regarded as conflicting with each other'. 'Ships of war [he wrote] spring from ships of burden, and the QUEEN's Service is connected with the Merchant Service by the closed ties'. The *Shipping and Mercantile Gazette* too campaigned on behalf of the SHS, and the *Lancet* continued its theme that the SHS should be offered part of the Greenwich Hospital; the writer claimed: 'The benefit to the merchant service [of facilities at Greenwich Hospital] would be great; to the [RN] the advantage [of a naval medical training-school comparable to the army medical training-school at Netley would be considerable].[43]

In a further tirade, the *Lancet* proclaimed: 'Are the Lords of the Admiralty aware that, whilst they refuse compliance with the wishes of the managers of the Hospital-Ship, many a fine fellow, whose blood had been shed in defence of his country, or whose strength had been wasted in spreading our commerce, is languishing, dying perhaps, for want of space within the condemned wooden walls of the *Dreadnought*?' Another claimant to space in Greenwich Hospital, the article continued, was the 'borough of Greenwich, [see below] which represents upwards of 150,000 people, and who have not a single hospital bed at their disposal nearer than the metropolis'. The *Lancet* then advocated a further approach to the Admiralty, and failing any action, 'an appeal to the Imperial Parliament'.[44]

In a further letter to the *Times* in March, 'Beta' again stressed the plight of the SHS which at that point had an annual income of 'about 9,000*l*' and an expenditure of 10,000*l*. He ended his letter: 'Sir, what shall be done for the [SHS]? The admiralty refuse them a part of the vacant Hospital, and hesitate to grant them, out of the 2,605,000*l*, a sum sufficient to build them a new hospital. The Board of Trade hold to their Acts of Parliament, and draw a profit from those Acts of 10,500*l* a year, to a large part of which in equity the [SHS] would seem entitled. And, to crown all, and illustrate the spirit in which our rulers regard an important class of the community, the Admiralty withdraw from the merchant service, the privilege, which by long years of usage has hardened into a right, of education for 150 or 200 of their children in the Greenwich Hospital Schools'.[45]

The relative success of the visit to Lord Derby (see above) had been followed by congratulatory messages from several sources. 'Beta' in a yet further letter 'briefly chronicle[d] the course of the agitation which [had] terminated with such success'; he pointed to the fact that this was 'not the first time that … Pakington had overridden the prejudices of his naval colleagues at the Board of the Admiralty', and he expressed the gratitude of merchant seamen to him. The *Lancet*, however, added a caution that 'it must now be the care and concern of the *Dreadnought* staff, executive as well as medical, to maintain on land that *prestige* in the minds of the public that has always been attached to their hospital afloat'. The writer also hoped that the SHS's *clinical* material could be utilised by the naval medical officers, making this 'a sort of naval Netley'.[46]

In a further update, the *Lancet* considered that: '… in fulfilment of Lord Derby's pledge, the Government have decided [this was a premature announcement as *The Times* was hasty to point out] to allot for the use of the *Dreadnought* the eastern front and south-east angle of the east wing of Greenwich Hospital [i.e. part of Queen Mary's Quarter see Figure 13.8]. This affords ample accommodation for three hundred men, with a kitchen equal to cooking for a much larger number, baths, laundries, and house surgeons' rooms. It is an admirably planned and spacious range of buildings, which we have reason to believe would make one of the most complete hospital establishments in the metropolis'. *The Times* meanwhile pointed out that Queen Anne's Quarter (see Figure 13.9) would be a superior site from the SHS's viewpoint; not only would it make a better hospital than Queen Mary's Quarter (conversion, for example, would be simpler), but it was situated on the river frontage.[47]

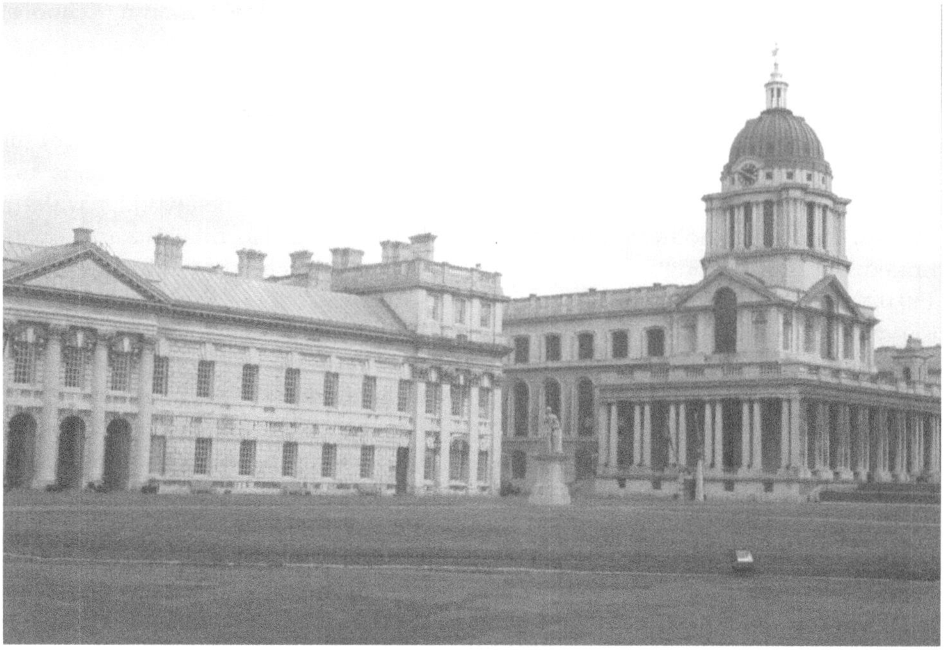

Figure 13.8: Queen Mary Quarter (right) of the Royal Hospital Greenwich [photograph: March 2000].

A hospital for the needs of Greenwich?

Having successfully negotiated (or so it seemed) a home for the SHS within Greenwich Hospital, various voices were raised in support of another portion of this building being made available as a hospital for the people of Greenwich (see above) – 'a vast manufacturing and ship-building population'; 'Greenwich [the report continued] with its neighbourhood has a population of about three hundred thousand, without a single bed for its sick and disabled and although it is no great distance from the metropolis, it is no unfrequent occurrence to have cases returned from London Hospital for want of beds'. This idea however, received a hostile reaction from HM Government. 'To divert any portion of Greenwich Hospital to such a purpose would be to sanction the application of the building to purposes directly contrary to the intentions of its founders'. And furthermore, it would be difficult to claim the space back should the RN need it! Mr (later Sir Charles) DuCane (1825–89) speaking in the House of Commons) 'could therefore hold out no hope that the Government would ever be likely to sanction any appropriation of the building for sick persons belonging to the borough of Greenwich'.[48]

The debate warms up

Despite the Prime-Minister's assurance, the Admiralty was far less enthusiastic about the Society taking over part of its 'empire'. An SHS minute dated March 1867

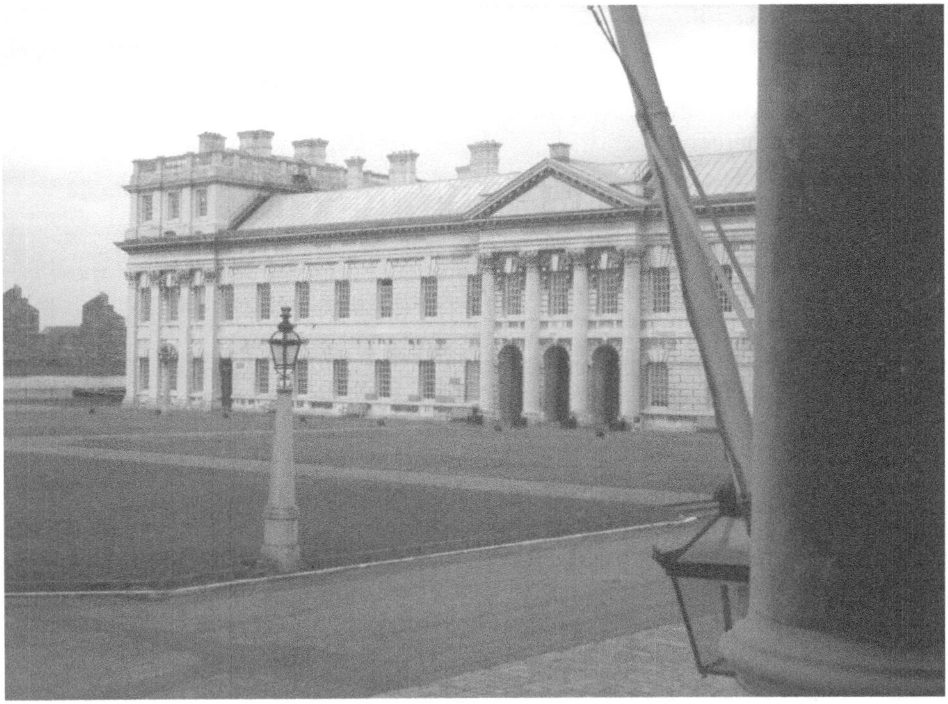

Figure 13.9: Queen Anne Quarter of the Royal Hospital, Greenwich [photograph: March 2000].

states that the Secretary 'had called at the Admiralty to ascertain when the Society could be put in possession of the portion of Greenwich Hospital assigned to it'. He was, however, merely given an appointment to meet the new First Lord of the Admiralty – Henry Corry (1803–73). A further minute two weeks later records: 'Read a letter from the Admiralty in reply to the Secretary's letter of the 25th ultimo – stating that their Lordships are prepared to lend to the Society a portion of Queen Mary's Ward sufficient for the accommodation of 300 patients with their Medical & other attendants – and adding, that their Lordships are unable to comply with the request that the Dreadnought should be given up to this Society and that the proceeds of her sale might be appropriated to its funds'.[49]

At this juncture 'The Secretary [of the SHS] received authority for the Committee to represent to the Admiralty that the operations of the Society must be carried on contiguous to the river and also to forward to their Lordships Dr H T L Rooke's statement in writing as to the impracticability of Queen Mary's Ward as a Hospital for sickness and disease'. The unsuitability [in Rooke's view] of Queen Mary's Quarter was re-emphasised in a further SHS minute: 'The Secretary was authorised to show this letter to DuCane and to state that the Committee would be quite willing to refer the question to any two or more Medical Officers belonging to the most distinguished hospitals'.[50] A fortnight later an SHS minute records: 'Read a letter from the Admiralty stating that Dr [J S] Bristowe [of St Thomas's Hospital]

& Mr [T] Holmes [of St George's][51] had been deputed to report whether Queen Anne or Queen Mary's Quarter would be best adapted for the Society'; the SHS Committee 'Ordered that Mr [George] Busk & the visiting Physicians be requested to visit Queen Anne and Queen Mary's Wards of Greenwich Hospital & report to the committee thereon'.

Queen Anne or Queen Mary?

Two subsequent reports to the SHS Committee outlined inspections of these two quarters. On 3 May: 'Read a letter from Dr [R] Barnes and one also from Dr [S H] Ward stating that they had gone over both Queen Anne and Queen Mary's quarters and that if the side partitions in the wards of the latter [could] be removed they should prefer that Quarter for the Society's Hospital. – Ordered that copies of these letters be given to Dr Rooke'.[52] The following week, Busk's report was read to the Committee: '... he considered that Queen Anne's wing at considerable Expense might be made available for the purposes of the Hospital but that with respect to Queen Mary's this was next to impossible. Admiral Sir W[illiam] Bowles [the SHS Chairman] promised to give a copy of this letter to one of the Lords of the Admiralty'. The minute continued: 'Read a letter from Dr Rooke reporting [in reference to the letters of the Visiting physicians] his further conviction of the impracticability of Converting Queen Mary's Wing to a proper Sick Hospital'.

A subsequent SHS minute dated 31 May records: 'The Chairman reported that in Company with Adml Sir Peter Richards [CB and] Busk – the secretary had waited upon Mr Corry [see above] the first Lord of the Admiralty by appointment yesterday afternoon – but that from ... Corry's having been considerably detained beyond the appointed time by a Cabinet Council Meeting, there was little time to speak to him – but he had given him a Memorandum on the subject of the importance of granting Queen Anne's quarter to the Society as the committee felt that otherwise the only course left to them would be to build a Hospital ...'. Meanwhile Busk (accompanied by Rooke) had taken a further close look at Greenwich Hospital; while he favoured Queen Anne's Quarter (after a great deal of alteration), he felt that *neither* option was ideal.[53]

Admiralty politics

Meanwhile, the *Times* was conscientiously covering this ongoing saga, but 'Beta' again entered the correspondence in April; he had formed the opinion that following the Prime Minister's promise (of five weeks previously) all was settled; 'We little knew the power of low intrigue' he continued '... the scanty remnant and successors of the privileged officers who once monopolized all the fairest portions of the Hospital buildings ... declared that the Merchant Seamen might be admitted, but good care should be taken that they were stowed away in the remotest corner of the Hospital.'...'The Admiralty knew perfectly well [that Queen Mary's quarter] cannot possibly be accepted by the Society'. He gave five cogent reasons (most of them geographical and/or structural – the emphasis being on *ventilation*); 'of all the quarters of the Hospital [he wrote it is], that which is most unsuited for the

[SHS], and that which in time of war the Admiralty could least well spare'. He was a convinced advocate of Queen Anne's quarter which he considered 'has all the advantages which [Queen Mary's quarter] lacks'. This letter drew a comment from Corry in the House of Commons; he spoke of 'the unfounded impression' that this letter was calculated to convey to the public, giving good reasons (or so he felt) for favouring Queen Mary's Quarter for use by the SHS. An anonymous writer in the *Shipping and Mercantile Gazette* considered Corry's statement 'cannot be regarded in any way satisfactory'.[54] Meanwhile, the *Lancet* continued with its campaign for Queen Anne's Quarter – which was in many respects more suitable (largely because it had a river frontage) for the SHS's requirements. *The Times* considered that Queen Mary's Quarter was structurally (and from the viewpoint of *ventilation*) unsatisfactory, but that the 'wards in the first floor of Queen's [sic] Anne's quarter ... are, in most respects similar to those of St Bartholomew's Hospital'.[55]

Further support for Queen Anne's Quarter was forthcoming in yet a further letter from 'Beta'. He began by commending the fact that the Admiralty had referred the matter to Mr (later Sir) John Simon (1816–1904)[56] (Medical Officer of the Privy Council) of the Board of Health; however, Simon declined the invitation (on the grounds that he had an 'excess of official business') and nominated instead Bristowe and Holmes (see above). The *Lancet* adjudged these gentlemen to be 'very fit persons for the present purpose', as they had recently reported on 'the sanitary condition of hospitals, throughout the country ...'. In a leading article entitled 'The rights and wrongs of the Greenwich Hospital question', the *Medical Times and Gazette* considered that Queen Anne's quarter had the advantage of a river frontage, but offered 'inferior accommodation'. This article also immediately poured scorn on the idea of a *resident* chaplain!

A rapid response from Rooke followed: 'Queen Anne's Quarter is [not] all we could wish', and he outlined the reasons for the SHS declining Queen Mary's Quarter. Not only was this not on the river, but the wards were 'subdivided by brick partitions, not removable without endangering the safety of the building'. An editorial comment pointed out that should the Society acquire Queen Anne's Quarter, the Admiralty would be unlikely to 'grant permission for erecting ... placards as the side of the *Dreadnought* presents'. In reviewing the subject once again, the *Lancet*'s writer pointed to the undoubted superiority of the kitchens, laundry, cellars and bathrooms of Queen Mary's quarter. It was also felt that whichever quarter was granted, considerable expenditure would be required and it might after all prove wise in the long-term to build their own hospital on the plot of land which the SHS had already purchased.[57]

Unexpected Support for Queen Mary's quarter

In an article published in early May, titled 'Scandal about Queen Anne', the *British Medical Journal* had some alternative views (*invited* comments were written by a 'distinguished authority'); if the sick patient was to be considered of paramount importance, Queen Mary's Block was the preferred option (for a general hospital), but from a staff viewpoint Queen Anne's quarter was undoubtedly superior! The writer felt that the former building was sufficiently close to the river, because a 'very large proportion of the *Dreadnought*'s patients do not reach Greenwich by river at all, but by land'. Overall, he felt that the SHS authorities had been unwise to request part of Greenwich Hospital, because they 'have abundant means with which to build a hospital of their own', and using their own plans.[58]

It must have come as a severe blow to the SHS to learn that Bristowe and Holmes (see above) had in the meantime also favoured Queen Mary's quarter (largely, but not entirely, because the *ventilation* there was better); a minute in May states that the Admiralty 'deemed [the report of these gentlemen] conclusively in favour of Queen Mary's Quarter [and that] it was advisable that someone on behalf of the society should go over that Quarter with the Director of Works [in order] to ascertain what work should be done, after which their Lordships would let the Committee know the Cost of the same'. The letter from the Admiralty together with the Bristowe and Holmes report, was published in full in the *British Medical Journal*.[59]

Shortly after this (June 1867) 'Beta' had another letter published in the *Times;* he referred to the decision of the First Lord of the Admiralty (Corry) six weeks previously to obtain the opinion of Simon to adjudicate on which part of Greenwich Hospital the SHS should occupy. The subsequent arbitration (he claimed) had been prearranged and the judgement had therefore miscarried; Simon's nominees (i.e. Bristowe and Holmes) had heard (he claimed) only one side of the dispute. 'Beta' maintained that structural alterations could in fact be made to Queen Anne's Quarter and that the Admiralty Director of Works (Major Clark RE [who was *not* a surveyor]) had misled the enquiry; the Inspector of Works of Greenwich Hospital (who *was* a qualified surveyor) had assured the SHS authorities that there would be no difficulty in making the necessary alterations. Two days later, Bristowe challenged Beta's views in the *Times*; this was *not* a simple matter he declared, and there were several views on the suitability of one or the other parts of Greenwich Hospital; for example, Barnes and Ward 'agree [he wrote] substantially in opinion with the Director-General and ourselves'. Furthermore, he considered that the assessment had been openly and fairly carried out; the admiralty had furnished all correspondence on *both* sides of the argument. Bristowe ended his letter by claiming that neither quarter was in his (and Holmes') opinion suitable for a General Hospital, and that the SHS authorities would do well to withdraw their application for part of Greenwich Hospital and 'devote all their energies to that which was the original plan – namely, the building of an entirely new hospital of their own, on some carefully selected site'.[60]

The SHS has doubts

The Committee of the SHS was clearly unhappy about the way the inspection had been carried out, and Kemball Cook (on behalf of the Society's Committee) wrote a further Memorial to the Secretary of the Admiralty: 'The Admiralty had discarded the SHS advice [he wrote], and *all* of the medical officers involved, together with … Sir Peter Richards, … should take the final decision.' But, their Lordships considered that the 'town of Greenwich should also be represented at such a Meeting'. After Richards declined to be present, it was decided *not* to call such a conference but 'the decision should be left to an officer selected by their Lordships'. However, they 'declined to entertain this proposal' and the Society instead nominated Mr Tatum, Senior Surgeon of St George's Hospital, and also protested 'against the intervention of the Inhabitants of Greenwich as wholly inadmissible'. In any event, the first resolution was passed unanimously, i.e. that 'neither Quarter could be converted so as to be in accordance with modern Hospital requirements'. The second resolution, giving the vote in favour of Queen Mary's was 'carried against the Society by a majority of one, the Parliamentary Representative for Greenwich voting against the Society, although declaring that he knew nothing whatever about Hospitals, or their wants'. Mr Suter, 'the Builder at Greenwich' (Kemball Cook wrote) had provided an estimate of the expense of converting Queen Mary's quarter into a General Hospital; it was likely to be £25,000 to £27,000. Since they would merely be 'tenants at will' this was an exorbitant sum. That of converting Queen Anne's quarter would have been only £10,000. The offer of Queen Mary's Quarter was therefore firmly 'turned down'.[61]

Urgency of removal

The urgency of the situation was admirably stressed in a letter to the *Times* by Dr Harry Leach (Medical Officer on the Hospital-ship).[62] The constant noise 'consequent upon the construction of iron barges in the immediate vicinity of this ship [he maintained was seriously affecting the medical management of] a patient dying of consumption or delirious from fever [and] the use of a stethoscope for the detection of chest disease is, under these circumstances, totally impossible'. He requested a decision on the relocation of the Hospital to 'the spacious [empty] wings of Greenwich Hospital' as a matter of the greatest possible urgency.[63]

Both Greenwich Hospital quarters are rejected

This unfortunate saga, beginning with an offer by the Prime-Minister of the day of accommodation in the Royal Hospital, and ending with the SHS 'reluctantly declining the Admiralty's offer of part of Queen Mary's quarter', was reviewed in the *Shipping and Mercantile Gazette*: 'The process by which this unworthy intrigue has been worked out deserves attention, and demands publicity' (the writer considered). Queen Anne's quarter was not offered because 'some five or six pensioned officials ... have snug quarters there and intend to hold to them if they can'. A minute in May records: 'Read a letter from Mr. Busk written after his perusal of the [Admiralty's] report – and one also from Dr Rooke thereon both stating that Queen Anne's was the only portion of Greenwich Hospital (except the *Infirmary* – see below) which could be made available for the Society's purposes'.

In any event, the SHS authorities were clearly furious with the content(s) of this report; in answer to a question from Mr Charles Norwood (1825–91) (MP for Hull) in the House of Commons, Lord (Henry) Lennox (1821–86) reiterated the facts of the case, and indicated that Sir Peter Richards and Sir Charles Trevelyan (1807–86) had been approached with a view to a further inspection, but both were too busy to undertake this task.[64]

The Infirmary becomes a distinct possibility

The SHS Committee meeting in August was attended by Norwood (see above). He reported that in a 'debate which he had originated in the House of Commons ... it had been proposed that the *Infirmary* [my italics]... be given up to the Society in lieu of either Queen Anne or Q. Mary's Quarter'. This proposal had apparently 'found much favour in the House'; he wanted to know therefore whether the SHS would accept the *Infirmary* provided the Admiralty offered it? This meeting, to which both Busk and Rooke had been invited, came to the unanimous decision 'to accept the Infirmary and Mr Norwood undertook to mention this to the Secretary of the Admiralty'.

At a later meeting, the Secretary reported that 'Mr Ayrton had told him that Lord ... Lennox (see above) had promised to refer to Mr DuCane's Committee now sitting at Greenwich Hospital on the Expenditure of the Infirmary &c., his suggestion made in the House of Commons on the 12th instant that the Infirmary be closed and the building be given to this Society in lieu either of Queen Anne or Queen Mary's Quarter – and that until the Committee had made its Report nothing further could be known on the subject'.[65]

However, the Admiralty were still keen to loan St Mary's Quarter, and an SHS minute dated 30 August states: 'Read a letter from the Admiralty dated 16th inst. stating that My Lords had received the Report of the Gentleman who met in conference to decide on the merits of Queen Anne's and Queen Mary's Wards at Greenwich Hospital and that they are of opinion that neither is well adapted for the purposes of a General Hospital for diseased Seamen, and that Queen Anne's Quarter appears to have been proved to be the least suitable. That My Lords are still prepared to repeat the original offer of Queen Mary's Ward if the Society consider it advisable to accept it.' The Secretary's reply, stated that as the Chairman and the majority of the Committee had left London (for the summer) the consideration of their Lordship's letter must be deferred for the present; this was approved! It is clear from the minutes that the Society was giving renewed consideration to Queen Mary's quarter; at a meeting in September the likely expenditure of adaptation of that building was considered; this was based on figures obtained by Rooke at the request of Bowles. At a specially summoned meeting later that month, these estimates were considered, but rejected on the grounds that the sum was too high. A minute in December refers to a bill for £21=00 from a Mr Suter of Greenwich (see above) 'in consideration of the Estimate he had made of the cost of adapting Queen Mary's Quarter of Greenwich Hospital to the use of this Society'. The Committee decided that this amount should be paid but only after Suter had submitted 'detailed items of his Estimate'.[66]

Lack of progress to date

In August 1867, the *Lancet* devoted a leading article to the future of Greenwich Hospital. This was based on an in-depth debate in the House of Commons reported in *The Times*. The controversy surrounding Greenwich Hospital had 'committed the future Lords of the Admiralty [the writer considered] to some definite course of action'. Much of the debate focused on the enormous 'expenditure at Greenwich Hospital', but the 'wings will soon be entirely empty; and we may remark, *en passant* that the [SHS] may then, if they think fit, [consider] the loan of the *infirmary* [my italics] with some hope of success'. But the future of the remainder of the vast building remained, at the time, undecided (a situation reminiscent of the debates of the 1990s); a school for girls, a local Greenwich Hospital, a Medical College for the naval service (a naval Netley) persistently championed by the *Lancet*? But Childers envisaged the establishment of a College for *both* services (i.e. the Army and the Navy) – a scheme which the *Lancet*'s writer considered, presented 'difficulties which are insurmountable'. The probability of the Society applying for the lease of the *Infirmary* was now taken up by the *Pall-Mall Gazette*, and was also reported in the *Times*.[67]

Serious reconsideration of building a *new* Hospital

It is clear that the SHS Committee were now disenchanted with negotiations with the Admiralty (which were leading nowhere) and were again exploring the '*new* Hospital' option. A minute in November 1867 records: 'The Secretary reported that he had only this morng. [sic] obtained the plan of the [SHS] Hospital Site which he had just ordered to be lithographed – but that he found it would be necessary to give with a Copy of it to Architects, definite instructions on various points as to the sort of Hospital required'. It was eventually arranged that 'Mr. McGrouther would bring with him to the Committee at their next Meeting, the Treasurer or Architect of Saint Thomas's Hospital (now building) to give the Committee some advice as to the course they should pursue'. At the next SHS Committee, a minute records: 'The Committee saw Mr [Henry] Currey (see Figure 13.10),[68] the Architect of Saint Thomas's Hospital now building – a plan of the site belonging to this Society was given him and he promised to go over the ground and give the Committee an outline sketch of what he might Consider the best mode of arranging a Hospital thereon and an estimate of the probable Expense of its Erection – the more detailed plan &c. could be afterwards gone into but should the Society get into any portion of the Royal Hospital at Greenwich – he would make no charge for the preliminary plan and estimate'. The Secretary was instructed not to give a second, or any further, publication of the Advertisement to the Architects for Competition drawings, and (as no plan of the site nor any Instructions had yet been given to anyone) it was 'Ordered that those gentlemen who had made enquiries, be informed that the Committee had made other arrangements'. Currey again attended – at a December meeting when he 'laid before them plans for a hospital on the Society's site and he read a statement explanatory whereof. Ordered that the same [i.e. the plans] do lie on the table for the consideration of the Members of the Committee for the next few

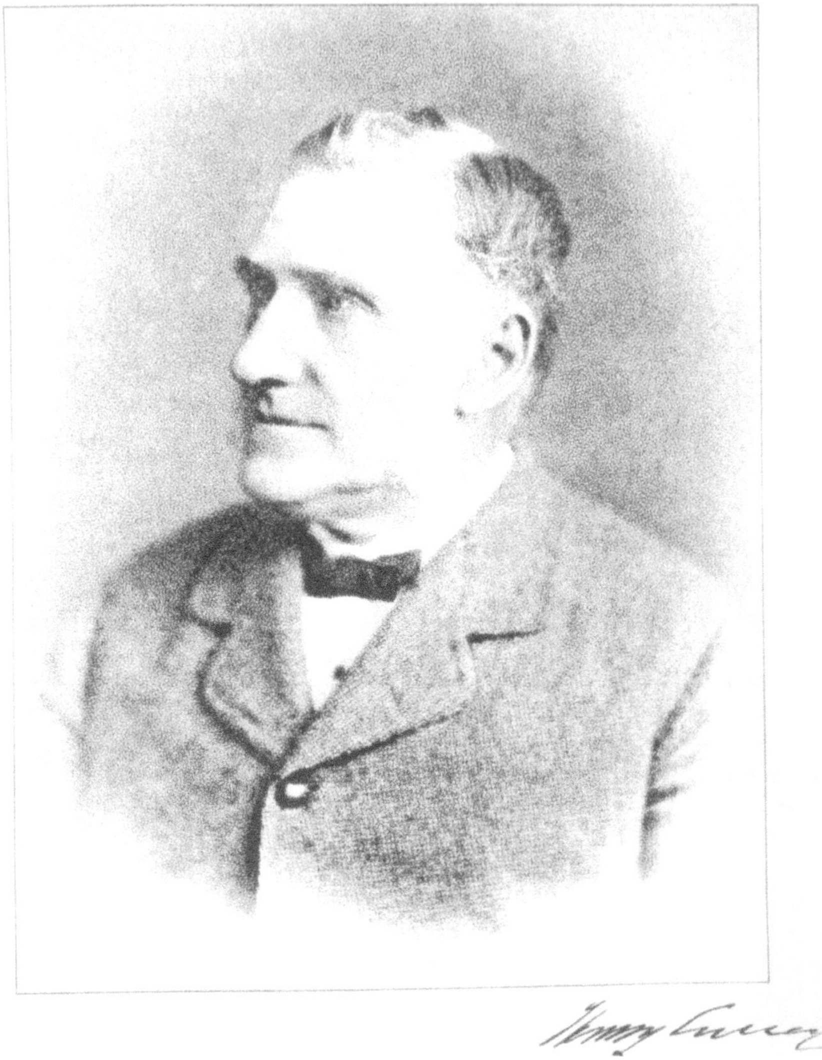

Figure 13.10: Henry Currey (1820–1900), the architect of the *new* St Thomas's Hospital. He designed a building to occupy the land purchased by the Society.

weeks'.[69] Unfortunately, these plans cannot be traced, and it is unknown whether they remain extant.

The Royal Hospital and its Infirmary are at last vacant

In August 1867, the *Lancet* drew its readers' attention to the fact the inmates of the Royal Hospital were costing £120=00 per head, in contrast to the London Hospitals averaging 'not more than £40'. It is 'proposed [therefore] to give the able-bodied the usual outdoor allowance, and to send the sick now in hospital to Haslar'. Such a move would leave the *Infirmary* (Figure 13.11) (which the SHS had already agreed to accept if offered) and the four Royal blocks vacant. This (i.e. the Infirmary) the report continued, 'with very limited alteration, [the SHS] can utilise and convert into efficient wards, obtaining within this portion of the building a river frontage and a ready "stair entrance" to the new *Dreadnought*.'

The potential offer of the Infirmary to the SHS was reported in the *British Medical Journal*; with this loan would be offered 'the plot of ground to the river walk, allowing [the SHS] access to the unused stabling and brewery which shut it from the river'. The *Lancet* for October 1867 also gave hope that the Infirmary would be made available; this however, depended on the 'forthcoming report of ... DuCane's Committee [which might] result in the total emptying of Greenwich Hospital, and so give the Admiralty an opportunity of offering ... use of the infirmary to the *Dreadnought* authorities'.[70] A *Lancet* reporter meanwhile continued with his familar theme that a naval medical school should be attached to the Seamen's Hospital.

The *raison d'être* of the DuCane Report had been to enquire into the management and expenditure of the hospital and its schools – with economy and efficiency to

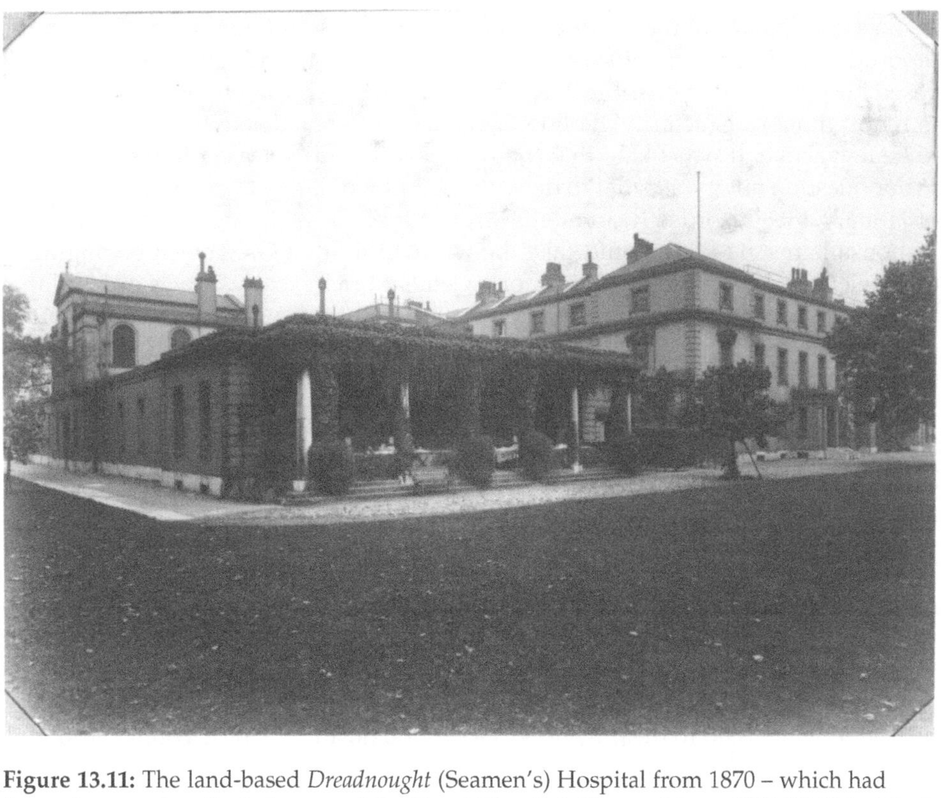

Figure 13.11: The land-based *Dreadnought* (Seamen's) Hospital from 1870 – which had formerly served as the Infirmary of the Royal Hospital, Greenwich – c.1900 [SHS Archive]. The single-storey building to the left is Somerset Ward, with the chapel above it.

the fore. Details of the present state of the infirmary are included in an appendix to the report – written by Bristowe and Holmes (see above); most patients, they wrote, were 'old bed-ridden men' (resembling those in a workhouse infirmary rather than an 'ordinary general hospital') who required a minimum of medical, but a great deal of nursing care. The patients included however, 'a small number (about 136 per annum) of accident cases, more or less severe, admitted from the neighbouring dockyards and elsewhere'.[71]

The possibility that the SHS would take over the Infirmary ('which would in no way interfere with future plans for the utilisation of the hospital proper') were endorsed in an anonymous article in the *Lancet* for December 1867; it reminded its readership that 'the clearance of Greenwich Hospital originated with, and was mainly carried out by the Liberal Government', and had been initiated by the Duke of Somerset. 'We are [he wrote] credibly informed that there is ample accommodation at Haslar [and] other naval hospitals for those decayed seamen who now occupy the helpless wards of this infirmary'. The writer also urged once again 'the establishment of a naval medical school [which 'would occupy but one of four wings of the Hospital] at Greenwich'.[72]

The events of 1867 summarised

A concise summary of the complex events of 1867 was laid out in the 47th Annual report. Kemball Cook emphasised that no decision concerning the site of a land-based hospital was yet possible 'but [the committee] earnestly hope soon to be able to report more satisfactorily'. Following a year of frenzied activity, 1868 promised to be less active. It was likely that the *Infirmary* would be leased to them, and the major question now, was what to do with their plot of land at Greenwich. A minute of January 1868 records: 'Read a letter from Mr Shalless stating that he knew of a responsible person who would take the waste ground at Greenwich belonging to the Society at Ten pounds a Month for a Cement brick factory. It was ordered that the offer be accepted should the Secretary find that there would be no brick burning to make a nuisance to the Neighbourhood nor using of the soil of the Hospital site for the manufacture of the bricks'.[73]

The future of the Royal Hospital is uncertain and the Queen Mary option remains viable

In March 1868, the *Lancet* continued its support for the SHS and a detailed report which referred to the continued under-utilisation of the fine buildings which had already appeared in the *Pall Mall Gazette*, was published in *The Times*. It was now intended, the *Lancet* recorded, to 'make extensive alterations in the buildings known as Queen Mary's and Queen Anne's Quarters, such as will render those portions of the building adapted to the purposes of a general hospital'. The account continued: 'we trust … that the grounds we have always advocated for the admission of the *Dreadnought* to Greenwich Hospital have been at length recognised'. In an update in April, the same journal recorded that in the DuCane report, which had already been presented to the Admiralty, there was a recommendation that 'those sailors and marines [i.e. RN *and* Mercantile Marines and members of the Naval Reserve] discharged from the service [due to] disablement, either by disease or injury, who are deprived, from want or length of servitude, of pensions' should be admitted to Greenwich Hospital. In addition (the writer continued with his former theme) is the suggestion that 'a Naval Medical School should be formed at Greenwich [in King William's quarter, i.e. to the east of Queen Mary's quarter], similar to the very excellent institution for the army at Netley'.[74]

Corroborating these impressions, the *British Medical Journal* provided more detail concerning the numbers of personnel involved: 'in 1866, there were 1468 ['invalid naval pensioners and men invalided from the naval service]' on the Register of the Naval Reserve in the Port of London. It was also recommended that the school should be increased to 1,000 by the addition of 200 boys.

The Times, the *Lancet* and the *British Medical Journal* all contained detailed coverage of the DuCane report, *before* official release of the document. *The Times* was especially damning – the report which, it claimed, had been composed of 'uninformed advisers (who lacked knowledge about the history of Greenwich Hospital)' unlike the Treasury, the Privy Council, the Colonial Office, and the Post Office who 'settle their own affairs at home'. Greenwich Hospital it maintained, was *very* costly when compared with other service and civil hospitals. The *Lancet* reminded its readership that 'the *Dreadnought* has been assigned no place or voice in the matter'. In their report, the *British Medical Journal* was on the whole congratulatory, although the writer had certain reservations concerning the 'selection criteria' for those suffering from disease 'attributable to the service'.[75]

In July, *The Times* devoted a further leading article to the *future* of Greenwich Hospital; this had been precipitated by a motion to the House of Commons from Alexander Cochrane-Baillie (1816-90). The recent report (the writer contested) sought 'to restore in some measure the vicious system [i.e. the 'monastic' institution] which the Duke of Somerset overthrew.'... 'Any Out-pensioner who ... needs the treatment of the Infirmary may by the existing rules become a life-tenant of Greenwich Hospital ... But the Committee propose to admit ... invalids discharged from the other naval hospitals without reference to possession of a pension or to length of service'.

But what are we to do with the vacant buildings (*The Times* asked)? 'The Infirmary and four 'quarters' of the Hospital together in cubic measure as nearly as may be five times the extent of St George's Hospital, while the number of patients is about the same'. The problem is to fill the vacuum with tenants who have a claim on the country, who will keep the building warm in time of peace, and be ready to vacate it, when the demand arises, in time of war'. The writer continued by recommending that the SHS be accommodated in these buildings: 'It would have cost the country nothing to give them the use of Queen Anne's Quarter ... But the Admiralty [remained] jealous of the merchant seamen, and there was no member in the House of Commons who had the industry to ascertain, or the energy to press the strength of their claim'. 'The best use [the writer concluded] will be to move into the vacant quarters the Marines from Woolwich, and with them the Woolwich Marine Infirmary'. An anonymous writer in the *Lancet* alluded to a speech by

Childers (see above) who in addition to showing that the DuCane report was flawed (in recommending reversion in part to a 'monastic institution'), criticised him for not pursuing the matter of a Naval School within the walls of Greenwich Hospital.[76]

The Admiralty continued with its policy regarding the Queen Mary option. A minute in September 1868 states: 'Read a letter from the Lords Commissioners of Her Majesty's Treasury in reply to the Society's letter of the 4th July last, stating that while their Lordships will be quite ready to assist as far as they are able, in providing accommodation for the requirements of the Society in Greenwich Hospital, they are not prepared to submit any vote to the House of Commons'.[77]

Extensive repairs were required to the *Dreadnought* Hospital-ship in August of that year (see Chapter 8); the patients were transferred to the *Belle-isle* – which had previously been used as a cholera-hospital moored off Deptford Creek. An anonymous writer to the *Lancet* concluded that it would 'be a subject of great regret if the repairs now proceeding on board the Dreadnought [ship] are likely to lead to a renewal of her lease of existence as a hospital ship'. 'There is now no doubt (he continued) that the Society should have accepted the quarter originally offered by the Government ...'.[78]

It is unclear whether these articles influenced the SHS Committee, but there is no doubt that at this stage they were having second thoughts about the unsuitability or otherwise of Queen Mary's quarter; a minute in November recorded the conclusions of a Sub-Committee set up on 17 July to reconsider this possibility; they felt that the Society should: (i) acknowledge the letter received from the Treasury (see above), thanking their Lordships for re-offering to accommodate them in Greenwich Hospital, and (ii) accept the offer of Queen Mary's quarter for use by the Society. 'Ordered [the minute continued] that the advice tendered by the Sub-Committee be adopted and that a letter be sent to the Treasury in Conformity thereto'. A subsequent minute in December recorded: 'Read a letter from the Admiralty acknowledging the receipt of the letter of the 4th November last stating that the Committee are willing to accept Queen Mary's quarter ... and in reply acquainting the Committee that the matter stands over for the decision of the New Board.[79]

The *Lancet* meanwhile was optimistic that the newly constituted Board (of the Admiralty) would take 'some definite line of action with regard to Greenwich Hospital': the 'present First Lord is strongly in favour of utilising part of that grand pile of buildings in the formation of a Naval Medical School, [but] the decks of the *Dreadnought* Hospital Ship can alone supply [adequate *clinical* material for their medical students]'.[80]

The events of 1868 summarised

A summary of the year's progress was provided in the 48th report of the SHS; at the end of 1868, Kemball Cook wrote: the Committee had 'been deliberating both upon the possibility of erecting a *new* building [for which the Treasury had ... declined to make a contribution], and ... upon the propriety of taking the [Queen Mary's] Quarter of Greenwich Hospital already offered – *without the expenditure of any large sum of money in alterations*. While the latter option would not be ideal, it would in fact provide a Building 'far more suitable for the Patients than is the *Dreadnought* [Hospital-ship]'.[81] The SHS Committee seemingly remained convinced, however, that Queen Anne's Quarter was preferable to either alternative!

Fruitful negotiations at last

Eighteen sixty-nine was the year of successful negotiation. *The Times* mentioned (a viewpoint subsequently taken up by the *Lancet*) in January of that year that it was the intention of Government 'to remove [next October] the infirm pensioners to the hospital at Netley', thus leaving the entire building free for 'military purposes' and thereby forming an institution which was 'common for the training of all men entering the medical branches of the public service, – a United Service Medical School for her Majesty's Naval and the British and Indian Army Services'. This move resulted from a visit by [Sir George] Trevelyan (1838–1928) of the Admiralty. Meanwhile, the *British Medical Journal* declared that 'We have reason to believe that the present Admiralty scarcely approve of the course of the late Board in carrying out the recommendation of … DuCane's Greenwich Hospital Committee by increasing the number of admissions from the out-port hospitals'.[82]

Much was meanwhile taking place with respect to the *governance* of Greenwich Hospital, and improved uses of its revenues; both Childers and (Sir George) Trevelyan addressed this subject in Parliamentary debates designed to introduce the Greenwich Hospital Bill. Trevelyan maintained that the 'Board of Admiralty … intended a reduction in the number of in-pensioners [some were to be sent to Haslar and Portsmouth] to such as could be accommodated within the walls of the *infirmary* [my italics]'. 'It was highly probable [he continued] that … the infirmary at Greenwich might not be required [after a short interval] for its present purposes. In such case would it not be well to hand that infirmary over to the [SHS]?' Childers concluded the debate, however: 'It was only proposed to give the Dreadnought the advantages of the infirmary in the event of its being required'. This debate (the Bill had superseded the DuCane report [see above] which had been presented to Parliament on 19 March the previous year) which was opened by Trevelyan was also recorded in detail in both the *Shipping and Mercantile Gazette* and the *Lancet*: 'no further admission [the *Lancet* writer reported] will be granted to the Infirmary … the patients now located therein will be pensioned off at the rate of 1s 6d per day, or allowed to remain, and that, when the building is vacant, it will be offered to the Dreadnought authorities'. 'The *Dreadnought* staff [he continued] will fail in a palpable duty if their exertions do not cause this hospital to become one of the best centres for the study of practical medicine in the metropolis or its suburbs'.[83]

The *Lancet* article concluded: 'We would suggest … that the infirmary … should be given up to the *Dreadnought*, and the main building be devoted to the care of the infirm and disabled sailors, as proposed by Dr SIBSON:[84] the Naval Medical School being the uniting bond between the two institutions'. The speech made by Trevelyan was communicated to the SHS committee at an April meeting: 'it appeared [read the minute] to be the intention of Her Majesty's Government (with the consent of Parliament) in the Expected Event of the Infirmary … becoming Empty, to grant the site of it to this Society in lieu of the Dreadnought. Read a letter from Mr Trevelyan (in reply to the Secretary's application) promising to send a copy of the Greenwich Hospital Bill when it had been laid upon the table of the House of Commons'. But, as the *Lancet* pointed out 'It is to be noticed that the claims of the [SHS] are not formally recognised in the Bill ...'. And later the same journal remarked: 'In case infirm and helpless seamen of the RN should not become in-pensioners in sufficient numbers to justify the maintenance of an establishment at Greenwich, the Admiralty propose to place the Infirmary and Somerset Ward at the disposal of the Committee of the *Dreadnought* Hospital ship'. The writer continued: 'We fear that the prospect of the *Dreadnought* Hospital being transferred to Greenwich is ... indefinitely postponed, and with it the foundation of a naval medical school, of which no mention occurs in the [Greenwich Hospital Bill]'.[85]

Two anonymous articles in the *Times* summarised the content(s) of the Bill (championed by Trevelyan, Childers and [Sir William] Adam (1823–81): 'The Bill ... gives permission to the Admiralty to permit Greenwich Hospital, or any part thereof, to be occupied and used temporarily for any public, charitable, or other useful purpose, but on condition that the buildings shall be at all times available for the purposes to which they would have been originally applicable'. Those pensioners remaining after October 'can comfortably be lodged within the infirmary', and every such applicant, if his claim is allowed, will be offered 'the infirmary or of residing with his friends'. A further anonymous contribution to the *Lancet* for June, was seemingly ambivalent on the subject of the 1869 Greenwich Hospital Bill, the second reading of which had been carried by a large majority; the writer was obviously pleased that the SHS was likely to be accommodated at Greenwich, and that an asylum was being provided for 'men whose health has been deteriorated by exposure in the service', but he was nevertheless opposed to 'cases requiring medical and surgical aid [being accommodated] at Haslar and Plymouth Hospitals' – which the DuCane Committee (whose evidence was taken in 1867) had also considered virtually impossible; 'at Haslar, especially [the writer continued], it would be difficult to separate acute from chronic cases, the treatment of whom is totally different'.[86]

Following further parliamentary debate, the Bill was read a third time and passed; it was accepted by the Lord's following limited debate, and the Act became law on 2 August 1869. The *Times* succinctly outlined the major content(s) of the new Act, and on 14 August the same newspaper devoted a leading article to the matter (see above).[87]

Greenwich Hospital and its Infirmary are eventually empty!

The Times carried a short report in September which recorded: '... all of the pensioners who have either friends to take care of them or who are not absolutely helpless and bedridden have availed themselves of the offer of leaving the institution, and ... the number left on the 1st of October next [1869] will be so reduced as to be easily accommodated in the Somerset Ward of the Infirmary, thereby leaving the whole range of the hospital and infirmary vacant, and at the disposal of the Admiralty'. Later that month, *The Times* confirmed these initial impressions; it also stated that 'the men who were about to leave the Hospital expressed themselves satisfied with the amount of the out-pension awarded to them'. The *Lancet* in mid-September stated that 'it is probable that by the end of the current month the hospital proper and the infirmary will be absolutely empty, and the *helpless* [my italics] patients who remain will be accommodated in the Somerset Ward. It is presumed that, if these conditions are fulfilled, the infirmary will be offered by the Admiralty to the [SHS], according to a suggestion made by Mr Trevelyan when the Bill was in progress'.[88]

THE PENSIONERS DEPART

In late September, *The Times* gave news of an event that must have been keenly awaited by the SHS: 'Yesterday afternoon [20 September] the final arrangement for the last batch of in-pensioners of Greenwich Hospital to leave that establishment under an offer from the Admiralty of augmented pensions, the *minimum* being 36/10s per annum, were arrived at, and beyond some 40 or 50 of the aged and helpless who are in the infirmary, today will witness the dispersion of those who have been its inmates'. The article added: 'The whole of the men who have thus accepted their discharge upon the increased allowance have left on the understanding that the Hospital will be open to them in the event of failing health ...'. The writer added that the number of re-entries were 'likely to be very few', and that 'those now under medical treatment will be moved to other naval establishments'.[89] On 2 October, the same newspaper carried a further leading article which began: 'Yesterday the walls of Greenwich Hospital were closed against the pensioners of the [RN]'. The same day the *Lancet* declared: 'At present there are under fifty old pensioners left, men without friends to receive them and incapable of undergoing removal to the Naval Hospital', and a week later it proclaimed 'The exodus from Greenwich Hospital has ceased, and there are now only about thirty bedridden inmates located in the Somerset Ward'.[90]

The Infirmary is at last loaned to the SHS

Although there was general optimism from the *Lancet* that the 'infirmary will [at last] be offered to the [SHS]', there were differing opinions on the fate of Greenwich Hospital overall! Various views were expressed in correspondence to *The Times*; one was that it should be used to educate 'the children of seamen of all grades in both the Navy and Commercial Marine', and another (from a retired Rear-Admiral) for 'the education of naval cadets' after which they should be sent to sea immediately, thus doing away with training ships. The idea of a Naval University of Greenwich (canvassed by the *Lancet* – see above) did *not* meet with general approval; a Captain in the RN felt for example, that this would undermine Portsmouth College, and furthermore that Greenwich was no place to establish a naval college. He was not alone; 'an old student of the RN College [at Portsmouth]' was strongly opposed to the idea of transferring the RN College from Portsmouth to Greenwich.[91]

The loan of the Infirmary was agreed by the Admiralty in late 1869; an SHS minute in mid-November recorded that the Admiralty would welcome an application from the Society for the loan of the infirmary. A further minute in January

1870 'contained the Admiralty's reply to that application: '... their Lordships are willing to lend the Society the Infirmary and Somerset Ward of Greenwich Hospital on lease at the Nominal Rent of One Shilling per Annum on Certain conditions therein stated – and adding that if these terms be Accepted by the Society their Lordships will instruct their Solicitor to prepare the necessary documents, and on the Completion to his satisfaction, their Lordships will be prepared to hand over the premises to the Society. Ordered [the minute continued] that the terms be accepted and that the Secretary do write in reply to this letter unconditionally accepting the loan of the building on the terms stated'. A Sub-Committee was immediately formed to administer the Hospital 'under the altered circumstances'; this to consist of 'Captn Hon. F Maude RN, Captn Vincent Budd, Captn R L Hunter, Captn Farrer, James McGrouther and Joseph Moore Esquires'.[92]

The fate of the main royal hospital buildings

By July 1871, the Admiralty had still not reached a clear decision, however, on the future of the main buildings; the Prime-Minister, now W E Gladstone[93] sent his apologies for absence from a meeting at Greenwich of local residents, but emphasised that it was important that these building were utilised. A fortnight later, a large deputation from Greenwich, Woolwich and Deptford called on Gladstone in order to discuss the matter further; however, once again no decision was forthcoming. *The Times* (quoting a *Graphic* article) hoped that 'some portion of the building will be devoted to the formation of a naval museum'.[94]

The events of 1869 summarised

The 49th report of the SHS (reviewing the previous year) pointed out that if utilised, considerable expenditure would have been required on alterations to either Queen Anne's or Queen Mary's Quarter. This was not, however, the case with the *Infirmary* [Kemball Cook explained] – 'a large building entirely separate from the main edifice – which was built, and to the present time has been used, for the same work as that carried out by this Society'. 'The Lords Commissioner's of the Admiralty [he continued] under the powers afforded them by the "Greenwich Hospital Act" of the last [Parliamentary] Session, have agreed to grant the Society the loan of the Infirmary (and the adjoining Somerset Ward) of Greenwich Hospital, at a nominal rental, upon conditions to which the Committee had previously signified their consent'.[95]

Removal to land at last

Thus, after more than five years of negotiation, with Kemball Cook at the helm, preparations for removal from Hospital-ship to land had been completed in January 1870. *The Times* reproduced a *Lancet* article of February advising its readership of the successful termination of the transactions, and giving an historical outline of the saga (thus ending almost half a century of Hospital-ships).

This article, however, continued that the 'crusade' for a Naval Medical School at Greenwich was *not* in fact to come about. This report was followed three days later by another leading article: Greenwich Hospital, it maintained, had 'outlived its time', and further, that 'the system, rules and customs of the establishment belonged to a bygone age'. The leader-writer stressed the length of time the SHS had had to negotiate before a final (satisfactory) settlement was forthcoming. The *Shipping and Mercantile Gazette* welcomed the Admiralty's decision, but at the same time regretted the long time-span of these transactions – which had cost the SHS a great deal of unnecessary expense, and had prolonged the agonies inflicted on patients on the Hospital-ships. This viewpoint was echoed by the *London Mirror*; 'Red-tapeism, as usual [it claimed] interfered with the settlement of the question'.[96]

Details of the lease (Figure 13.12) were formally accepted in early March; an SHS minute records: 'Read a letter from the Solicitor to the Society returning the draft lease. The Secretary was instructed to return the same to the Admiralty Solicitor [G H Bristow] asking (as he had already done) that the term of 21 years be altered to 99 – that it be suggested that the Fire Insurance be Effected in the name of the Treasurer of this Society for the time being as well as in that of the Solicitor of the Admiralty – and that the blank as to the amount of insurance be filled up for £10,000'. A month later a further minute records: 'The Secretary reported that possession was given to him, on the 1st instant on behalf of the Society, of the Infirmary of Greenwich Hospital – together with the charge of twenty patients [19 according to the *Lancet*] on behalf of the Admiralty and that [Harry] Leach [the Resident Medical Officer – see above] was attending to them.[97]

Actual removal of the patients from the *Dreadnought*-ship to the Infirmary and Somerset Ward of Greenwich Hospital took place on 13 April (see above). The *Lancet*

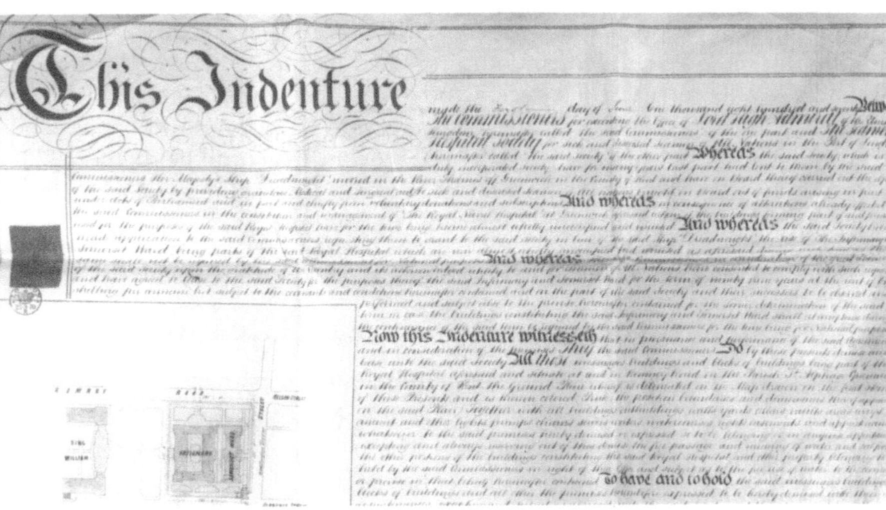
This Indenture
Between
Whereas
And whereas
And whereas
Now this Indenture witnesseth
To have and to hold

Figure 13.12: The lease (from the Lords Commissioners of the Admiralty) of the Infirmary and Somerset Ward of The Royal Hospital, Greenwich to the SHS – dated 1 June 1870. [SHS Archive].

remarked ('… though located at Greenwich, the institution … derives its status from the city and port of London') [and] that although facilities in the new venue were excellent, … the wards are very small, and unless some structural changes are made, efficiency will be purchased at the cost of a very large nursing staff'.

Details of the new *Dreadnought* Hospital were outlined in *The Times*, which later that year described the new institution as 'a great boon to the suburb and the south-east district'. The cost of removal had, however, been substantial; the *Lancet* estimated it at £1,990. The *British Medical Journal* also gave details of the new venue, which it anticipated would accommodate about 300 patients: 'The eastern wing will be devoted to medical, and the western to surgical cases, and the single-storey wing [Somerset Ward], will form an admirable casualty and out-patient department'. The writer predicted that accident cases from Greenwich, Woolwich, Charlton, Blackheath, and Deptford would all be sent to the *Dreadnought* rather than to Guy's or St Thomas's.[98]

The land-based hospital

Some 18 months after the removal, *The Times* reported favourably on the transition from ship to land; 'on medical and sanitary grounds, the change is a very decided improvement. The present quarters … consist of 88 wards, most of which have but three beds each, instead of three wards … containing collectively about 200 beds'. This article also emphasised that the removal had involved the SHS in considerable expenditure (see above).

The 51st SHS report contained reference to improved *nursing* in the new premises. The first step was to appoint a Matron; 'it is the source of satisfaction [Kemball Cook reported], that in electing Miss T. U. COLLINS, – a gentlewoman of experience both as a Nurse and a Matron – the Committee have secured the performance of highly important duties in a most conscientious and satisfactory manner'. The report then recorded that the team of nurses had had to be increased from 9 (one male and 2 females on each of 3 decks), to 17 (one male and 16 females).[99]

Kemball Cook had held the title of Secretary (with the addition of House-Governor in 1870) for approximately 25 years (from 1849 until he died on 27 June 1874), and it was largely due to his zeal and enthusiasm that removal from the last of the hospital-ships to land ultimately came to fruition.

Disposal of the Society's land in East Greenwich

Figure 13.13 shows a legal document giving details of a proposed auction of the SHS land (acquired in 1865–6) in 1870. Preceding the production of this document, correspondence had taken place between Kemball Cook and the Auctioneers; it was decided to attempt to auction the entire plot of land owned by the Society rather than sell it as smaller lots. The SHS (through Kemball Cook) had decided to put a £10,000 'reserve price' on the sale, but regrettably there were no bidders and despite various offers, the land remained unsold until 1880 – by which time Kemball Cook had died (*see* Chapter 12).[100]

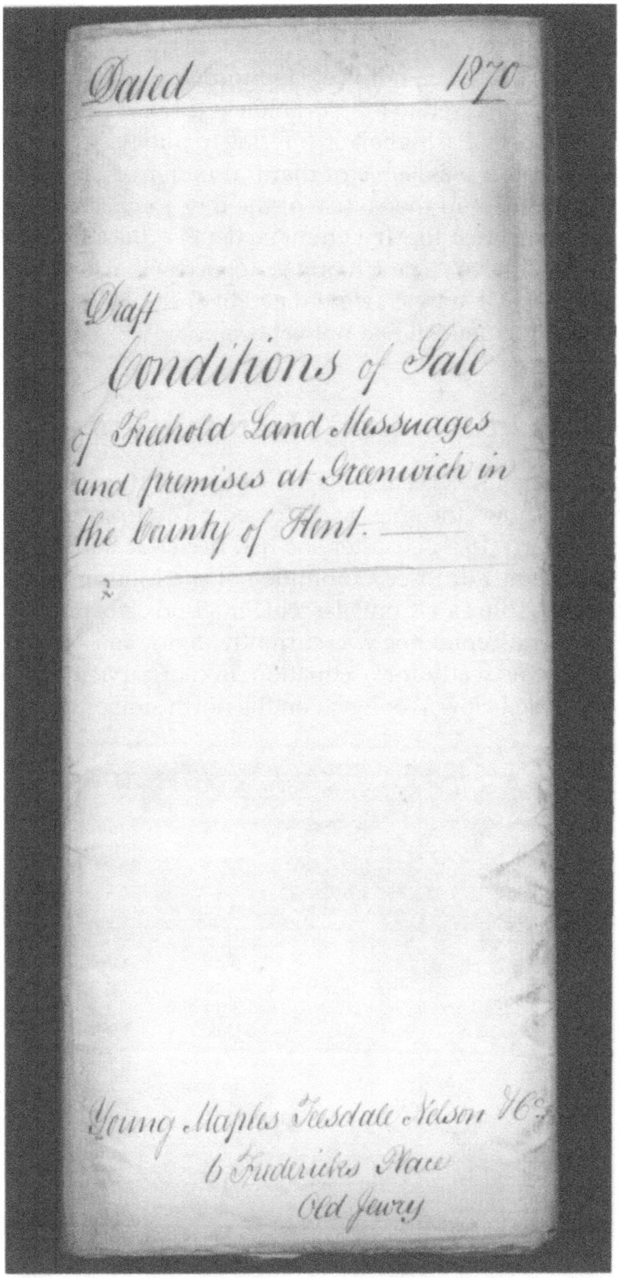

Dated 1870

Draft

Conditions of Sale

of Freehold Land Messuages and premises at Greenwich in the County of Kent.

Young Maples Teesdale Nelson & Co

6 Fredericks Place

Old Jewry

Figure 13.13: Document (dated 1870) referring to the proposed sale, by auction, of the land in East Greenwich owned by the SHS. [SHS Archive].

In January 1880 an SHS minute states that Burdett – who had taken over the Secretaryship - had 'given refusal of the *Hospital site* at East Greenwich for £10,000, to Messrs Stone & Co. Coppersmiths of Deptford until that day 8th inst.' Following this, he read a letter addressed to Messrs Shalless & Budds by a Solicitor, Mr Durant of 5 Guildhall Chambers, Basinghall St. offering to purchase the site for £9,500 cash. After some discussion it was '*Ordered* that if no offer of £10,000 cash be received from Messrs Stone & Co. in the course of the day, the Secretary be authorised to offer the land at that price to Mr Durant's clients – the offer to hold good until Tuesday 13th inst inclusive'. The Chairman reported that the negotiations for the sale of the land at East Greenwich were stated by the Solicitor to be 'all progressing favourably but that the deposit had not yet been paid'.[101]

Future of the *Dreadnought* Hospital-ship

Thus, after approximately 13 years, the SHS removed from the last of the hospital-ships. Figure 13.14 shows the ship being towed away from her familiar moorings. It was decided in early 1871, i.e. after she had been vacated by the SHS for about a year (by the General Purposes Committee of the Metropolitan Asylums Board [MAB]), to fit out the ship as a 'Convalescent Small-pox Hospital' at the Admiralty's expense, as a small-pox epidemic was currently raging in London.

The ship, which was ready for occupation, in that capacity by 8 May 1871, was 'moored off, or a little below Woolwich on the north side of the river', a site which

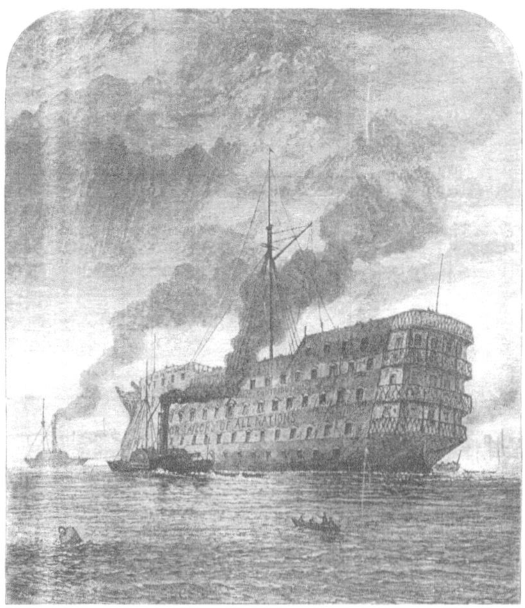

Figure 13.14: Engraving showing the last of the hospital-ships being towed from her moorings in Greenwich Reach having served for a short time as a smallpox hospital. [*Ill. London News* 1872; 30 November: 1].

did not meet with universal approval of the residents of Greenwich![102] Initially there were 200 inmates, but although the *Lancet* was unhappy about a further 50 being accommodated, the *British Medical Journal's* correspondent was far more enthusiastic: 'The arrangements under which the patients are sent from the small-pox hospitals at Stockwell, Homerton, and Hampstead, to the *Dreadnought* Hospital Ship off Deptford creek, continue to work well… The duration of their stay on board varies from nine to twenty days'.[103]

In September, the *Lancet* however carried the following notice: The 'Dreadnought' Committee of the [MAB] have arranged to close the vessel finally for the reception of small-pox convalescents on the 14th prox.' During the five month period, '1021 cases [had been] taken on board [and] three deaths only [had] occurred'. It is the … intention of the Board [the writer continued] to keep the *Dreadnought* for any epidemic emergency that may arise'. A later issue of the *Lancet* considered that an advertisement for the 'sale [by the Hackney Vestry] of the temporary hospital for small-pox was very ill-timed'; the writer had in mind the possibility of another cholera epidemic – for which isolation facilities would be urgently required. He was also conscious of difficulties involved in *disinfection* of the ship from small-pox.[104]

In 1872, the *Illustrated London News* recorded the removal of the *Dreadnought* from her moorings (see Figure 13.14) – where she and her predecessors, had 'occupied a position off Deptford, almost immediately opposite the Isle of Dogs, [for] more than half a century', to Chatham.[105]

The land-based *Dreadnought* (Seamen's) Hospital: internal problems

By mid-1872, the *new* Seamen's Hospital (situated by this time for over two years in the former *Infirmary* of Greenwich Hospital) had become well-established. However, not everyone was satisfied with its administration. For example, the *Lancet* remarked that '… while the great hospitals of the [RN] have for the last three years [i.e. since mid-1869, been run by a single] medical officer in place of [a] captain-superintendent, the [SHS was] making progress in exactly the opposite direction, a layman being appointed to supervise the medical men'. The anonymous writer remarked that 'when the old *Dreadnought* was in use the senior medical officer was the superintendent …' Now, he continued, 'the Secretary of the Society (Kemball Cook), who formerly resided in London had persuaded the old naval officers … to appoint him as house governor'. This arrangement certainly did *not* meet with the approval of the medical officers; indeed, one house-surgeon (Swan) had resigned in consequence; 'no professional man [the writer continued] will submit to such treatment from a lay committee'. In a subsequent issue, the *Lancet* writer recorded: 'We understand that the stipend of the house-governor exceeds that of the whole medical staff [which amounted to a salary] with residence of £600 a year'.[106]

A year later, the same journal again referred critically to this matter in an annotation: 'changes [the writer informed its readership had] taken place in the staff, not in the administration' – four medical officers had apparently been 'dismissed from duty' in the previous 18 months. The writer was also critical of the matron's role; an infected nurse had caused three cases (two of them fatal) of erysipelas. This event, upon which an opinion from the medical staff had *not* been sought, had apparently resulted in the resignation of a large number of nursing staff. The means by which finances were being conducted was yet another matter for comment.[107]

The fact that there were no *medical* members of the SHS Committee of Management was also the subject of an anonymous article in the *Lancet*; the views of a former house-surgeon had precipitated this report. At a quarterly Court of Governors in January 1874, Capt. the Hon. F Maude, RN (and others) 'strongly opposed' a suggestion (by Dr Carr, an Honorary life-governor) that the 'visiting physicians and the senior resident officer should have seats on the board'. Later that year the same journal was able to record: '[The SHS] have given the professional administration of their hospital into the hands of their chief professional officer, they have abolished the obnoxious title of house-governor, and have relegated the secretary (Kemball Cook) to his proper post – that of regulating and improving the financial aspects of this very admirable institution'.[108]

The 1875 Annual General Meeting found the Society 'in by no means a flourishing state as to funds'. Burdett had by this time been appointed Secretary, and the *Lancet* report appealed to the SHS Committee to 'make a special appeal to the *public* [my italics] without delay'. A subsequent article in the same journal emphasised that 'though housed in Admiralty buildings [the Society] receives no financial aid from the Government', a theme which was reiterated in subsequent Annual Reports. Later that year, *Land and Water* reiterated the *Lancet* writer's view, and gave its readership a further summary of the *history* of the SHS; it also referred to a fund-raising campaign launched in April of that year.[109]

Other problems following removal

The years 1876–80 saw the consolidation of the *new* venue with Burdett at the helm! That the SHS received no Government support was repeatedly re-emphasised by the *Lancet*'s anonymous reporter; in 1877, he suggested that the only means of major fund-raising was to set up a 'floating receiving house in the Thames'; this might 'not only prove a good advertisement, but would also be a great convenience to the [acutely] sick sailor'. The charity eventually attracted funding from the Hospital Sunday Fund (no doubt due to the influence of Burdett).

The 1880 report stressed how the patients (seamen) themselves had made a significant contribution (£1200, or approximately 1/10) to the running costs of this institution. '"Poor Jack" [the writer continued], in one way at least, sets a worthy example to the working classes on shore whose wages, as a rule, far exceed his'.[110] The *Lancet* for 1880 however, took a totally unsympathetic stance, and concentrated on the vast cost of maintaining an *inappropriately positioned land-based hospital*'. The writer criticised the site of the establishment (which was not well equipped as a *general* hospital) and was *not* in a good position for the sick sailor, who had to cross the river to get there! 'No wonder [he concluded that] increasing numbers of sailors seized with sudden and severe illness apply for admission at the hospitals on the side of the river on which the docks are situated'. 'It appears [he commented that] the [SHS] holds an invested capital of £112,000, besides the use of the hospital premises rent-free from the Government'. With this vast wealth and its failure to meet the needs of the sick sailor 'we do not [he claimed] think the Committee can make a very serious claim on private charity'.[111]

Contemporary *medical* reports compiled by Johnson Smith (see Chapters 12 and 15) also received detailed coverage in the *Lancet*. Overall, widespread interest in the charity – especially following removal to land – was documented; the most impressive advance was perhaps a sharp decline in sepsis due to '... antiseptic (Lister's) treatment adopted since 1874 ...'.[112]

References and Notes

1 Anonymous. Leading article. *Times, Lond* 1869; 14 August: 9; Anonymous. The Greenwich Hospital Acts. Vict. 1865; cap 88 89: 5 July and Vict. 1869: cap 44: 2 August; From the foundation of Greenwich Hospital (in 1696) until 1834, every Merchant Seaman was (by an Act of Parliament of 1695) compulsorily compelled to contribute sixpence each month to the Treasury – for which nothing in the case of the mercantile marine, was received in exchange; **Silas Kemball Cook** (1818–1874): *See* Chapter 12.

2 50th Annual Report. In: *An account of the origin and progress of the Seamen's Hospital Society for sick and diseased seamen of all nations, in the Port of London, Greenwich, S.E. (late Dreadnought.). Supported by voluntary contributions. Established 1821, Incorporated 1833.* London: E A Reeves. 1871: 15–19; Anonymous. Leading article. *Times, Lond* 1869; 2 October: 6; Council of Management Minutes: 9: 209.

3 *Op cit.* See note 2 above (Minutes) 8: 403.

4 **George Busk**, FRCS, FRS (1807–86): *see* Chapter 12.

5 **Henry Turner Lane Rooke**, MD (1824–70): *see* Chapter 12.

6 **Robert Barnes** FRCP (1817–1907): *see* Chapter 12.

7 **Stephen Henry Ward** FRCP (1819–80): *see* Chapter 12.

8 F Nightingale. *Notes on Hospitals: being two papers read before The National Association for the Promotion of Social Science, at Liverpool, in October, 1858 with evidence given to the Royal Commissioners on the state of the Army in 1857* London; J W Parker & Son 1859: 108.

9 *Op cit.* see note 2 above (Reports). 44: 17–22.

10 S K Cook (ed). Seamen's Hospital Society. *Copy of three letters received by the Committee.* Greenwich: Seamen's Hospital Society 1864: 10 [SHS Archive].

11 *An Act for incorporating the Members of a Society, commonly called the 'Seaman's (sic) Hospital Society' and their successors, as therein mentioned and provided; and for the better enabling them and empowering them to carry on the charitable and useful Designs of the same Society.* Guliemi IV. Regis 1833: 6 May; *Op cit.* see note 2 above (Minutes) 8: 416.

12 *Op cit.* see note 2 above (Minutes). 9; Anonymous. The Seamen's Hospital Society. 1865 *Lancet*; i: 245.

13 Conveyance of Hereditaments at Greenwich in the County of Kent. *The Commissioners of Greenwich Hospital to The Seaman's (sic) Hospital Society.* Draft. Young Maples Teesdale & Young, 6 Fredericks Place, Old Jewry. 1865; 11 May: 5 [SHS Archive].

14 J W Nickols to S K Cook. 1865: 12 January: 1; 19 January: 1; 26 January: 1; 2 February: 1 [Greenwich Hospital Archive, PRO Kew ADM/66/45].

15 Morden College, Blackheath, had been founded in 1695 by Sir John Morden (1623–1708) who was a member of the Boards of the Turkie and East India Companies – and a prosperous city of London merchant and philanthropist – to provide homes for 40 merchants who had 'demonstrated their ability in the business world but who had

failed through no fault of their own' or in the original words: for 'poor Merchants ... such as have lost their estates by accidents, dangers and Perills of the seas or by any other accidents, ways or means in their honest endeavours to get their living by Merchandizing'. The college building was designed by Sir Christopher Wren. Over the years, Morden College (which now houses 400 individuals) has become an important Charitable Foundation owning a great deal of land in Greenwich and its surroundings [*see also*: Joyce P. *Patronage and poverty in Merchant Society : The History of Morden College Blackheath 1695 to the present*. London: Gresham Books 1982: 106; Anonymous. *Morden College : a brief guide* 6th ed. London: Trustees of Morden College 1995: 36.]

16 *Op cit.* see note 2 above (Minutes). 9: 430, 447.

17 Morden College. Minutes 5 (1851–1870) 1865; 12 July: 473.

18 *Ibid*. 1866; 7 March: 490.

19 Conveyance of Houses and Land at Greenwich in the County of Kent. *The Trustees of Morden College to the Seaman's (sic) Hospital Society* Draft. Young Maples Teesdale & Nelson. 1866; 31 December: 12 [SHS Archive].

20 W Bowles to the Right Honourable the Lords of Her Majesty's Treasury 1865; 6 March: 1 [SHS Archive]; see also *Op cit.* see note 2 above. 1865; 83 March: 432–434; S K Cook to F Peel. 1865; 2 June; S K Cook to HM Treasury. 1865; 1 July: 2 [SHS Archive]. [*See also:* A Lambert. Bowles, Sir William (1780-1869) In: H C G Matthew, B Harrison (eds). *Oxford Dictionary of National Biography*. Oxford: Oxford University Press 2004; 6: 967–9].

21 See note 2 above (Reports). 45; 17–21.

22 *Op cit.* see note 2 above (Minutes). 9: 495.

23 Anonymous. Leading article. *Times, Lond* 1865; 31 May: 11; Anonymous. Leading article. *Shipping and Mercantile Gazette* 1867; 10 June: 5; Anonymous. Leading article. *Times, Lond* 1868; 15 April: 9; Anonymous. Leading article. *Times, Lond* 1868; 20 July; 8–9; Newell P. *Greenwich Hospital : a Royal Foundation 1692–1983*. London: Greenwich Hospital 1984: 278; G C Cook. Changing rôle(s) for the Royal Hospital, Greenwich. *Historia Hospitalium* 2000; 22: 35–46.

24 W Carr, H C G Matthew. Childers, Hugh Culling Eardley (1827–1896) In: H C G Matthew, B Harrison (eds). *Oxford Dictionary of National Biography*. Oxford: Oxford University Press 2004; 11: 443–6. Anonymous. Greenwich Hospital. *Times, Lond* 1865: 21 March: 8; Anonymous. Parliamentary Intelligence: Greenwich Hospital. *Times, Lond* 1865; 26 April: 6; *Op cit.* See also note 23 above.

25 *Op cit.* see note 23 above. Anonymous. Leading article. *Shipping and Mercantile Gazette* 1865; 31 May: 5.

26 Anonymous. Parliamentary Intelligence: House of Commons. The Greenwich Hospital Bill. *Lancet* 1865; i: 608; Anonymous. Greenwich Hospital. *BMJ* 1865; i: 576.

27 [Surgeon, RN]. Greenwich Hospital Pensions. *Lancet* 1865; i: 639. P Chilcott. Pakington [*formerly* Russell], John Somerset, first Baron Hampton (1799–1880) In: H C G Matthew, B Harrison (eds). *Oxford Dictionary of National Biography*. Oxford: Oxford University Press 2004; 42: 434–7.

28 *Op cit.* See note 21 above.

29 *Op cit.* See note 2 above (Minutes) 8. 1865; 26 April 6: Anonymous. The mercantile marine and Greenwich Hospital. *Lancet* 1865; i: 576; [Justitia] The Merchant Seamen and Greenwich Hospital. *Times, Lond.* 1865; 8 May: 6; 1865; 22 May: 9. 'Justitia' was the pseudonym of John Arthur Roebuck (1801–79), a prominent barrister and politician of the time.

30 Anonymous. Leading article. *Times, Lond* 1865; 8 May: 10; F Lean. The merchant seamen and Greenwich Hospital. *Times, Lond* 1865; 16 May: 6.

31 [Vigil]. Greenwich Hospital. *Times, Lond* 1865; 8 June: 11; Anonymous. Greenwich Hospital Fund. *BMJ* 1865; i: 629; Anonymous. Greenwich Hospital Bill. *Times, Lond* 1865;

9 June: 7; 14 June: 8; 20 June: 9–10; 28 June: 8; J Parry. Graham, Sir James Robert George, second baronet (1792–1861) In: H C G Matthew, B Harrison (eds). *Oxford Dictionary of National Biography.* Oxford: Oxford University Press 2004: 23: 204–10; A Lambert. Milne, Sir Alexander, first baronet (1806-1896). *Ibid*; 38: 285–8; G C Boase, H C G Matthew. Cave, Sir Stephen (1820–1880) *Ibid*; 10: 602.

32 Anonymous. Parliamentary Intelligence. *Times, Lond* 1865; 30 June: 6; Anonymous. Leading article. *Times, Lond* 1865; 28 September: 8; Greenwich Hospital Act. 1865 28° and 29° Vict c 88, 89. 1865; 5 July: 417–425.

33 Anonymous. The Greenwich Pensioners. *Times, Lond* 1865; 27 September: 10; C Dickens. Greenwich Pensioners. *Times, Lond* 1865; 20 June: 6; Anonymous. Greenwich Hospital. *BMJ* 1865; ii: 596.

34 *Op cit.* see note 32 above; *Op cit.* see note 2 above (Minutes). 1865; 21 July: 458; 28 July: 459; Anonymous. Greenwich Hospital. *Times, Lond* 1865: 25 October: 10.

35 *Op cit.* See note 2 above (Minutes). 9: 477; *Op cit.* see note 28 above; Anonymous. The uses and abuses of Greenwich Hospital. *BMJ* 1866; ii: 655.

36 See note 2 above (Reports). 46: 16–20; *Op cit.* See note 20 above.

37 Anonymous. What should be done with Greenwich Hospital? *Lancet* 1866: i: 128–9; Anonymous. Leading article. *Shipping and Mercantile Gazette* 1866; 6 Feb: 5.

38 S K Cook to the Lords Commissioners of the Admiralty: The memorial of the committee of the Seamen's Hospital Society. 1866; 5 March: 1 [SHS Archive]; *Op cit.* See note 2 above (Minutes). 9: 490–94.

39 *Op cit.* See note 2 above (Minutes). 9: 496; Anonymous. Leading article. *Shipping and Mercantile Gazette* 1866; 15 March: 5.

40 Anonymous. The eventualities of Greenwich Hospital. *Lancet* 1866; ii: 585–86; *Op cit.* see note 35 above; Anonymous. The Greenwich Estimates. *Lancet* 1867; i: 238.

41 **Edward George Geoffrey Smith Stanley**. Fourteenth Earl of Derby (1799–1869) served as Prime Minister in 1852, 1858–9 and 1866–8. He came from a Lancashire family of Whig magnates, and was a keen race-goer. He had inherited the Earldom in 1851. [*See also*: G M Thomas, *The Prime Ministers from Robert Walpole to Margaret Thatcher* London: Secker & Warburg. 1980: 124–7; A Hawkins. Stanley, Edward George Geoffrey Smith, fourteenth earl of Derby (1799–1869) In: H C G Matthew, B Harrison (eds). *Oxford Dictionary of National Biography.* Oxford: Oxford University Press 2004; 52: 178–87].

42 *Op cit.* See note 2 above (Minutes). 9: 557–8; Anonymous. The use of Greenwich Hospital. *Times, Lond* 1867; 5 March: 12; Anonymous. Leading article. *Shipping and Mercantile Gazette* 1867; 5 March: 5. [*See also*: W D Rubinstein. Northcote, Stafford Henry, first earl of Iddesleigh (1818–1887) In: H C G Matthew, B Harrison (eds). *Oxford Dictionary of National Biography.* Oxford: Oxford University Press 2004; 41: 141–50].

43 [Beta]. The Dreadnought and Greenwich Hospital. *Times, Lond* 1867; 22 January: 7; Anonymous. Leading article. *Times, Lond* 1867; 22 January: 9; Anonymous. Leading article. *Shipping and Mercantile Gazette* 1867; 23 January: 5; Anonymous. The abuses of Greenwich Hospital. *Lancet* 1867; i: 86.

44 Anonymous. *Lancet* 1867; i: 217.

45 [Beta]. The Seamen's Hospital Society. *Times, Lond* 1867; 5 March: 12.

46 *Ibid.* 1867; 6 March; 5; Anonymous. Greenwich Hospital. *Lancet.* 1867; i: 309.

47 Anonymous. Greenwich Hospital. *Lancet.* 1867; i: 861; Anonymous. Greenwich Hospital. *Times, Lond* 1867; 5 April: 9.

48 Anonymous. The future of Greenwich Hospital. *Lancet* 1867; i: 368; Anonymous. Greenwich Hospital. *Times, Lond* 1867: 15 March: 4; Anonymous. Greenwich Hospital. *Lancet* 1867; i: 378–9.

49 *Op cit.* see note 2 above (Minutes). 1867; 9: 22 March: 2; 1867; 5 April: 5–6. [*See also*: E J Feuchtwanger. Corry, Henry Thomas Lowry (1803–1873) In: H C G Matthew, B Harrison (eds). *Oxford Dictionary of National Biography.* Oxford: Oxford University Press 2004; 13: 506–7].

50 *Ibid.* 10: 7.

51 **John Syer Bristowe** FRCP FRS (1827–95) was a physician at St Thomas's Hospital, London. He was born in Camberwell, and educated at Enfleld, King's College School, and St Thomas's Hospital – where he spent most of his career, serving as Full Physician from 1860 until 1892. His main interests were in neurology and public health. At the RCP, he served as Senior Censor and gave the Croonian and Lumleian lectures. [T H Pennington. Bristow, John Syer (1827–1895) In: H C G Matthew, B Harrison (eds). *Oxford Dictionary of National Biography.* Oxford: Oxford University Press 2004: 7: 687–8]. **Timothy Holmes** FRCS (1825–1907) was educated at Merchant Taylors' School, Pembroke College, Cambridge and St George's Hospital. He subsequently held many positions at the Royal College of Surgeons and the Royal Medical Chirurgical Society [Anonymous. *Plarr's Lives* 1930; I 554–5; D'A Power, C Kerslake. Holmes, Timothy (1825–1907) In: H C G Matthew, B Harrison (eds). *Oxford Dictionary of National Biography.* Oxford: Oxford University Press 2004; 27: 805–6].

Bristowe and Holmes travelled widely in the UK inspecting hospitals; they had written various reports on public health matters for the Privy Council – especially on the construction and sanitary conditions of hospitals throughout the country. Bristowe & Holmes also wrote a joint report '*On the Hospitals of the United Kingdom and their administration*'.

52 *Op cit.* See note 2 above (Minutes). 10: 8, 9–10: 10–11.

53 *Op cit.* See note 2 above (Minutes). 10: 15; Anonymous. The *Dreadnought* and Greenwich Hospital. *Lancet* 1867 i: 579–580.

54 [Beta]. The Admiralty and Greenwich Hospital. *Times, Lond* 1867; 11 April: 10; Anonymous. Parliamentary Intelligence: Greenwich Hospital. *Times, Lond* 1867; 13 April: 5; Anonymous. Leading article. *Shipping and Mercantile Gazette* 1867: 15 April: 5.

55 Anonymous. Greenwich Hospital. *Lancet* 1867; i: 465–6; Anonymous. The Dreadnought and Greenwich Hospital. *Times, Lond* 1867; 15 April: 5.

56 **(Sir) John Simon** KCB FRS (1816–1904) was one of the great sanitary reformers of the nineteenth century. Educated at St Thomas' Hospital, London, he later became medical officer of the General Board of Health (1855–8), and of the Privy Council under the Public Health Act (1858–71). He later became Chief Medical Officer of the Local Government Board (1871–6). [See also: R Lambert. *Sir John Simon 1816—1904 and English social administration.* London: Macgibbon & Kee 1963: 669; C Hamlin. Simon, Sir John (1816–1904). In: H C G Matthew, B Harrison (eds). *Oxford Dictionary of National Biography.* Oxford: Oxford University Press 2004; 50: 660–3].

57 [Beta]. The Admiralty and Greenwich Hospital. *Times, Lond* 1867; 16 April: 7; Anonymous. Greenwich Hospital and the 'Dreadnought'. *Lancet* 1867; i: 457–8; Anonymous. The rights and wrongs of the Greenwich Hospital question. *Medical Times and Gazette* 1867; i: 414; H T L Rooke. The Greenwich Hospital question. *Medical Times and Gazette* 1867; i: 453; Anonymous. Greenwich Hospital and the 'Dreadnought'. *Lancet* 1867; i: 524.

58 Anonymous. Scandal about Queen Anne. *BMJ* 1867; i: 513.

59 Anonymous. The *Dreadnought* and Greenwich Hospital. *Lancet* 1867; i: 579–580; *Op cit.* see note 2 above (Minutes) 1867: 24 May: 13; Anonymous. The *Dreadnought* and Greenwich Hospital. *BMJ* 1867; i: 616.

60 [Beta]. The Dreadnought and Greenwich Hospital. *Times, Lond* 1867; 11 June: 9; Bristowe JS. The Dreadnought and Greenwich Hospital. *Times, Lond* 1867; 13 June: 6.

61 S K Cook to the Secretary, the Admiralty. 1867; 12 October: 2 [SHS Archive]; Anonymous. The 'Dreadnought' and Greenwich Hospital. *Lancet* 1867: ii: 526. [*See also*: Anonymous. Tatum, Thomas (1802–1879) *Plarr's Lives* 1930; ii 383].

62 **Harry Leach** MRCP (1836–79) *see* Chapter 12. [See also: G C Cook. Leach, Henry (1836–1879) In: H C G Matthew, B Harrison (eds). *Oxford Dictionary of National Biography.* Oxford: Oxford University Press 2004; 32: 950–1; G C Cook. Harry Leach MRCP (1836–1879); control of scurvy in the British Mercantile Marine, and first Port Medical Officer for the City of London. *J Med Biog* 2000; 8: 133–139].

63 H Leach. The Dreadnought Hospital. *Times, Lond* 1867; 8 July: 10.

64 Anonymous. Leading article. *Shipping and Mercantile Gazette* 1867; 25 October: 5; *Op cit.* see note 2 above (Minutes). 1867; 24 May: 13–14; Anonymous. Greenwich Hospital. *Times, Lond* 1867; 17 August: 7; Anonymous. Medico-parliamentary: Greenwich Hospital. *BMJ* 1867; ii: 167. [*See also*: F M L Thompson. Lord Henry Charles George Gordon-Lennox (1821–1886) In: H C G Matthew, B Harrison (eds). *Oxford Dictionary of National Biography.* Oxford: Oxford University Press 2004; 33: 368; G C Boase, D Washbrook. Trevelyan, Sir Charles Edward, first baronet (1807–1886) In: H C G Matthew, B Harrison (eds). *Oxford Dictionary of National Biography.* Oxford: Oxford University Press 2004; 55: 323–4].

65 *Op cit.* See note 2 above (Minutes). 10: 27, 28.

66 *Ibid.* 10: 30, 32, 33, 47.

67 Anonymous. The future of Greenwich Hospital. *Lancet* 1867; ii: 163; Anonymous. Greenwich Hospital. *Times, Lond* 1867; 6 August: 6 & 7; Anonymous Greenwich Hospital. *Times, Lond* 1867; 15 August: 9.

68 **Henry Currey** (1820–1900) had prepared plans for the new St. Thomas' Hospital by 13 June 1865 on similar lines to those of the French hospital Lariboisiére. This hospital was planned to take 588 beds, and the foundation stone was laid by Queen Victoria on 13 May 1868. The fact that this was also a difficult site for which to plan, might have been the Society's reason for inviting his advice and expertise. [*See also:* E M McInnes *St Thomas' Hospital* London: Cerge Allen & Unwin 1963: 230; G C Cook. Henry Currey FRIBA (1820–1900): leading Victorian hospital architect, and early exponent of the 'pavilion principle'. *Postgrad Med J* 2002; 78: 352–9]

69 *Op cit.* see note 2 above (Minutes). 10: 43, 44, 49.

70 Anonymous. The future of the Royal Hospital and the 'Dreadnought', Greenwich. *Lancet* 1867; ii: 202; Anonymous. The solution of the Greenwich Hospital question. *BMJ* 1867; ii: 129; Anonymous. The 'Dreadnought' and the Greenwich Hospital. *Lancet*; ii: 526; *Report of the Committee appointed to inquire into the present system of management of Greenwich Hospital and Schools, with minutes of evidence and appendix. Presented to the House of Commons by Command of Her Majesty.* London: Her Majesty's Stationery Office 1868.

71 J S Bristowe, T Holmes. Report on the Infirmary of Greenwich Hospital. *In : Report of the Committee appointed to inquire into the present system of management of Greenwich Hospital and schools, with minutes of evidence and appendix.* London: Her Majesty's Stationery Office 1868: 102–103. [*See also: Op cit.* See note 51 above.]

72 Anonymous. The future of Greenwich Hospital. *Lancet* 1867; ii: 711. [*See also:* W F Rae, H C G Matthew. St Maur (*formerly* Seymour), Edward Adolphus, twelfth duke of Somerset (1804–1885) In: H C G Matthew, B Harrison (eds). *Oxford Dictionary of National Biography.* Oxford: Oxford University Press 2004; 48: 665–6].

73 *Op cit.* See note 2 above (Reports). 47 16–20; note 2 above (Minutes) 10: 54.

74 Anonymous. Greenwich Hospital. *Lancet* 1868; i: 328; Anonymous. Greenwich Hospital. *Times, Lond* 1868; 19 March: 9; Anonymous. Greenwich Hospital. *Lancet* 1868; i: 447.

75 Anonymous. The official report on Greenwich Hospital. *BMJ* 1868; i: 332; Anonymous. *Times, Lond* 1868; 15 April: 9; Anonymous. *Lancet* 1868; i: 475; Anonymous. Greenwich

Hospital. *Lancet* 1868; i:631; Anonymous. The Medical Reports of Greenwich Hospital. *BMJ* 1868; i: 404; Anonymous. Greenwich Hospital. *BMJ* 1868; i: 509.

76 Anonymous. *Times, Lond* 1868; 20 July: 8–9; Anonymous. *Lancet* 1868; ii: 119.

77 *Op cit.* See note 2 above (Minutes) 10: 100.

78 Anonymous. Seamen's Hospital Society. *Times, Lond* 1868; 20 August: 9; Anonymous. Seamen's Hospital Society. *Lancet* 1868; ii: 266.

79 *Op cit.* See note 2 above (Minutes) 10: 106–107, 114.

80 Anonymous. The Admiralty, Greenwich Hospital, and the 'Dreadnought'. *Lancet* 1868; ii: 836.

81 *Op cit.* See note 2 above (Reports). 48: 15–19.

82 Anonymous. *Times, Lond* 1869; 21 January: 9; Anonymous. Greenwich Hospital. *Lancet* 1869; i: 140; Anonymous. Greenwich Hospital. *BMJ* 1869; ii: 78. [*See also*: P. Jackson. Trevelyan, Sir George Otto, second baronet (1838–1928) In: H C G Matthew, B Harrison (eds). *Oxford Dictionary of National Biography*. Oxford: Oxford University Press 2004; 55: 333–7].

83 Anonymous. Greenwich Hospital. *Times, Lond* 1868; 6 March: 6; Anonymous. Greenwich Hospital. *Times, Lond* 1868; 28 April: 6; Anonymous. *Shipping and Mercantile Gazette* 1868; 28 April: 5; Anonymous. *Lancet* 1868; i: 610–611.

84 **Francis Sibson** (1814–76), FRCP FRS initially came from Edinburgh, treated cholera patients in the 1831–2 epidemic and after this resumed his medical training at Guy's and St Thomas' Hospitals, London. He subsequently became a consultant physician at St Mary's Hospital. Sibson also served on the senate of the University of London and held office in the British Medical Association. [*See also* K Brown. Sibson, Francis (1814–1876). In: H C G Matthew, B Harrison (eds). *Oxford Dictionary of National Biography*. Oxford: Oxford University Press 2004; 50: 493–4].

85 *Op cit.* See note 2 above (Minutes). 10: 139–140; Anonymous. Greenwich Hospital. *Lancet* 1869; i: 694–659; Anonymous. Greenwich Hospital. *Lancet* 1869; i: 723.

86 Anonymous. Greenwich Hospital. *Times, Lond* 1869; 18 May: 9, and 19 May: 9; Anonymous. *Lancet* 1869: ii: 16. [*See also*: S Lee, H C G Matthew. Adam, William Patrick (1823–1881). In: H C G Matthew, B Harrison (eds). *Oxford Dictionary of National Biography*. Oxford: Oxford University Press 2004; 1: 218–9].

87 Anonymous. Greenwich Hospital Bill. *Times, Lond* 1869; 25 June: 7–8, 30 June: 8, and 17 July: 5; The Greenwich Hospital Act 1869. An Act to make better provision respecting Greenwich Hospital, and the application of the revenues thereof. 1869: 2 August: Chap 44 & 45, 32 & 33 Vict: 265–268; Anonymous. Greenwich Hospital. *Times, Lond* 1869; 11 August: 4; *Op cit.* see note 2 above (*Times*).

88 Anonymous. Naval and military intelligence. *Times, Lond* 1869; 10 September: 7; Anonymous. Greenwich Hospital. *Times, Lond* 1868; 16 September: 4; Anonymous. *Lancet* 1869: ii: 419.

89 Anonymous. Greenwich Hospital. *Times, Lond* 1869; 21 September: 4.

90 *Op cit.* see note 2 above (Reports). Anonymous. Greenwich Hospital. *Lancet* 1869; ii: 486 and 519.

91 F Summerly. The use of Greenwich Hospital. *Times, Lond* 1868;4 October: 8; G H P White. Greenwich Hospital. *Times, Lond* 1869; 22 October: 10; E Field. The naval university. *Times, Lond* 1871; 6 October: 6; [An old student of the RN College]. Greenwich or Portsmouth? *Times, Lond* 1871; 18 October: 3.

92 Anonymous. The utilization of Greenwich Hospital. *Times, Lond* 1871; 28 July: 5; Anonymous. The utilization of Greenwich Hospital. *Times, Lond* 1871; 11 August: 12; Anonymous. Greenwich Hospital. *Times, Lond* 1871: 19 August: 5.

93 *Op cit.* See note 2 above (Minutes). 10: 172, 185.

94 **William Ewart Gladstone** (1809–94) served as British Prime Minister from 1868–74, 1880–85, 1886, and 1892–94. His father had been a Liverpool merchant who made a great deal of money from the slave trade. Educated at Eton and Christchurch, Oxford, he became a noted Greek Scholar; he also devoted a great deal of energy to 'reforming' young London prostitutes; *Op cit.* See note 41 above (Thomas): 147–153. [*See also*: *Gladstone.* London: The Hambleton Press. 1998: 302; H C G Matthew. Gladstone, William Ewart (1809–1898). In: H C G Matthew, B Harrison (eds). *Oxford Dictionary of National Biography.* Oxford: Oxford University Press 2004; 22: 383–409.]

95 See note 2 above (Reports). 49: 15–19.

96 Anonymous. Greenwich Hospital and the Dreadnought. *Times, Lond* 1870; 4 February: 4; Anonymous. *Times, Lond* 1870; 7 February: 9; Anonymous. Leading article. *Shipping and Mercantile Gazette* 1870; 4 February: 5; Anonymous. The 'Dreadnought' Seamen's Hospital. *London Mirror* 1870; 12 February: 156.

97 *Lease of The Infirmary and Somerset Ward of The Royal Hospital at Greenwich in the County of Kent.* The Lords Commiss^{s} of the Admiralty to the Seamen's Hospital Society. Dated 1 June 1870: 4 [SHS Archive]; *Op cit.* see note 2 above (Minutes) 1870; 9: 11 March: 193; 8 April: 206; Anonymous. Seamen's Hospital Society. *Lancet* 1870; i: 560–561; *Op cit.* see note 62 above.

98 *Op cit.* see note 2 above; *Op cit.* see note 97 above (*Lancet*); Anonymous. The 'Dreadnought' on land. *BMJ* 1870; i 415; Anonymous. Our sick sailors. *Times, Lond* 1870; 22 April: 4; Anonymous. The Seamen's Hospital. *Times, Lond* 1870; 22 November: 8; Anonymous. Seamen's Hospital Society. *Lancet* 1871: i: 205.

99 Anonymous. The Seamen's Hospital. *Times, Lond* 1871; 18 December: 5; *Op cit.* see note 2 above (Reports): 51 1872: 18–21.

100 Draft – *Conditions of Sale of Freehold Land Messuages and Premises at Greenwich in the County of Kent.* Young Maples Teesdale Nelson & Co. 6 Fredericks Place, Old Jewry 1870: 10 [SHS Archive]; Shalless & Coppinger (Auctioneers, Valuers and Estate Agents) to The Seamen's Hospital Society. 1870; 13 July: 2; Cook SK to Nelson RR 1870; 23 July 2; Hardwick PC to Young Maples 1870; 25 July: 2; Hardwick PC to Young Maples, Teesdale 1870; 29 July: 3; Shalless & Coppinger to The Seamen's Hospital Society 1870; 6 August: 2; Shalless & Coppinger to the Seamen's Hospital Society 1870; 11 August: 2; Shalless & Coppinger to The Seamen's Hospital Society 1870; 16 August: 2, SK Cook to Messrs Young, Maples & Co 1870: 17 August: 1; *Op cit.* see note 2 above (Minutes) 1874: 9: 26 June: 407–8.

101 *Op cit.* See note 2 above (Minutes) 10, 11: 225–227, 231.

102 Anonymous. The 'Dreadnought' small-pox hospital. *Lancet* 1871: i: 545; Anonymous. The 'Dreadnought' convalescent hospital. *Lancet* 1871: i: 623; Anonymous. Greenwich Hospital. *Lancet* : i: 624.

103 Anonymous. The 'Dreadnought' small-pox hospital. *Lancet* 1871; i: 725; Anonymous. The Dreadnought convalescent hospital. *BMJ* 1871; i: 564.

104 Anonymous. The 'Dreadnought' small-pox convalescent hospital. *Lancet* 1871; ii: 408; Anonymous. Disused small-pox hospitals. *Lancet* 1871; ii: 588.

105 Anonymous. The Dreadnought Hospital-ship. *Illustrated London News* 1872; 61: 510.

106 Anonymous. The Seamen's Hospital, Greenwich. *Lancet* 1872; ii: 56; Anonymous. The Seamen's Hospital. *Lancet* 1872; ii: 235.

107 Anonymous. Annotation. *Lancet* 1873; ii: 459–460.

108 Anonymous. Seamen's Hospital Society. *Lancet* 1874; i: 100; Anonymous. The Seamen's Hospital. *Lancet* 1874: ii: 639.

109 Anonymous. The Seamen's Hospital Society. *Lancet* 1875; i: 249; Anonymous. The Seamen's Hospital. *Lancet* 1875; i: 555; Anonymous. Seamen's Hospital, Greenwich. *Lancet* 1877; i: 289; Anonymous. The Seamen's Hospital. *Lancet* 1878; i: 248; Anonymous.

The Seamen's Hospital Society. *Lancet* 1879; ii: 824–5; Anonymous. The Seamen's Hospital, Greenwich. *Land and Water* 1875; 25 December: 499–500.

110 *Op cit.* see note 109 above; Anonymous. 'Time nihil'. *Lancet* 1879; i: 205–6; Anonymous. The Seamen's Hospital. *Lancet* 1880; i: 813–4; *Op cit.* See note 2 above (Reports) 59: 9–16.

111 Anonymous. Annotation. The Seamen's Hospital Society. *Lancet* 1880; ii: 705.

112 Anonymous. The Seamen's Hospital. *Lancet* 1877; I: 921; Anonymous. The Seamen's Hospital. *Lancet* 1878; i: 164; *Op cit.* see note 109 above.

Chapter 14

Expansion of facilities – at the *Dreadnought* and further afield

During the half-century 1870–1920, the 'Merchant Navy of the world' expanded significantly: for example, 'In 1860 the Mercantile Marine of the principal European maritime countries, and of the [USA, comprised] 10,806,642 tons'; around 1880, 'it consisted of 14,490,038 tons'. Obviously, coupled with this massive expansion, there was a sharp increase in the number of sailors requiring medical attention. There was a timely reminder of the overall importance of the Mercantile Marine in the 80th Annual Report (1900) published the following year:

> … since the abolition of the transports maintained by the Admiralty, the carrying of troops between England and His Majesty [Edward VII]'s possessions abroad has entirely been effected in British Merchant ships … during the present War in South Africa, … the Commander-in-Chief himself and his Army of upwards of a quarter of a million men, together with their impedimenta of horses, ordnance, ammunition, and stores, engineering plant and appliances, have been carried by sea a distance of 7,000 miles.[1]

Towards the end of the period under review in this chapter (1870–1914), the 94th Report likened 'This new and greater struggle [The Great War 1914–18]' to that at the time of the foundation of the [SHS] – which had taken place in the wake of another 'great European war (the Napoleonic War[s])'.

> The line of demarkation between the RN and the Merchant Service [was however] more strongly marked than a hundred years ago, but the men who man our transports and carry on our commerce have fully borne their share of danger alike with those wounded in battle with the Empire's enemies. In this time of war stress the voluntary Hospitals of England have proved more than ever their efficiency and their value; among them the Dreadnought stands high.

This report also drew attention to the crucial part which the SHS had played during the first year of the war:

> The Admiralty immediately accepted two hundred and twenty-five beds in the Hospitals of the Society, and over one hundred wounded

> men have been received besides those who have fallen victim of disease largely consequent upon exposure and hardship.

The 1909 Report stressed that the Society (which '[received] no State aid beyond the use of The Dreadnought Hospital ...') was 'not only the oldest but the largest Corporation for giving to our Seamen what is essential to their hard calling – skilled treatment when they are stricken down by accident or disease, and a haven of rest until they are fit to return to duty'. Finance was, as formerly, to the fore (although during the latter part of this period, the Kings' Fund – founded by Sir Henry Burdett – frequently came to the Society's assistance); it was decided in late 1892 to compare the cost per patient treated at the *Dreadnought* hospital with the major London Hospitals. This was favourable, the cost per occupied bed being £65=4=4 compared with >£100 at most of the London hospitals.[2]

Incidentally, the death of one of the greatest social reformers of the nineteenth century the Rt Hon the 7th Earl of Shaftesbury KG (1801–85), a Vice-President of the Society, is recorded in the Committee of Management minutes; this was followed by a notice of a National Memorial.[3]

Administrative office

When the Society became land-based in 1870 – *see* Chapter 13 – the SHS (temporarily) abandoned its central London office (*see* Chapter 12), and administration was relocated to the *Dreadnought* Hospital itself. However, in 1890 a new office was opened in the *city*, at 24 Budge Row (off Cannon Street). This was used as the Boardroom from 1890 until 1897; meetings alternated with Greenwich; following this, the venue seems to have been let by the Society, although suitable tenants proved difficult to find. Probably on account of cost, the building was later abandoned.

Beginning in 1898, meetings alternated between Greenwich and the Institute of Chartered Accountants, Moorgate Place, Moorgate Street, EC. At a meeting on 11 November 1904 reference to 'negotiations ... in regard to the first floor at 13a Cockspur Street [off Trafalgar Square]' was made. It was resolved that these offices 'be taken on lease ... at a rental of £375 per annum ...'; the furniture was subsequently bought by the Society for £110. The first meeting of the Committee in these new premises was convened on 24 March 1905. On 12 May 1905 the 'back office' was offered for letting to the Royal Waterloo Hospital for Children and Women at £100 annually, and a further £20 for use of the boardroom. On 24 May the following year, a further minute records that these offices be 'let to the Atlantic Union at £150 per annum for three years'. The Cockspur Street offices do *not* therefore seem to have been a great success, and the last occasion on which the Management Committee met there was on 9 May 1907. They were subsequently let to Mr Philip Yorke for £100 per annum (in November 1908).

The Board Room of the Marine Society was at that time investigated, while negotiations for another room at the Institute of Chartered Accountants were made later that year. It is clear that by March 1909 the Society was anxious to be 'relieved' of the lease of the Cockspur Street building; this was accomplished in May, although legal proceedings were not completed until April 1910.[4]

The *Dreadnought* Hospital

Figure 14.1 shows a plan of the ground-floor of the *Dreadnought* Hospital in 1892. As already indicated in Chapter 13, this building had been established in 1763–8 as the Infirmary of the Royal Hospital, with accommodation for up to 256 patients. In 1760, James ('Athenian') Stuart (the architect) had been appointed Surveyor, and the major catalyst to the erection of this long desired infirmary was the sudden availability of funds at the conclusion of the Seven Years War. The Somerset Ward (which included the Chapel – John Yenn was at that time the surveyor) to the west, had been added in 1808 and the West Wing, destroyed by

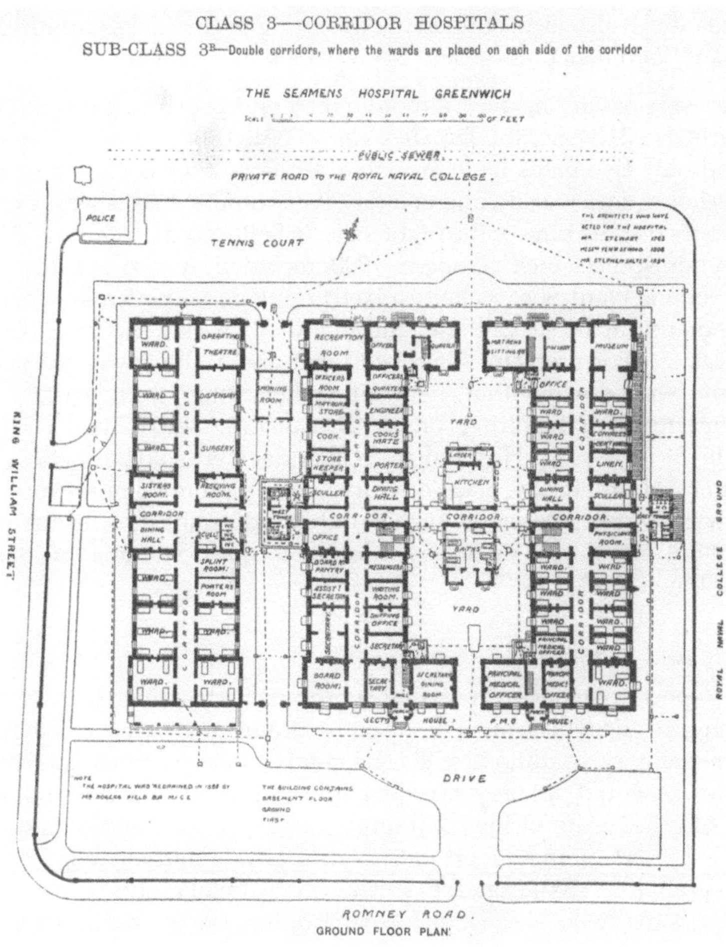

Figure 14.1: The ground-floor of the *Dreadnought* Hospital in 1892 [H C Burdett. *Hospitals and Asylums of the World : Their Origin, History, Construction, Administration, Management and Legislation; With plans of the Chief Medical Institutions Accurately Drawn to a Uniform Scale in Addition to Those of All the Hospitals of London in the Jubilee Year of Queen Victoria's Reign*. London: J & A Churchill 1891, 1893; 1–4: 701, 348, 944, 463].

fire on 1 October 1811, was soon rebuilt. The West Wing (surgical) housed the Northumberland Ward on the first floor, and the Ranlett Ward (Chapters 15 and 21) on the second. In the East Wing (medical), the first floor housed Middle-East ward, and the second the nurses' quarters.

A former probationer nurse has recorded her recollections of the *Dreadnought* in 1902:

> There were still a few old naval pensioners in the wards, as well as a patient who had actually worked on the last of the hospital-ships. A few beds, consisting of 'low iron frames with canvas lashed on to them' from the last of the ships remained on Somerset Ward. The out-patient department consisted of two rooms near the main entrance to Somerset Ward, which also incorporated the operating theatre at its entrance. The Ranlett Ward [Chapters 15 and 21] was then in 'full swing'.

The nurses were of varying ages; although the London teaching hospitals declined to take girls of <24 years, the *Dreadnought* accepted 21 year olds. Nurses shared rooms, and only two baths were available. Off-duty time consisted of two-hours daily, four-hours once weekly, and one-day every month. Lights were extinguished at 22-00 hours (i.e. the time of the night-sister's first round).[5]

Other reminiscences include one of 1900, recorded by a former night-sister on Northumberland Ward. She recalled a mixed population of patients – Scandinavians, Greeks, Indians, Japanese, Chinese, and many others. Enteric fever (Chapters 11 and 16) was a major problem; she related that one of the house-physicians died, and that she 'went down with it', being nursed by Sister Middle-east.[6]

Many, but not all of the fittings on the '*Dreadnought*'-ship (Chapter 13) had been removed to the land-based Hospital; the remainder were sold by auction.[7] An initial problem to face Burdett – the SHS Secretary (always a shrewd purveyor of financial matters) was the rateable value of the land-based establishment; the position is clearly set out in a letter (signed by Burdett) to the Committee of Management – dated 20 June 1876.

The fabric and other facilities

The 63rd Report (together with several subsequent ones) referred to a very costly undertaking, i.e. the replacement of the entire drainage system – which had undermined the 'sanitary condition' of the hospital, which 'with cholera threatening these shores ... would not only have jeopardised the patients' lives but have been dangerous to the health of the community at large'. The Landlords of the property, i.e. the Lords Commissioners of the Admiralty, undertook to meet the cost by making 'a grant [of £1500] from the Greenwich Hospital funds'.[8]

The Report for 1899 referred to further trouble, i.e. the decadent state of the *Dreadnought* building itself; this was an *old* structure and amongst urgent problems the following were listed:

i) New floors were required throughout the building;
ii) Certain partition walls should be removed: (this was rendered possible by generous contributions from the King's Fund – see below);

iii) The hot-water system required remodelling;
iv) The roof needed extensive repairs;
v) The nurses' quarters needed remodelling; and
vi) Hydraulic lifts were necessary.

These repairs and alterations were estimated to cost between £15,000 and £20,000, for which the Lords Commissioners of the Admiralty were again successfully approached for a contribution. The east wing required a good deal of structural attention in the first decade of the twentieth century; the King's Fund as usual helped out.[9]

A further item of expenditure was the 'introduction of Electric Light to the … Hospital …'. Electricity was obviously required for the 'Rõntgen Ray apparatus', and the Medical Staff had 'pointed out the great advantage from a health point of view, of Electric Light over Gas'.[10]

These 'improvements' and structural changes (including alterations to the 'Out-Patient Department and … the Mortuary' as well as introduction of isolation facilities) at the *Dreadnought* were of course necessary, and came at a propitious time for 'the establishment of the London School of Clinical Medicine [LSCM] (*see* Chapter 19); this was to open its doors to students in early 1906 – as envisaged in the 1905 Report. The financial implications outlined in that Report – an initial capital outlay of £300 and 'an annual expenditure of about £1,000' – were surely a gross underestimate![11]

Owing to expansion within the hospital (e.g. the Rõntgen Ray, sterilisation, and Anaesthetic departments) 'the buildings at Greenwich were by the early 20th century becoming extremely congested'; the Lords Commissioners of the Admiralty had apparently declined permission for extended buildings. The 86th Report continued:

> … in future it will be necessary to obtain additional accommodation in some way, and it has been suggested that if a site could be provided in the vicinity of the Hospital where the Nurses could reside, and where an adequate Out-Patient department could be arranged, it would set free sufficient space in the Dreadnought Hospital to enable the patients in the wards to be treated with the latest modern requirements.

It was estimated that such a project would cost 'something over £20,000'.[12]

In 1899, the Society's architect, Keith Young, produced a report recommending enlargement of the wards. Until then, the small wards of the original infirmary had been retained, but Florence Nightingale, amongst others, had advocated far larger wards (the 'pavilion principle') which provided greater *ventilation*. The appropriate changes, with removal of many of the partitions, were made possible by further generous support from the King's Fund.[13]

Other developments

A significant development (the LSCM to the fore) was the amalgamation of the *Dreadnought*, and Miller Pathological Departments (Chapter 19). This came about in 1911.[14]

The existent Greenwich horse-ambulance was, by 1900 deemed unsatisfactory and 'worn out'; it was sold later that year to the Petersfield Isolation Hospital for £15=00. A later minute (10 November 1905) records the repair of the replacement ambulance for £15=4=0, and on 11 October 1906 the SHS Committee approved '15/= a week [this was later increased to 20/= per week] for horsing the ambulance, instead of 8/= per journey'.[15]

Another matter (the Society has always been a predominantly Christian foundation) was the construction of a *new* Chapel over the central section of Somerset Ward (at an estimated cost of £1,281); it was subsequently dedicated by the Lord Bishop of Rochester on 16 October 1885. At a later date it was resolved that a stained-glass window be erected in this chapel in memory of John Lyddeker (*see* Chapter 7). Following this, a request by the PMO (Johnson Smith) for a window to 'commemorate the services of Mr Rooke and Dr Harry Leach' (Chapters 12 and 15) was made.

Improved conditions for the patients

The Reports for 1877 and 1878 emphasised greater comfort for the *inmates* [my italics]; a campaign was launched, by the Chairman, to obtain (by donation) 250 pictures to 'interest the patients and [hence] to make them cheerful and contented' which would adorn the wards and thereby 'increase the comfort of the inmates'.

The wards in Somerset Wing (Annie Zunz) had been newly constructed and were officially opened on 20 July 1910. Noise, was a further problem; that caused by the tramways outside the *Dreadnought* was a major problem which was partly solved by replacing the centre of the roadway with 'wood pavement'![16]

The question of 'incurable' patients (i.e. those hospitalised for ≥2 months) was repeatedly raised; they were apparently *removed*, but to where is not stated in the minutes![17]

Landsmen, women and children

The contentious matter of whether to treat 'minority' groups (landsmen, women and children who numbered about 300 of the in-patients annually in 1894 and 1895) in a Marine Charity (such as the *Dreadnought*) received recurrent attention in the Annual Reports; it was felt however, that because the nearest general hospital (to Greenwich), with the exception of the Miller, was several miles away, together with the fact that many of these individuals suffered from accidents and were therefore designated *emergencies*, 'it would be an act of inhumanity to send [them away]'.

The question of admission of females to the *Dreadnought* Hospital, was aired in the Committee of Management minutes; it was 'Ordered that Female cases of Accident brought to this hospital be admitted – but treated in a Ward exclusively devoted to them'. Regarding admission of women to the Albert Dock Hospital (ADH), a meeting held on 13 September 1895, ruled: 'that women *in extremis* [my italics] or in exceptional cases [only] were to be admitted and a report [should be] made to the Committee at the first opportunity'.

In June 1908, 'It was resolved that a letter [should] be written to the Medical Officers calling their attention to the fact that Landsmen, Women and Children are *not* [my italics] objects of the care of the [SHS]'. Subsequent meetings echoed this sentiment, especially with regard to Out-Patients.[18] This continuing debate led to a demand for a precise definition of a *seaman*; the chairman (P A Nairne) stated that:

> a Seaman is a man who either is at sea, or engaged in shipping, or who has been at sea the working portion of his life. A man who has been at sea for a short period and given it up and become a landsman, is no longer a Seaman.[19]

In 1901, the Society received a letter from the Women's Liberal Federation suggesting that women should be 'allowed to sit upon the Committee of Management'. But as in most other establishments at that time, this (potential) move was shelved.[20]

Extension of facilities to other parts of 'dockland'

For almost half a century, between removal of *clinical* facilities to dry-land (in April 1870) until the outbreak of the Great War, the SHS experienced a period of sustained growth. Table 14.1 summarises those facilities available in 1905 (i.e. 35 years after removal to land). First, came the creation of two dispensaries – with out-patient facilities – close to the relevant docks (see below). Many felt that the newly opened Tilbury Docks (in 1886) also warranted facilities – see below. The Branch (*ADH*) was opened in 1890 (following a detailed SHS Report); this establishment – located between the Royal Albert and Royal Victoria Docks – had, like its parent hospital, both in-patient and out-patient facilities. It was here that Patrick Manson (1844–1922) (Chapter 18), already on the Consultant Staff of that institution, together with

Table 14.1: The Society's establishments in 1905.

Category of establishment	*Institution*		*Date opened*
Hospital	(i)	*Dreadnought* Seamen's Hospital, Greenwich. 250 beds and Out-patient Dept (Hospital open 24 hours per day).	April 1870
	(ii)	The Albert Dock Hospital, E. (ADH) 50 beds and Out-patient dept (Hospital open 24 hours per day)	June 1890
Dispensary	(iii)	East & West India Docks Dispensary, East India Dock Road, E. (Open daily [except Sunday] from 9 am to 10 am and 12.30 pm to 1.30 pm)	October 1880
	(iv)	Dispensary for Seamen, Gravesend (open daily [except Sunday] from 9.30 am to 10.15 am).	June 1887
School	(v)	The London School of Tropical Medicine (LSTM) (situated at the ADH)	October 1899
	(vi)	The London School of Clinical Medicine (LSCM) – Post Graduate (situated at the *Dreadnought* Hospital)	1906

much 'political' support from the Secretary of State for the Colonies – the Rt Hon Joseph Chamberlain, launched the London School of Tropical Medicine (LSTM) in 1899. Establishment of the LSTM was considered of enormous importance, and dominated the affairs of the Society throughout the following decade; it was also to occupy a substantial amount of space in subsequent minute-books.

With the LSTM project firmly and successfully launched, attempts were made by Manson (and others) to found the LSCM (Chapter 19) – to utilise *for teaching purposes* the wealth of *clinical* material available at Greenwich – at the land-based Dreadnought Hospital. Manson, by this time, rapidly approaching retirement – he would be 65 in 1907 – was clearly adamant that this school should be completed as a matter of urgency. Unfortunately, this venture was to be shrouded by financial problems. This event (which necessitated another significant expansion in the number of consultant staff, as well as substantial alterations to the hospital buildings) also came to dominate the Society's affairs – and is reflected in subsequent *Minute Books* (and *Annual Reports*) during the first decade of the twentieth century. At the turn of the century, therefore, the Society maintained two hospitals (the 'flagship' establishment at Greenwich, and the *ADH*) and two dispensaries (Table 14.1; Figure 14.2). In addition it overlooked the LSTM and also the LSCM (situated at the *Dreadnought* itself).

The Great War (1914–18) brought many disruptions. The 94th Report stated:

> ... many members of the Medical, Nursing and Lay Staff have left to serve their country both abroad and at home. We who cannot go [the writer continued] envy them the power to give active service to the Empire.

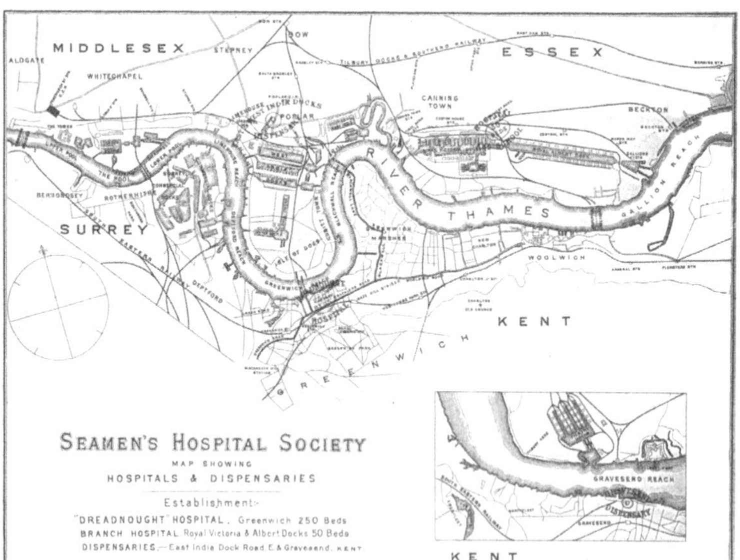

Figure 14.2: Map, showing the extent of the SHS 'Empire' in 1900; the two hospitals, and two dispensaries are shown. [Annual SHS Report, 1900].

The LSTM therefore had to be slimmed down; not only had many of its staff joined the Armed Services, but student numbers at the two schools declined dramatically. The impact on the newly established LSCM was nothing short of catastrophic; Manson had completely retired by the end of hostilities and the project therefore lacked a 'driving force'; the war had virtually heralded the total collapse of what appeared a promising postgraduate enterprise. The sole viable component to survive was the pathological department (Chapter 19).

The dispensaries

WELL STREET

In January 1880, the possibility of establishing a Dispensary on the *north* side of the Thames was addressed; the Chairman of the Committee of Management moved:

> That in the interests of Seamen, for whose benefit the Hospital was established, the time appears now to have arrived when a sub-committee should be appointed with instructions to ascertain and report, whether it may not be advantageous to extend the Society's usefulness by the formation of a Dispensary for Out-patients in the vicinity of the large docks situated on the North side of the Thames.

A sub-committee, set up on 12 March, approved the idea, and considered that such a Dispensary should be established 'in the neighbourhood of the East India Dock Road', near the Sailors' Home at the 'premises in Well Street known as the Destitute Sailors' Asylum'. At a subsequent meeting, the Chairman reported 'that the Committee of the Sailors' Home had agreed to let a portion [of the asylum] to the Hospital for the proposed Dispensary at a nominal rental of £1 per annum'.

The 60th Report recorded that 'the Committee in early October 1880 had opened a Dispensary in Well Street, London Docks (which was strictly to provide 'free relief of *bonâ fide* seamen who produce evidence of having been at sea within three months of the date at which they first apply for treatment'), which would of necessity 'entail a large additional expenditure annually'.[22] The *raison d'etre* for expanding *clinical* facilities was 'spelt out' in detail in that Report:

> that [area is] the centre of the district where sailors chiefly lodge when ashore, and this situation has been specially selected with the view of doing as much good as possible. [The Report continued]: a portion of the Destitute Sailors Asylum had been let to the hospital authorities … at a nominal rent … . The situation of the [*Dreadnought*] has obliged out-patients who require only casual relief to lose no time and incur expense (*6d* a visit) because of its distance from the docks. There is reason to fear than many seamen have in consequence resorted to quacks and unqualified practitioners at the risk of health and a waste of money. The establishment of This Dispensary [the report emphasised], will remove many of these evils, while it will confer substantial benefits not only on seamen, but upon owners and captains, to whom the proper

> treatment of seamen when sick, and their healthy condition, are of the first importance.

This Dispensary had only out-patient facilities (Figure 14.3), and in the event of in-patient treatment being required, the sailors would be transferred to the *Dreadnought* Hospital by a 'special conveyance provided for that purpose'.

The following report recorded that instead of morning opening it had been decided to open 'from the forenoon to the afternoon'; this would allow 'a man [to go to the Docks] in the morning ... to seek a ship for his next cruise ... and to [come] back to his home for his dinner, and to the Dispensary, if necessary'. At a meeting held in 1881, it is minuted that: 'The proof of a notice regarding the Well St. Dispensary was submitted. It was amended, adopted and ordered to be printed & distributed amongst the Ships as they arrived in the River'.[23]

In May 1882, the surgeon to the Well St. Dispensary (George Makins FRCS) resigned after 18 months in the post; the reason is not stated. His successor was Mr Ernest Little MRCS, who seems to have been somewhat erratic in his hours of attendance, as was his colleague, Mr Leadbeater!

GRAVESEND

The 66th Annual Report alluded to the opening of Tilbury Docks (see also Chapter 2); a Sub-Committee had visited Gravesend, and the members were of the opin-

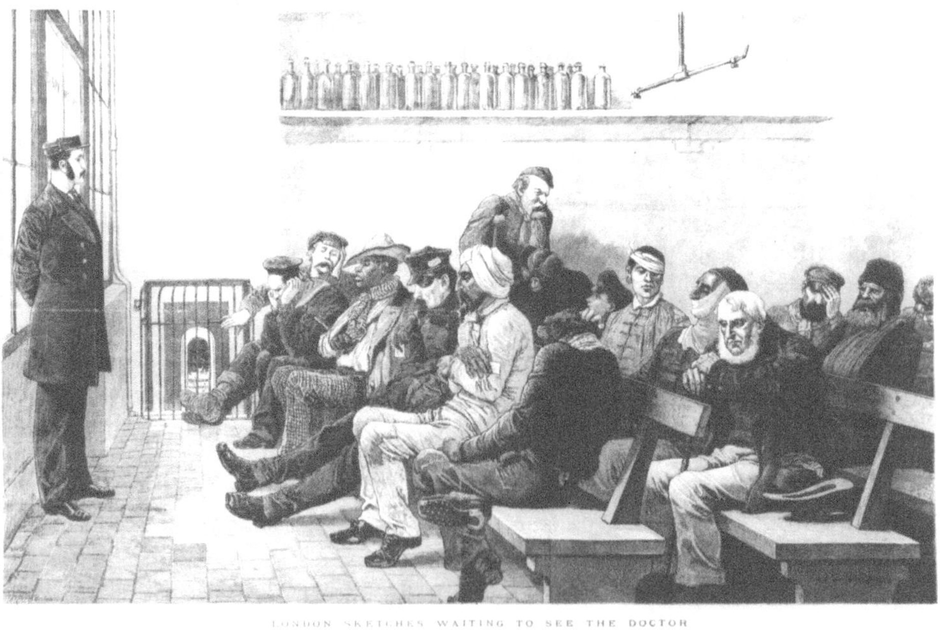

Figure 14.3: Engraving showing the waiting room (for out-patients) at the Well Street Dispensary [*Illustrated London News*].

ion that a Dispensary should be opened there: 'advantage should be taken [the report stated] of rooms in a building belonging and attached to the Sailors' Home at Gravesend, close to the public landing-place on the banks of the Thames ...'. This Dispensary was opened in June 1887. Here too, there was uncertainty concerning the most suitable opening hours – the morning or afternoon? The former seemed more favourable! The surgeon there was Onslow Robert Richmond; he served until 1896 – when his health 'broke down' – after having completed nine years of service. A change in opening time was instituted in 1898; it was changed from 11am–11.45am to 9.30–10.15am, or 'so long as it may be necessary for patients to be seen'. There seems at that time to have been a great deal of continuing uncertainty regarding use of the term 'landsman' (see above); the surgeon to the Gravesend Dispensary (in 1907) classified 'Waterman, Lightermen [and] Fishermen ... as Landsmen'![24]

EAST INDIA DOCK ROAD

The 1891 Annual Report contained the following note: 'In consequence of the large number of Sailors now congregating in the neighbourhood of the East and West India Docks [it had been decided to remove the Well Street Dispensary – to which fewer patients were at that time attending] to 51, East India Dock Road [EIDR] – on 15 September 1891.'

At a meeting in June 1890, it was therefore agreed to close the Well Street Dispensary 'on the 24th inst.'. However, at a meeting on 26 March 1891 it was felt that this institution was still viable, and an inspection indicated that during the previous year, 416 (i.e. 23%) of the *new* cases were suffering from VD. A year later the Committee of Management ultimately decided that if it could be acquired 'at a rent not exceeding £50 per annum', the facility in EIDR would be more suitable than the Well St. site. The offer was accepted on 'a three years repairing lease'. By June 1894, the 'old tenant of 51 East India Dock Road had left' and the premises were let to a new one at £2=16=0 per month. Here also, there are several reports in the minutes of late attendance by the Medical Officers.[25]

Mr Walter Fowler FRCS, who had been Medical Officer of the Well Street Dispensary, was therefore dismissed (together with his Dispenser). He then became Honorary Consulting Surgeon to the EIDR Dispensary, and arrangements were made for an additional Medical Officer appointed to the newly opened ADH to attend daily at 12.00 until 2.00pm. It was not until 1897 in fact, that the EIDR Dispensary ultimately had its own Medical Officer. The following year Mr J Ralph Prior, Surgeon to the EIDR Dispensary resigned on grounds of ill health, and the next year his successor Mr Frank Morris MRCS also resigned. In 1899, 'certain repairs and alterations to the drains and sanitary arrangements [at this Dispensary] were demanded by the Sanitary Inspector of the Board of Works for the Limehouse District. By this time, the property was apparently in a 'very dilapidated condition'. The 1901 Annual Report contained the following statement:

> ... No. 51, East India Dock Road [which in 1898 had been reported to be in a very poor condition structurally [had] been sold by the Society's landlords, and the Society must [therefore] vacate the premises at an early date. [The SHS Committee had therefore] entered into an agreement to

> rent for £60 per annum suitable accommodation ... in the new buildings of the Seamen's Mission, in Jeremiah Street, East India Dock Road.[26]

Two years later, Mr W H J Oxley, MRCS, a general practitioner of 119 East India Dock Road, was appointed *not* as Surgeon, but as medical officer, but whose attendances also proved somewhat erratic. In 1906, the opening hours of the EIDR Dispensary were again changed, this time to 9–10am, and 12.30–1.30pm.

The Albert Dock (Branch) Hospital

An important development was recorded in the 1888 Annual Report; the Superintendent of the East and West India Dock had requested the Society's Management Committee to 'establish a branch or cottage hospital at Tilbury (i.e. on the north bank of the Thames). This led to the formation of a Special Committee (chaired by P A Nairne) to examine 'the entire question of providing additional hospital accommodation for mariners in the Port of London'. This Committee, which reported in October 1888, concluded, however, that 'the largest number of seafaring men congregating in any one place in the Port of London unprovided with medical or surgical aid [was not at Tilbury but] in the vicinity of the Albert and Victoria Docks'; they recommended therefore, that 'steps be forthwith taken for establishing a branch hospital with twelve beds and an out-patient department in that locality'. Furthermore, the Well Street and Gravesend Dispensaries should 'be retained for the present'. This conclusion was accepted by the Management Committee, and it was estimated that the building would cost about £3000, with annual maintenance of about £1000. This development led to the foundation of the first Branch Hospital (ADH) (see below).

A Special General Court of Governors '[was] requested to authorise the General Committee to take upon lease from the London and St Katherine Dock Co. such land, at such rent, upon such terms and for such period as may be considered necessary for the erection of a Branch Hospital at the Albert and Victoria Docks'. A meeting held on 22 March 1889 approved proposed plans for the ADH, but was unhappy about the extent of the rental of £100 per annum (from the Dock Co.); if this could be reduced to £50 per annum, the Special Committee had permission to proceed and tenders (to be examined by the General Committee at their meeting on 10 May) sought.[27]

The *raison d'etre* for a Branch Hospital (ADH) was clearly stated in the 69th Report:

> The shipping of the Port of London now extends over such a vast area, that a single hospital, no matter where situated, cannot of itself render adequate medical and surgical assistance at all the great centres where seafaring men congregate. At the present time [1889], Seamen arriving at the Victoria and Albert Docks suffering from serious ailments, have to be conveyed a distance of between two and three miles, often at great danger and suffering to the patient, before Hospital accommodation can be obtained ... . Sufficient land has been rented from the London and India Docks Joint Committee immediately between the two Docks

[the Royal Albert and Victoria], and over two-and-a-half miles from the nearest Hospital.[28]

LAYING THE FOUNDATION STONE, AND OPENING THE ADH

Ceremonial arrangements for 'Laying [the] Foundation Stone of the New … Hospital at the Royal Victoria and Albert Docks [in Connaught Road, designed by Mr Keith D Young, FRIBA (1848–1929)]' were set out in a brochure published by the SHS in 1889. HRH Prince George of Wales, K.G. (later King George V) (1865–1936) duly arrived by 'Special Train [from Fenchurch Street Station] at the Central Station, Royal Albert Dock, at 3.55 on Monday 15 July 1889'; there, he was received by the Chairman [of the SHS, Frederick Cleeve Esq., R.N., C.B.] and a Deputation of the Committee of Management … and proceeded to the Hospital site by carriage'; the route was 'lined by the 15th Middlesex Rifle "Volunteers", the "Boys" of the Royal Hospital School Greenwich, the Crews of the Steamships belonging to the Peninsula and Oriental Steam Navigation Company, Messrs. Donald Currie & Co., Messrs. Geo. Thompson & Co., Messrs. Lamport & Holt, the General Steam Navigation Company, and other lines of "vessels" frequenting the Port of London'. The 'European sailors [wore, the programme continued] the Uniforms of the various Lines, the Lascars and the Orientals …Eastern costume'; '… steamships, sailing ships and steam yachts to the number of over one hundred [were] decorated with flags'.

The Prince was unfortunate enough to arrive 'in a heavy downpour of rain', but the Stone was duly laid at 4.00pm after prayers (led by the Lord Bishop of Colchester) together with a loyal address – given by the Chairman; the Hospital was being designed (the brochure continued), to 'accommodate twelve Patients, together with a Medical and Nursing Staff, and there [was also to] be an Out-Patient Department'. Owing to the fact that it was the *only* Hospital within three miles, it was envisaged [according to the Chairman] that 'accidents occurring in the Docks, and urgent cases arriving in vessels' would be attended to; attached to the Hospital, was to be 'a Horse Ambulance, for removal of Patients from their vessels'.[29]

The Hospital (Figure 14.4) contained: 'two general wards [one on each of two floors] of five beds each, an isolation ward of two beds, and two rooms which [could] be used as additional or spare wards if occasion should require'; there was also an 'out-patient waiting room, with a consulting-room' and a Dispensary, Kitchen, Store, etc. as well as 'Quarters for the Medical Staff and Matron, and Bedrooms for the Nurses and Female Servants', a mortuary, post-mortem room and an ambulance house had been built in the grounds. The first storey was 'of yellow brick with red facing, and the upper stories and roof [were] covered with red tiles'. The intention was that 'the beds … be used for the retention of urgent or special cases, all others being transferred by ambulance to [the *Dreadnought* to which the hospital was 'in telephonic communication'].[30]

The ADH was officially opened by HRH the Prince (1841–1910) (the future King Edward VII) and Princess (1844–1925) of Wales, at 2.30pm on Tuesday 24 June 1890. They had boarded the Steamer 'HM Stanley' (named after the high profile African explorer who had 'rescued' David Livingstone [1813–73]) at 1.30pm at Westminster Pier, and were met at the Landing Stage by 'the President [of the

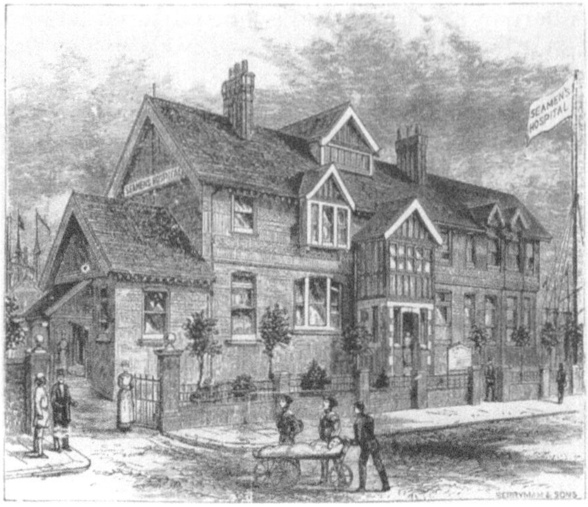

Figure 14.4: The original Albert Dock (Branch) Hospital (ADH) – opened in 1890 [Courtesy, Wellcome Library, London].

SHS, Admiral H.R.H. the Duke of Edinburgh (1844–1900)], the Committee of the Hospital, and the Authorities of the Docks'. Following prayers (again led by the Bishop of Colchester) and a loyal address (by the President) TRH duly declared the Hospital open and; following this, Her Royal Highness consented to a ward being named 'the "Alexandra" Ward'.[31]

The newly-opened establishment was immediately an outstanding success; it served the Royal Docks personnel – as well as the *tropical* discipline from 1899 (see below) – until it was noted in 1935, that the foundations of the hospital were subsiding (Chapter 20). In the first six months there were 230 in-, and 938 out-patients, of whom 91 were transferred to the *Dreadnought*. A 'considerable number [were] Lascars from the P. and O. Steam Navigation Company, and British India Steam Navigation Company'.[32]

LATER DEVELOPMENTS AT THE ADH

The Secretary (Michelli) negotiated in 1895 with the London and India Joint Committee for a reduction in the rent (from £50 [see above] to a peppercorn rate) for the plot of land on which the ADH stood; this, together with the use of waste land adjoining the hospital (on the north side), was agreed.

In late 1896, expansion of the ADH out-patient facilities was considered necessary'; it was minuted that: '... though the number [of out-patients is] increasing ['almost entirely in cases of accident and emergency'] there is no special increase since the charge of 2d has been made to each Out-Patient at the Poplar'. The following January, a sub-committee (chaired by P A Nairne) recommended (in a printed report) major expansion of out-patient accommodation at the ADH, together with ten extra beds (to make a total of 26), a ward kitchen, additional sleeping accommodation, and a physician/surgeon's side room. A subsequent meeting at which the architect (Young) and the engineer (Herbert Birkett) were also present agreed these and other additions – providing a total of 32 beds. The cost of the new buildings was estimated at 'about £7,500 and the piling £1,200'.

It is clear from the Annual Reports and Board Minutes, that by 1896 (i.e. six years after its opening) the ADH was hopelessly inadequate from the point of view of size – both from an in-patient and out-patient perspective; the annual total of those 'relieved' had rapidly overtaken that of the *Dreadnought* itself. In consequence, a Sub-Committee, set up to look into the matter, recommended 'that 10 [additional] beds be added to the [ADH], and that adequate Consulting Rooms, Waiting Rooms, &c., be added to the Out-patient department'. The erection of a new wing, was considered 'an imperative necessity', despite the fact that it would entail additional expenditure to the tune of £400 per annum. The 1897 Report recorded, 'To make the enlargement effectual it [would be] necessary to add 20 beds and a new Out-Patient Department, at a cost of upwards of £8,000'.[33]

In August 1900, the Port of London requested 'a strip of land at the Southern boundary of the [ADH] site'; this was granted, but they sought 'a piece of land to the East of the Hospital in lieu thereof'.

A 'tropical school' on the ADH site

Although there were significant financial implications, the request (from Joseph Chamberlain's office) to found the LSTM at the ADH (Chapter 18) arrived at an opportune moment for the SHS. In early 1898, a Sub-Committee was set up to consider whether the Society would sponsor a School of Tropical Medicine; this Committee reported to the Committee of Management on 15 April, that a School should in fact be set up and situated at the ADH (where 78% of the 'tropical' cases in the care of the SHS had been located in the previous six months – 1 September 1897 to 28 February 1898). The 1898 Annual Report stated, however, that 'An increase [in the number of beds to 30] would *not* fully meet the demand, and this Committee expressed the opinion that if a School for the study of Tropical Diseases is to be formed, the Hospital should not contain less than 45 beds'.

The 78th Report recorded that: 'The new Wing will contain two large wards, and the School buildings will be equipped with the usual laboratories, class rooms, and sleeping accommodation for students'. It was estimated that this extension of hospital facilities, together with the creation of a 'properly equipped medical School' would cost 'upwards of £16,000 [towards which the Colonial Office had 'agreed to contribute £3,500'], together with an amount estimated at £1000 per annum' for maintenance, and the Foreign Office an undisclosed sum. H.M. Secretary of State for India had donated a further £1000. In 1900, an amended estimate from the architect showed 'that the cost of adding a room to the Operating Theatre and making various alterations in the roof will raise the cost by £807'.[34]

The foundation of the LSTM of course represented, a major change in tack for the SHS: the Society had until then been solely a *service* organisation, whereas creation of the LSTM would add a *teaching* component. The 79th report commented: 'The establishment of the [LSTM] marks a new feature in the development of the

Society, for it is the first occasion on which a serious effort has been made to place the valuable teaching material which exists in the Hospitals of the Society at the disposal of Medical Science'.

The fact that the SHS had undertaken this *teaching* role in addition to its *service* commitment, proved to be a contentious matter. At a meeting on 14 April 1905, Mr Silas Waymouth RN protested 'against the [LSTM] being worked as an integral part of the [SHS]'. He proposed furthermore that '… the union between the Society and the School should be dissolved'; but on 'a show of hands this resolution was lost by eight votes to two'.

This school, it was recorded, was to be managed by a LSTM Committee consisting of 'Members of the Committee of Management [of the SHS], Members of the Medical and Surgical Staff [of the ADH] and Teachers in the School [Chapter 18], with power to recommend to the [SHS] Committee of Management candidates for election as Teachers and Lecturers in the School, and also to recommend the adoption of such Bye-Laws and Regulations as they may from time to time consider necessary for the proper government of the School'. In the *new* wing were to be several 'named Beds':

The Nairne Bed
The Coote Bed
The American Victoria Jubilee Bed
The P. & O. Bed
The Lady Strathcona Bed
The Sir William Maxwell Cot
The Sir Donald Currie Bed.[35]

But by 1903, the structural condition of the 'older portion of the [ADH]' was already giving cause for concern (see also Chapter 20); the 83rd Report continued: 'the piling [had] been found to be defective, and in some places quite rotten [and] it will be necessary to under-pin the building and put in steel piles and girders. This will entail a cost of, probably, £3,000'. This matter was addressed in several subsequent Annual Reports and was paid for, in part, by a further donation from the King's Fund. The state of the foundations (especially In the north wing) of the 'older portion' also gave repeated cause for concern, and this was also frequently minuted.[36]

Enlargement of the ADH meant that other additions were also necessary: 'for sanitary reasons, a new Mortuary [had to be constructed, and it was also necessary] to reconstruct the Kitchen'. The probable cost of these new buildings was estimated at £8,000. Also, to meet the requirement(s) of the rapidly growing LSTM, it was deemed 'absolutely necessary to increase the Laboratory Accommodation, to provide a suitable Library, Lecture Hall, and also additional Sleeping Accommodation' at an estimated cost of £5,000. By this time, the LSTM had become a viable enterprise, and additional expense on the ADH was inescapable; the 1903 Annual Report recorded: '… a sum of about £4,000 is required to meet the expenditure on the new Out-Patient department [with a 'waiting room [accommodating] over 50 patients; a room for the Out-Patient Physician or Surgeon; an examining room where bandaging can be done and minor injuries attended to. A new Dispensary is also attached, and for the first time adequate accommodation [will be provided for the Dispenser] and an Isolation Ward [with] accommodation for two patients'. This work was completed in June 1904.[37]

Other matters involving the two hospitals

Rotation of staff

In a revolutionary move, the Society's Committee resolved at a meeting on 11 December 1903 that 'two [of the] Physicians at Greenwich [Drs Rankin and Hewlett] and a Physician at the Branch Hospital [ADH, Dr Andrew Duncan] should rotate between the two Hospitals'.[38]

MANSON'S VIEWS ON STAFFING AND PATIENT CARE AT THE ADH

In late 1893, Manson considered, in a letter to the SHS Committee of Management, that:

- i) Junior doctors at the ADH should be selected by [the] Staff at that hospital, and not the *Dreadnought*;
- ii) black and white patients should be separated;
- iii) black attendants should be provided; and
- iv) the windows [at the ADH] were not properly fitted.'

The last of these suggestions was apparently supported by the PMO; the remainder were *not* approved.[39]

PAYING PATIENTS

The question of Paying Patients in beds endowed by Austen Chamberlain's Fund at the ADH was raised at a meeting in December 1913; the decision was that patients with a *tropical disease* were expected to pay an amount in accordance with their circumstances.[40]

STRUCTURAL DAMAGE TO THE ADH

On 6 July 1898, a severe explosion damaged the ADH and nine individuals (five of whom subsequently died) were seriously injured.

RESULT OF AN INQUEST

In August 1903 a letter was read from the West Ham Coroner relating to a man who had been brought to the ADH following an accident; he died 15 minutes later without having been seen by a doctor. The jury at the inquest 'thought [that] 20 minutes rather a long time to wait in an accident Hospital before a patient is seen'.[41]

THE BOER WAR

During the South African War (1899–1902), beds at the ADH were offered for 'sick and wounded soldiers'.

THE SAMARITAN FUND

This fund was founded in the period under review, with a gift of £740 from George Sturge. The objective was to enable the Committee of Management to provide clothing for those in need, and also rail and boat fares to any location in the UK. If it were not for the fund, it was concluded, sailors would find themselves strangers (without money or a home) in the Port of London.[42]

CHRISTMAS FESTIVITIES

Christmas continued to be a time of celebration at the Society's institutions. As in the Hospital-ship days, special Christmas entertainment was put on (Figure 14.5); activities are recorded both in the Society's minutes, and also in several contemporary newspapers and journals.

A Hospital for the Tilbury Docks?

With the inauguration of the Tilbury Docks in 1888 (see above) an urgent need for a Branch Hospital there had already been aired (see also Chapters 2 and 20). A minute of the Committee of Management (before the ADH was opened) states:

> A letter dated 6th January [1888] was read from the directors of the East and West India Dock Co. inviting this society to establish a branch Hospital at Tilbury and offering a building there as a temporary Hospital. It was resolved that the letter be referred to the Finance Sub-Committee with power to add any other member of the General Committee to the Sub-Committee for the consideration of this subject and to report to the Committee. And that the same Sub-Committee should also consider whether it would be desirable to have a branch Hospital or Dispensary near any of the large Docks either in addition to or in lieu of the Dispensaries at Well street and at Gravesend.

At a follow-up in 1891, the Dock Company again offered 'free of cost' a 'substantial brick building' with transfer of their subscription to the Gravesend Hospital to the SHS. Due to the fact that the Society had, the previous year opened the ADH, they again stalled on the grounds that finances were inadequate for a further extension.

A later letter from the London and India Docks Joint Committee (January 1892) indicated that they were now prepared to 'place at the disposal of the Society … £390=12=1 towards preliminary expenses'. This led to the formation of a Provisional Local Committee which reported on 10 June 1892: '… if assured of adequate local support, the Society will, ere long be able to open a Branch Hospital at Tilbury Dock [with 'at least 12 beds'] on the lines of that opened a year or two hence at the Royal Albert Dock'. It was estimated that 'the cost of maintenance [would] be about £1000 per annum, of which one half [would] have to be raised locally'. The matter was referred to a Special Committee.

An 'offer [had therefore been made] of a suitable building [originally erected as dwelling accommodation for Dock workers] entirely free of cost, together with a

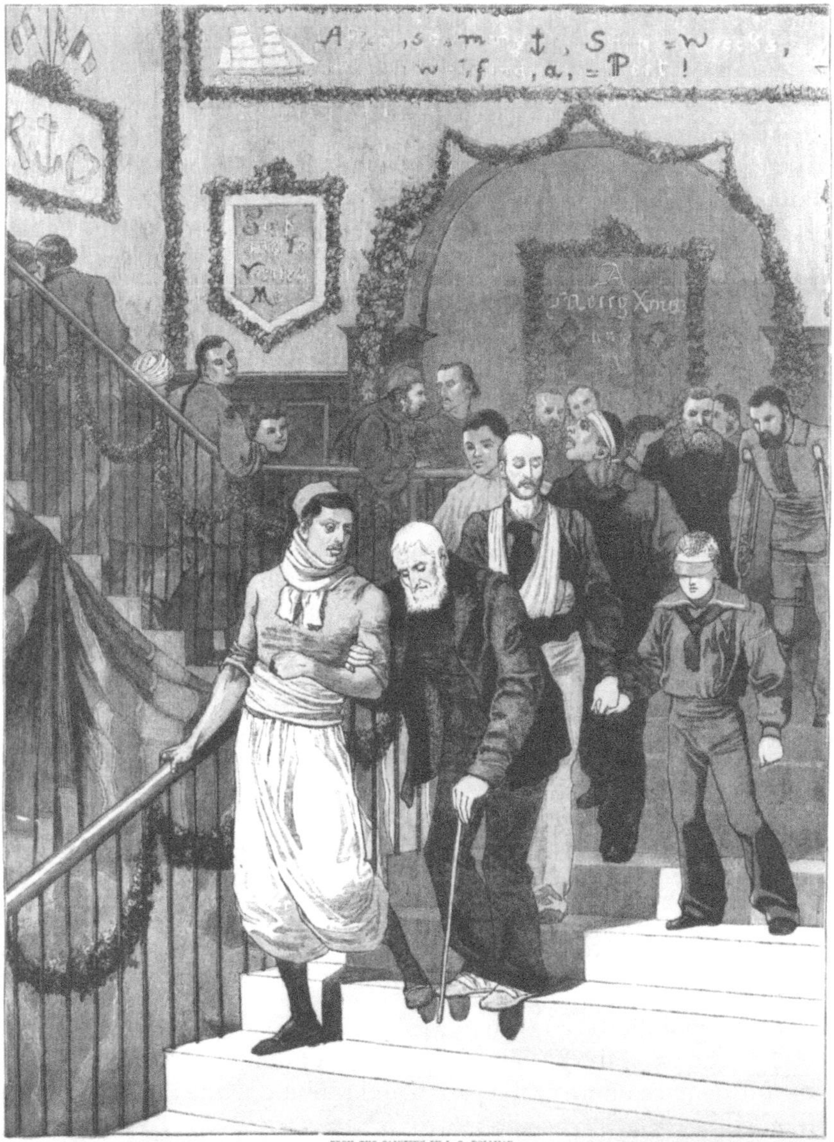

FROM THE PAINTING BY J. C. DOLLMAN

CHRISTMAS DAY AT THE SEAMEN'S HOSPITAL, GREENWICH—COMING DOWN TO DINNER"

Figure 14.5: Engraving showing Christmas festivities at the Dreadnought hospital in 1876 [*Illustrated London News* 1877: 6 January].

sum of £390 towards the preliminary expenses'. The overriding problem was the *cost* of maintenance, it being estimated that this would amount to about '£1,000 or £1,200 [annually]'. The SHS Committee therefore once again procrastinated (primarily due to the precarious state of the Society's finances), but in 1894 decided *against* proceeding with the project.

On 27 April 1894, a Committee of Management minute recorded a meeting which the Secretary had attended regarding 'a Cottage Hospital [erected by Mr Passmore Edwards – a prominent philanthropist – in 1894] in the Tilbury District'; an offer of this building, which adjoined the Tilbury Docks, had been made by Edwards. It is clear that the Committee, which now had two alternatives, was again 'dragging its feet'. The Chairman (The Hon Sydney Holland – later to become the secretary of the [Royal] London Hospital) and Secretary (Mr A Borer) of the Tilbury Dock Hospital were enthusiastic about joining forces with the SHS in November 1903, but again no definite decision was taken. There was however an understandable drawback with the Tilbury Hospital 'takeover'; it was intended to admit 'landsmen, women and children equally with sailors'; a retrospective breakdown of Patients treated at the Tilbury Hospital during 1901, indicated that 63 were landsmen, women and children whereas only 19 were seamen!

Nothing concrete was apparently done until 1904. Then, renewed negotiations with the President of the 'Passmore Edwards Cottage Hospital at Tilbury' took place. The Tilbury question had in fact come to a head; a printed memorandum was discussed at a meeting on 8 April, giving two options: (i) the Passmore Edward 'Cottage Hospital' – which would put seafarers first – 'about 70% [were] seamen or men directly connected with the sea, while only 5% [were] women' but this hospital had no 'Out-Patient Department, [or] Isolation Ward, and no accommodation for a Resident Medical Officer', *or* (ii) the Tilbury Hospital (which was open to 'all and sundry'). A decision was ultimately taken by the Board in favour of the Passmore Edwards alternative, so this hospital had ultimately 'won the day' (Chapter 20)![43]

The Society's rôle immediately prior to the Great War (1914–18)

The 92nd Annual Report highlighted the part played by the SHS with the war approaching:

> ... the Corporation carries on two great Imperial undertakings. The care of the Seamen of the Empire in their hour of illness and suffering, and the furtherance of medical research and training in the [LSTM] and the [LSCM].[44]

The following year, the Report recorded:

> A decrease has taken place in the number of patients treated by the Society [which is] almost entirely accounted for by the reference of trivial cases in the Dispensaries and Casualty Departments to panel doctors under the Insurance Act [of 1911, which did not affect the major work of the Hospitals]; and it has not brought about a reduction in expenditure. The Sailor needs Hospital treatment as much as ever, and he can only get it in future, as in the past, by the sympathy and help of generous friends.[45]

References and notes

1 62nd Annual Report: 82: 11–12; 80: 19.
2 *Ibid*. 89: 14; 94: 11; Committee of Management Minutes 12: 156–161; 13: 478, 523; 15: 227, 238, 242.
3 *Op cit*. See note 2 above (Minutes) 11: 195, 207; J Wolffe. Cooper, Anthony Ashley-, seventh Earl of Shaftesbury (1801–1885). In: H C G Matthew, B Harrison (eds). *Oxford Dictionary of National Biography*. Oxford: Oxford University Press 2004; 13: 223–7.
4 *Op cit*. See note 2 above (Minutes) 12: 7–8, 473; 13: 119, 225; 14: 214; 15: 2,20, 34, 70, 73–74, 169, 212, 222; 14: 122, 135, 136, 139, 143, 154, 156, 162, 171, 176–77, 253, 308, 339, 343, 363, 394, 417, 430, 432, 434, 435, 481, 484, 486, 493; 15: 7, 13, 19.
5 [AM]. The Dreadnought Hospital thirty years ago: by one of the probationers. *SHS Quart Mag* 1933; 5 (1): 20.
6 [EEF]. At the "Dreadnought" in 1900. *SHS Quart Mag* 1934; 6 (i): 14; [*See also:* [WVI]. In a Seamen's Hospital: patients from every corner of the globe. *SHS Quart Mag* 1936; 8 (4): 14–15].
7 J Bold. *Greenwich: an Architectural History of the Royal Hospital for Seamen and the Queen's House*. London: Yale University Press 2000: 207–221; *Op cit*. See note 2 above (Minutes) 9: 210.
8 *Op cit*. See note 2 above (Minutes) 9: 535–537; 11: 78. *Op cit*. See note 1 above 63: 11.
9 *Op cit*. See note 1 above 79: 23–24. [*See also*: *Op cit*. See note 2 above (Minutes) 15: 227, 238, 242].
10 *Op cit*. See note 1 above 82: 22. [*See also*: *Op cit*. See note 2 above (Minutes) 13: 487–488; 14: 435].
11 *Op cit*. See note 1 above 85: 23–24.
12 *Ibid*. 86: 14.
13 *Ibid*. 64: 9–10; *Op cit*. See note 2 above (Minutes) 11: 151, 161–162, 171–172; *Op cit*. See note 7 above.
14 *Op cit*. See note 2 above (Minutes) 15: 60, 65–66, 172.
15 *Ibid*. (Minutes) 13: 232, 239, 273, 299; 14: 214, 267, 403, 411.
16 *Op cit*. See note 1 above. 57: 14; 58: 15; 60: 13.
17 *Op cit*. See note 2 above (Minutes) 10: 477, 484, 489; [*See also:* G C Cook. *Victorian Incurables: a history of the Royal Hospital for Neuro Disability, Putney*. Spennymoor: The Memoir Club 2004: 272; G C Cook. Caring for 'incurables': the 150th anniversary of the Royal Hospital for Neuro-disability, Putney. *Postgrad Med J* 2004 80: 426–30; G C Cook. *The incurables movement: an illustrated history of The British Home*. Oxford: Radcliffe Publishing 2006].
18 *Op cit*. See note 1 above; 74: 14; 75: 13; 76: 14; 77: 20; 78: 20; 81: 21. [*See also: Op cit*. See note 2 above (Minutes) 14: 379, 388, 411–412, 468; 15: 53; *Op cit*. See note 7 above].
19 *Op cit*. See note 2 above (Minutes) 14: 402.
20 *Ibid*. 13: 394.
21 *Ibid*.
22 *Op cit*. See note 2 above (Minutes) 10: 232, 238, 251–253, 267–268, 269–270, 279, 350, 421; 11: 48, 75, 103; 12: 13, 45, 48, 54–55, 84–85, 87–88; *Op cit*. See note 1 above. 60: 10–11.
23 *Op cit*. See note 1 above. 61: 11–12.
24 *Ibid*. 66: 11; 67: 8. [*See also*: *Op cit*. See note 2 above (Minutes): 12: 2–3, 6, 7, 439; 13: 78; 14: 237, 241, 342, 345].
25 Op cit See note 1 above 71: 12; *Op cit*. See note 2 above (Minutes) 12: 79, 83, 93–94, 223, 231, 234, 249, 267, 282, 283, 328, 357, 361; 13: 8, 42–43, 131, 201–202, 204, 213–214, 232, 243, 270, 273; 14: 1, 22, 237, 340, 375.
26 *Op cit*. See note 1 above. 81: 21.

27 *Ibid.* 68: 16; [*See also*: *Op cit.* See note 2 above (Minutes) ('Hospital accommodation at the Docks') 11: 1–4, 430].
28 *Op cit.* See note 1 above 69: 10–11. [*See also*: *Op cit.* See note 2 above (Minutes): 11: 429, 449–450, 494; 12: 248, 329–330, 351, 419–420, 434–435, 445, 490–491; 13: 78–79, 228–229, 229–230, 299, 310–311; 14: 44, 227; 15].
29 Anonymous. 1889. The Seamen's Hospital Society. *Illustrated London News* 1889 27 July, 115; *Op cit.* See note 2 above (Minutes) 11: 474–77. [*See also*: G C Cook, A J Webb. The Albert Dock Hospital, London: the original site (in 1899) of Tropical Medicine as a *new* discipline. *Acta Tropica* 2001: 79: 249–255].
30 *Op cit.* See note 1 above. 70: 10–12.
31 *Op cit.* See note 29 above (Cook, Webb); Anonymous. The Seamen's Hospital Society. *Illustrated London News* 1890 28 June, 819; Anonymous, The Seamen's Hospital Society. *Lancet* 1890 i, 1337; *Op cit.* See note 2 above (Minutes) 12: 12–13; [*See also*: F Driver. Stanley, Sir Henry Morton (1841–1904) In: H C G Matthew, B Harrison (eds). *Oxford Dictionary of National Biography.* Oxford: Oxford University Press 2004: 52: 214–20].
32 G C Cook. *From the Greenwich Hulks to Old St Pancras: a history of tropical disease in London.* London, Athlone Press 1992. 63–66, 163–217; *Op cit.* See note 1 above, A W Clarke. Tropical Medicine; facilities in London. *Times, Lond* 1927 1 October 6.
33 *Op cit.* See note 1 above. 76, 77.
34 *Op cit.* See note 1 above 72: 11; 78 [*See also:* G C Cook. 'Tropical' cases admitted to the Albert Dock Hospital in the early years of the London School of Tropical Medicine. *Trans R Soc Trop Med Hyg* 1999; 93: 675–77].
35 *Op cit.* See note 2 above (Minutes) 14: 64,172.
36 *Op cit.* See note 1 above. 83: 19–20. [See also *Op cit.* See note 2 above (Minutes) 15: 39, 52, 62.]
37 *Ibid.*
38 *Op cit.* See note 2 above (Minutes) 15: 2, 23, 26.
39 *Ibid.*
40 *Ibid.* 14: 19. [*See also*: *Op cit.* See note 32 above (Cook)].
41 *Op cit.* See note 2 above (Minutes). 11: 372, 12: 77–78, 114, 142–146, 148, 274, 293, 297; 14: 28–29, 35, 76, 86; 15: 213.
42 Anonymous. The Samaritan Fund. *SHS Quart Mag* 1933; 5 (1): 19.
43 *Op cit.* See note 1 above 84: 21; A J A Morris. Edwards, John Passmore (1823–1911). In: H C G Matthew, B Harrison (eds). *Oxford Dictionary of National Biography.* Oxford: Oxford University Press 2004; 17: 941–3.
44 *Op cit.* See note 1 above 42: 11.
45 *Ibid.* 93.

Chapter 15

The Society's expanding staff 1870–1914

The non-medical staff from the removal to land (in 1870) until the outbreak of the Great War in 1914 are summarised in Table 15.1. The advent of the London School of Tropical Medicine (LSTM) in 1899 (*see* Chapter 18), and soon afterwards the London School of Clinical Medicine (LSCM) in 1906 (*see* Chapter 19) necessitated substantial expansion in the Society's Consultant staff – both for *clinical* and *teaching* purposes. Manson was closely involved in both projects. Table 15.2 summarises additions (with dates) to the SHS medical staff between 1870 until the formation of the LSTM in 1899.To achieve this expansion, Manson arranged: (i) recruitment of several close colleagues (with tropical medicine connections) to the Albert Dock Hospital (ADH) (they were subsequently given *joint* contracts to work both in that hospital and also the *Dreadnought*), and (ii) importation of several eminent and well established physicians and surgeons who had had no previous experience with the SHS, who were subsequently based at the *Dreadnought* Hospital to add strength to the LSCM – both from a teaching and also a 'political' viewpoint.

For biographical details of Doctors Budd, Barnes, Ward, Leach and Mr Busk – see Chapter 12; because his career overlapped with the early days of the 'land-based' *Dreadnought*, the latter days of Leach's life are covered in this chapter. Several physicians joined the staff of the Dreadnought Hospital immediately after removal to land and prior to the advent of the LSTM and LSCM.

Administrators

Chairman of the Committee of Management

Little is known of most of these men, although they were, in most cases, highly influential in shaping the Charity.

LE BRETON

Mr Francis Le Breton was a member of the Committee for 19 years; in the last five of these (1869–74) he served as Chairman. Le Breton resigned on 22 May 1874 due to 'advanced age'. He was 'in command', therefore, when clinical facilities were removed from the last of the hospital-ships to the Infirmary of the Royal Hospital. He died in 1880.[1]

Table 15.1: The non-medical personnel who served the *Dreadnought* after removal to land (1870) until the outbreak of the Great War in 1914.

Patron:	18[70]–1901	Queen Victoria (1819–1901)*
	1901–1910	King Edward VII (1841–1910) & Queen Alexandra (1844–1925)
	1910–[14]	King George V (1865–1936) & Queen Mary (1867–1853)
Vice-Patron:	18[70]–1901	HRH The Prince of Wales (1841–1910) KG KT
	1889–92	HRH Prince George of Wales (1865–1936) KG
	1892–99	HRH The Duke of York (1865–1936) KG KT
	1899–1900	HRH The Duke of Cornwall & York, (1865–1936) KG KT KP
	1912–[14]	Admiral HSH Prince Louis of Battenberg (1854–1921) GCB GCVO KCMG
President:	18[70]–76	Vacant
	1876–1900	Admiral HRH The Duke of Edinburgh RN (Duke of Saxe-Coburg & Gotha) KG KT KP (1844–1900)
	1900–05	Vacant
	1905–11	His Grace the 9th Duke of Marlborough (1871–1934) KG
	1912–[14]	Admiral HSH Prince Louis of Battenberg (1854–1921)
Chairman, Committee of Management:	18[70]–74	Francis Le Breton, Esq. (18?–80)*
	1874–85	Joseph Moore, Esq. (18?–89)
	1885–89	Frederick Cleeve, Esq. (18?–1905)
	1889–95	Admiral the Hon. Francis Egerton (18?–94)
	1895–98	Vacant
	1898–[14]	P A Nairne (1840–1921)
House-Governor & Secretary/Secretary:	18[70]–74	S Kemball Cook (1818–74)*
	1874–80	H C (later Sir Henry) Burdett (1847–1920)†
	1880–87	W T Evans
	1887–19[14]	P J Michelli (1853–1935)†
Assistant Secretary:	1880–82	P J Michelli (1853–1935)†
	1882–1906	Walter Adams (?–1905)
	1906–08	D G Buckle
Chaplain:	18[70]–70	J J W Harris
	1870–76	W F Mothersole
	1876–80	Francis Tofts
	1880–82	H de Castro Collyer
	1882–99	H T Heffell
	1899–1900	Brooke Lambert (Vicar of Greenwich)
	1901–?	S M Bardsley

Table 15.1 – *continued*

Treasurer:	18[70]–81	H S Thornton, FRS
	1881–1901	J Deacon
	1901–[14]	Col R Williams
Matron:	1871–74	Miss T U Collins
	1874–82	Mrs M Brown
	1882–95	Miss A G Cooke
	1885–19[14]	Miss A M Hall MBE
Collector/Visiting Agent:	18[70]–74	Henry Swift
	1874–78	A C Stopford
	1878–80	R S Bunnett
	1880–96	Walter Adams
	1896–19[14]	G H Hamilton
Collector/Agent for Ships & Shipping/ Secretary to Shipping Department:	1874–75	F M Sims
	1875–77	F M Balfour & E Worthington
	1877–19[14]	E Worthington
Dispenser/and Electrician:	1881–82	C E Davies
	1882–86	H Puntan
	1886–1908	T Hart

*See also Chapter 12; +KCB 1897, KCVO 1907; †Knighted 1921.

MOORE

Mr Joseph Moore (*see* Figure 15.1) was elected to that office on 26 June 1874, having already served on the Committee for six years. After presiding for twelve years, he too resigned 'in consequence of increasing years' in 1886. Moore died in 1889.[2]

CLEEVE

Mr (later Sir) Frederick Cleeve RN KCB who had experienced distinguished service in the Royal Navy, was elected Chairman in 1886, having served on the Committee since 1871; however, he resigned on 12 July 1889, having served for eighteen years. Cleeve was especially involved in the foundation of the ADH in 1890, and also in the 'establishment of the Dispensaries at the London Docks and Gravesend'. Overall, he had been connected with the Society for 34 years, when he died in 1905.[3]

Table 15.2: Medical and surgical staff of the *Dreadnought* (1870–1914).

Physicians:

Name:	*Visiting Physician:*[+]	*Consulting Physician:*
G Budd, FRS (1808–82)	–	18[70]–80*
R Barnes (1817–1907)	18[70]–70	1882–1904*
S H Ward (1819–80)	18[70]–75	1875–80*
J H Jackson, FRS (1835–1911)	18[70]–71*	–
R E Thompson (1834–1912)	1871–73	–
C H Ralfe (1842–96)	1873–80*	–
H Leach (1836–79)	1875–79	–
J Curnow (1846–1902)	1879–99	–
R E Carrington (1853–87)	1880–86	–
(Sir) R Quain FRS (1816–98)[†]	–	1882–96
H T Griffiths (1853–1905)	1886–88	–
J Anderson (1840–1910)	1888–99	–
Dermatologist:		
(Sir) Malcolm Morris (FRCSE)[‡] (1849–1924)	–	
Electrical Department:		
S Barker	19?–09	–
A H Pirie	1909–11	–
W Stewart	1911–?	–

Surgeons:

Name:	*Assistant Surgeon:*	*Surgeon:*	*Visiting/ Consulting Surgeon:*[§]	*Consulting Surgeon:*
G Busk, FRS (1807–86)*	–	1839–18?	1854–	18[70]–86
W J Smith (1840–1912)*	18[70]–70	1871–81	–	1905–1912
HTL Rooke (1824–70)*	–	18[70]–70	–	–
R Rendle (18?–1907)	–	–	1873–74	–
J N C Davies-Colley (1842–1900)	–	–	1874–80	1886–1900
(Sir) G R Turner (1855–1941)	–	–	1881–99	–
W Turner (1870–1944)	–	–	1895–1934	1934–44
Surgeon to Out-patients:				
J B Christopherson (1868–1955)				
Ophthalmic Surgeons:				
DS Gunn (1862–1939)	1891–1899			
L V Cargill (1866–1955)	1899–19[14]			
Dental Surgeon:				
J Warburton Brown	1901–1902			

*See also Chapter 12.

[+]After 1891, this title was changed to physician.

[†]Physician Extraordinary to Queen Victoria (from 1889); created baronet on 10 February 1891.

[‡]Appointed KCVO in 1908.

[§]After 1891, the term Surgeon was usually applied to this category.

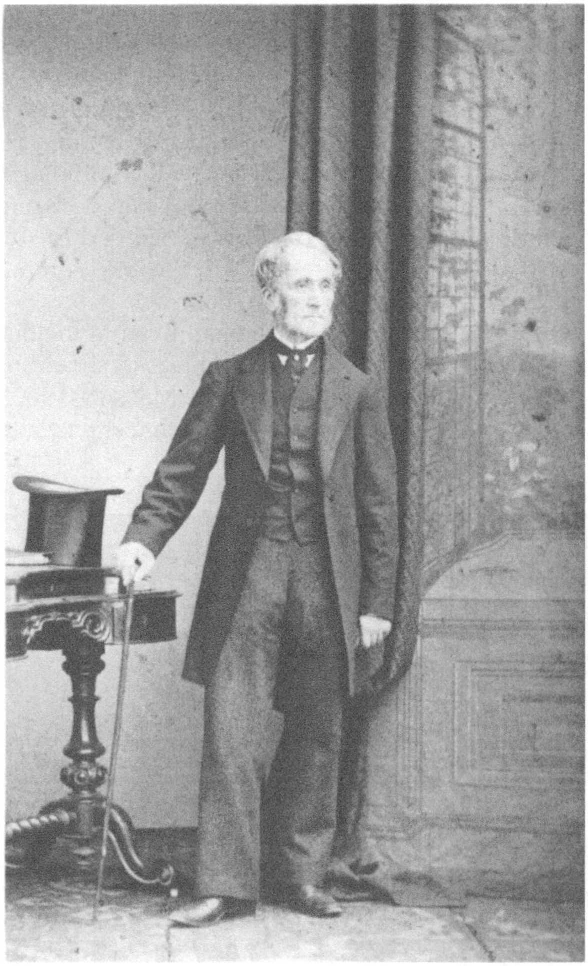

Figure 15.1: Joseph Moore, Chairman of the SHS Committee of Management (1874–86). [SHS Archive.]

EGERTON

Admiral the Hon Francis Egerton took over the Chairmanship (having 'acceded to the unanimous request of his colleagues') in 1889, having already been a member of the Committee for ten years. He had in fact initially joined the Committee in 1866, but shortly afterwards was 'ordered [away] on active service'. He was to die in office on 15 December 1895 (i.e. after six years as Chairman).[4]

NAIRNE

A two-year 'interregnum' in the Chairmanship followed, during which time the Committee of Management meetings were chaired by the Deputy-Chairman – P A Nairne.

P A (later Sir Perceval) Nairne (1841–1921) (*see* Figure 15.2) was Chairman from 1898–1921. The fifth son of Captain Alexander Nairne, RN (1785–1866), a distinguished naval officer (he had served in the battle of Copenhagen) who himself had been a member of the Committee of Management from 1836–66), he was educated at Clapham Grammar School, and subsequently became a Solicitor. In 1864 Nairne was admitted into a firm (W & R Baker) which ultimately became Baker and Nairne. He was a 'survivor' from the hospital-ship days, and thus presided over the *expanding* Society. When the LSTM was founded (in 1899), Nairne also became Chairman of the School Committee. He became a prominent freemason, being Worshipful Master of his Lodge on two occasions.

The Camberwell Borough Council (Nairne had lived in the district for most of his life) apparently decided, after his death, that a road should be named Nairne Grove. He died on 10 December 1921. According to Manson-Bahr, Nairne, who was a very conservative man, was 'a staunch, modest, almost retiring figure, wise and steadfast in council'. He was also a keen yachtsman.[5]

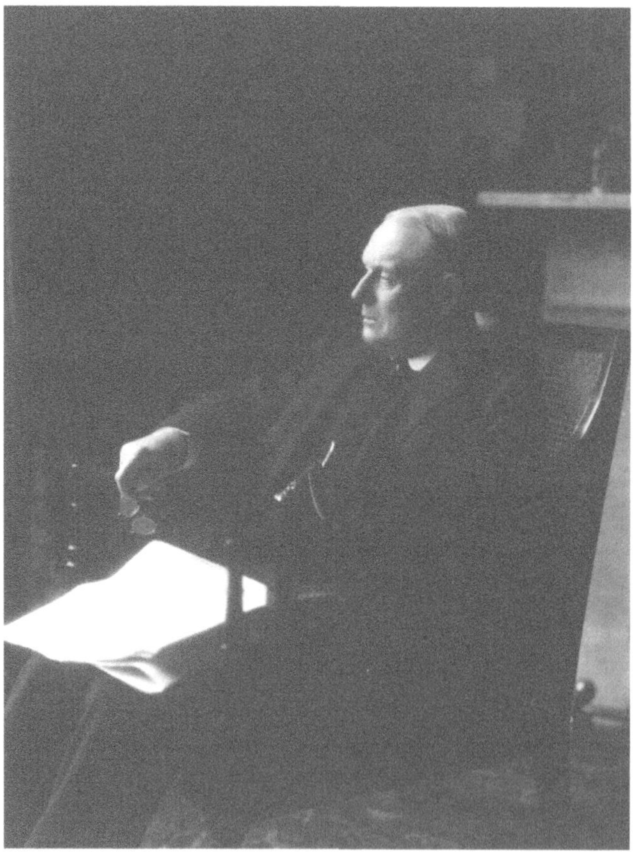

Figure 15.2: P A (later Sir Perceval) Nairne (1841–1921), Chairman of the SHS Committee of Management (1898–1921), and Chairman of the LSTM Committee (1899–1921). [SHS archive.]

Secretaries

This era was dominated by two great Hospital Secretaries; They were: H C (later Sir Henry) Burdett KCB KCVO (1897–1920) and P J (later Sir James) Michelli CMG (1853–1935); while the former was Secretary for only a relatively brief period (six years), the latter retained that position for forty years – from 1887 until 1927; he was also Secretary of the LSTM from its foundation in 1899 until 1924 – when it ceased to come under the auspices of the SHS. The term House Governor, added in 1870, was abandoned after Kemball Cook's death in 1874.

BURDETT

Burdett (*see* Figure 15.3) was arguably the greatest of the Society's secretaries, despite the fact that he held that position for a mere six years. At the 1881 Annual General Meeting, the First Lord of the Admiralty, Lord Northcliffe, presented

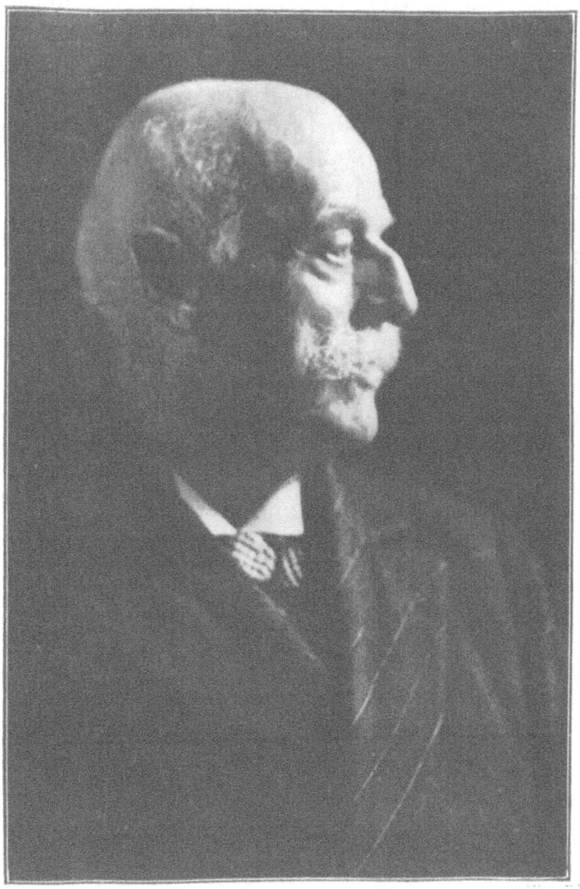

Figure 15.3: H C (later Sir Henry) Burdett (1847–1920), Secretary of the Society (1874–80). [Courtesy, Wellcome Library, London.]

him with a 'beautifully illuminated address' to mark his valuable services during the previous six years and the 'advances made in the administration during his period of office'. His work was *not*, Northcliffe emphasised, 'confined' to the *Dreadnought* (Seamen's) Hospital, for he had also 'organised the Home Hospital movement, produced the standard work on the Cottage Hospital, served as a Special Commissioner of the *Sanitary Record*, and contributed valuable papers to the *Transactions* of the Sanitary Institute'; simultaneously he had completed medical education (in Birmingham and London) necessary for a qualification in medicine.

Later that year, the honorary medical and resident officers of the *Dreadnought* presented Burdett with a carved oak library table as a mark of esteem, and in recognition of 'their appreciation of his successful labours during the period he [had] had the management of Greenwich Hospital'. Regarding Burdett's philanthropic endeavours, the Prince of Wales (later King Edward VII) (1841–1910) considered: ' … for what Mr Burdett has done for the great charitable institutions of this country, his name will always go down to posterity, and will remain as at present a household word'. Before he joined the Society in 1874 (he was elected as Secretary on 25 September 1874), Burdett had served for six years as Secretary of the Queen's Hospital, Birmingham, and after his resignation from the Society in 1880, he became Secretary to the Share and Loan Department of the London Stock Exchange, where he remained for 17 years (until 1897).

Burdett had shrewd financial and managerial skills – which made him extremely valuable to the Society. He was also a great hospital administrator and believed passionately in the value of the Voluntary Hospital system (and its charitable background), and was author of numerous books, including *Burdett's Official Intelligence* and *Burdett's Hospitals and Charities*. He also wrote a massive four-volume work, *The Hospitals and Asylums of the World*. He was founder and editor of the weekly journal *The Hospital*. He was also a pioneer of nurse-training and founded the (Royal) National Pension Fund for Nurses. Burdett was also one of the originators of the Hospital Sunday Fund. He also founded the *Home Hospitals Association*, the *Hospitals Association* (later the *British Hospitals Association)*, The League of Mercy, and the King Edward VII Fund for London. He was a champion of the Cottage Hospital. Burdett died of 'heart failure' at his home in Porchester Square, London on 29 April 1920.[6]

MICHELLI

P J (later Sir James) Michelli CMG (1853–1935) (Figure 15.4) served the Society for a total of 57 years. He had been appointed Steward of the *Dreadnought* Hospital in 1878, and was its Secretary from 1887 until 1927, and later its Treasurer. From 1899 until 1924, when he handed the post over to the Governing Body of the LSHTM, he was also Secretary of the LSTM. He was, according to P H Manson-Bahr, 'a loveable, ingenuous, noble-hearted and loquacious Irishman'. Michelli was also President of the Hospital Officers' Association (1905–6), and of the Hospital Officers' Club (1906–9). He died on 3 April 1935. A bed in the *Dreadnought* Hospital was later named after him.[7]

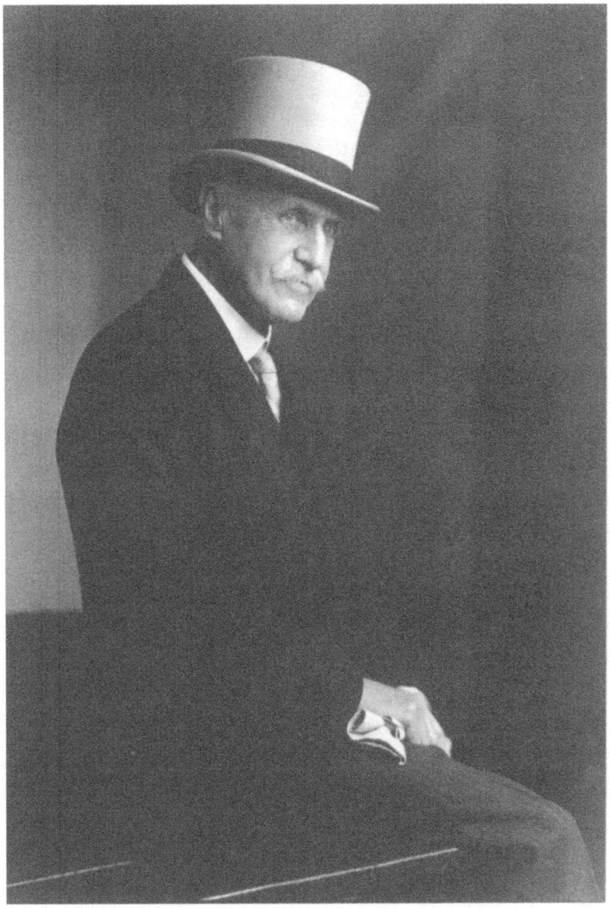

Figure 15.4: P J (later Sir James) Michelli (1853–1935), Secretary of the Society (1887–1927) and Secretary of the LSTM (1899–1924). [Courtesy, Wellcome Library, London.]

TRACEY

Another highly influential member of the Board of Management during this period was Admiral Sir Richard Tracey KCB (1837–1907). He served as Deputy-Chairman between 1901 and 1907. He later became President of the Royal Naval College, Greenwich.[8]

Medical staff

Table 15.2 summarises the medical staff, ie before the expansion necessitated by the formation of the LSTM and the LSCM, in 1899 and 1905, respectively.

Physicians

THOMPSON

Reginald Edward Thompson FRCP (1834–1912) was a Visiting Physician to the *Dreadnought* Hospital from 1871 until 1873. Educated at Brighton College, Trinity College, Cambridge, and St George's Hospital, London, he graduated MB Cantab in 1860 and MD in 1863. In 1862 he passed the MRCP, and was elected FRCP in 1868. The year after graduation, he accompanied Viscount Milton on a shooting expedition to the 'far Canadian North-West', where there were 'herds of buffalo and unsubdued tribes of Indians ... still in possession of the prairies of Alberta and Saskatchewan'. This incidentally led to a further expedition (led by Milton and Dr W B Cheadle) which was apparently instrumental to 'the inception and construction of the Canadian Pacific Railway'.

Back at St George's (as a medical registrar) he dealt with numerous patients suffering from typhus (Chapter 11); having contracted the infection himself, he reported his own illness in the *St George's Hospital Reports* for 1866. The following year he wrote about typhoid fever, and described the differences between these two infections. In 1869, he wrote on rheumatic pericarditis; in the same year he was elected Assistant Physician, and in 1880 Full Physician to the Brompton Hospital for Consumption – on retirement, in 1894, becoming Consulting Physician. He wrote on the occurrence of phthisis in families based on cases under his care at the Brompton Hospital, and which was published in '*Family Phthisis*'. He was also Secretary and Vice President of the Royal Medical and Chirurgical Society. In November 1911 he suffered an intra-cranial vascular episode, and died on 10 September 1912. He had married a daughter of Professor Augustus de Morgan (a mathematician) in 1874, and there were two sons of the marriage.[9]

RALFE

Charles Henry Ralfe FRCP (1842–96) served as a Visiting Physician to the *Dreadnought* Hospital from 1873 until 1880. Born in India, and following the death of his father (who was killed in action at Fort Sauger), he became a pupil at the Bath United Hospital, later removing to King's College London, and obtaining the MRCS in 1863. His first appointment was as House Surgeon to the Female Lock Hospital, and in late 1863 he entered Gonville and Caius College, graduating in natural science with honours, and ultimately obtaining an MD. Following a spell in general practice in Doncaster, he moved to London, settling in Queen Anne Street. He was then employed at the Charing-cross Hospital and published a handbook on Physiological Chemistry in 1873; following this, he became Demonstrator of Physiological Chemistry at St George's Hospital.

At Greenwich, Ralfe apparently made important in-roads into the *chemistry* of scurvy. He was elected FRCP in 1878, and on 2 June 1880, he was appointed Assistant Physician to the London Hospital, and although never a full physician, he was given the title of Consulting Physician on his retirement in May 1896. In 1879 he published a joint report on 'Pyaemia, Septicaemia, and Purulent Infection'. He also wrote a 600 page text on '*Diseases of the Kidney*'. For many years, he was on the staff of *The Lancet*. He had 'shown a tendency to glycosuria, that increasing scourge of modern life', for some years, and this was later complicated by 'a severe outbreak of carbuncles and boils'. About 18 months before his death, Ralfe developed pulmonary tuberculosis, and despite moving (after premature retirement) to the fresh air of the village of Billericay, Essex he died on 26 June 1896. Ralfe had been twice married, his first wife having died in 1873; there were no children.[10]

LEACH

Henry (Harry) Leach MRCP (1836–79): the greater part of Leach's career with the Society – most of it on the third of the Hospital-ships – has been outlined in Chapter 12. In 1873, i.e. when the *clinical* facilities had been land-based for about three years, he resigned from the Society and on 24 July 1873 was appointed first Port Medical Officer (PMO) for the City of London. Although he seems to have retained this position to the time of his death (in 1879) he had returned to the SHS, as Visiting Physician, in 1875.

As PMO, his major task was to preserve the metropolis from potential threats of disease conveyed by the incoming sailors. He was in effect the preventive medicine physician from Teddington Lock to the Nore – some 88 miles! Soon after his appointment, he had 'to guard against a threatening epidemic of cholera'. He also had to deal with an outbreak of scarlatina ('scarlet fever') – in the school-ship *Worcester* – smallpox, typhoid fever (on the reformatory ship *Cornwall* moored off Purfleet), together with the threat of imported yellow fever and plague. These were all major 'challenges' to this newly appointed PMO.

The onerous duties of Port Health Officer in Leach's day have been succinctly summarised by Willoughby in the *SHS Quarterly Magazine;* the two essential facts to be ascertained were: (i) had there been any illness (or deaths) during the voyage of the incoming vessels, and (ii) were all on board in a fit state at that time. All potentially infective cases, e.g. plague and smallpox, were immediately removed to the Port Sanitary Hospital at Denton, while non-infectious (e.g. most 'tropical' and venereal) cases were directed to one of the Society's hospitals.

Leach's terminal illness began in 1875 with an haemoptysis. Despite two spells in South Africa (with his wife) his pulmonary tuberculosis failed to arrest, and he died at his home in Westminster on 26 November 1879 at the age of 43 years.[11]

CURNOW

John Curnow FRCP (1846–1902) was appointed Visiting Physician to the SHS (an appointment which received very little coverage in his obituary notices) in 1879. He had qualified MRCS and MB (London) in 1870 having entered King's College Medical School as a student in 1864; in 1871, he was awarded the MD (with gold medal). A year before, he had been appointed demonstrator in anatomy at King's College, and in 1873, he succeeded to the Chair of Anatomy (a post which he held until 1896); in this year he also passed the MRCP examination. At King's College Hospital, Curnow was successively Assistant Physician (1874), Physician to Outpatients (1882) and full Physician (1890). In 1896, he was elected to the Chair of Clinical Medicine – which he held until his death. Elected FRCP in 1878, he delivered the Goulstonian Lectures to the Royal College of Physicians in 1879. Between 1883 and 1896, Curnow was Dean of the Medical Department at King's College Hospital. For his last 25 years he was on the staff of *The Lancet*.

In 1899, Curnow resigned from the SHS on the grounds that he was opposed to the foundation of the LSTM (by Manson and Chamberlain) at the ADH (*see* Chapter 18); at the *Dreadnought* Hospital, he had 'used the opportunities afforded him ... to become familiar with many of the phases of tropical disease'. George Turner (see below) who also resigned in 1899, recalled these events some 30 years later:

> 'At the time of the institution of the School for Tropical Medicine at the Albert Docks, the committee of the [SHS] made and published their plans without consulting the staff of the Dreadnought. Although they advertised the fact that we were all to teach, the only medical officer who was consulted was one physician [Patrick Manson] not connected with the parent institution, and this was done secretly. I do not want to rake up an old controversy, but as a result of the committee's high-handed proceedings the whole of the medical staff of the Dreadnought resigned [this is in fact an exaggeration], and feeling in the medical profession was for a time so strong that it was difficult to find any one to fill their places.'[12]

Curnow never married; he died suddenly from 'acute pneumonia ... and syncope' at the age of 56 years.[13]

CARRINGTON

Robert Edmund Carrington FRCP (1853–87) was a Visiting Physician to the Society from 1880 until 85. Educated at the King's School, Gloucester, Gloucester Infirmary and Guy's Hospital, he had a brilliant student career. Having passed the MRCS in 1875, he became House-surgeon and resident obstetrician at Guy's; he was then elected demonstrator in anatomy (a post he held from 1877 until 82), and during this appointment he suffered a severe attack of typhoid fever. In 1882 he published a *Manual of Dissections* for students. He passed the MB, followed by the MD London and MRCP examinations in 1878 and 1879 respectively; a year before his premature death, he was elected FRCP. In 1883, having previously served as medical registrar and demonstrator of pathology at Guy's, he was appointed Assistant Physician and head of the Skin Department. The positions at Guy's which he held at the time of his death (he died '... suddenly and unexpectedly' on 16 March 1887 from 'double pleuro-pneumonia, possibly resulting from septicaemia acquired whilst ... performing a post-mortem examination') were: Senior Assistant-Physician, Senior Demonstrator of Pathology, Curator of the Museum, editor of the *Guy's Hospital Reports*, and Sub-dean of the Medical School.[14]

QUAIN

(Sir) Richard Quain Bt. FRCP FRS (1816–98) (*see* Figure 15.5) was Consulting Physician to the SHS from 1882–96. Born at Mallow, County Cork, his early education was undertaken at the Diocesan School at Cloyne; for five years he was

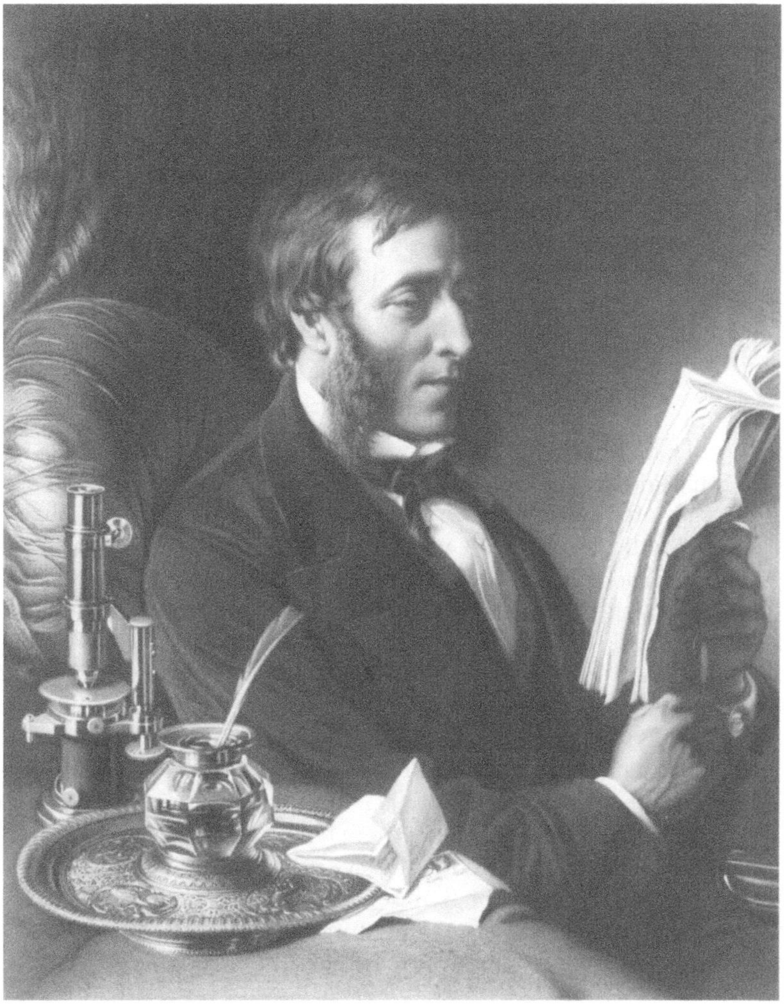

Figure 15.5: (Sir) Richard Quain Bt FRCP FRS (1816–98), Consulting Physician to the Dreadnought (1882–96). [Courtesy, Wellcome Library, London].

apprenticed to a surgeon-apothecary at Limerick. Quain's medical training was at University College Hospital (UCH) London; after graduating MB in 1840, and MD two years later, he held house appointments at UCH, and in 1848 and 1855 he was elected assistant-physician, and full Physician, respectively. In 1875 he was made a Consulting Physician at the Brompton Hospital, and also at Greenwich, and at the Royal Hospital for Consumption at Ventnor. At the RCP, he was Lumleian Lecturer (1872), Senior Censor (1877), Harveian Orator (1885), and Vice-President (1890). He was also president of the Harveian Society (1853) and the Pathological Society (1869), and Chairman of the Pharmacopoeia Committee of the General Medical Council (GMC). From 1891 until his death, Quain was President of Council of the

GMC. He was also a member of the Senate of the University of London. In 1865, he took part in a Royal Commission (chaired by Earl Spencer) on Rinderpest (Cattle Plague). Quain was Editor of the *Dictionary of Medicine* – first published in 1882, with a second edition in 1894.

In 1891 Quain was appointed Physician-Extraordinary to Queen Victoria, and given a baronetcy. His patients included: Millais, Landseer, the Carlyles and Charles Dickens. In 1854 he married Isabella Agnes (only daughter of Captain George Wray of the Bengal Army); they had four daughters. A year or so before he died, he suffered from a malignant disease (unspecified) which necessitated several surgical operations. He died at his house in Harley Street on 13 March 1898 after an illness lasting one year.[15]

GRIFFITHS

Herbert Tyrrell Griffiths (1853–1905) was a Visiting Physician to the SHS from 1886 until 1888. Educated at Eton, Trinity College, Cambridge and St George's Hospital, London, he graduated MA and MD, in 1879 and 84 respectively. In 1881 he 'passed ... into the Indian Medical Service'; he was Herbert Exhibitioner and Martin Medallist at the Army Medical School, Netley. Shortly after arriving in India however, he found the life 'uncongenial to him' and resigned his commission. Following this, he was successively House-Physician and Medical Registrar at St George's Hospital, Physician's Assistant at the Brompton Hospital for Consumption, and Clinical Assistant to the Central Throat Hospital; he was also Surgeon to the Kensington Dispensary. He then entered General Practice (although many felt that a 'career as a Consultant Physician was virtually guaranteed') and served most of his subsequent career in Kensington Square; in early 1905, he moved (following retirement from medical practice) to Preston Candover where he died on 3 November from pleuropneumonia. Griffiths had married a daughter of Sir Richard Garth, and had three children. He resigned from his SHS appointment in 1888, after he had suggested that the Honorary Staff of the Society should receive a 'pecuniary Honorarium'; furthermore, he complained that the nursing standards at the *Dreadnought* Hospital were substandard (see also Chapter 17)![16]

ANDERSON

John Anderson FRCP CIE (1840–1910) served as a Visiting Physician to the SHS from 1888 until his resignation, with Curnow, Turner and Gunn, in 1899 when the LSTM opened (see Chapter 18). He received his medical training at St Andrew's University, qualifying with the MRCS (1861) and LSA (1862) diplomas. Following house appointments at the Royal Infirmary, Manchester, he entered the Army Medical Service in 1864; he subsequently served in India with the Royal Artillery; and on return to England, he underwent further studies at Edinburgh University and the Royal Military College, Camberley. In 1880, he returned to India as personal physician to the Marquis of Ripon - who subsequently became Viceroy. On retirement from the Army, he was appointed to the SHS and King Edward's Hospital for Officers; he also became a lecturer on tropical diseases at St Mary's Hospital, Paddington. Some seven months before his death, he 'was attacked ... with a grave form of paralysis (right-sided hemiplegia and aphasia – presumably a thrombotic stroke – from which he never recovered …'. Anderson married and had four children.[17]

MORRIS

(Sir) Malcolm Alexander Morris KCVO (1849–1924) (*see* Figure 15.6). Educated at St Mary's Hospital, London, Berlin and Vienna, Morris was the first dermatologist to be appointed to the Society's staff. As well as serving the SHS, he was surgeon to the Skin Department at St Mary's Hospital, London. Morris was also Chairman of the Institute of Hygiene and the British Federation of Medical and Ethical Services, and Vice-President of the National Council for Combating Venereal Diseases. Morris was a senior figure in the dermatology and venereal disease world.[18]

Surgeons

SMITH

William Johnson Smith FRCS (1840–1912). Smith's early days with the Society (on the last of the Hospital-ships) have been related in Chapter 12. Following removal to land, he was to play a major role in the surgical activities of the SHS. He was Principal Medical Officer (PMO) from 1873 until 1904 (when he retired), his immediate predecessors in this post being H T L Rooke (who had occupied the

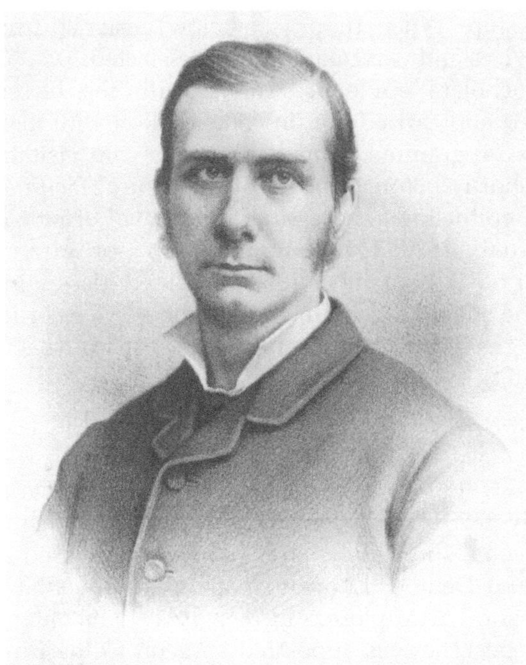

Figure 15.6: (Sir) Malcolm Morris (18?–1924) – first dermatologist to the *Dreadnought*. [Courtesy, Wellcome Library, London.]

post for 11 years (1859–70) followed by Harry Leach (from 1870 until he resigned to become Medical Officer to the Port of London in 1873). He was also Surgeon to the ADH. Smith was instrumental in collecting data for successive Medical Reports (from 1870 until 1905); these valuable documents outline the diseases encountered at the *Dreadnought* Hospital and ADH between those dates. He also wrote: '*A medical and surgical help for Shipmasters and Officers in the Merchant Navy: including first aid to the injured*' London: Charles Griffin & Co Ltd 1895: p333. This book went to a second edition in 1900. Smith also contributed a paper on 50 cases of *Hepatic Abscess* managed by the Society between 1870 and 95, and a chapter in Allbutt & Rolleston's book – *System of Medicine* 1909. He died at Kenley, Surrey on 26 November 1912.[19]

ROOKE

Henry Turner Lane Rooke (1824–70) was a surgeon to the SHS during the crucial period of removal from the last of the hospital-ships to dry land. He had been a student at King's College, London (in 1846 he obtained the MRCS and LSA) and graduated from Edinburgh University with an MD in 1848. In September 1848, Rooke was appointed junior medical officer to the *Dreadnought* hospital-ship (under Busk, whom he succeeded in 1854). However, shortly after taking up this appointment he took part in the Crimean War (1854–6) as a surgeon on the civil medical staff (thus resigning his SHS appointment). After the conclusion of hostilities, he returned to Britain, took a short course at the Dublin Rotunda, and entered general practice at Wisbech, Cambridgeshire. When Tudor (see below) resigned from the Society he again offered his services and was unanimously re-elected.

During the 1866 cholera epidemic, Rooke, with the blessing of the SHS Committee, organised and carried out (in collaboration with his colleague Harry Leach – see above) a programme of medical ship-to-ship visitations on the river Thames. However, shortly before removal of the clinical facilities to dry-land he developed a lingual epithelioma, necessitating removal of part of his tongue by James Paget in February 1870. This tumour rapidly spread and he died at the *Dreadnought* hospital on 17 September 1870. A stained glass window was subsequently erected in the chapel to 'commemorate the services of *Dr Rooke* and [his colleague] *Mr Harry Leach*, who had been for a great many years Members of the Hospital medical staff …'.[20]

RENDLE

Richard Rendle FRCS (?–1907) was a Visiting Surgeon at the *Dreadnought* hospital for a brief period only, 1873–4. He received his medical training (and subsequently became a house-surgeon, surgical registrar (where he 'devised an inhaler' – *see: Lancet* 1871: i: 634) and Demonstrator of Anatomy at Guy's Hospital and qualified with the MRCS and LSA diplomas in 1868; in 1871 he obtained the FRCS. In addition to his SHS post, he was appointed surgeon to the Royal Infirmary for Women and Children, Waterloo Road, and RMO at the Brompton Hospital for Consumption. Following his resignation, he 'took medical charge of an emigrant ship bound for Queensland, Australia'. There, he remained and became Medical

Officer to the Lying-in Hospital and Hospital for Children as well as Health Officer for Brisbane and RMO of the Government Hospital, Freemantle. Rendle later practised at Taringa, near Brisbane. He died at Kingaroy (Taringa), Queensland on 10 August 1907.[21]

DAVIES-COLLEY

John Neville Colley Davies-Colley (formerly John Neville Colley Davies) FRCS (1842–1900) served the Society well; he was a Visiting Surgeon from 1874–80, and subsequently Consulting Surgeon (1886–1900). Davies was educated at King's College School, London, and Trinity College, Cambridge (where he was a pensioner and later a scholar). In 1864 he graduated BA (and in the same year entered Guy's Hospital), afterwards becoming a Fellow of both Trinity and St Catherine's Colleges. In 1868 he obtained an MB (Cantab), and MA in 1867. He was appointed Surgical Registrar and Tutor at Guy's; following this he became Lecturer on Experimental Philosophy and Demonstrator of Anatomy. In 1872, Davies-Colley was appointed Assistant Surgeon at Guys, and in 1880 full Surgeon; there he adopted Listerian principles. He was an examiner in anatomy and surgery for both the RCS and Cambridge University. As a young man he was a good athlete and oarsman. Davies-Colley married the daughter of Thomas Turner, Treasurer of Guy's; two sons also obtained the FRCS diploma, whilst their daughter became the first female Fellow of the RCS. In November 1899, 'cancer of the liver' was diagnosed but he 'continued imperturbably at his work'. He died at his country house in Pulborough, Sussex on 6 May 1900. [22]

TURNER (GEORGE)

(Sir) George Robertson Turner KBE, FRCS (1855–1941) was a Visiting Surgeon to the *Dreadnought* from 1880 until 1899, when together with Curnow, Anderson and Gunn he resigned (see Chapter 18). He received his medical training at St George's Hospital, London; during his younger days, he was an accomplished athlete, having played rugby football for England against Scotland in 1876. After qualification in 1877 (with the MRCS and LSA diplomas), he obtained the FRCS in 1880. Turner lectured on anatomy and surgery at St George's and after his resignation from the SHS became a Full Surgeon at that hospital, having been elected Assistant Surgeon in 1887. Later, at the onset of the Great War (1914–1918) he was appointed Consultant to the Admiralty with the (temporary) rank of Surgeon Rear-Admiral; he received a CB and KBE in 1917 and 1919 respectively, for his services at the naval hospitals at Chatham and Plymouth. Following the Gallipoli (see also Chapter 20) evacuation, he sailed to Malta to assist in the repatriation of 700 wounded soldiers. Turner wrote an autobiography (*Unorthodox Reminiscences*; London: John Murray, 1931), and also *Mary Stuart – Forgotten Forgeries* 1933. Turner married and had five children.[23]

TURNER (WILLIAM)

William Turner FRCS (1870–1944). When Johnson Smith transferred from the *Dreadnought* to be a Consulting Surgeon at the ADH (in 1895), William Turner was added to the consultant staff. After education at King's College School, King's College London, and King's College Hospital – where he was a pupil of Lord Lister – Turner qualified (MRCS) in 1893. At his teaching hospital he served as House Surgeon, House Physician, Demonstrator of Anatomy, and Surgical Registrar; following this he served for a short time on the MAB's smallpox ships. Although appointed, in August 1897, Assistant Physician to Westminster Hospital, he soon afterwards volunteered for active service in South Africa with the Imperial Yeomanry, where he was surgeon at the base hospital at Deelfontein (1900), and Medical Officer in charge of the Branch Hospital at McKenzies Farm (1900–1). Back at the Westminster Hospital, he was surgeon and lecturer in clinical surgery, and subsequently held the post of Senior Surgeon for eleven years. During the Great War (1914–18), Turner served at the 4th London General Hospital with the temporary rank of Major, RAMC. He was also on the staff of King George Hospital for Officers, the 22nd American Red Cross Hospital, and Mrs Mitchison's Hospital at Clock House, Chelsea. On his retirement (in 1934) he was elected Consulting Surgeon and Vice-President of the Westminster Hospital. As well as being Consulting Surgeon to the *Dreadnought* (he had been Visiting Surgeon from 1895 to 1934) he was also Consulting Surgeon to King Edward Memorial Hospital, Ealing; the Royal Hospital for Diseases of the Chest, Maidenhead Hospital, and the London Brighton and South Coast Railway. In 1904, Turner married Lily, only daughter of J K Hamilton of Tavistock; they had one son.[24]

CHRISTOPHERSON

John Brian Christopherson CBE FRCS FRCP (1868–1955) was Surgeon to Outpatients. He qualified from Caius College, Cambridge and St Bartholomew's Medical School in 1893. As well as becoming Surgeon to the *Dreadnought* Hospital, he was Assistant Surgeon to the ADH. He had had considerable experience of tropical medicine (especially schistosomiasis) in the Sudan. He later joined the staff of the London Chest Hospital. Christopherson married the daughter of Joseph Ormerod, physician to Barts.[25]

GUNN

Donald Stilwell Gunn FRCS (1862–1939) was educated at University College London and, after qualification in 1883, he served as an assistant demonstrator of anatomy, and house physician at the Great Northern Hospital. He was later house surgeon at Moorfields, and then surgeon to the Royal Westminster Ophthalmic Hospital, the Sick Children's Hospital and the *Dreadnought* Hospital. He retired in 1902 and, due to failing health, moved to South Africa. During the Great War he was a temporary surgeon in the Royal Navy. He died unmarried in London on 14 March 1939.[26]

CARGILL

Lionel Vernon Cargill FRCS (1866–1955) (see also Chapter 20) was educated at King's College London and became house surgeon to Lord Lister. He was then

Surgical Registrar at the Royal Eye and King's College Hospitals; he was elected assistant surgeon to the former in 1896 and to the latter in 1899, the same year in which he was appointed ophthalmic surgeon to the SHS. Cargill served in both the South African and the Great Wars. He also had many other interests, amongst which was the Mastership of the Society of Apothecaries in 1939-40. Cargill was married and had three daughters.[27]

Staffing the three dispensaries

As recorded in Chapter 14, SHS Dispensaries were opened at Well Street, (later covering the East and West India Docks), and Gravesend. These were usually manned by relatively junior doctors who in most cases stayed for only a year, or so (*see* Table 15.3). However, an exception was Walter Fowler, who after serving for three years at the Well Street Dispensary, was appointed Consulting Surgeon to the East India Dock Road Dispensary; he served in this capacity from 1892 until his death at Bendigo, Australia, in 1917 (see below).

FOWLER

Walter Fowler FRCS (1858–1917) received his medical training at Guy's Hospital – from 1879, until qualification with the MRCS (1883) and LSA (1884) diplomas. Prior to this he had studied at Caius College, Cambridge where he both graduated in the Natural Science Tripos and obtained the Tancred Medical Studentship. After a spell as Obstetric Resident at Guy's, he started practice in Birmingham (in 1885); however, on the death of his father (who practiced in Bishopsgate Street, London, EC) in 1886, he moved to 12 Old Burlington Street and started practice at 36 Finsbury Pavement. In 1889, he was appointed Surgeon to the SHS, and Pathologist to the Central London Throat and Ear Hospital. Probably on account of impending illness, he moved (with his wife and two young children) to Echuca, Victoria, Australia in 1892 – where for nine years he pursued private practice. In 1900, or thereabouts, he was appointed RMO at Bendigo Hospital and became 'one of the leading provincial surgeons' in the state of Victoria.[28]

Table 15.3: Staff of the Society's Dispensaries (1870–[1914]).

Well Street Dispensary	Gravesend Dispensary	East India Dock Road Dispensary
Surgeon:	*Surgeon*:	*Surgeon*:
C E H Cotes (1880–)	O R Richmond (1887–96)	J R Prior (1897–99)
W Fowler (1886–89)	C E Robbs (1896–19[14])	F Morris (1899–1900)
		K Steele (1900–01)
		W H F Oxley (1901–[14])
		Consulting surgeon:
		W Fowler (1889–1917)

Opening of the London School of Tropical Medicine (LSTM) in 1899 (see also: Chapter 18)

Physicians

MANSON

(Sir) Patrick Manson GCMG FRCP FRS (1844–1922) (Figure 15.7). Manson was in fact appointed physician to the ADH (but not the *Dreadnought*) in 1892. After his pioneering work on mosquito-involvement in the transmission of lymphatic filariasis, in Amoy, China, it was his intention to retire to Scotland in 1889 – the country of his birth. In 1883, Manson had moved from Amoy to Hong Kong where as well as developing a large private practice, he had founded the University and Medical School of Hong Kong.

Born at Oldmeldrum, Aberdeenshire and educated at the Gymnasium and West End Academy, Aberdeen, he had entered Aberdeen University in 1860, graduating MB, CM in 1895, and MD a year later. In 1886, he received an honorary LLD from Aberdeen University.

Due to financial losses after return from China, he found it necessary to resume paid employment – in London. Whilst at the ADH, Manson visualised *Plasmodium* spp. (originally demonstrated by Laveran in Algeria in 1880). Extrapolating from

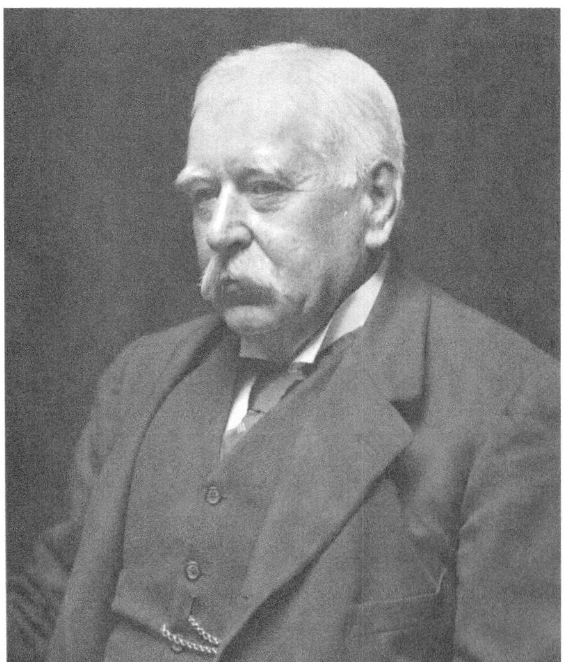

Figure 15.7: (Sir) Patrick Manson FRCP (1844–1922), Consulting Physician to the ADH and 'the father of modern tropical medicine'. [Courtesy, Wellcome Library, London.]

his work on filariasis, in 1896 Manson developed a mosquito-malaria hypothesis; this, propounded in three Goulstonian Lectures to the Royal College of Physicians, undoubtedly influenced Ronald Ross (1857–1932) in his research in India in 1897–8.

In London, Manson also began giving public lectures on tropical disease, and published widely on *tropical medicine* – culminating, in 1898, in his classical work: *Tropical Disease: a manual of diseases of warm climates*. In addition to his ADH appointment, Manson was appointed physician and medical adviser to the Colonial Office (in 1897); it was here that he established a close liaison with the Secretary of State for the Colonies – the Rt Hon Joseph Chamberlain (1836–1914) who was at that time embarking on a scheme to boost medical care for British expatriates in the tropics – especially in West Africa.

It was largely due to Manson's influence that (i) the LSTM was founded at the ADH, and (ii) that several physicians and surgeons with intimate knowledge of *tropical medicine* were appointed to its staff (*see* Chapter 18). He was later to take a leading role in the foundation of the LSCM in 1906 (*see* Chapter 19). Manson finally retired in 1912 and died on 9 April 1922. He had married Henrietta Isabella, second daughter of Captain Ptolemy Thurburn RN in 1875; they had three sons and three daughters.[29]

Establishment of the LSTM obviously necessitated expanding the staff of the ADH (most of whom were expected to teach) and the following were appointed. Table 15.4 summarises medical staffing of the ADH – *after* the LSTM opened in 1899.

HEWLETT

Richard Tanner Hewlett FRCP (1865–1940) was a Visiting Physician to the Society from 1899–1908. He had qualified MRCS in 1889, and graduated MB in 1890, and MD in 1892. After house-appointments at his teaching hospital (King's College) he served there for three years (1891–4) as Demonstrator in Bacteriology. He then became bacteriologist to the Jenner (later Lister) Institute of Preventive Medicine, and from 1901–25 occupied the Chair of Bacteriology at King's. With the SHS, Hewlett became Physician (1899), Director of Pathology (1908) and ultimately Consulting Pathologist. Throughout these years, however, he apparently 'kept in touch with the clinical side of medicine'. At the LSTM, Hewlett lectured (for > 30 years) on bacteriology, and in the Great War (1914–18) also acted as pathologist to the Richmond War Hospital. He was extremely interested in the application of bacteriology to hygiene and public health. Hewlett was twice married; and had three sons and two daughters from the first, and three sons from the second. Latterly, he was 'burdened with a painful affliction' and died at Greenwich on 10 September 1940.[30]

DUNCAN

Andrew Duncan FRCP FRCS (1850–1912) was a Visiting Physician to the Society from 1899 until his death in 1907. Educated at Cholmeley School, Highgate and King's College, London (where he was apparently an outstanding student); he qualified with the MB (Lond) from King's College Hospital (in 1874). Following this, he held junior appointments at his teaching hospital, Charing Cross, St Mary's, the

Table 15.4: Staff of the Albert Dock Hospital (ADH) (1890–19[14]).*†

Physicians:	
P Manson	1892–1907 (Consulting Physician, from 1912)
R T Hewlett	1899–1908 (Director of Pathology, from 1908)
A Duncan	1899–1907
G Rankin	1899–19[14]
F M Sandwith	1912–[14]
C W Daniels	1912–[14]
Surgeons:	
W J Smith	1895–1902 (Consulting Surgeon, from 1901)
W Turner	1896–19[14]
J Cantlie	1899–1906
J B Christopherson	1899–1902
L H McGavin	1902–[14]
A Evans	1902–06
C C Choyce	1905–1919
Ophthalmic Surgeon:	
D S Gunn	1898–99
Dental Surgeon:	
K W Goadby	1901

Stanhope Street Dispensary and the *Dreadnought* Hospital, Greenwich. He obtained the MD (Lond) in 1875. Duncan also studied at Vienna, Strasbourg and Berlin, and passed the FRCS examination in 1877. A year later, he entered the Bengal Medical Service (IMS) as a surgeon; he won the Parkes Medal at the Army Medical School, Netley, in 1885. He was involved in the Afghan War (1878–80) under Lord Roberts and was seriously wounded at Charasiab. Duncan also served in the Hazara campaign (1891). He received none of the civil appointments normally granted to promising IMS Officers – probably due to a paper he had written in 1885 – *'The Unsanitary Tendencies of the State Sanitation'* in which he 'censured the chief sanitary officers of India'; this appeared in book format in 1888 as: *'The prevention of disease in tropical and sub-tropical campaigns'* – London: J & A Churchill: 396.

Duncan retired (with the rank of Lieutenant-Colonel) on 1 February 1900 ('much damaged in strength and constitution'), settled in London and was elected to the staff of the ADH, and the Westminster and Western General Dispensaries; he was a lecturer on tropical medicine at the LSTM and the Westminster Hospital. For many

*In 1899, the Medical Staffs of the *Dreadnought* and Albert Dock (many appointed to boost the teaching staff of the LSTM) Hospitals amalgamated, i.e. following the resignation of J Curnow, J Anderson, G R Turner and D S Gunn.

†From 1900, the *Academic* staff of the LSTM were listed separately.

years, he was a collaborator on the literary staff of *The Lancet*. In 1908, Duncan published: '*A Guide to Sick nursing in the Tropics*'. He died after 'a long illness' in London on 17 October 1912. All his obituarists refer to the fact that he should have been far more widely recognised; the fact that he was *not* was largely associated with his forthright approach, and downright opposition to the 'establishment'.[31]

RANKIN

Guthrie Rankin FRCP (1854–1919) was Physician to the *Dreadnought* Hospital between 1899 and 1917, when he resigned and was made a Consulting Physician to the Society. Rankin (a 'kindly Scot') studied medicine at Glasgow University and graduated MB (Glasgow) in 1880; two years later he proceeded to the MD. For 15 years he had been a general practitioner – at Kilmarnock and later Warwick, where he was also Physician to the Dispensary and Cottage Hospital. In addition to his SHS appointment, he was Physician to the Royal Waterloo Hospital for Children and Women; Rankin also lectured on medicine at the LSCM – which he took a prominent part in founding in 1905. Rankin had married in 1883, and died on 14 September 1919 at Helford, Cornwall - his west country home.[32]

Later *medical* additions to the staff of the LSTM were: F M Sandwith and C W Daniels (see below).

Surgeons

CANTLIE

James Cantlie FRCS KBE (1851–1926) (*see* Figure 15.8) was appointed to the ADH in 1899 and held the position of Surgeon there until 1906. Cantlie was born at Dufftown, Banffshire, and educated at Milne's Institution and, like Manson, Aberdeen University; after graduation with honours in natural science in 1871, he proceeded to Charing Cross Hospital, qualifying in medicine in 1873. In 1877 he became Assistant Surgeon at his teaching hospital and obtained the FRCS. In 1887 Cantlie took the diploma in public health and travelled to the Far East, where he was one of the founders of the College of Medicine for Chinese Students at Hong Kong; he served there as Dean for seven years. By his friendship with Sun Yat Sen, a former student and first President of China, he apparently exerted considerable influence over that country. He also took part in the Egyptian Cholera Expedition of 1883. In 1885, he had written: '*The degeneration of Londoners*', in which he deprecated the neglect of physical training and fresh air.

After return to London in 1897, Cantlie became Surgeon to the ADH (see above), and from 1898 was both the inaugurator and first editor (with WJ Simpson) of the *Journal of Tropical Medicine*. From 1885 until 1888 he had commanded the Volunteer Medical staff Corps in London, and became chief surgeon to the Metropolitan Division of the *St John's Ambulance Brigade*; in 1914 he founded the College of Ambulance in London. With Manson and Chamberlain he had a prominent role in the establishment of the LSTM. He was made KBE in 1918. Cantlie married Mabel, daughter of Robert Barclay Brown, and had four sons.[33]

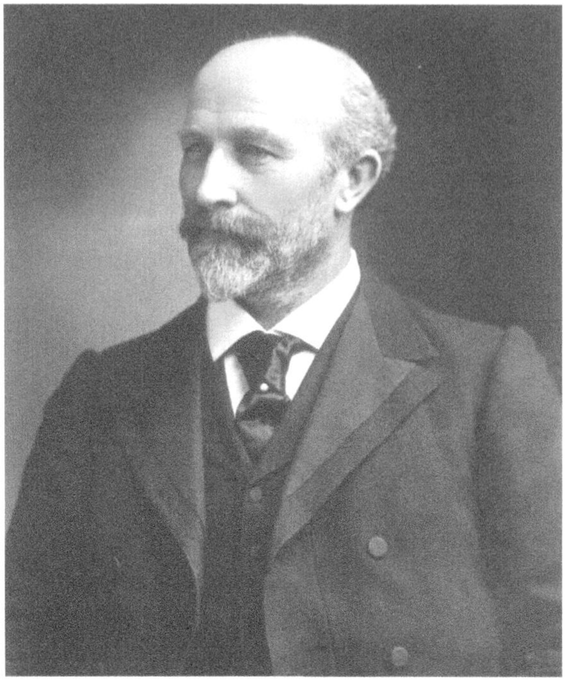

Figure 15.8: (Sir) James Cantlie FRCS (1851–1926), Surgeon to ADH (1899–1906). [Courtesy, Wellcome Library, London].

MCGAVIN

Following the appointment of these three physicians and a surgeon in 1899, there was a brief hiatus – in fact until 1902, when another surgeon was added to the Consultant staff: Lawrie Hugh McGavin FRCS CBE (1868–1932). He was born in Calcutta, educated at Fettes College, Sandhurst and Guy's (from 1893) from which he qualified in 1898. He obtained the FRCS in 1890, and became Surgeon to the Women's Hospital, Soho, and the North-West London Hospital. McGavin was appointed Surgeon to the *Dreadnought* Hospital in 1902, and later became a Consulting Surgeon. During the Great War (1914–18) McGavin was unfit for active service; however, he continued his work in civilian practice. He was Surgeon to King George's Hospital, the Endsleigh Hospital for Officers, as well as the Michie Red Cross Hospital. He married in 1892 and had three daughters.[34]

Later appointments

SANDWITH AND DANIELS

The LSTM was opened in 1899 (see Chapter 18); Manson was to 'mastermind' two further appointments of close colleagues as physicians to the LSTM – Sandwith and Daniels (*see* Table 15.4); however, they were not appointed until 1912.

Fleming Mant Sandwith FRCP CMG (1853–1918) (*see* Figure 15.9) was born at Belgaum, India and educated at Charterhouse and St Thomas's Hospital, London. Following qualification in 1876 (with the MRCS and LRCP diplomas, he was appointed surgeon with the National Aid Society's Ambulance – serving in the Turko-Serbian War; Sandwith undertook similar duties with the Stafford Horse Ambulance during the Turko-Russian War (1877–8). Following a short period in practice at Wandsworth, he travelled to Egypt to 'fight a cholera epidemic' in 1883; there, he subsequently became Vice-Director of the Egyptian Public Health Department, instigated various hospital reforms, served as physician to the Kasr-el-Ainy Hospital in Cairo, and was Professor of Medicine at the Cairo Medical School (1890–1904). During the South African War (1899–1902), he served as Senior Physician to the Imperial Yeomanry Hospital, Pretoria. During 1888, Sandwith wrote a series of articles which were published in the *Lancet* on dengue fever. He also wrote: '*Medical Diseases of Egypt*' and '*Egypt as a Winter Resort*'.

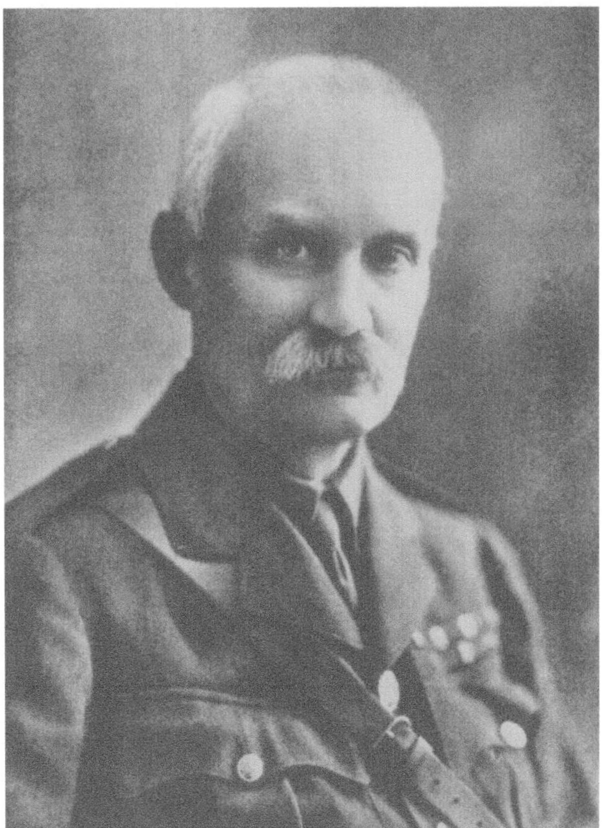

Figure 15.9: Fleming Sandwith FRCP (1853–1918), Physician to ADH (1912–19). [RSHTM Archive].

In 1904, he moved to England and became a lecturer at the LSTM; from 1907 he was also a lecturer at St Thomas's Hospital. In 1912, Sandwith was appointed Physician to the ADH (Manson had then retired to Ireland), but his career there was interrupted by the Great War (1914–18) when he became a Physician to King George's Hospital, and Consulting Physician (with the temporary rank of Colonel) to the East Mediterranean Force. Sandwith subsequently became Senior Physician to the ADH. He was twice married and had two sons and two daughters.[35]

Charles Wilberforce Daniels (1862–1927) (*see* Figure 15.10) had a distinguished tropical career. Educated at Manchester Grammar School and Trinity College, Cambridge, he graduated BA with first-class honours in natural sciences in 1883. He undertook medical training at the (Royal) London Hospital. Following junior appointments at the London, and Queen Charlotte's Lying-in Hospital, he joined the Colonial Medical Service in 1890. He was posted (for four years) to Fiji – where he made careful observations on dysentery. Next came British Guiana, where he impressed Manson with his work on lymphatic filariasis; as a result of this, he was sent by the Royal Society (RS) to confirm (or refute) Ross's claim to have solved the mode of transmission of malaria in 1899.

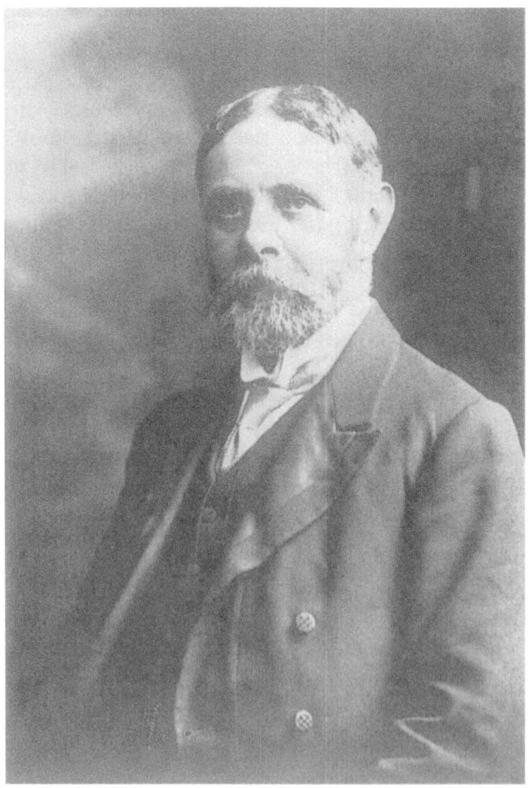

Figure 15.10: Charles Wilberforce Daniels FRCP (1862–1927), Physician to the ADH. [Courtesy, Wellcome Library, London].

After a spell in Nyasaland (now Malawi) as a member of the RS's commission on Blackwater Fever; he returned to England, and became Superintendent of the LSTM. However, in 1903 he was persuaded to take (temporarily) the post of Director of the new Institute of Medical Research at Kuala Lumpur. Back in London, and after a further period at the LSTM, Daniels retired from the Colonial Service and entered private practice. He was appointed Physician to the ADH, and from 1920 the Hospital for Tropical Diseases; he lectured on Tropical Medicine at the London and St George's Hospitals, and the London School of Medicine for Women. In 1912 he succeeded Manson as Medical Advisor to the Colonial Office. Daniels died after a long 'neurological' illness at the ADH on 6 August 1927.[36]

Opening of the London School of Clinical Medicine (LSCM) in 1906 (see also Chapter 19): expansion of the *Dreadnought*'s consultant staff

The implementation of another new initiative (Chapter 19) necessitated a further significant expansion of the Society's staff – both involving patient care and post-graduate teaching. Several of the most eminent London physicians and surgeons were approached. Table 15.5 summarises those who accepted the 'challenge'.

Physicians

DUCKWORTH

Sir Dyce Duckworth Bt FRCP (1840–1928) (*see* Figure 15.11) was appointed physician to the Society in 1905, and continued in that capacity until his death, although he gave up active work in 1917. Educated at the Royal Institution School and the

Table 15.5: Staff of the London School of Clinical Medicine (LSCM) (1905–[4]): additions to the clinical staff.

Physicians:	
Sir Dyce Duckworth Bt	1905–[14]
(Sir) Frederick Taylor	1905–[14]
(Sir) John Rose Bradford Bt	1905–[14]
(Sir) Sydney Russell-Wells	1908–[14]
Surgeons:	
Sir William Bennett	1905–1911(Consulting Surgeon, from 1912)
(Sir) Mayo Robson	1905–06
A Carless	1905–08
A H Evans	1905–07
(Sir) E Rock Carling	1911–[14]
C C Choyce	1912–[14]

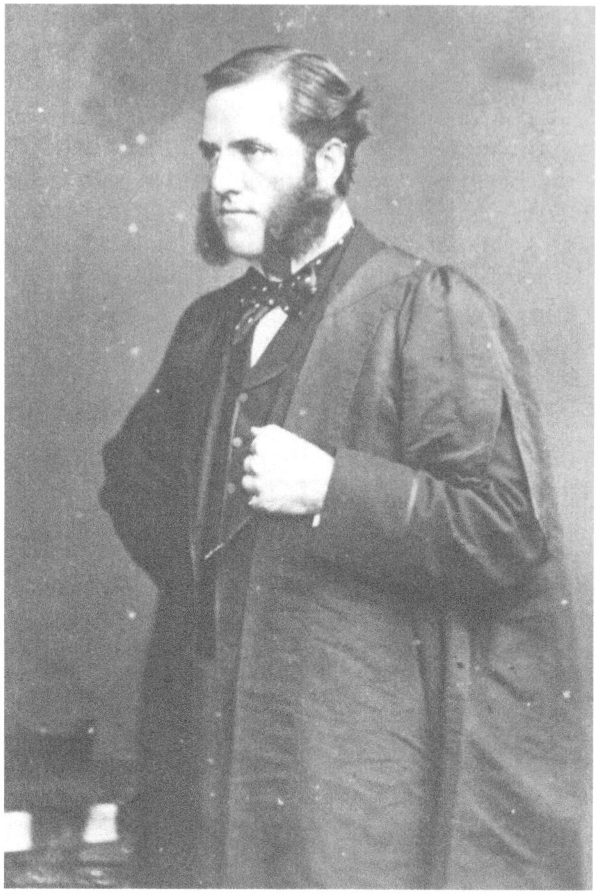

Figure 15.11: Sir Dyce Duckworth Bt FRCP (1840–1928), Physician to the Dreadnought (1905–28). [Courtesy, Wellcome Library, London].

Royal Infirmary Medical School, Liverpool, and Edinburgh University, he qualified in 1862 with the MRCS diploma, and obtained the MD degree with honours the following year. Duckworth served as a resident house physician at the Edinburgh Royal Infirmary, and in 1864 entered the Naval Medical Service (for which throughout his life he apparently 'retained a special affection') as an Assistant Surgeon in which he was posted to Stonehouse Hospital, Devonport; however, after one year, he resigned his commission to become Medical Tutor at St Bartholomew's Hospital, and was appointed Assistant Physician there in 1869.

From 1870 until 1875, Duckworth was in charge of the Skin Department at Bart's. In 1883 he was made a full physician and continued in that capacity until his retirement in 1905, i.e. when he joined the *Dreadnought* staff. At the RCP, he was Lumleian Lecturer (1896), Harveian Orator (1898), Senior Censor (1903), and Treasurer (1884–1823). Having been knighted in 1886, he was created a baronet in 1909, and served as Honorary Physician to HRH The Prince of Wales (later King

Edward VII) from 1890 until 1901. He was said to be an orthodox exponent of the *art* of medicine. He wrote a *Treatise on Gout* in 1889. Throughout his life, he was 'a champion of the nursing profession'. Duckworth was apparently an extreme Tory and a High Church Anglican; he 'opposed in no uncertain terms ... the emancipation of women' (he felt that 'the proper place for them was at home, or at most as nurses'). Duckworth was twice married: from the first he had a son and daughter, and from the second, two sons.[37]

TAYLOR

(Sir) Frederick Taylor Bt FRCP (1847–1920) was educated at Epsom College and Guy's Hospital; he qualified MRCS and MB in 1868, and two years later proceeded to the MD and became a Demonstrator in Anatomy at Guy's. In 1873, he was elected Assistant Physician and, in 1885, Physician. From 1874 until 1884 he was joint editor of the *Reports*, and during that period until 1888 he was Dean of Guy's Medical School. As well as serving on the staff of the SHS, he was physician to the National Hospital for Diseases of the Heart, the Evelina Hospital for Children, and the Royal School for Deaf Children. At the RCP, he was Censor (1904–5), Lumleian Lecturer (1904), Harveian Orator (1907 and 1910), and President (1915–18) in succession to Sir Thomas Barlow; he did not seek re-election in 1918 due to the onset of his (mortal) illness. He was also President of the Royal Society of Medicine. In 1917, he was created a baronet. Taylor was the author of *The Practice of Medicine* (1890) which went to an eleventh (and last) edition in 1918. In 1907 he became Consulting Physician to Guy's. He married in 1884 and had two sons and a daughter.[38]

BRADFORD

(Sir) John Rose Bradford Bt FRCP FRS (1863–1935) (*see* Figure 15.12) was educated at University College School and UCL – where he graduated with a first-class BSc in zoology in 1883; he qualified in medicine from UCH in 1886, and served as a house-physician there. Bradford was elected Assistant Physician (and obtained the MD) in 1889, and held a similar position at the National Hospital for the Paralysed and Epileptic, Queens Square (1893–6). In 1894, he was elected FRS for clinical research (most of which was neuro-physiological). In 1895 until 1903 he was Professor-Superintendent of the Brown Institution, and subsequently Professor of Materia Medica at UCL; he afterwards succeeded to the chair of medicine, and the Holme Lectureship in Clinical Medicine. Bradford was a Full Physician at UCH in 1897. In 1898, he published *Clinical lectures on Nephritis*, and in later years contributed to: Allbutt and Rolleston's *System of Medicine*, and Allchin's *Manual of Medicine*. He then became a full-time administrator: member of the governing body (and chairman) of the Lister Institute (1899–1918), biological secretary to the Royal Society (1908–15), and organiser of a centenary celebration to mark the birth of Lister.

Between 1905 and 1919, Bradford was a Physician to the SHS, and from 1912 to 1924 Senior Medical Advisor to the Colonial Office. He became a close friend of Sir David Bruce (1855–1931) (who had carried out pioneering work on brucellosis and trypanosomiasis), and in 1907 he became a member of the tropical diseases committee of the Royal Society; in 1908, he inaugurated the Sleeping Sickness Bureau

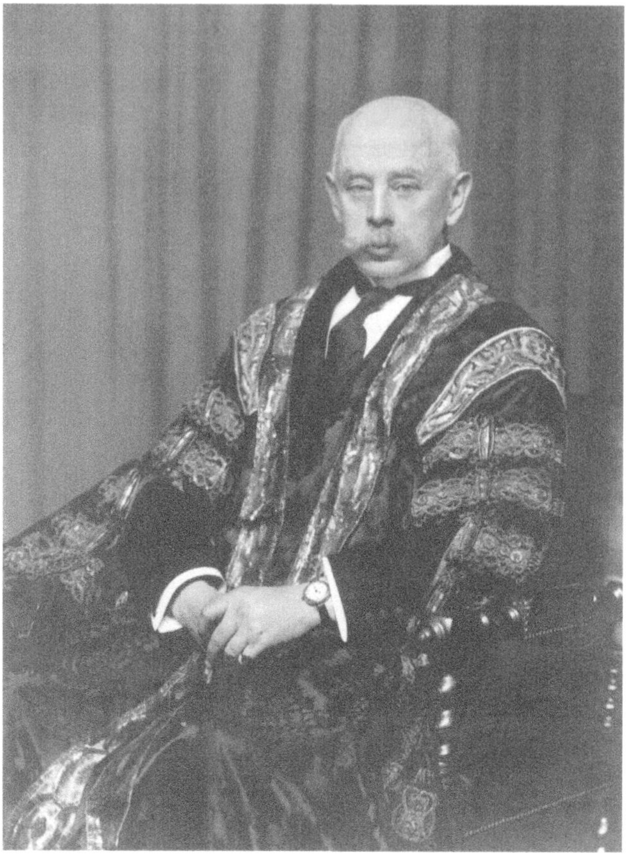

Figure 15.12: Sir John Rose Bradford Bt FRCP (1863–1935), Physician to the *Dreadnought* (1905–1919). [Courtesy, Wellcome Library, London].

– which later became the Tropical Diseases Bureau of the London School of Tropical Medicine. He was also connected with the King Edward VII's Hospital Fund for London, and with the UCL executive committee. Bradford was largely instrumental in establishing the Beit Trust Fellowships.

He stood (unsuccessfully) for the parliamentary seat in the University of London. From 1926 until 1931 he was PRCP; he had previously been Goulstonian (1898), Lumleian (1904), and Harveian (1926) lecturer, and had previously served as Senior Censor. Throughout the Great War (1914–18) Bradford served in France with the British Expeditionary Force as a Major-General in the Army Medical Service. In 1911, he was appointed KCMG, and in 1931 created a baronet. He married in 1899 but did not have children.[39]

RUSSELL-WELLS

(Sir) Sydney Russell-Wells FRCP MP (1869–1924). Originally Sydney Russell Wells, he was educated at the Dorset County School, the Royal College of Science (where he was 'devoted to chemistry') and University College London; he graduated BSc in 1889. After qualification (with honours) in 1893 with the London MB at St George's Hospital, he held several junior appointments there. In 1904 and 1909 he was elected Assistant Physician and Physician, respectively, of the National Hospital for Diseases of the Heart. At the SHS, he was elected to corresponding positions in 1906 and 1908, respectively. Between 1906 and 14, he lectured at the LSCM. At the University of London, Russell-Wells was a member of Senate from 1903 until his death, chairman of council for external students (1908–19) and Vice-Chancellor (1919–22). He was elected to parliament (as a conservative) for the University of London constituency in 1922. Russell-Wells married in 1895, and had a son and two daughters. He died suddenly following a myocardial infarction on 14 July 1924.[40]

Surgeons

BENNETT

(Sir) William Henry Bennett FRCS (1852–1931) (*see* Figure 15.13) was educated privately and at Weymouth College; he entered St George's Hospital in 1869, where he was a founder of the *Student's Journal and Hospital Gazette* in 1873. He obtained

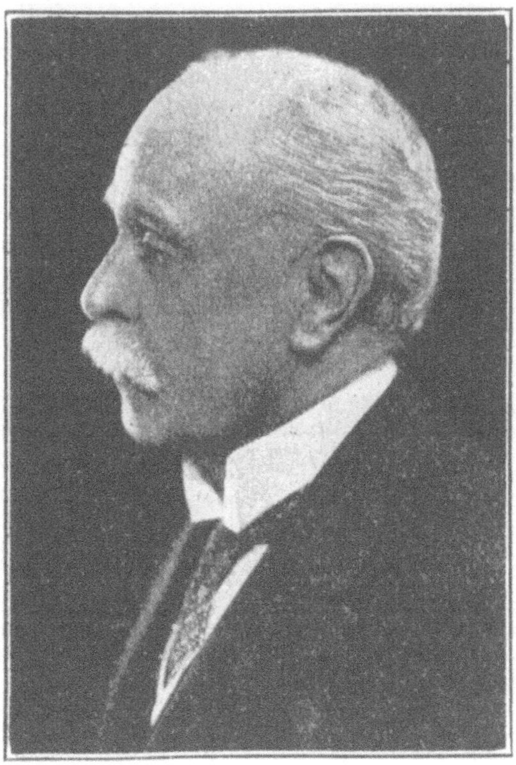

Figure 15.13: Sir William Bennett FRCS (1852–1931), Surgeon to the *Dreadnought* (1905–11). [Courtesy, Royal Society of Medicine].

the FRCS in 1877. In 1880 he was elected Assistant Surgeon to St George's, and Surgeon seven years later – succeeding Timothy Holmes (1825–1907); on retirement in 1905 he was made Consulting Surgeon, Governor, and a member of the House-Committee. He was also surgeon to the SHS, the Hospital of St John and St Elizabeth, the Grosvenor Hospital for Women and Children, and the Belgrave Hospital for Children. At the RCS, Bennett was examiner in anatomy (1884–93), and a member of the Court of Examiners (1897–1902). He undertook services to the sick and wounded on their return from the Boer War. During the Great War (1914–18) he resigned all appointments in order to 'devote his energies to the service of the British Red Cross and the Order of St John'. Bennett was appointed surgeon to King Edward VII Hospital, and was subsequently a Vice-President of the SHS. He walked with a slight limp following poliomyelitis in early life. He was twice married but had no children.[41]

MAYO-ROBSON

(Sir) Arthur William Mayo-Robson FRCS (1853–1933) was educated at Wesley College, Sheffield, and the Leeds School of Medicine where he had a distinguished student career. He qualified (MRCS) in 1874 and was appointed demonstrator of anatomy (at Leeds); between 1876 and 1886 he was a lecturer in that subject. Having passed the FRCS examination in 1879, he was made Assistant Surgeon to the General Infirmary, Leeds, and in 1884 became a Surgeon there; he also held the posts of lecturer in pathology (1886), and teacher of operative surgery (1888). From 1890–99 he was Professor of Surgery at the Yorkshire College, Victoria University (the forerunner of the University of Leeds). In 1902, he moved to London. When the Great War began in 1914, he served in France with a Field Ambulance (he had joined the Territorial Force in 1908 and later organised a hospital for the French army); he later saw service in Gallipoli and Egypt, and had the rank of temporary Colonel, Army Medical Service.

Following the war, Mayo-Robson, who had by now hyphenated his name, became a member of the consultative medical council at the War Office; he was also appointed surgeon to the SHS, and King Edward VII Hospital, Windsor. Mayo-Robson retired from practice and pursued his major recreational activities: travel, fishing and big game shooting (he was accidentally 'shot in both thighs' near Nairobi, Kenya). At the RCS, he was Hunterian Professor of Surgery on three occasions (1897, 1900 and 1904), member of council (1893–1910), Bradshaw lecturer (1904) and Vice-President (1902–3 and 1904–5). He 'had a marked influence on the younger generation of surgeons' (which included [Baron] Moynihan [1865–1936], who was his house-surgeon in 1887–8). He was a prolific author – many of his publications were directed to surgery of the biliary system and pancreas. Early in his career his work had beem mostly gynaecological. Twice married, there were three daughters of his first marriage.[42]

CARLESS

Albert Carless FRCS CBE (1863–1936) was educated at Carrington Lodge, Richmond; King's College School; King's College; and King's College Hospital. He qualified with the MB and BS degrees in 1886 and 1887, and in 1888 obtained the MS and FRCS. After serving as house surgeon at King's College Hospital, he was elected Assistant Surgeon in 1889 – serving under Lord Lister. He was appointed Surgeon in 1898, and from 1902–18 was Professor of Surgery at King's College. During the Great War (1914–18) he had a distinguished career in the Army Medical Service, becoming Consulting Surgeon to Eastern Command. 'The guiding motive of [his] life was [apparently a] deep and abiding interest in evangelical religion'; he was Medical Director of Dr Barnardo's Homes. In 1898 he published a *Manual of Surgery*. Carless married and had two sons – both of whom were killed in action.[43]

EVANS

Arthur Henry Evans FRCS (1872–1950) was educated at Neath Proprietary School and Westminster Hospital – learning biology from HG Wells. He qualified in 1895 with the MRCS, LRCP diplomas, and served as house-surgeon at his teaching hospital, and later at Liverpool. In 1897 he took the MB and BS degrees, and in 1898, the MD; he had obtained the MS degree in 1901. He 'saw active service with the Imperial Yeomanry Field Hospital' in South Africa, where he was taken prisoner. Following the Boer War, Evans was elected Assistant Physician to Westminster Hospital (1902), subsequently becoming a Full Surgeon, and on retirement in 1937 Consulting Surgeon. As a surgeon his interests ranged from orthopaedics to thoracic and thyroid surgery (at the Royal Hospital for Diseases of the Chest). He also served on the staff of the *Dreadnought*, the Royal Masonic Hospital, the London Temperance Hospital (he was a life-long total abstainer), and the Royal Bethlem Hospital. During the Great War, he served (in England) as Captain (RAMC). There were three sons (two became surgeons) of his marriage in 1908. He died on 20 March 1950 after suffering from 'progressive Parkinsonism'.[44]

ROCK CARLING

(Sir) Ernest Rock Carling FRCS (1877–1960) qualified with the London MB, BS with a gold medal in 1901. He served, whilst still a student, with the Imperial Yeomanry Field Hospital in the South African (Boer) War – having entered Westminster Hospital in 1895. Prior to this he had been educated at the Royal Grammar School, Guildford, and King's College, London. He became FRCS in 1904. In 1906 (after serving as house-surgeon and demonstrator in anatomy) he was appointed to the *Dreadnought* and Westminster Hospitals; he also served as Consulting Surgeon to Chislehurst, Watford, and Hornsey Hospitals and was later Consultant to the King Edward VII Convalescent Home for Officers at Osborne. During the Great War he served in Flanders and France, initially as a Captain RAMC(T), but later as a Major and Surgical Specialist.

After the war, he became a pioneer in the use of radium at Westminster Hospital; he also became Dean of the Medical School, and had an important rôle in the planning and development of the *new* Westminster Hospital (of which he was later elected Vice-President). During the 1939–45 war, Carling was Consultant Adviser to the Ministries of Health and Home Security. Following that war he took part in the Ministry's survey of the Hospital Services; Carling also served on many

Committees (some connected with atomic energy) and Trusts. He was a member of the MRC. He married and had two sons.[45]

CHOYCE

Charles Coley Choyce FRCS CMG CBE (1875–1937) was a New Zealander, educated in Auckland (Grammar School and University – from which he graduated BSc in 1896). In 1897 he left New Zealand and entered the University of Edinburgh (from which he graduated MB, ChB in 1901). Choyce became house-surgeon to the Leicester Infirmary, and the *Dreadnought* (under William Turner – see above) in 1902. In 1905, Choyce was appointed Medical Superintendent of the *Dreadnought* (in succession to W J Smith [see above]); here he became Assistant Surgeon (1907) and teacher of operative surgery (1907), Senior Surgeon (1912) and (on his retirement due to ill-health in 1919) Consulting Surgeon. He was Dean of the LSCM (1907), and surgeon to in-patients at the ADH. At the Royal Northern Hospital, Choyce was Surgeon to Out-Patients. During the Great War, he was OIC 18th General Hospital, a Lieutenant-Colonel (RAMC) and Consulting Surgeon to the Egyptian Expeditionary Force. When demobilised (in 1919) he was appointed first director of the new surgical unit at University College Hospital (UCH), and in January 1920 Professor of Surgery in the University of London. Failing health began in 1926 and he died on 2 April 1937 at UCH. Choyce married in 1903 and had a son and a daughter. He was a keen sportsman, excelling at rugby football and cricket. His most important literary contribution was a '*System of Surgery*', published in 1912 (3rd ed 1932).[46]

Nursing Staff

During much of this period (1870–1914), nursing was dominated by a long-serving Matron, Miss Alice Mary Hall. It was she who wrote to Florence Nightingale in 1901 concerning nursing in the South African war(s); a treasured possession of the Society is a short letter received from Miss Nightingale in 1901 (*see* Figure 15.14).

> 10, South Street [–,] Park Lane, W. [–,]
> December 17th 1901
>
> Dear Madam
>
> Many thanks for your very kind letter. I am delighted that Bertha Sutcliffe has passed for South Africa. And I trust God willing, that she may fulfil her duties as a Nurse should do. It is very kind of you to ask to see me – And I shall be most happy. I am sorry that I am engaged all this week: but I could see you next Monday if that would be quite convenient to you at five (5) o'clock.
>
> With kind regards, [–,] yours very faithfully[–,] Florence Nightingale[47]

(a) 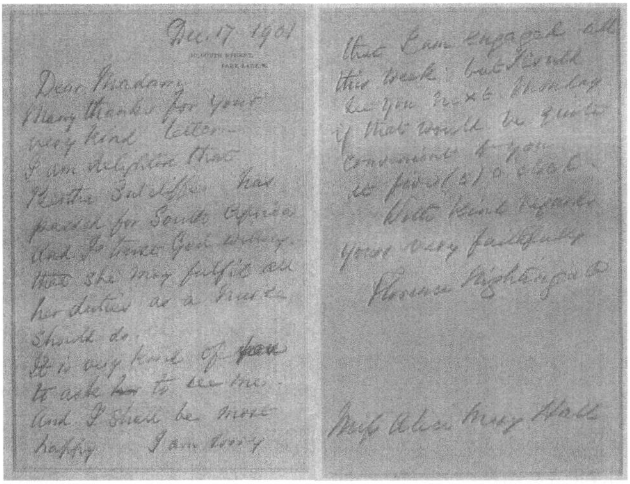

Dec 17 1901

10 South Street, Park Lane W.

Dear Madam

Many thanks for your very kind letter

I am delighted that Nurse Sutcliffe has passed for South Africa and I trust God willing that she may fulfil all her duties as a Nurse should do.

It is very kind of ~~you~~ to ask ~~her~~ to see me. And I shall be most happy. I am sorry that I am engaged all this week; but I would see you next Thursday if that would be quite convenient to you at five (5) o'clock.

With kind regards

yours very faithfully

Florence Nightingale

Miss Alice Mary Hall

(b) 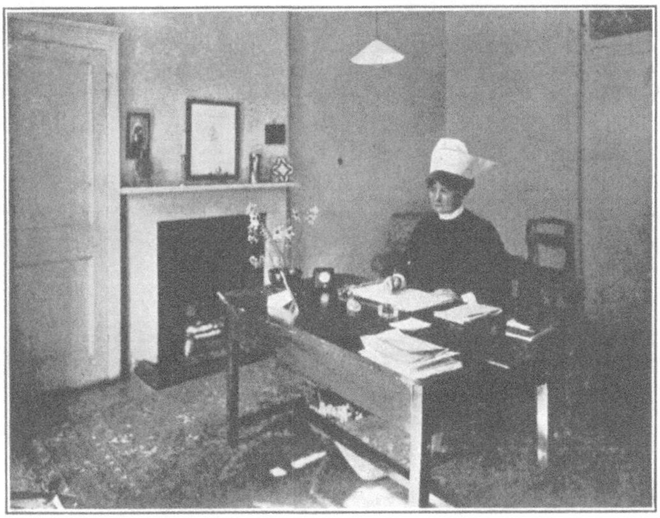

Figure 15.14: (a) Letter (dated 17 December 1901) from Florence Nightingale (1820–1910); in reply to one from the *Dreadnought*'s Matron, Miss Alice Mary Hall (b).

References and Notes

1 *Annual Reports*, 54 and 60.
2 *Ibid*. 54, 66 and 69.
3 *Ibid*. 66, 69 and 85.
4 *Ibid*. 69 and 75.
5 *Op cit*. See note 1 above: 81; *Who Was Who 1916–28*: 267; C S Nairne. Perceval Alleyn Nairne (1841–1921). In: John Nairne (1711–1795) (Minister of Anstruther Easter) and his descendants. McCorquodale & Co Ltd: private circulation. 1931: 39–41; Anonymous.

A fragment of Old Greenwich; Seamen's Hospital Society property at Highbridge. *SHS Quart Mag* 1932; 4(1): 11–12; P Manson-Bahr. *History of the School of Tropical Medicine in London 1899–1949.* London. H K Lewis. 1956: 125–6.

6 Anonymous. *Times, Lond* 1920; 30 April: 9; Anonymous. *Lancet* 1920; i 1029–1030; Anonymous. *BMJ* 1920; i: 657; *Op cit.* See note 1 above: 60; G C Cook. Henry Charles Burdett (1847–1920): outstanding hospital administrator, successful Secretary of the Seamen's Hospital Society, and notable philanthropist. *J Med Biog* 2001; 9: 195–207; F Prochaska. Burdett, Sir Henry Charles (1847–1920) In: H C G Matthew, B Harrison (eds). *Oxford Dictionary of National Biography.* Oxford: Oxford University Press 2004; 8: 741–3.

7 *Op cit.* See note 1 above: 68; Anonymous. *Lancet* 1935; I: 874; Anonymous. *BMJ* 1935; i: 808; Anonymous. Half-a-century devoted to hospitals: Sir James Michelli's remarkable career. *SHS Quart Mag*. 1935; 7(2): 9–10; [*See also*: *Op cit.* See note 5 above (Manson-Bahr): 126–127]; Anonymous. The Michelli bed. *SHS Quart Mag.* 1937; 9 (4): 14–15.

8 Anonymous. A friend to naval and merchant seamen – Admiral Sir Richard Tracy, KCB. *SHS Quart Mag* 1934; 6 (1): 7.

9 Anonymous. *Lancet* 1912; ii: 797; Anonymous. *BMJ* 1912; ii: 749; *Munk's Roll* 4: 166; *Op cit.* See note 1 above: 53.

10 Anonymous. *Lancet* 1896; ii: 135; Anonymous. *BMJ* 1896; ii; 47; Anonymous. *Munk's Roll* 4: 258–9.

11 H Willoughby. The work of a Port Health Officer. *SHS Quart Mag* 1930; 2 (4): 4–7; G C Cook. Harry Leach MRCP (1836–1879): control of scurvy in the British Mercantile Marine, and first Port Medical Officer for the City of London *J Med Biog* 2000; 8: 133–139.

12 G Turner. *Unorthodox Reminiscences.* London: John Murray 1931; 90. [*See also*: G C Cook. Dr Patrick Manson's leading opposition in the establishment of the London School of Tropical Medicine: Curnow, Anderson, and Turner. *J Med Biog* 1995; 3: 170–177].

13 Anonymous. *Lancet* 1902; ii: 174-7; Anonymous. *BMJ* 1902; ii: 226–7; Anonymous. *Munk's Roll* 4: 255–6; *Op cit.* See note 1 above: 79. [*See also*: *Op cit.* See note 12 above (Cook)].

14 Anonymous. *Lancet* 1887; i: 653; Anonymous. *BMJ* 1887; i: 699–700; Anonymous. *Munk's Roll* 4: 299; *Op cit.* See note 1 above 67.

15 Anonymous. *Times*, Lond 1898; 14 March: 10; Anonymous. *Lancet* 1898; i: 16–20; Anonymous. *BMJ* 1898; i: 793–5; Anonymous. *Munk's Roll* 4: 63-4; R Davenport-Hines. Quain, Sir Richard, baronet (1816–1898) In: H C G Matthew, B Harrison (eds). *Oxford Dictionary of National Biography.* Oxford: Oxford University Press 2004; 45: 651–3.

16 Anonymous. *Lancet* 1905; ii: 1513–4; Anonymous. *BMJ* 1905; ii: 1377; *Op cit.* See note 1 above 68.

17 Anonymous. *Lancet* 1910; ii: 87; Anonymous. *Munk's Roll* 4: 384; *Op cit.* See note 1 above 68 and 79. [*See also*: *Op cit.* See note 12 above (Cook)].

18 Anonymous. *Medical directory* London: J & A Churchill 1920; 274.

19 Anonymous. *Plarr's Lives* 1930; ii: 325–6; C C Choyce. Dr Johnson Smith: a famous Dreadnought Surgeon. *SHS Quart Mag* 1935; 7 (1): 12.

20 Anonymous. *Lancet* 1870; ii: 453; [*See also:* Committee of Management Minutes: 11: 161–162].

21 Anonymous. *Lancet* 1907; ii: 1063; Anonymous. *Plarr's Lives* 1930–51; ii: 221.

22 Anonymous. *Lancet* 1900; i: 1475–6; Anonymous. *BMJ* 1900; i: 1201–2; Anonymous. *Plarr's Lives* 1930–51; 1: 324–5.

23 Anonymous. *Lancet* 1941; i: 526; Anonymous. *BMJ* 1941; i: 610; Anonymous. *Plarr's Lives* 1953; 790–1. [*See also: Op cit.* see note 12 above (Cook)].

24 Anonymous. *Lancet* 1944; i: 645; Anonymous. *BMJ* 1944; i: 671; *Plarr's Lives* 1953; 791–2. [*See also: Op cit.* See note 5 above (Manson-Bahr): 141].

25 Anonymous. *Plarr's Lives 1952–64*: 75–6; A Crichton-Harris. Undercurrents on the Nile: the life of Dr John B Christopherson (1868-1955). *J Med Biog* 2006; 14: 8–16.
26 Anonymous. *Plarr's Lives 1930–51*: 358–9.
27 *Ibid. 1952–64 : 67–8.*
28 *Ibid. 1930*; i: 415.
29 Anonymous. *Times, Lond* 1922; 10 April: 15 & 16; Anonymous. *Lancet* 1922; i: 767–769; Anonymous. *BMJ* 1922; i: 623–626 & 702–703; [*See also*: P H Manson-Bahr, A Alcock. *The life and work of Sir Patrick Manson* 1927: 274; Anonymous. The father of tropical medicine. *SHS Quart Mag* 1929; 1: 35–38; R Ross. *Memories of Sir Patrick Manson* 1930: 26; Manson-Bahr. *History of the School of Tropical Medicine in London (1899–1949)* 1956; 328; P Manson-Bahr. *Patrick Manson: the father of tropical medicine* 1962: 192; G C Cook. *From the Greenwich Hulks to Old St Pancras: a history of tropical disease in London* 1992: 68–79; London: Athlone Press; J W W Stephens, M P Sutphen. Manson, Sir Patrick (1844–1922) In: H C G Matthew, B Harrison (eds). *Oxford Dictionary of National Biography*. Oxford: Oxford University Press 2004; 36: 553–5].
30 Anonymous. *Lancet* 1940; ii: 407; Anonymous. *BMJ* 1940; ii: 400; *Munk's Roll* 4: 476–7; Anonymous. *Nature, Lond* 1940; 26 October. [*See also*: *Op cit.* see note 5 above: (Manson-Bahr):138].
31 Anonymous. *Lancet* 1912; ii: 1185–6; Anonymous. *BMJ* 1912; ii: 1258; *Munk's Roll* 4: 483–4; Anonymous. *Plarr's Lives* 1930: 1: 354–5. [*See also*: Op cit see note 5 above (Manson-Bahr) 142–4.
32 Anonymous. *BMJ* 1919; ii: 428–9; *Munk's Roll* 4: 493.
33 Anonymous. *Nature, Lond.* 1926; 117: 832; Anonymous. *Lancet* 1926; i: 1121–2; Anonymous. *BMJ* 1926; i: 971–2; Anonymous. *Plarr's Lives* 1930: i: 192–3. [*See also*: *Op cit.* See note 5 above (Manson-Bahr): 142–4; J Cantlie Stewart. *The quality of mercy: the lives of Sir James and Lady Cantlie.* London: George Allen & Unwin. 1983: 277; M Harrison. Cantlie, Sir James (1851–1926) In: H C G Matthew, B Harrison (eds). *Oxford Dictionary of National Biography.* Oxford: Oxford University Press 2004; 9: 962–4].
34 Anonymous. *Lancet* 1932; ii: 1030; Anonymous. *BMJ* 1932; ii: 901; *Plarr's Lives* 1930; i: 507; Anonymous. In memoriam: Hugh Lawrie McGavin, CBE, FRCS. *SHS Quart Mag* 1932; 4 (4): 10.
35 Anonymous. *Lancet* 1918; i: 347–8 and 754; Anonymous. *BMJ* 1918; i: 273; Anonymous. *Munk's Roll* 4: 423–4. [*See also: Op cit.* See note 5 above (Manson-Bahr): 145–6].
36 Anonymous. *Lancet* 1927; ii: 361; Anonymous. *BMJ* 1927; ii: 287–81, 329; *Munk's Roll* 4: 529–30. *Op cit.* See note 5 above P Manson-Bahr: 162–165. [*See also*: G C Cook. Charles Wilberforce Daniels (1862–1927): underrated pioneer of tropical medicine. *Acta Tropica* 2002; 81: 237–50].
37 Anonymous. *Times, Lond* 1928; 21 January: 12; Anonymous. *Lancet* 1928; i: 210–211; Anonymous. *BMJ* 1928; i: 161–162; Anonymous. *Munk's Roll 4:* 179-180; A E Garrod, P Wallis. Duckworth, Sir Dyce, first baronet (1840–1928) In: H C G Matthew, B Harrison (eds). *Oxford Dictionary of National Biography.* Oxford: Oxford University Press 2004; 17: 41–2.
38 Anonymous. *Lancet* 1920; ii: 1226–7 and 1279; Anonymous. *BMJ* 1920; ii: 954–5; *Munk's Roll 4*: 268–9.
39 Anonymous. *Times, Lond* 1935; 8 April: 16; Anonymous. *Lancet* 1935; i: 906–908; Anonymous. *BMJ* 1935; i: 805–807 and 857; Anonymous. *Munk's Roll* 4: 391–3; T R Elliott, T O'Neill, Bradford, Sir John Rose, baronet (1863–1935) In: H C G Matthew, B Harrison (eds). *Oxford Dictionary of National Biography.* Oxford: Oxford University Press 2004; 7: 186–7.
40 Anonymous. *Lancet* 1924; ii: 138; Anonymous. *BMJ* 1924; ii: 134; Anonymous. *Munk's Roll* 4: 582–3.

41 Anonymous. *Lancet* 1932; i: 58; Anonymous. *BMJ* 1932; i: 80–1; Anonymous. *Plarr's Lives 1953*: 69–70.
42 Anonymous. *Lancet* 1933; ii: 948–9; Anonymous. Br med *J* 1933; ii: 761–2; Anonymous. *Plarr's Lives 1953*: 546–8.
43 Anonymous. *Lancet* 1936; i: 1097; Anonymous. *BMJ* 1936; i: 963; *Plarr's Lives 1953*: 131–2.
44 Anonymous. *Lancet* 1950; i: 647; Anonymous. *BMJ* 1950; i: 791; *Plarr's Lives 1953*: 264–5.
45 Anonymous. *Lancet* 1960; ii: 213–5; Anonymous. *BMJ* 1960; ii: 313–4; Anonymous. *Plarr's Lives 1970*: 68–69; S Cade. Carling, Sir Ernest Rock (1877–1960) In: H C G Matthew, B Harrison (eds). *Oxford Dictionary of National Biography*. Oxford: Oxford University Press 2004; 10: 133–4.
46 Anonymous. *Lancet* 1937; i: 902–3 and 957; Anonymous. *BMJ* 1937; i: 787–8; Anonymous. *Plarr's Lives 1953*: 146–7; [A D]. Professor Charles Choyce: the passing of a great surgeon. *SHS Quart Mag* 1937; 9(2): 14–15.
47 Anonymous. Alice Mary Hall, MBE *SHS Quart Mag* 1937; 9 (4): 16; [*See also*: F Nightingale to A M Hall 1901: 17 December: 1 [SHS Archive]; Anonymous. A letter from Florence Nightingale. *SHS Quart Mag* 1938; 10(2): 22; *Ibid*. Anonymous. Alice Mary Hall, MBE 1937; 9 (4): 16].

Chapter 16

Diseases encountered by the Society 1870–1914

In this chapter, I attempt to highlight those diseases which occupied the time and skill of the Society's physicians and surgeons from 1870 until the outbreak of the Great War in 1914.

Overall, the half-century *after* the Society's facilities were removed to land, was less spectacular from a strictly *clinical* viewpoint than was the case in the days of Hospital-ships (*see* Chapter 11); scurvy in the Mercantile Marine had been brought substantially under control (due largely to the SHS initiative with Harry Leach at the helm), and the last major visitation of cholera had taken place in 1853–4, although a less severe one occurred in 1866. The health of merchant seamen was however, constantly undermined by other problems – e.g. *accidents* and *venereal disease* (and its numerous complications).

The 1879 *Annual Report* asked: 'Has the Society provided a hospital, a convalescent institution, and [also] a home for sick and destitute Seamen of all nations? ... delegated to the Managers in the Act of Incorporation, dated 6th May 1833'. 'Undoubtedly [this report continued] it has fulfilled this threefold duty'; regarding the second of these roles 'some who have required sea air have been sent to Bognor through the kindness of the Merchant Taylor's Company, others to Brighton, or to Seaford, their expenses ... being paid by the Society'. On an almost apologetic note, the 53rd Report (1873) had recorded:

> It must be borne in mind that from lack of room and other causes the Committee are unable to accommodate *every* [my italics] Seaman who falls sick in the Port of London ['this Hospital is no local Institution for the Port of London'], in addition to the large number sent from the different ports, and in consequence many Sailors find their way into Guy's, the London, and Poplar Hospitals.

In September 1886, the following was minuted:

> ... the *police authorities* should *be informed* at the earliest-opportunity of the *number of any cab* that might *bring a case* of [infectious disease] to the *Dreadnought* Hospital. The Secretary was instructed to direct that the *number of every cab and its driver* which brought a patient to the Hospital should in all instances be entered in the case Book and to request the PMO to inform him at the earliest possible opportunity of all cases of

> *contagious or infectious* disease brought to the Hospital in a public conveyance with a view to the request of the Commissioners of Police being complied with.

In 1907/8, the Society made plans to establish its own *isolation ward* for infectious disease in general, largely due to the fact that sailors could *not* be managed at Metropolitan Asylums Board (MAB) hospitals; however, this could not be implemented immediately as a result of financial problems. *Cost* of satisfactory management was a constant challenge, as the 53rd Report recorded: 'The very nutritious diet, often including large quantities of wine and brandy, which has to be provided during a patient's usually slow recovery from the effects of a bad accident, sufficiently indicates the expense necessitated in the treatment of accidents ...'.

The spectrum of disease was still broad however, as the 76th Report documented:

> 'Mariners suffer greatly from pulmonary and other diseases of the chest, brought on by cold, exposure, and climatic influences; from storm and shipwreck they suffer accidents and bodily injury ...'.

A persisting problem (which is repeatedly highlighted in the Reports and Minutes) was how many landsmen, including women and children should be cared for – bearing in mind that the SHS had been set up exclusively for the care of sick and injured seafarers. The 1894 Report recorded: '... many of [the Landsmen, Women and Children] are suffering from accidents and emergencies which it would be an act of inhumanity to send from the doors ...'. Several others refer to the fact that the Society's Hospitals are a long distance (with the exception of the Miller) from a *general* hospital – 'there being no Hospital nearer than London Bridge'.[1]

Tuberculosis

In all walks of life 'phthisis' was in the period under review a major killer; it was, however, a particularly serious affliction in the Mercantile Marine, poor ventilation in the forecastle being a risk factor. This disease was by no means, however, confined to the seafarer himself; the staff – both medical and nursing were also vulnerable. Harry Leach (Chapters 12 and 15), one of the physicians, died of this disease. In February 1909, an SHS nurse developed tuberculosis: 'Nurse Lynn, the Senior Nurse of the [ADH] had contracted phthisis and ... arrangements had been made for her admission to the Ventnor [Isle of Wight] Hospital for Consumption'. And some two years later, an SHS minute referred to the condition of Nurse Munro who had been admitted to the Brompton Hospital Sanatorium, Frimley with phthisis; she subsequently made a temporary recovery, and ultimately resumed her duties at the *Dreadnought* hospital. However, all was *not* well, and a subsequent minute (in 1912) recorded that under treatment 'at the Ventnor Consumption Hospital [she] had developed serious symptoms and it was feared [she] was in a critical condition'. In consequence she was discharged from the hospital, and the Society undertook to maintain her in rooms at Ventnor. A later minute indicates that one of the Laboratory Assistants also, was suffering from phthisis and had been sent to a sanatorium.[2]

In the late nineteenth century, sanatoria became 'fashionable'. Although the causative agent of tuberculosis (*Mycobacterium tuberculosis*) had been identified by Robert Koch (1843–1910) in 1882, it was not until almost 60 years later that an effective chemotherapeutic agent (streptomycin) was introduced to combat this infection. During these years, numerous sanatoria were established throughout Britain and other countries, the underlying rationale being that a 'change of air' to, for example, the dry, warm Mediterranean littoral or various alpine resorts (affordable by the wealthy) had led to beneficial results. John Coakley Lettsom (1744–1815), a fashionable Quaker physician (who had founded the Medical Society of London in 1773) had in fact introduced exposure to 'open air' for patients suffering from scrofula at the Royal Sea Bathing Infirmary, Margate as early as 1791. A similar strategy for patients suffering from 'pulmonary phthisis' had been initiated between 1840 and 1843, by George Bodington (1799–1882) at Sutton Coldfield. However, it was not until the latter days of the nineteenth century that 'open-air' treatment for this disease had become a 'respectable' option; even then it was available only to the wealthier members of society.

The Society's physicians were in fact pioneers of this new technique in seafarers. They introduced 'open-air' treatment of this infection in the 'Ranlett' ward (see Figure 16.1) situated on the roof of the West Wing of the *Dreadnought* hospital. The 1901 Report recorded:

> Consumption, or as it is now more generally known Phthisis, has stricken down many a sailor … The [SHS] Committee … are glad to record that they have received from the Medical Staff of the Dreadnought Hospital a gratifying Report, showing that the method of treating their patients on the *out-door system* [my italics] has been conspicuously successful ….

The first mention of 'open-air' treatment for 'phthisical patients' had in fact been minuted in April 1900: 'The Medical Council [of the SHS] having drawn the attention of the Committee to the subject of erecting shelters on the west roof of the

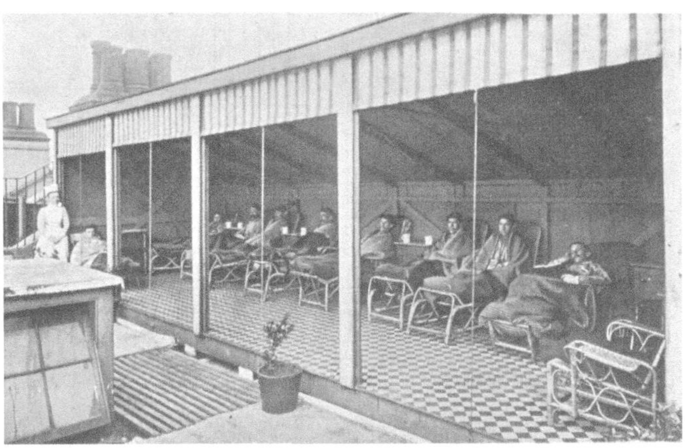

Figure 16.1: The 'Ranlett' ward – for open-air treatment of phthisis – was situated on the roof of the West Wing of the *Dreadnought* Hospital, Greenwich. [SHS Archive].

Dreadnought Hospital ... it was resolved that the House Visitors be asked to report on the subject after consultation with the PMO and Physicians'. This was duly carried out with the result that 'four wards upon the Upper West Floor, now used principally as sleeping accommodation for Porters, be equipped as Medical Wards and that four other Wards be closed to Patients and the space thus vacated be used for the accommodation of the staff'. In December 1901 'it was resolved that [the PMO's report on this topic] be printed and circulated and made part of the Medical Report of the year'. And an update in early 1904 indicated that the Society's Committee were satisfied with 'the success of the out-door treatment at Greenwich and ordered that [the physicians] report be printed with the Annual Medical Report'.

Figure 16.2 summarises data on admission rates (and deaths) from 'pulmonary phthisis' recorded in successive General Reports between 1890 and 1906; the mean annual admission rate was 103, with an in-patient average of 24. Five successive Reports summarise the *Dreadnought* experience with the *new* 'open-air' technique (which took from 80–90 days), from 1900 to 1905; in every case, *M. tuberculosis* had been demonstrated in a sputum-sample. Table 16.1 summarises the results; mean mortality-rate was approximately 11%, which was markedly lower than that using orthodox measures (see above). Furthermore, general improvement in the overall state of 'well-being' was noted to be more common in those undergoing 'open-air' treatment. Clearly, this study would not stand up to present-day scientific scrutiny; how for example were cases selected for 'open-air' treatment? And owing to difficulties involved in monitoring the health of seafarers, there was little (if any) long-term follow-up. However, the result was in keeping with con-

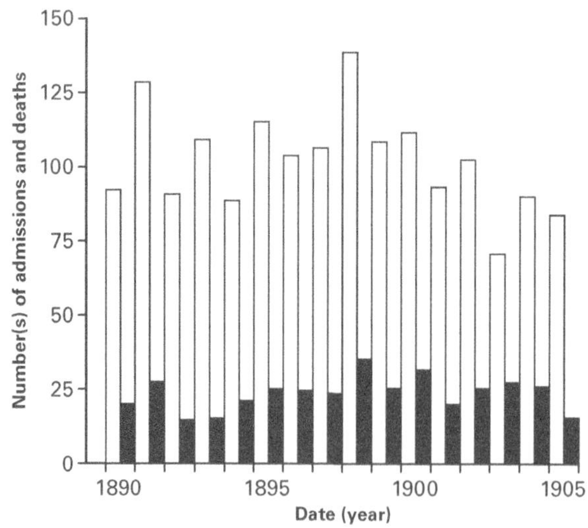

Figure 16.2: Number(s) of cases of 'pulmonary phthisis' admitted to the *Dreadnought* Hospital, Greenwich (white columns) between 1890 and 1905. Numbers of deaths are shown by black columns. Mean mortality rate, 23.6%.

Table 16.1: Annual number of admissions (and deaths) resulting from 'pulmonary phthisis' (1900–1905) using the 'open-air' technique.

Date (year)	*No. admitted for treatment*	*No. remaining under treatment*	*No. deaths.*	*% deaths**
1900–01	45	11	6	13.3
1901–02	56	9	7	12.5
1902–03	48	10	6	12.5
1903–04	57	10	6	10.5
1904–05	52	12	4	7.7

* Mean mortality rate = 11.3%

temporary opinion in the *civilian* population, leading to the evolution of sanatoria for patients in many parts of Britain. Although some general hospitals (Sheffield Royal Infirmary and the Royal Berkshire Hospital, Reading are two examples) had begun accepting patients with 'pulmonary phthisis' as early as 1899 such institutions were exceptional. It was also impossible to find accommodation for long-term (convalescent) management following a period of 'open-air' treatment at the *Dreadnought* Hospital.[3]

The author of the 1901 *Dreadnought* experience concluded:

> When it is considered that a large proportion of Phthisical cases reach the Dreadnought in a poor state of general health, and often with the disease already far advanced, we venture to think that the results have not been unsatisfactory, and we trust the Governors will consider that they justify the facilities they were good enough to afford us for carrying out this plan of [open-air] treatment.

This experience of the SHS physicians must therefore have engendered a good deal of optimism for 'open-air' treatment in 'pulmonary phthisis', which was to last until the 1960s when anti-tuberculosis chemotherapy was widely introduced.

The 1901 report (see above) continued: 'During the year the Committee received an offer [via the Prince of Wales' Hospital Fund] of a Home [to accommodate 30 or 40 patients] in the Isle of Wight which might be used for convalescent or Phthisical patients'. However the Society declined this offer on the grounds of expense.

In early 1905, the Physicians of the *Dreadnought* felt that 'segregation of Phthisis' should be considered, and 'it was resolved that the Visitors be requested to meet the Physicians with a view to an extension of the open-air treatment if possible'. The 90th *Report* stated: 'The phthisical patients generally occupy a bed for at least three months, sometimes a year, while the Greenwich Hospital pensioners, of whom there are now six, often remain the rest of their lives.' And the *Report* three years later, recorded: 'Public attention has recently been especially called to the treatment of Tuberculosis … . The Committee wish to point out that twenty beds are devoted [to this disease]'.[4]

Scurvy

As already related in this book (*see* Chapter 11), this disease had been brought largely under control in the latter days of the hospital-ships, effective legislation being introduced in 1867, and implemented on 1 January 1868. However, when the Society became land-based in 1870, cases of scurvy were still being referred to the *Dreadnought*. The 1870 Report for example (see above), recorded 51 cases that year, of whom 30 were from British and the remainder from foreign ships; however, since 20 October 1870, no case of scurvy had been admitted to the *Dreadnought* hospital. That was not the end of the saga, however; 40 cases (24 from British and 16 from foreign vessels) were admitted during 1871, the same number (30 from British and 10 from foreign vessels) the following year, but a mere 11 (nine from British and two from Russian vessels) in 1873.[5]

By the early twentieth century this deficiency disease had been largely eliminated from both the RN and the mercantile marine. But even then, although it was generally accepted that scurvy (in most cases there was 'a history of a very prolonged sea-passage') resulted from a lack of dietary vegetables and lime (or lemon) juice, other factors were still under consideration. Johnson Smith's 1883 medical report, for example, contained a conclusion reached by Mr Gray (Board of Trade), Dr Collingridge (Port of London Sanitary Committee) and Dr WH Neale (medical officer to a recent Arctic expedition) to the effect that scurvy could not be prevented by 'lime-juice, of *itself*'; a 'meat [rather than] a vegetable diet [it was concluded, was necessary] for prevention.' This misconception had doubtless arisen from widespread use of lime juice, with its far lower ascorbic acid content, rather than lemon juice which was largely based on economy.[6]

Cholera

The last time London was severely afflicted by the Asiatic cholera had been in 1853–4 (Chapter 11). A foreboding of *new* epidemics (the cause was still *not* known with any degree of certainty) was constantly in the minds of all and sundry. Hence, the medical staff of the SHS was always alert to the possibility of a new 'visitation'. As late as 1893, the 73rd *annual report* stated: 'Though seriously threatened by an outbreak of Cholera, this calamity has been happily averted, and not a single case, even of a suspicious nature, was received; ... but a whole ward was held in readiness with every requisite for the immediate treatment of this disease'.

Over 20 years earlier (in 1871) an SHS Minute documented correspondence from the House Governor and Senior Medical Officer 'asking what was to be done with any Cholera case applying for admission; it was 'Ordered that the House Governor [Kemball Cook] take such steps as he may deem best in the matter'! At the following meeting, the matter was again raised, and a letter was read from Dr Buchanan of the Medical Department of the Privy Council; he ruled that 'he was anxious to induce the authorities who have districts along the river below bridge to join in Employing an officer [he named Harry Leach as a suitable candidate] who should examine into the recurrence of any cases of cholera and take the needful steps for preventing the spread of the disease from any such cases …'. However, a further letter (also from Buchanan) indicated 'that an arrangement had been made whereby cholera cases would be received on board the Dreadnought'. After further correspondence, a letter was received from the Town Clerk of the Corporation of London … promising that 'Cholera Cases should *not* [my italics] be sent [to the Dreadnought]'.

In 1883, the MAB contacted the Society's Committee asking whether in the event of a '*cholera* emergency arising' they would be prepared to '*assign beds* for the treatment of 12 male and 12 female patients?'. Before coming to a decision the Committee decided to ask the PMO (Johnson Smith) what steps were taken during the 'last visitation of *Cholera*'. The decision was that owing to pressure on the beds, they were 'not prepared to set Beds aside solely for the reception of landsmen'. In August 1884, the PMO compiled a report on the management of a potential cholera outbreak in London and/or on the Thames: in it, he advocated prompt admission of any case entering the Port of London; sailors would be managed either in a prepared ward ('in as isolated a position as possible') at Gravesend or at the *Dreadnought*, while landsmen would fall under the aegis of the MAB. As a result, the PMO prepared an '[isolation] room for five patients in Upper East (South) [ward]'.

The following year (1884), 'The Chairman [of the SHS] drew attention to a paragraph … in the "Times" regarding the approach of *Cholera* to the Metropolis; it was, however, resolved to leave this matter 'to the discretion of the [PMO]'. Again, in 1892, it was felt by many that cholera was again on its way to London. A minute recorded: '30 beds had been set aside on N.W. floor for the receipt of cholera patients … The venereal cases that were under treatment on N.W. floor had all been discharged, except 6 and these would at once be sent away or treated on other floors in the event of a cholera case being admitted.'

And a year later, with the continuing threat of cholera re-emerging: 'Arrangements had been made to keep some of the wards in Upper West vacant and to retain them in case of need in the same way as last year'. It was however reported that, as yet, no cases even of a suspicious nature had been seen. Nothing was heard hereafter of the Asiatic cholera in London and it remained a *nineteenth-century* catastrophe with three major visitations![7]

Typhoid (enteric fever)

Enteric fever is repeatedly mentioned in the Society's minutes. In December 1877 a minute of the SHS Committee of Management made it clear that all cases of typhoid fever admitted to the *Dreadnought* should be reported: seamen to the Port of London Sanitary Authority, Deptford, and landsmen to the 'Local Health Authorities of the District from which the patients came'.

Typhoid was always a threat to the *staff* (as well as to patients) of the Society's Hospitals, several cases (with significant mortality) being minuted amongst the nursing staff. In 1899, a nurse (who had been in the employ of the Society since 1896) died of typhoid fever contracted at the ADH, and in 1901 a Ward Sister at the *Dreadnought* contracted the infection. In April 1903 another nurse was reported as being seriously ill (she duly recovered) and in late 1912 another nurse at the *Dreadnought* died of this disease; she too, had contracted the infection from a patient.[8]

Scarlet fever (Scarlatina)

Today, scarlet fever (a Streptococcal infection) is rare, and does not produce a significant mortality-rate, largely because the causative organism has lost its virulence. This disease at that time necessitated the destruction of clothing, for which the SHS felt obliged to compensate.

In 1898, one of the House Surgeons at the ADH 'contracted scarlet fever [and was] sent to the Islington Fever Hospital'; fortunately, he fully recovered. Another victim was a laboratory assistant at the ADH. This infection was certainly no respecter of rank, for the surgeon to the East India Dock Road Dispensary (Dr Oxley) was 'laid up' with scarlet fever in May 1906! In December 1896, the SHS Committee however approved of 'visitors under the age of 15 being excluded from the wards [while the infection was prevalent] in the neighbourhood of Greenwich'. [9]

Diphtheria

A minute of March 1888 records: 'The Secretary was instructed to convey to the PMO the opinion of the Committee that when possible it is advisable not to admit cases of Diphtheria'. A later report documented diphtheria (contracted from a patient) in a nurse at the *Dreadnought* Hospital; this resulted in a 'letter [being sent to] the Medical Practitioners in the neighbourhood informing them that cases of diphtheria and other infectious diseases were not admissible to the Seamen's Hospital, Greenwich'; such patients should in fact be cared for in 'one of the hospitals under the [MAB]'.[10]

Influenza

In January 1890, a minute recorded: '... that 9 Nurses had been warded suffering from influenza'.[11]

Plague

Yersinia pestis infection (plague) was not a major problem either in the Hospital-ship days, or at the land-based *Dreadnought* or Albert Dock Hospital. However, it remained a potential threat as the following extract (from a report by the PMO – Johnson Smith) to the Committee of Management in 1900 makes clear:

> On Thursday, July 26th [1900], at 8.30p.m., a lascar was received from the [ADH] with an intimation from the Resident Medical Officer of this Institution that the history of the case and the symptoms presented by

this patient suggested the necessity of submitting him to close observation and strict isolation. On the following day at 1.30 p.m. after a short absence from the hospital, I saw this patient and found that the case had been properly and fully dealt with as one of a very infectious character. In the course of the afternoon Dr. Collingridge, the Medical Officer of Health for the Port of London, to whom the case had been reported was present with me, and we … came to the conclusion that the general condition of the man and symptoms he presents indicated rather some local disorder (suppurating gland in groin) than any infectious disease.

On the following morning (Saturday, July 28th) the Patient was decidedly better, but in consequence of a report on previous cases in the same ship Dr Collingridge thought with myself that it would be advisable to remove this man to the Port of London infectious Hospital at Gravesend. This removal was effected on the same date at 10.30 p.m., the Patient, in the course of a day or two having been seen by Dr Bulstrode of the Local Government Board, It was thought well by both Dr Collingridge and myself to postpone the removal of this patient until after sunset as during the day and evening the pier and its approaches were crowded by excursionists.

The Patient, Dr. Collingridge informs me, has since made very favourable progress and is now apparently well. The only indication of the nature of his disease, and this I regard as a very clear and decided one, is the fact that a careful and prolonged examination of the discharge from the bubo [swollen lymph gland] revealed the undoubted presence of the specific bacillus of bubonic plague [*Yersinia pestis*].

Dr Hewlett, Physician to the Seamen's Hospital and assistant Director at the Institute of Public Medicine, was enabled to report this on Tuesday, July 31st.

The following is an abstract of suspicious cases observed at the [ADH]. All these men, [who were] the subject of the above report, came from the crew of the SS *Rome* P. & O.:

July 12 [1900]. Francis Borette, Admitted July 12th, Died July 15. Treated as cases of enteric fever. On post mortem examination no signs of this disease found.

July 22. A Lascar died suddenly on board the "Rome". Body taken to [ADH]. On post-mortem examination no indication of disease except acute congestion of the brain which condition was also observed in proceeding case (F Borette).

July 24. Lascar, admitted with fever (temperature 104° Farenheit). This Patient progressed favourably for a time but as he developed a swollen and inflamed gland in the groin, the discharge from which contained in abundance the specific organism of plague [*Y. pestis*], he was transferred on July 27th to the Infectious Hospital at Gravesend. This man, like the patient sent from Greenwich, has done well.[12]

Trichinosis (trichiniasis)

Forty-three cases of a then unknown infection occurred between 23 September and 23 October 1879, on a reformatory school-ship lying off Purfleet (see Figure 16.3) – several miles downstream from Greenwich. A total of 14 of these boys had in fact been admitted to the *Dreadnought* Hospital – 10 on 1 October, and four on 6 October.[13]

They were first considered by Leach (like those in a previous outbreak in October 1875) to be caused by *enteric fever* (see above) which originated from the 'fouling of the water-supply with excremental matter from a patient sick of the malady'. It became widely felt that the 'outflows of the metropolitan sewage ... at Crossness and Barking' were responsible for this disease. However, doubts about this diagnosis soon arose and 'the Committee of the ship [applied] to the Home Secretary for additional skilled assistance [to investigate] the outbreak'. One of the Medical Inspectors employed by the Local Government Board – W H Power FRS (1842–1916) (see Figure 16.4)[14] – was directed to visit the ship. He was immediately

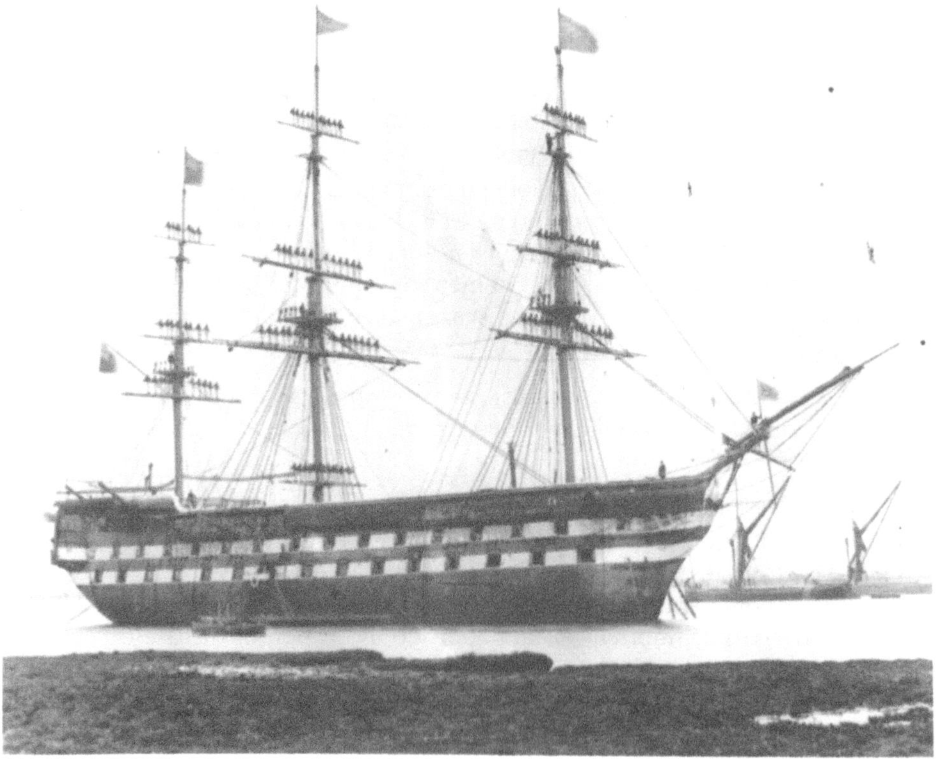

Figure 16.3: The *Cornwall* reformatory school-ship moored off Purfleet; she had originally (in 1815) been named the *Wellesley* but was renamed in 1868 – when her rôle was changed. The ship was subsequently sunk by enemy action of 24 September 1940. [Reproduced from the National Maritime Museum archive, with permission].

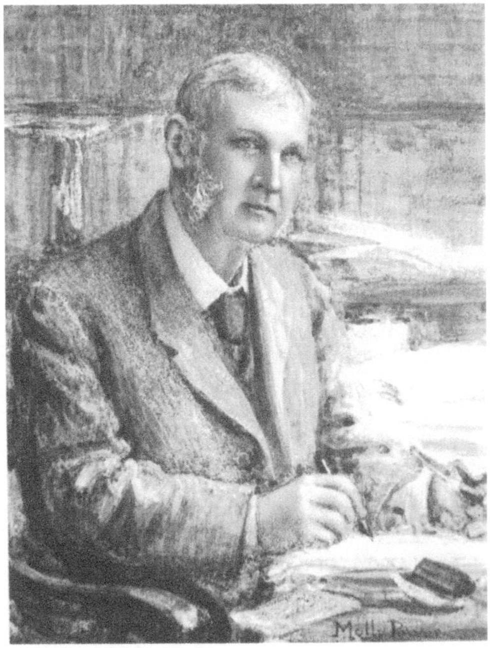

Figure 16.4: W H Power FRS (1842–1916): Medical Inspector to the Government Board. [Courtesy, The Wellcome Library, London].

suspicious that the disease was not enteric fever, but trichinosis (trichiniasis)*, and an 'application was made to the Home Secretary for permission to exhume [after burial two months earlier] the body of the only youth who had died [on the eighteenth day of illness] of the malady'. Power's suspicion was confirmed

*Historically, larvae of *Trichinella spiralis* had first been identified in *Homo sapiens* in a patient under the care of George Leith Roupell FRS (1797–1854) (*see* Chapter 12) at St Bartholomew's Hospital, London in 1834. The 21-year-old James Paget FRS (1814–1899), then a first-year medical student, witnessed this autopsy, and he was probably the first to record the 'whitish specks ... scattered throughout the muscles' of this middle-aged Italian man. The discovery was in fact recorded by Paget at the Abernethian Society on 6 February 1835, and Owen's paper (see below), which was read at the Zoological Society, followed 18 days later. However, Paget's discovery was publicised (and a definitive report subsequently written) by Richard Owen FRS (1804–1892); he is now widely regarded, almost certainly erroneously, as the discoverer of the larval form of *T. spiralis*. Priority in this discovery subsequently became the subject of heated correspondence both in the leading medical journals and also *The Times* newspaper. Reports in 1866 concentrated initially on cases of the infection in Germany, although a Guy's Hospital case (in 1828) was brought to the fore; Cobbold (see below) referred his readers to the works of Virchow, Leuckart and Pagenstecher for accurate descriptions of this parasitosis, but this correspondence concluded that Paget should be given credit for the discovery. Further reference to the controversy arose in 1882 (i.e. soon after the *Dreadnought* outbreak had been reported). Claims by Owen that he should be given credit for the initial discovery were at that time vehemently dismissed by Cobbold.

at this post-mortem, and ingestion of 'certain American pork' was incriminated aetiologically. *The Lancet* considered that '... people in this country have hitherto had a remarkable immunity to [the acute form of trichinosis] – an immunity which, it is to be feared, since the large and increasing importation of foreign pork, is becoming a thing of the past'.[15]

Committee Minutes dated 10 October 1879 recorded:

> The Secretary having reported the admission [to the *Dreadnought* Hospital, Greenwich] of 10 boys from the Cornwall training ship *Ordered* that a sub committee be appointed consisting of Messrs Joseph Moore [Chairman], J R Edridge and Captain Budd to confer with the committee of the Training Ships on the Thames with the view to making permanent provision for the isolation and treatment of sick boys on such vessels ....[16]

The *British Medical Journal's* correspondent recorded: 'the only previous [recognised] outbreak of trichinosis [in England had occurred] at Workington, Cumberland, in April 1871 [and was] caused by eating the flesh of a home-fed pig'. This information was corroborated by Thomas Spencer Cobbold FRS (1828–1886) (see Figure 16.5)[17]

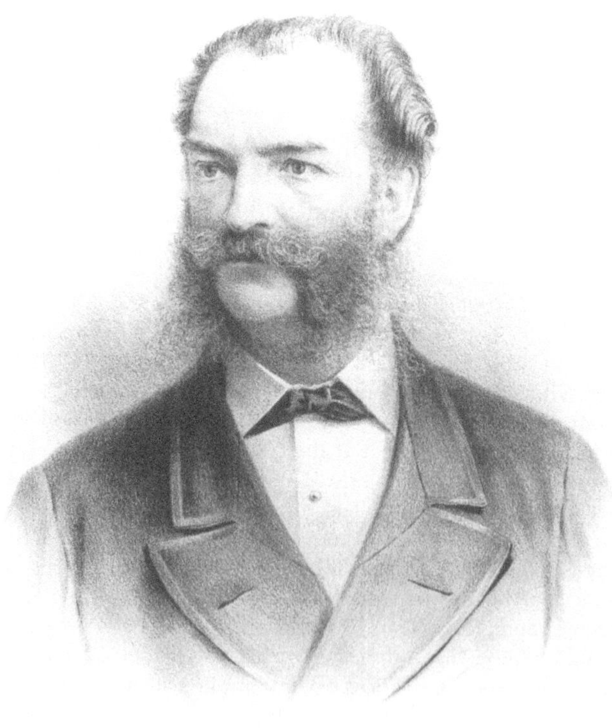

Figure 16.5: Thomas Spencer Cobbold FRS (1828–86): leading authority on helminthic diseases. [Courtesy, The Wellcome Library, London].

(see below) in a letter to that journal. Curiously, however, he (Cobbold was unquestionably the most distinguished helminthologist in England at that time) expressed doubt about the diagnosis of the *Cornwall* cases; he concluded that the disease was *not* caused by *T. spiralis* but by 'an unknown form of nematode parasite', and that 'we ought rather to look to an indifferent water-supply than to diseased meat as the primary source of the outbreak'. Not too surprisingly, an anonymous correspondent in *The Lancet* was critical of Cobbold's opinion; however, these conclusions were upheld by W L Dickinson (who had apparently detected the first (recognised) outbreak of trichinosis in Britain – at Workington [see above]. The reason(s) for Cobbold's scepticism remains unresolved, and the bulk of evidence must have supported trichinosis (trichiniasis) as the cause of this outbreak.

An anonymous writer (who emphasised the potential seriousness of the infection) proceeded to recommend adequate cooking of all pork – whether 'trichinised or not'; outbreaks of trichinosis on the European continent were due, he considered to the flesh being inadequately cooked, 'an unpleasant habit [which was] common in many parts of Germany of eating pork, particularly in the form of sausages, more than half raw'. 'Uncooked pork or ham [he wrote] is excessively dangerous, and should never be eaten by any person who respects his health or his life ...'.

The matter was deemed to be of sufficient importance to be raised in the House of Lords (by Lord Thurlow [1838–1916]) on 19 February and 23 March 1880. After a brief delay, the Power report (the author was ably assisted by Mr Mortimer de Brent) was published; the thoroughness of the investigation, which demonstrated beyond doubt that the outbreak was caused by 'salt (trichinised) pork', was praised by anonymous writers in both the *Lancet* and *British Medical Journal*. A careful histological examination of the exhumed body (by Dr Robert Cory) had disclosed 'trichinae ... largely in the muscles, particularly in the diaphragm, some fully grown and *one wandering and living*, others in different stages of less development, and considerable numbers of brood trichinae ... beneath the under-surface of the mucous membrane of the intestine'. The boys' food had apparently been prepared (in bulk) separately from that of the officers on board the *Cornwall* 'who escaped illness', the suspect meat being 'American pork' ... obtained from a firm in Bristol [consisting] solely of 'belly-pieces, and therefore of parts of many pigs, and of those parts most likely to be infested with trichinae'. How many of the cases formerly diagnosed as 'enteric fever' had in fact been caused by trichinosis, these writers asked!

Details of the unfortunate outbreak were succinctly summarised in the General Report of admissions to SHS establishments published in 1880; trichinosis, it recorded, 'has frequently been observed on the Continent, particularly in Germany and in the Netherlands, but very rarely in this country [England]'. That fortunate situation (for Britain) still pertains today![18]

Venereal Disease

In the middle of the nineteenth century (in 1864), Busk[19] had described to an expert committee, the various forms of sexually-transmitted disease to afflict merchant seamen (*see* Chapter 11). In the latter days of the century (i.e. following removal to land), Johnson Smith had also collected figures for sexually-transmitted disease; these were published in successive 'Medical Reports' (from 1876 until 1906).[20] The 93rd *Annual Report* (1913) stated that a total of 25 beds (at the *Dreadnought*) were reserved for venereal disease, a degree of attention 'almost alone among general Hospitals'.

In 1891, there was apparently concern that VD could be transmitted in baths (a matter which was raised again in 1907). This led to the Society's Committee expressing the opinion 'that there should be a special bath set apart for venereal patients'.[21]

Treatment in the years under review was not without problems. The cost of 'Salvarsen' (used for syphilis) was considerable, as is clear from a minute of February 1914:

> The [SHS] Medical Council reported that £187 had been spent upon Salvarsan at the Dreadnought Hospital [£82 had been paid by patients]. It was approved that 'Landsmen and patients other than Seamen' should pay for their treatment, and that 'contributions offered by Seamen [be] accepted.

And a later minute records: '… a fee of 7½ guineas [was] paid to Mr Wilson Hake, Ph.D. the Chemical Analyst, for work in connection with an enquiry into the death of a patient who had been under treatment with Salvarsen or "606" in the Dreadnought Hospital'.

Smallpox

This highly contagious disease (variola) was obvious from a diagnostic viewpoint (the only confusion being with chickenpox [varicella]) and had always been a problem faced by the Society. It had (since the foundation of the SHS) been an infection which had to be removed from the *Dreadnought* (or ADH) wards – either afloat or on shore – as a matter of urgency.

In the early days of the Society, cases (following diagnosis) were immediately transferred to the Smallpox Hospital at St Pancras, or after July 1850 its successor at Highgate Hill.[22] An amicable relationship had existed with the surgeon there– James Furness Marson, FRCS (?–1877)[23] – despite the fact that the SHS had to pay for admissions (and burials) resulting from direct referral (*see* Chapter 11); the Society was *not* willing, however, to pay for cases which found their way to the Smallpox Hospital by other means. The SHS had given an annual donation of 10 guineas to the hospital; in addition, a further donation of £20=00 was made in 1849 due to the fact that in the previous year, 45 cases had been referred from the Society.

Friction between the two organisations had begun in 1854 (*see* Chapter 11); Marson had written to the SHS Superintendent asking him to remove a man (a 'South Sea Islander, ignorant of the English language') referred by the *Dreadnought* staff, otherwise he would refuse admission of *all* subsequent cases. Both Marson and the Secretary to the Smallpox Hospital (Cliff) emphasised that they were unhappy with the 'arrangements between the two hospitals'. This disquiet had led to an ultimatum from the Smallpox Hospital setting out *their* terms for referral of cases to the Smallpox Hospital. By 1870 the relationship had deteriorated still further, and cases of the disease had to be transferred elsewhere. In 1876, for example, referrals were to Stockwell Hospital; the following year to the Smallpox Hospital, Old Kent Road, and (temporarily) to the Deptford Hospital.

This policy (re-emphasised in a letter to the Local Government Board in May 1876 and again in May 1881) of *not* managing patients with smallpox at the *Dreadnought* Hospital led to frequent skirmishes with the authorities during the 50 years under review. The case of a man suffering from the infection, who travelled 'by Mail train from Newcastle' to Greenwich is documented in the Committee minutes; it was decided to report the case to the Board of Trade, and to emphasise that this disease was 'not received in this Hospital'. The matter was taken up by Mr (later Sir) John Simon[24] of the Medical Department of the Privy Council. On another occasion, the Clerk to the Greenwich Union called attention to 'cases of smallpox having been referred to the Workhouse after being refused admission to [the *Dreadnought*]'. At a later meeting (in 1876) 'the Chairman informed the Surgeon that it was the wish of the Committee that in future in doubtful cases [there had apparently been some diagnostic difficulty in a case admitted to the *Dreadnought*] the patient should not be admitted, but that steps should be taken to have such cases removed by Ambulance to the Stockwell Hospital'.

The case of a 'colored seaman' sent to the Smallpox Hospital, Old Kent Road, who subsequently died of the infection was the subject of a further communication (in April 1877) – this time from the Clerk to the Greenwich Board of Guardians. The patient had *not* been sent directly to the Smallpox Hospital and the writer suggested that he 'was a source of public danger whilst going from the [*Dreadnought*] to the Relief Office and waiting at the latter place'. As a result it was resolved by the SHS Committee of Management that cases of smallpox should be temporarily kept at the *Dreadnought* until the Ambulance arrived – but with two recent cases this had taken 3½ and three hours, respectively, because the Society had 'had to provide a horse and driver for the ambulance'.

However, 'temporary detention' was discontinued shortly afterwards, and at a later meeting (November 1879), 'The Chairman explained that by clause 16 of the Poor Law Act [of] 1879 the [MAB] have power to provide all necessary ambulances for the removal of [cases suffering from an infectious disease]'. In 1884, letters were read from the Town Clerk, of Guildhall, and the Clerk to the Greenwich Union concerning a man with smallpox who was refused admission to the *Dreadnought*, and instead directed to the Smallpox Hospital, Deptford; rather than accept this advice, he returned to the *Dreadnought* the following day.

Later that year, a plan was produced for an 'isolation house' in the vicinity of the *Dreadnought*, which would in effect be a transit centre for smallpox (and other infectious) cases whilst awaiting the arrival of an ambulance. In the event, this failed to materialise, but a room 'in the basement of the Hospital' was identified which would 'meet the wishes of the [MAB] until … arrival of an Ambulance'.

A year later, two members of the *Dreadnought* staff contracted smallpox. The course of events is graphically described, together with a delay in getting an ambulance from the fever hospital at Hither Green, but with a more satisfactory result from New Cross![25] In 1897 'The P.M.O. reported [to the Committee] that there had been an outbreak of Small Pox [affecting five cases] on the Middle East Floor of the [*Dreadnought*] Hospital'.[47]

In November 1901, due to an 'epidemic of Small Pox in London', the PMO warned that 'it might become advisable to close the Hospital to patients' friends ...'. In the following January, he, in conjunction with the Secretary, was 'empowered to exclude Visitors until the necessity for such exclusion shall have passed'. This restriction seems to have remained in operation until early May the following year. Overall management at Greenwich (including the vaccination programme) during this epidemic earned praise from the Medical Officer of Health (MOH) for the Borough of Greenwich. The matter of smallpox affecting sailors *specifically*, was frequently aired. In 1881 for example, a minute states:

> A letter was read from Dr Collingridge, *Medical Officer* to the *Port of London*, in which he stated that the cases of *smallpox* which had occurred amongst sailors were extremely few and not sufficient in number to justify the Committee in going to the expense of a *floating Hospital*. The question of *vaccinating sailors* was ordered to stand over for the report of the P.M.O. of the [*Dreadnought*].

Smallpox at the ADH

In February 1895, the PMO reported an outbreak of smallpox at the ADH ('seven inmates of the hospital [three of them 'servants of the Society' and the remainder patients, were] attacked'); it 'spread so rapidly throughout the building as to threaten a serious interference ... with the working of this institution'. Both wards and the outpatient department were closed. This outbreak seems to have had its origins in a Lascar admitted from the S.S. *City of Cambridge*; as soon as he developed the exanthem he was transferred to a fever hospital. Fortunately, all but one of those affected had been vaccinated, and they were removed to a fever hospital. Spread was prevented by 'vaccination and ... disinfection of the ward and bed-linen'.

'Tropical' cases at the LSTM

The *clinical* component for the major activities of the London School of Tropical Medicine (see Chapter 18) were based at the ADH. In order to boost the number of cases of *tropical* cases (primarily for teaching and research purposes), those fitting this category were transferred from the *Dreadnought* hospital; this amongst other factors, led to considerable dissatisfaction (and subsequent resignations) amongst the consultant staff of the parent institution.[27]

Although a great deal of research into 'tropical' diseases was carried out by the LSTM staff at the ADH – both at that hospital and abroad – the *concentration* of 'exotic' cases was sparse. Although there is reference in the Committee minutes to leprosy, schistosomiasis, filariasis, sprue, oriental sore, beri-beri and pellagra, most of these cases originated abroad, and *not* at the ADH.[28]

Contemporary SHS reports give details of the diagnoses of patients admitted to the ADH in the early days of the LSTM. In 1891 for example, there were 217 medical and 287 surgical admissions (2419 out-patients were seen that year); six cases had been brought in dead, demise being caused by: drowning (2), fractured skull (2), 'enteric' (1), and 'heart disease' (1). Beginning in 1897, 'tropical cases' (67 that year) were categorised separately; *deaths* were included under *medical* admissions. From 1898 until 1905 a 'breakdown' of the diagnoses of the 'tropical' cases was published; in 1898 (i.e. the year *before* the LSTM opened) 35 admissions were due to malaria, 20 dysentery, 12 beri-beri and 11 from a miscellany of causes; phthisis and 'enterica' (typhoid fever), were classified under the umbrella of 'medical cases'.[29]

Figure 16.6 summarises 'tropical', medical, and surgical admissions since the ADH was opened, and during the early years (1899–1905) of the LSTM. Most cases at the LSTM were of *Plasmodium* spp infection (Table 16.2), beri-beri (which is rarely encountered today), and dysentery (most cases of which did not have a 'laboratory diagnosis'). The mean annual number of *Africans* admitted to the ADH during the years 1899–1905 was 15 (range 10–18), while that of *Asiatics* was 111 (range 93–129); corresponding annual number of 'landsmen' was 228 (range 209–259). Table 16.2 summarises the diagnoses of the '*tropical* cases' during the seven years from the opening of the LSTM, and Table 16.3 gives contemporary diagnoses of cases of *Plasmodium* spp infection. From these statistics it is clear that the amount of 'tropical

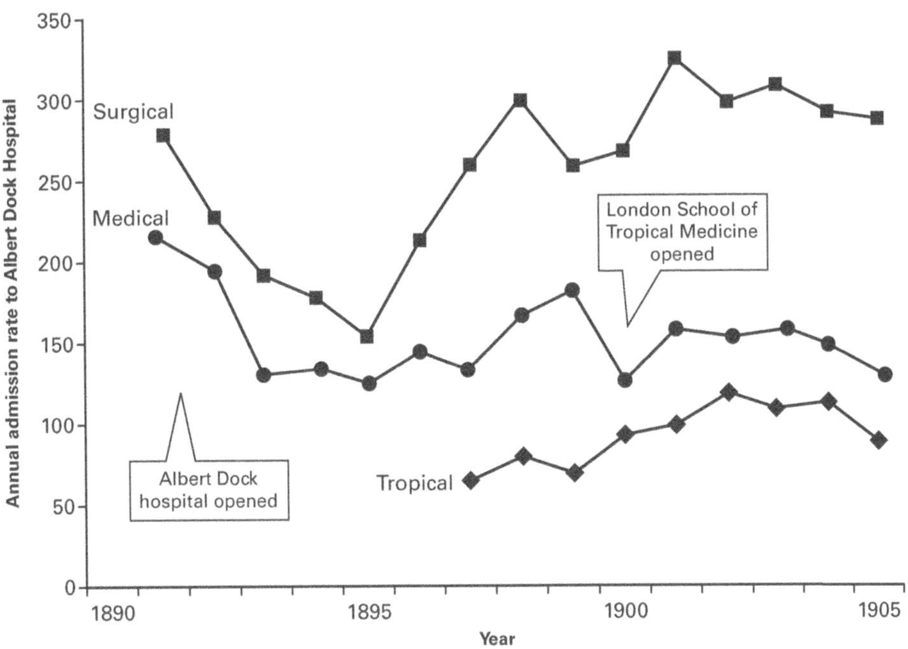

Figure 16.6: Admissions to the Albert Dock Hospital (ADH) from 1891–1905. Total 'tropical', medical, and surgical admissions are shown, for each year for which records are available.

Table 16.2: Contemporary diagnoses of 'tropical' admissions to the ADH.

Date (year)	*1899*	*1900*	*1901*	*1902*	*1903*	*1904*	*1905*
Viral							
Hepatitis/perihepatitis	–	–	3	6	1	2	2
Bacterial							
'Malta Fever'	2	2	2	2	–	1	1
Plague	–	2	–	–	–	–	–
Leprosy	1	2	2	–	–	2	1
Relapsing fever	–	–	–	–	–	–	2
Tropical sprue	–	–	2	4	8	4	6
Bacterial/protozoan							
Dysentery – acute	15	20	15	9	6	12	4
– chronic	11	5	12	14	22	12	12
– 'amoebic'	–	–	–	–	1	–	–
Protozoan							
'Malaria'	24	32	37	41	25	34	26
Kala-azar	–	–	–	2	2	3	1
Trypanoromiasis	–	–	–	1	2	–	5
Hepatic abscess	2	6	4	2	1	10	6
Helminthic							
Ankylostoma duodenale	–	–	–	1	3	1	6
Fillariasis	–	4	3	1	1	5	1
Guinea worm	3	8	4	6	5	1	–
Schistosoma spp	–	–	2	9	1	1	–
Taenia solium	–	–	–	–	1	–	–
Hydatidosis (of lung)	–	–	–	–	1	–	–
Nutritional							
Beri beri	13	13	16	23	23	26	16
Scurvy	4	–	–	–	–	–	–
TOTAL	75	95*	102	122**	110	115	89

*includes 1 case of 'tricophyton' infection.
**includes 1 case of 'granulomatous disease.

medicine' at the ADH was limited (this hospital dealt first and foremost with injuries sustained in the docks – see above); during the period under surveillance the mean admission rate for '*tropical*' cases was <2 per week, which must have been extremely disappointing from a teaching/research viewpoint.

Table 16.3: Contemporary diagnoses of *Plasmodium* spp admissions to the ADH.

Date (year)	*1899*	*1900*	*1901*	*1902*	*1903*	*1904*	*1905*
'Malignant' [P *falciparum*]	4	15	12	13	5	11	11
Blackwater fever	–	2	2	2	6	2	1
Benign tertian [P *vivax*]	5	3	4	8	1	9	13
Double benign tertian	–	2	5	5	4	–	–
Benign tertian + 'malignant'	–	–	–	1	–	–	–
Double benign tertian + 'malignant'	–	–	–	1	–	–	–
'Benign quartan'	–	1	2	–	2	4	1
Triple quartan	–	–	2	1	1	–	–
Double benign tertian +'quartan'	–	–	–	1	–	–	–
Post-malarial jaundice	–	–	–	1	2	–	–
Malarial cachexia	–	3	5	2	1	6	–
Unclassified	8	–	–	–	–	–	–
History, but no parasitological confirmation	7	6	5	6	3	2	–
TOTAL	24	33	37	41	25	34	26

These low figures probably justify, retrospectively, the opinion of several of Manson's leading 'opponents', that the Royal Victoria Hospital, Netley – which contained much 'clinical material ... afforded by invalided soldiers from India, China, and other tropical and sub-tropical stations in all parts of the world' (or possibly the Royal Victoria hospital at Haslar) would have been more suitable venues for the creation of the LSTM. Manson had, however, been appointed to the staff of the ADH seven years before the LSTM was opened! In the light of these facts, it is possible to better understand the acrimonious correspondence between Manson (who of course had Joseph Chamberlain's backing – see Chapter 18) and his 'opponents'. Did Manson (already a physician at the ADH) therefore make the correct decision in the interest of 'tropical medicine', or was he acting primarily from self-interest?[30]

Amoebiasis

An illness indisputably of tropical origin in seafarers, was *invasive hepatic amoebiasis*. It is now impossible (with the availability of modern chemotherapy) to appreciate how lethal was this disease 100 years ago. During a 25-year period in the late nineteenth century (1870–95) (i.e. shortly before the LSTM was established), 50 cases of hepatic abscess were admitted, and managed at one of the two SHS institutions. These patients had been admitted under several SHS physicians/surgeons (Chapters 15 and 18): J Curnow (11), S H Ward (7), J Anderson (6), H Griffiths (6), P Manson (4), C Ralfe (4), R E Carrington, H Leach, W J Smith and R Thomson (1 each); in eight cases the identity of the admitting physician/surgeon is not stated (case histories of 12 of these had been recorded elsewhere). Although it was generally termed 'tropical liver abscess' or 'abscess of the liver', a house physician (Dr C W Windsor) at the *Dreadnought* wrote that because a 'specific organism [had recently been described, the condition should] more accurately [be] called, 'Amoebic Abscess of Liver'. He also gave a lucid description of 'Amoeba Dysenteriae or Coli'.

Peak incidence was between 30–39 years (range: 17–56 years). Twenty-seven were of English nationality, but many other ethnic groups were represented (five were 'Hindoos' and two African). Thirty were Able Seamen, five Lascars and one a 'Landsman'. In 45, 'hepatic suppuration' was deemed to be present, 'such as is rarely met with, except in those who have visited tropical regions, or suffered from dysentery'. In two, it was apparently unclear whether the 'abscess' had *originated* in the liver or elsewhere, and in three there was 'metastatic suppuration' – resulting from either pyaemic or septicaemic infection. Seventeen underwent *surgical* drainage. Twelve were discharged *cured* and 38 died (post-mortem examination was carried out in 34) as a result of their disease. In those who recovered, the abscess had been drained surgically in eight, and had 'burst into the lung' in four. Of the fatal cases, the 'abscess' had burst into the peritoneal cavity – causing fatal peritonitis – in four, had 'perforated the diaphragm' in two, and ruptured into the right pleural cavity in three; the stomach, transverse colon and right kidney were the site(s) of perforation in other cases.

An association between liver abscess and dysentery had already been recorded by several observers; Curnow claimed that one of his patients (a Lascar) was unique because 'this [was] the first occasion [that the] co-existence [of *amoebae dysenteriae* in 'pus' from a liver abscess and dysenteric stool] has been demonstrated in this country [i.e. England]'. In 15 with a single hepatic 'abscess', intestinal ulceration was noted at post-mortem in eight (53%), whereas four gave a 'clear history of dysentery'. Twelve out of 20 with 'multiple hepatic abscess' had intestinal ulceration demonstrated at post-mortem examination; a further four gave a history of dysenteric attacks. Regarding aetiology, Windsor (see above) considered:

> At present, it is impossible to say what is the definite action of the amoeba, or by which path it ascends from the intestine to the liver, whether by the lymphatics or by the vascular system; but it has been supposed that at first numerous small abscesses are formed, which ultimately coalesce to form the large single abscess.

Little can be added to that conclusion more than a century later! It is salutary to recall that now the mortality rate, which approached 80%, should (by administration of one of the 5-nitroimidazole compounds – followed [when available] by diloxanide furoate) be virtually zero.[31]

Nosocomial infections

There are few references to hospital-acquired infection in the Committee of Management minutes. However, in October 1902 'the Visitors suggested that the large lower ward [of the *Dreadnought* Hospital] should be cleaned after a case of Erysipelas [had been managed there], but [as a result of] a letter … from Dr W. G. Ross giving the opinion of the two Surgeons, the subject was deferred'. However, the following year the subject of 'surgical' infections seems to have been taken seriously for 'The Medical Council [ruled] that so far as possible patients with cellulitis and other septic conditions will be isolated'.[32]

Smith's report for 1877 was accompanied by a table showing numbers of deaths resulting from pyaemia and erysipelas during a 22-year period (1854–1876). There was at that time great emphasis (by Florence Nightingale [1820–1910] amongst others) on these two important hospital-associated infections; the design and status of hospitals was assessed on the prevalence of those two entities. Smith pointed to a decline in mortality following removal to the *Caledonia* in 1856; however, after removing the clinical facilities to land there had been an *increase* in 'pyaemic' deaths; this, he considered, was due to an increase in the numbers of *landsmen* treated. This author correctly predicted that with the more widespread introduction of the 'antiseptic method' numbers of cases of pyaemia and erysipelas would decrease.[33]

Accident and Surgical admissions

The 66th Annual Report (1886) recorded: 'During the year [there have been many cases] of sickness caused by exposure after shipwreck admitted to the Wards, some of these patients being picked up in open boats at sea, and forwarded to the Seamen's Hospital by the British Consul at the first port at which the rescuing vessel touched'.[34]

Another example of urgent *surgical* management followed an explosion on a British India Associated steamer, an account of which is to be found in the 70th *Annual Report* (1890): '… one European (the second Engineer) and six Lascars were fearfully scalded [with the result that] they all ultimately died, four of the Lascars dying within the first 24 hours'.[35] And a further example of the devastating result(s) of an explosion (this time on the SS *Manitoba* in 1898): 'nine persons treated in the ward [of the ADH] were so seriously injured that three succumbed within 24 hours, and ultimately four only survived'.[36]

In the days of the hospital-ships, surgical practice during the winter months had been dominated by 'treatment of Lascars for severe frost-bite and gangrene'; things seem to have improved in the period under review in this chapter.

Comparison of afflictions of seafarers with those in the land-based population (1870–1914)

In 1867 (i.e. three years before removal to the land-based Hospital), Harry Leach,[37] (see also Chapter 12) resident Medical Officer on the Hospital-ship, provided a valuable insight into the health of sailors in the merchant service. The following year he published *The Ship Captain's Medical Guide* – which has since gone through numerous editions – and remains in use today; this was 'written solely for the use of Masters and Mates of vessels at sea', and covered 'accidents and diseases that occur[ed] on board ship ...'. It also emphasised how cases could 'be best treated by a non-professional man'. The entry regarding 'Ague, or intermittent fever [most cases were undoubtedly caused by malaria]' illustrates the clarity of Leach's advice:

> This disease, in one form or other, occurs chiefly in China, the West Indies, and on the west coast of Africa. A violent chill, followed by great heat, the whole attack lasting from two to eight hours, are sufficiently distinct symptoms, and two things are to be done before you can commence any satisfactory treatment – 1st see that the bowels are well opened with a dose of black draught; 2ndly find out as exactly as is possible the hours at which the chill fit usually begins. This will, with some care, be almost always ascertained. Having succeeded in fixing the time, give your patient 10 grains of quinine in a little water two hours before the expected attack. Repeat this twice, and, if unsuccessful in stopping the fit, or lessening its severity, increase the dose to 15 grains. Having stopped the chill fit completely, keep up this large dose three times afterwards, two hours before the expected attack, and give the man, besides these large doses, 3 grains of quinine three times a day, making him take this last prescription at least a week after all signs of the disease have passed away.[38]

Successive medical reports – compiled by Smith[39] – provide a valuable insight into the major health problems experienced by the seafarer of the late nineteenth and early twentieth centuries. The ADH (Chapter 14), situated on the northern bank of the River Thames had been opened in 1890; here, the emphasis was on *surgical* diseases – until the London School of Tropical Medicine (LSTM) was founded on that site in 1899. Although the Society obviously did not deal with *all* cases of disease in merchant seamen in the Port of London, details of morbidity and mortality experienced in these two hospital(s) must inevitably reflect the disease pattern in this class of men generally.

Classification of disease(s) in merchant sailors, and others treated at the Society's hospitals

There had, Smith wrote, been a notable increase in the number(s) of Lascars (See Figure 16.7) treated in the early years of the survey (1875–1905); by 1879 'so many as forty-one Hindoo sailors were admitted'. In his report for 1876, Smith drew attention to an 'apparently undue proportion of firemen and cooks' amongst the 878 medical and 1167 surgical admissions during the previous year, a fact to be reiterated in subsequent reports. Hospital relief had in 1875 been 'afforded to 113 persons ['landsmen'] not connected with the navigation of ships or river craft' – most having suffered accidents (they were therefore *surgical* cases) – usually in the vicinity of Greenwich.

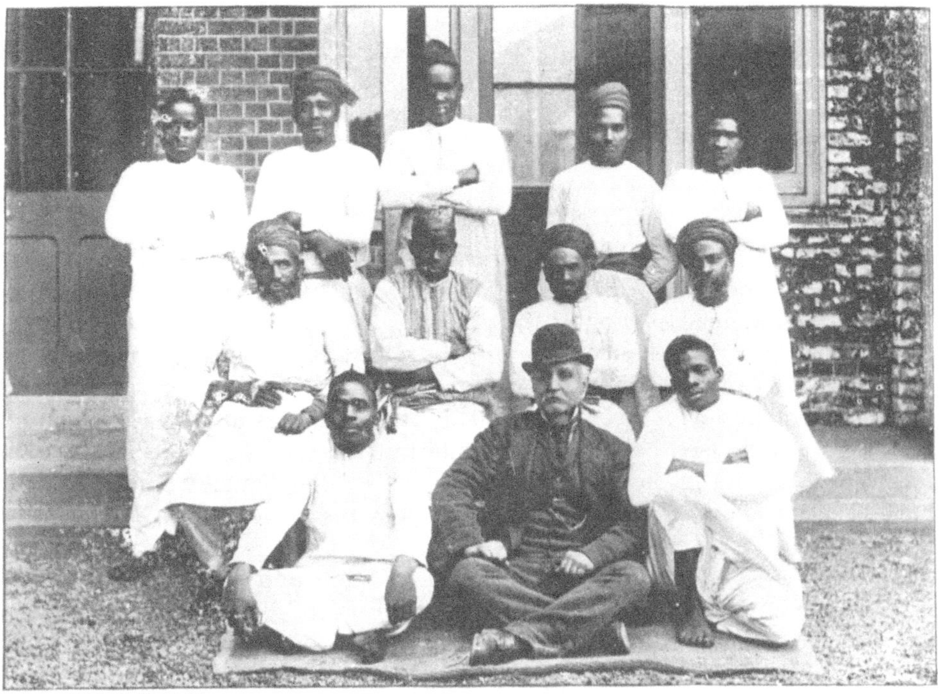

Figure 16.7: Group of *Lascars* outside the ADH in 1899. [SHS Archive].

In 1879, 24 women and children were treated out of a total of '156 persons living on land'; treatment of this group ('special cases') remained a contentious issue, being frequently discussed at SHS Committee meetings (see above), but the 1881 report emphasised that this 'class' did not exceed 15% of the *outpatient* total. In the following year, 177 were on-shore labourers, and 67 women and children; '233 … not associated in any way with shipping' were treated during 1882. With regard to admission of women, the 1885 report recorded a *decrease* in numbers treated as a result of 'improved hospital accommodation in the district [which] will probably become more marked in future'. Despite this, the vast majority of admissions were of seafarers from the Mercantile Marines of 'all nations'.[40]

In 1891 Curnow,[41] together with Smith, jointly attempted a *classification* of *medical* diseases admitted to the *Dreadnought Hospital* (>550 cases annually, compared with >750 *surgical* admissions) which were a major problem to the seafarer. This analysis (based on 7,718 admissions) covered the previous decade. They divided the diseases into: (i) *common* disorders (dominated by phthisis – nearly one-seventh of the whole [see below]), but also including: chronic rheumatism (a result of 'constant exposure to wet and cold, and from a poor diet'), 'cardiac valvular disease', pleurisy, pneumonia and chronic albuminuria – probably in most cases caused by long-standing renal disease) which afflicted both seafarers *and* also those on land (i.e. in the immediate vicinity of Greenwich); and (ii) *rarer* diseases, which had a greater prevalence in the seafarer, in comparison with residents of England, in their clientele at the *Dreadnought* Hospital: 'ague', 'enteric fever' (most cases were probably typhoid or paratyphoid), dysentery (or bloody diarrhoea), liver abscess (see above) and aortic aneurism(s) – the latter being attributed to 'syphilis [and] the mere strain of work'.[42]

MEDICAL DISEASES RESTRICTED TO THE SEAFARER

Figure 16.8 summarises the major *medical* admissions to the Society's hospitals between 1875 and 1905 which were considered more common in the merchant service than the general (English) population. Out of 1,546 cases of 'ague' (see above) only four died. However, mortality rate(s) from the other 'tropical' diseases was substantially higher; 68 out of 1,020 cases of 'dysentery', and 93 out of 859 of 'enteric fever' (see above), died. The prognosis for thoracic aneurism and liver abscess (see below) was significantly worse': 84 out of 242 of the former, and 19 out of 36 cases of the latter died. (Incidentally, Smith seems to have been uncertain of a connection between syphilis and aneurism of the thoracic aorta).

A downward trend in admissions caused by 'ague' and dysentery is apparent in Figure 16.8 – in the former case, widespread use of quinine and in the latter increasing recognition that a contaminated water-supply was relevant in aetio-

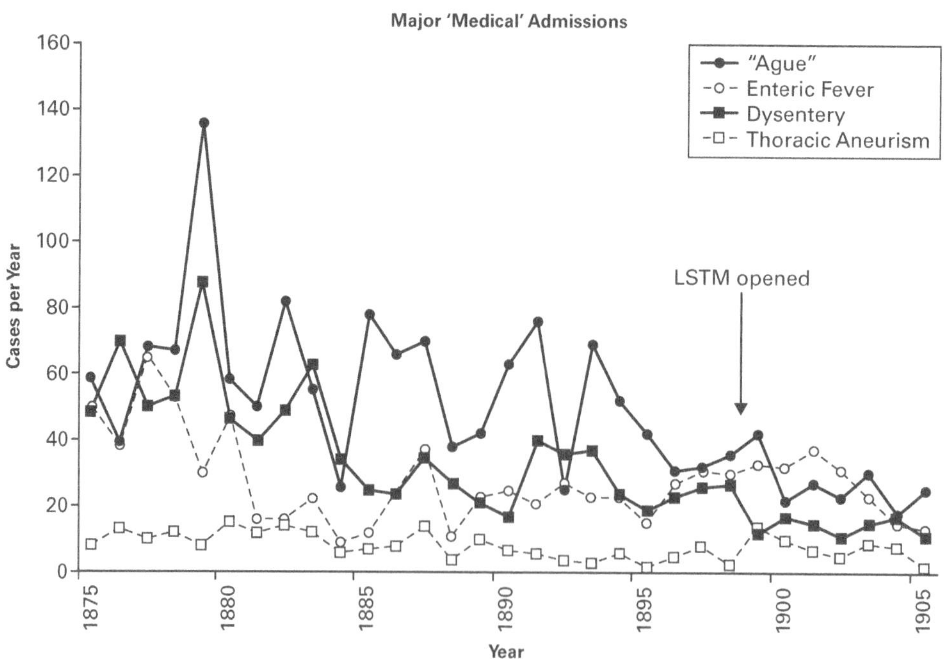

Figure 16.8: Diagnoses of leading 'medical' admissions to the *Dreadnought* and Albert Dock Hospitals between 1875 and 1905. Opening of the London School of Tropical Medicine (LSTM) at the Albert Dock Hospital in 1899 is indicated.

pathogenesis; foodstuffs were then disinfected. Regarding 'enteric fever' the admission rate during 1875 was boosted by cases from the *Cornwall* training-ship. In 1879, a minor outbreak of trichinosis occurred in boys from this training-ship (see above).[43]

The 1883 medical report referred to the regrettable entry into London of infectious disease – due to the fact that cases 'are still allowed to pass into the Port without very stringent action being taken by the Customs Authorities at Gravesend'; the quarantine regulations were being flouted, and the chief offenders in most cases were 'those in charge of foreign vessels or small coasting craft'. On the question of *transmission* of disease, Smith concluded in his 1879 report, obviously with the outbreak of trichinosis (see above) in mind, that 'should unfortunately any future epidemic of zymotic [infectious] disease occur in a training-ship, the authorities of that Institution might be able to retain the patients in some building or floating hospital quite apart, but still at no very great distance from the school.'

SURGICAL DISEASES RESTRICTED TO THE SEAFARER

Figure 16.9 summarises major *surgical* admissions to the *Dreadnought Hospital* between 1875 and 1905; these were dominated by sexually transmitted disease(s) (see above); from 1890, cases of gonorrhoea were recorded separately. In early 1878, the Committee of Management had ruled that 'applicants suffering from such forms of venereal disease [VD] as were not disabling or very severe [including those with 'mild venereal disorders and primary syphilis'] should be treated as out-patients and not as hospital inmates'. Smith's 1881 report however, referred to a decision to revert to the former system, but with certain modifications and restrictions [although it was exceedingly difficult to decide which were serious and/or mild cases of VD], and arrangements made that all such cases be treated in an isolated part of the Hospital, under the nursing control of male attendants'. Most leg ulcers were probably syphilitic in origin (although some had undoubtedly resulted from minor injuries), and urethral stricture was undoubtedly in most caused by gonococcal infection.[44]

DISEASES SIMILAR IN PREVALENCE IN THE SEAFARER AND THE 'ENGLISH POPULATION'

The *common* diseases were those considered by Curnow and Smith to be of similar prevalence in the seafarer to that in the English population, in and around Greenwich. In the 1881 report, Smith emphasised that 16 out of 26 deaths resulting from tuberculosis ('phthisis') (see above) had occurred in '*foreign* [my italics] seamen'; this disease was the major overall cause of medical morbidity and mortality throughout the period covered in this chapter. Smith had also commented in his 1876 report on the undue prevalence of 'chronic rheumatism' (89 cases) (see above).[45]

During 1875 (which was a fairly typical year), 104 patients died; the medical and surgical death rates were 8% and <3% of admissions, respectively), a reduction in

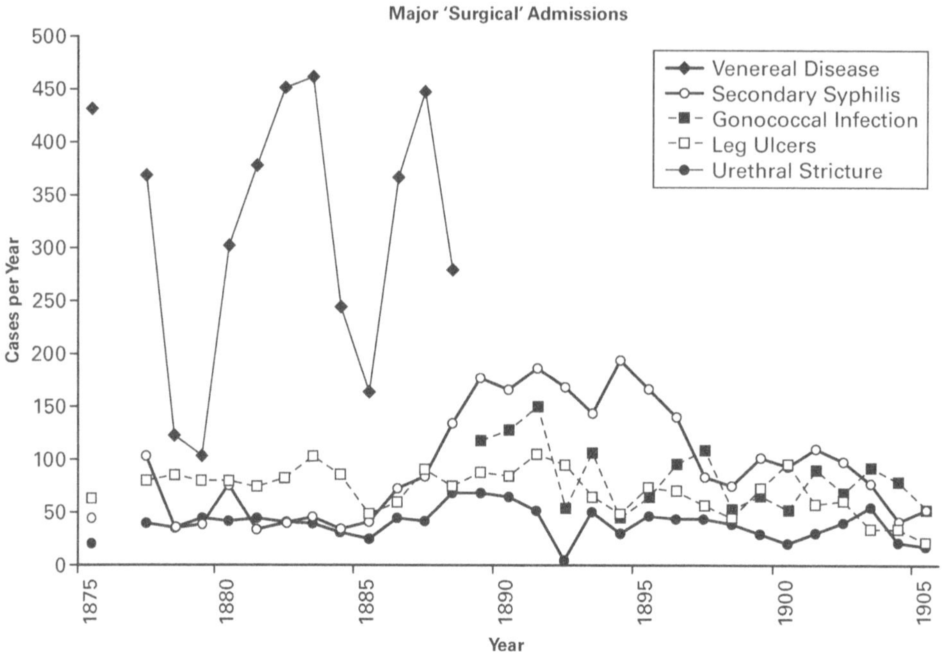

Figure 16.9: Diagnoses of leading 'surgical' admissions to the *Dreadnought* and Albert Dock Hospitals between 1875 and 1905. Most are probably all short or long-term manifestations of venereal disease (either syphilis or gonorrhoea).

mortality in the surgical wards probably being a result of '... Professor [Joseph] Lister's[46] plan of local treatment ...' together with improved sanitary conditions in the hospital. These mortality rates should, Smith wrote, be viewed against one of approximately 9% in the 'London General Hospitals'. There were, he considered, several reasons for these relatively encouraging figures:

i) lack of factories in the immediate vicinity of Greenwich,
ii) allocation of more beds for surgical (one-third were occupied by venereal diseases resulting from the 'peculiar temptations to which sailors are exposed') than medical cases,
iii) protection from 'cold and bad weather',
iv) availability of a large numbers of beds (compared with most hospitals) in relation to daily numbers of patients, and
v) the admission of numerous 'trivial' cases.

By 1880, 107 (5.9%) of the total number of admissions terminated in death; this comprised 11% of medical, and <2% surgical cases; the underlying reason(s) for this disparity is not clear.[47]

Overall assessment of the Society's value in the early 20th century

The inestimable value of the Society to the health of sailors in the Mercantile Marine is succinctly summarised in the 92nd Annual Report (1912):

> The true history of the Dreadnought and [ADH] is not to be found in impersonal statistics, but among the thousands of sailors scattered all over the world, who have found in the wards relief of pain and renewed health ... Seamen who have met with accidents at sea, far from the possibility of proper care and attention, or who have contracted diseases inseparable from the work in the Tropics, have received the special treatment which the neglect of their injuries or the obscurity of their disease necessitated, treatment which only the largest and most modern Institutions can supply. Simpler and less serious cases have been given unwearied attention and nursing coupled with an experienced appreciation of the Sailor's particular needs.[48]

References and notes

1 Annual Report: 50; 53; 76; 79.
2 Committee of Management Minutes. 14: 412; 15: 52, 57, 126–7, 221.
3 G C Cook. Early use of 'open-air' treatment for 'pulmonary phthisis' at the Dreadnought Hospital, Greenwich, 1900–1905. *Postgrad Med J* 1999; 75: 326–327; *Op cit.* See note 1 above. 81: 1901: 19; *Op cit.* See note 2 above. 13: 252, 257–8, 391; 14: 50, 154; R T Hewlett, G Rankin. Report on the open-air treatment of phthisis at the Dreadnought Hospital, Greenwich. From the 1st November, 1900, to the 30th October, 1901. In: *Tables of cases under treatment at the Hospitals and Dispensaries of the Seamen's Hospital Society in 1901.* London: E G Berryman & Sons 1902: 1–4; G Rankin, R T Hewlett. *Ibid.* 30th October, 1901 to the 30th October 1902. 1903: 22–25; R T Hewlett, G Rankin. *Ibid.* 1st November, 1902, to the 30th October, 1903. 1904: 21–24; R T Hewlett, G Rankin. *Ibid.* 1st November, 1903, to the 30th October, 1904. 1905: 21–24; *Ibid.* Anonymous. 1st November, 1904, to the 30th October, 1905. 1906: 22–24.
4 *Op cit.* See note 1 above: 50: 70, 90: 14.
5 *Ibid.* 51: 18; 52: 18; 76: 15.
6 W J Smith (ed). *A General Report of the cases under treatment at the Seamen's Hospital, Greenwich, together with an analysis of the medical (and surgical) cases.* Greenwich: Seamen's Hospital Society. 1876–1891; G C Cook. Disease in the nineteenth-century merchant navy: the Seamen's Hospital Society's experience. *Mariner's Mirror* 2000; 87: 460–471; G C Cook. Scurvy in the British Mercantile Marine in the 19th century and the contribution of the Seamen's Hospital Society. *Postgrad Med J* 2004; 80: 224–29.
7 *Op cit.* See note 1 above. 73: 11; *Op cit.* See note 2 above. 9: 283, 284–6, 287, 381; 11: 24, 103, 110–11, 114, 118, 132; 12: 155, 229.
8 *Op cit.* See note 2 above. 10: 89–90; 12: 33, 162; 13: 200, 369, 521; 15: 134.
9 *Ibid.* 12: 444; 13: 120, 131, 256, 401; 14: 252.
10 *Ibid.* 11: 383; 12: 484.
11 *Ibid.* 11: 495.

12 *Ibid.* 12: 279–81.
13 G C Cook. Outbreak of trichinosis (trichiniasis) – contracted in London in 1879. *Postgrad Med J* 2001; 77: 62–63.
14 A Hardy. Power, Sir William Henry (1842–1916). In: H C G Matthew, B Harrison (eds). *Oxford Dictionary of National Biography.* Oxford: Oxford University Press 2004; 45: 146–7.
15 S E Gould. *Trichinosis.* Springfield, Illinois: C C Thomas 1945: 356; D I Grove. *Trichinella spiralis* and trichinosis. In: *A history of human helminthology.* London: CAB International, 1990: 571–595. F Bruschi, R D Murrell. New aspects of human trichinellosis: the impact of new *Trichinella* species. *Postgrad Med J* 2002; 78: 15–22.
16 *Op cit.* See note 2 above. 10: 209–210.
17 G T Bettany, P Osborne. Cobbold, Thomas Spencer (1828–1886). In: H C G Matthew, B Harrison (eds). *Oxford Dictionary of National Biography.* Oxford: Oxford University Press 2004; 12: 281.
18 Anonymous. Medico-parliamentary. *HOUSE OF LORDS – Thursday, February 19th. Trichinosis. BMJ* 1880; i: 497. Anonymous. Trichinosis. *Lancet* 1880; i: 376–7; Anonymous. Medico-Parliamentary. HOUSE OF LORDS – *Tuesday March 23rd. Trichinosis on Board the Cornwall Training-Ship. BMJ* 1880; i: 497; *Op cit.* See note 13 above; W J Smith. *A General Report of the cases under treatment at the Seamen's Hospital, Greenwich, together with an analysis of the medical and surgical cases.* Greenwich: Seamen's Hospital Society 1880: 5–7.
19 **George Busk** FRS (1807–87) (see also Chapter 12) was appointed to the SHS in 1831, having served that Society as an apothecary from 1830. He became successively, Assistant Surgeon (1832), Resident Surgeon (1837), Surgeon (1841), Visiting Surgeon (1854) and Consulting Surgeon (1866).
20 *Op cit.* See note 2 above. 12: 66,68; 14: 320; 15: 63, 226.
21 *Op cit.* See note 1 above. 73: 12.
22 *Op cit.* See note 2 above. 4: 384, 349; 6: 295; 7: 241, 254, 512; [see also: G C Cook. Dr William Woodville (1752–1805) and the St Pancras Smallpox Hospital. *J Med Biog* 1996; 4: 71–78].
23 **James Furness Marson** FRCS (?–1877) was surgeon to the Smallpox and Vaccination Hospital – firstly situated at St Pancras, and latterly in Upper Holloway. He was also principal Vaccinator of the National Vaccination Establishment (*see* Chapter 12). (See also: J F Marson: Observations on the co-existence of variola and scarlatina, with remarks on the co-existence of other eruptive fevers. *Medico-Chir Trans* 1847; 30: 14–9; On smallpox and vaccination. Analytical examination of all the cases admitted during sixteen years, at the Smallpox and Vaccination Hospital, London; with a view to illustrate the pathology of smallpox, and the protective influence of vaccination, in degrees varying according as the vaccination has been perfectly or imperfectly performed. *Medico-Chir Trans* 1853; 36: 359–89).
24 C Hamlin. Simon, Sir John (1816–1904): In: H C G Matthew, B Harrison (eds). *Oxford Dictionary of National Biography.* Oxford: Oxford University Press 2004; 50: 660–3.
25 *Op cit.* See note 2 above. 9: 253, 256, 258, 519, 523–4, 526, 529, 537; 10: 48–9, 69–71, 93, 186, 213–4, 341–2, 350; 11: 87, 103, 106, 175–7; 12: 316–7, 473; 13: 383, 394, 430, 452; 14: 305, 373, 375, 378–9, 381.
26 *Op cit.* See note 1 above. 75: 12.
27 G C Cook. *Op cit. see* note 6 above (Smith). [*See also*: G C Cook. Doctor Patrick Manson's leading opposition in the establishment of the London School of Tropical Medicine: Curnow, Anderson, and Turner. *J Med Biog* 1995; 3: 170–77].
28 G C Cook. 'Tropical' cases admitted to the Albert Dock Hospital in the early years of the London School of Tropical Medicine. *Trans R Soc Trop Med Hyg* 1999; 93: 675–77.
29 *Op cit.* See Note 6 (Smith), 20 and 22 above.

30 P Hoare. *Spike Island: The memory of a military hospital.* London: Fourth Estate 2001: 417; P T Marsh. Joseph Chamberlain: *Entrepreneur in Politics.* New Haven, London: Yale University Press 1994: 725.

31 C W Windsor. Note of the Amoeba Coli. In: W J Smith (ed). *A General Report of the cases under treatment at the Hospitals and Dispensaries of the Seamen's Hospital Society.* Greenwich: E G Berryman & Sons 1895: 38–40; G C Cook. Invasive amoebiasis one hundred years ago: the Seamen's Hospital Society's experience (1870–95). *Trans R Soc Trop Med Hyg* 1999; 93: 220–21; P Manson. Abscess of the liver. In: *Tropical diseases: a manual of diseases of warm climates.* London: Cassell and Co Ltd, 1898: 343–378.

32 *Op cit. see* note 2 above. 13: 468, 496.

33 *Op cit. see* note 6 above (Smith); Pyaemia and erysipelas (both resulting from bacterial infection) were in the mid and late nineteenth-century considered 'markers' of standards of ventilation, sanitation and hygiene in hospitals. Florence Nightingale (1820–1910) was amongst those to used these indices to assess the merits of respective hospitals [see also: F Nightingale. *Notes on hospitals: being two papers read before the National Association for the Promotion of the Social Sciences at Liverpool, in October 1858. With evidence given to the Royal Commissioners on the State of the Army in 1857.* London. John W Parker & Son]. See also: Anonymous. Sites and construction of hospitals. *Builder* 1858; 16: 577–8; Anonymous. Construction of hospitals – the ground plan. *Builder* 1858: 16: 609–610; Anonymous. Hospital construction – wards. *Builder* 1858; 16: 641–643.

34 *Op cit.* See note 1 above: 66.

35 *Ibid.* 70: 11.

36 *Op cit.* See note 1 above: 78.

37 **Harry Leach** MRCP (1836–79); See also Chapters 12 and 15.

38 Anonymous. Report on the hygienic condition of the mercantile marine, and on the preventable diseases of merchant seamen. *BMJ* 1867; i: 36–7, 64–66, 89–91, 120–122, 147–148; H Leach. *Report on the hygienic condition of the mercantile marine, and on the preventable diseases of merchant seamen.* London: AM Walker, 1867: 32; H Leach. *The Ship Captain's Medical Guide.* 2nd ed. London: Simpkin, Marshall, and Co. 1868: 93.

39 **William Johnson Smith** FRCS (1840–1912); see also Chapter 12. In 1863 he was appointed Assistant Surgeon, and in 1871 Surgeon to the *Dreadnought* (Seamen's) Hospital, Greenwich. He later became Surgeon to the ADH. In 1905, Smith retired as Surgeon and Principal Medical Officer, and was thereafter a Consulting Surgeon to the ADH.

40 W J Smith (ed.). *A General Report of the cases under treatment at the Hospitals and Dispensaries of the Seamen's Hospital Society together with an analysis of the medical and surgical cases.* Greenwich: E G Berryman and Sons. 1892–1895; Anonymous. Seamen's Hospital Society. *Tables of cases under treatment at the Hospitals and Dispensaries of the Seamen's Hospital Society.* London: E G Berryman & Sons. 1897–1906; G C Cook, A J Webb. The Albert Dock Hospital, London: the original site (in 1899) of Tropical Medicine as a *new* discipline. *Acta Tropica* 2001: 79: 249–255.

41 **John Curnow** FRCP (1846–1902) qualified with the MB (and gold medal) from King's College Hospital in 1870; a year later, he was awarded the MD degree of the University of London, and elected FRCP in 1878. From 1878 until 1897, he was a physician to the *Dreadnought* Hospital, Greenwich; in 1899 (together with three colleagues) he resigned in opposition to the creation of the London School of Tropical Medicine at the ADH. He died suddenly (probably as a result of pneumonia) at the age of 56 years. [*See also*: G C Cook. Doctor Patrick Manson's leading opposition in the establishment of the London School of Tropical Medicine: Curnow, Anderson, and Turner. *J Med Biog* 1995; 3: 170–177].

42 J Curnow, W J Smith. Naval and military hygiene: *Statistics of Medical Cases admitted into the Seamen's Hospital, 1880–89. Lancet* 1891; ii: 452.

43 *Op cit.* See note 6 above (Smith), 20 and 22.
44 *Ibid.*
45 *Ibid.*
46 **Joseph Lister** (later 1st Baron) (1827–1912) introduced antiseptic treatment to surgery, and was therefore one of the pioneers of the 'germ-theory' of disease. [See also: R J Godlee. *Lord Lister*. London: Macmillan 1917: 686; C Lawrence. Lister, Joseph, Baron Lister (1827–1912). In: H C G Matthew, B Harrison (eds). *Oxford Dictionary of National Biography*. Oxford: Oxford University Press 2004; 33: 979–84].
47 *Op cit.* See notes 6 (Smith), 20 and 22 above.
48 *Op cit.* See note 1 above. 82: 11.

Chapter 17

Nursing and nurse-training at the *Dreadnought* and ADH: establishment of a school on Nightingale lines

Florence Nightingale (1820–1910) is usually given credit for initiating modern nurse-training, at St Thomas's Hospital in 1860, despite a great deal of hostility from the medical hierarchy of the day. The part played by Elizabeth Fry (1780–1845) should also not be forgotten. However, it is important not to overlook the contributions of doctors to these reforms – which started in the earlier part of the nineteenth century.

In addition to a comprehensive course in medical and practical nurse-training, every probationer under Nightingale had her own room and uniform. Eleven years later, Guy's Hospital also reformed its nursing arrangements, and a single nurse was allocated to every 12 patients; nurses' pay was increased to £20 annually, plus board and uniform. Other London teaching hospitals were, however, slow to implement Nightingale's reforms.[1]

Nightingale's views on disease in the mercantile marine

Nightingale was, in the light of her experiences at Scutari in the Crimean War, far more interested in the health of soldiers than sailors. However, in 1867 she was already engaged in a correspondence on health in the mercantile marine with her brother-in-law, Captain (later Sir) Harry Verney. The first letter (all were written from: 35 South Street, Park Lane, London, W.) seems to refer to the mercantile marine rather than the RN, but adds little light on the subject:

> My dear Capt. Verney
>
> The enclosed is a subject which interests me very much & to which I have indirectly paid some attention – I would gladly look over it now – but I am sure it would do little purpose as you can give me so little time & I am very busy. I hope you will let me see it in proof when I will read it carefully.[2]
>
> F.N.

However, this was followed five days later with one, which seems to relate to the SHS:

> My dear Capt.Verney
> I think your 'Society' for the 'Merchant Seamen' a noble thing to do & done in the best manner. I have carefully read (& shown to Dr. Sutherland[3]) your 'Sketch' [which does not seem to have survived]. We make only the enclosed suggestions
> Ever yours truly
> F. Nightingale[4]

And a week later she wrote:

> My dear Capt. Verney
> I think, with you, that the best thing to do with my suggestions will be to leave them out of the Appendices[sic]. Your Report is a practical one – that is the beauty of it. I wrote, as you are aware, merely in obedience to a request – merely to submit points for the practical consideration of your Committee. That (viz. practical consideration) is the end of the whole matter. I now merely add: – One principal *cause of the high Sick & Death Rates among Merchant seamen* [my italics] is their wretched accommodation. The more useful attention you draw to this, viz. the best sanitary arrangements on board ship for crews – the better. To get drawings & models from practical people – is a course which has succeeded in similar things.
> Ever yours
> F. Nightingale[5]

It is patently clear from this correspondence that Nightingale herself (some years before the 'germ-theory' of disease had been widely accepted, and in keeping with the great sanitary reformers of the nineteenth century, which were led by Thomas Southwood Smith [1788–1861]), was adamant that, coupled with poor ventilation, the sanitary conditions on board merchant ships were totally inadequate. These factors, she considered, promoted disease (and death) in seafarers.

The SHS began training nurses in 1877 – principally for their own purpose(s). Obviously, nurses had played a crucially important rôle in patient care in the hospital-ship days, but no formal training had been provided. In the latter days of the hospital-ships, many *Dreadnought* nurses had been male; they earned 21 shillings weekly compared with a woman's eight; ordinary female nurses received six shillings weekly, i.e. one third that of the messengers (the Society's lowliest servants). Nursing standards (there was much dishonesty, drunkenness and idleness) were appallingly lax during the latter days of the hospital-ships.[6]

In theory, female nurses had been acceptable since 1825 – when the SHS changed its 'men-only' rule – but few served on the ships, conditions being unacceptable. In fact, amongst reasons for removal to land was the lack of adequate facilities for the nursing staff – and hence the difficulty of recruitment; this had been stressed by the *medical* staff (Chapter 13). The surgeon, H T L Rooke (1824–70) (as well as other members of the medical staff) on board the *Dreadnought*, considered, for example, that conditions on board the hospital-ships (including rooms to which they could 'retire') were so inadequate for female nurses that good ones simply would not seek employment there. There were also difficulties associated with getting to and fro from the shore. Lack of adequate ventilation – close to the heart of Nightingale in her *Notes on Hospitals* – in the hospital-ships was also dominant in the minds of the physicians and surgeons.[7] When the Society became land-based, the nursing 'establishment' had been increased from one male and two females for each of three decks, i.e. a total of nine nurses, to 'one male nurse, and sixteen females' (17 in all).

Nursing at the *Dreadnought* soon after removal to dry-land

A Surgeon's Report soon after removal to land contained the following disquieting reference to nurse staffing:

> For some months past the proportion of severe to mild Cases has increased and, as is indicated by the increasing death rate, there has been a larger proportion in the cases under treatment of acute and severe disease. Under these somewhat altered conditions & also for other reasons, I think it right to express the opinion that the *Nursing Staff is not satisfactory* [my italics]. I would beg therefore to suggest, that, an enquiry on your part into the condition of this department, with a view to some change & improvements might materially increase the efficiency of the Medical Service. *Ordered.* That a Sub-Committee consisting of the Chairman, & MR T.R. Edridge be appointed to enquire into the present condition of the Nursing Department & to report.[8]

At a later meeting, a report of this Sub-Committee was duly read (and adopted):

> Your Committee have held two Meetings and have taken the evidence of the Visiting Physician, DR Harry Leach, the Visiting Surgeon, MR N. Davies-Colley, the Surgeon & the Matron upon the present arrangements of the Hospital. They have further had before them the details of the nursing systems of other metropolitan & Poor Law Hospitals and they find; – 1st That the number of Nurses to patients at the Seamen's Hospital is relatively smaller than at any other similar institution. 2nd That since the closing of the Upper West Ward there have been comparatively few patients sufficiently convalescent to render, as formerly, any useful assistance in the work of the wards. 3rd That the women, who have been employed hitherto, are on the whole of an inferior class, lacking in intelligence & otherwise ill-fitted for the performance of the important duty of nursing. 4th That the nurses at the Seamen's Hospital are not as well paid as those at other metropolitan Hospitals.
>
> Your Committee are of opinion that inadequate pay is at the root of the evil & they recommend that the wages of the nursing staff be increased

from a minimum of £15 & a maximum of £20 per annum as at present; to a minimum of £20 rising £1 annually to the maximum of £25 per annum, for fully trained nurses.

They further consider that it is desirable the nursing staff should be increased from its present number, 15 to 17, & they recommend that this shall be effected in the following manner. That the nursing staff shall consist of 13 fully qualified nurses and, 4 Probationers, and that the remuneration of the latter be at the rate of £12 for the first year, £15 the second, & £18 the third year, uniform being found them. They further recommend that the Sisters shall be entitled in future to an increase of wages, after five years service; & that at the expiration of this period (five years) a sister's wages shall increase from £30, rising to £1 per annum to £35. The Committee estimate that eventually these changes in the nursing department will entail an extra expenditure of £170 per annum but the Committee suggest that the new system shall be gradually introduced so that the immediate increase in the expenditure will not exceed £103 per annum. This increase will only be temporary as, by introducing probationers, the Committee have ascertained, that at the end of six months the expenditure will be reduced to £79. The Committee further recommend that every probationer nurse, who is approved after a month's trial, shall be required to enter into an agreement, to remain in the service of the Society for a period of three years, that is to say until her training is complete.

Jos Moore [Chairman of the S.H.S.,] [–,] Fred[k] Cleeve[9]

Several subsequent reports also record that all was not well at that time with nursing at the *Dreadnought*.[10]

Female nurses (see Figures 17.1 and 17.2) had in fact become vital to the Society; from 1870, women (and also children) from the local populations of Greenwich, Blackheath, Deptford and the surrounding districts all used the *Dreadnought* Hospital.[11]

The need for a competent matron also soon became apparent, as the minutes make clear:

> The [SHS] Committee [in 1871] [were] of opinion that a Matron should be added to the Staff of the Hospital who should be qualified to appoint, and exercise direct control over, the female nurses and servants. That her salary should be *£60* per annum besides board and lodging. That she should be a Member of the Church of England – from 30 to 45 years of age, and either single or a widow without family. Considering the great importance of getting a person thoroughly adapted to the various duties that would devolve upon the Matron – the Sub Committee [considered] it advisable that she should be selected by the House Governor, subject to approval of the Committee, and on probation for Three months.[12]

Six weeks later:

> The House Governor & Secretary [M[r] Silas Kemball Cook[13]] soon reported that he had Selected Miss [T.U.] Collins as in his judgement the

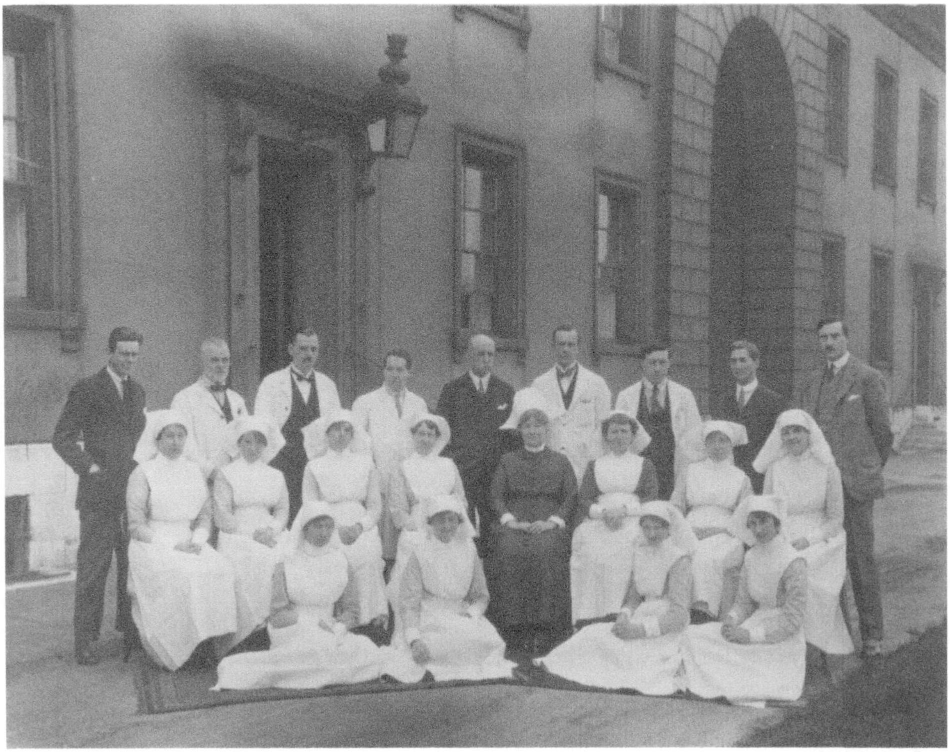

Figure 17.1: Nursing, and junior medical staff of the Dreadnought Hospital – early 20th century. [SHS Archive].

> most Eligible of all the Candidates for the Office of Matron. The minutes continued: 'Ordered that Miss Collins be appointed Matron on trial for three months'.

Collins soon used her influence in persuading the Society to appoint several female nurses as her deputies.[14] Regarding pay:

> Read a letter from the Matron to the House Governor recommending that £18 per annum with an increase of £1 a year up to £20 should be the pay for Nurses of Experience and £15 a year rising £1 a year for women who have not been trained. The House Governor reported that such a scale would put their Hospital in as good a position as others as regards pay to Nurses. Ordered that their recommendation be Carried out under the direction of the House Governor.

In addition, Collins was responsible for disposing of a good deal of 'dead wood'. The male doctors (who dominated the medical scenario at the *Dreadnought*) seem, however, to have found some difficulty in adapting to Collins' new strategies.[15]

The 'status' of the nursing profession in the 1870s was indeed at a low ebb! A memorandum shortly after the appointment of Collins emphasises the poor qual-

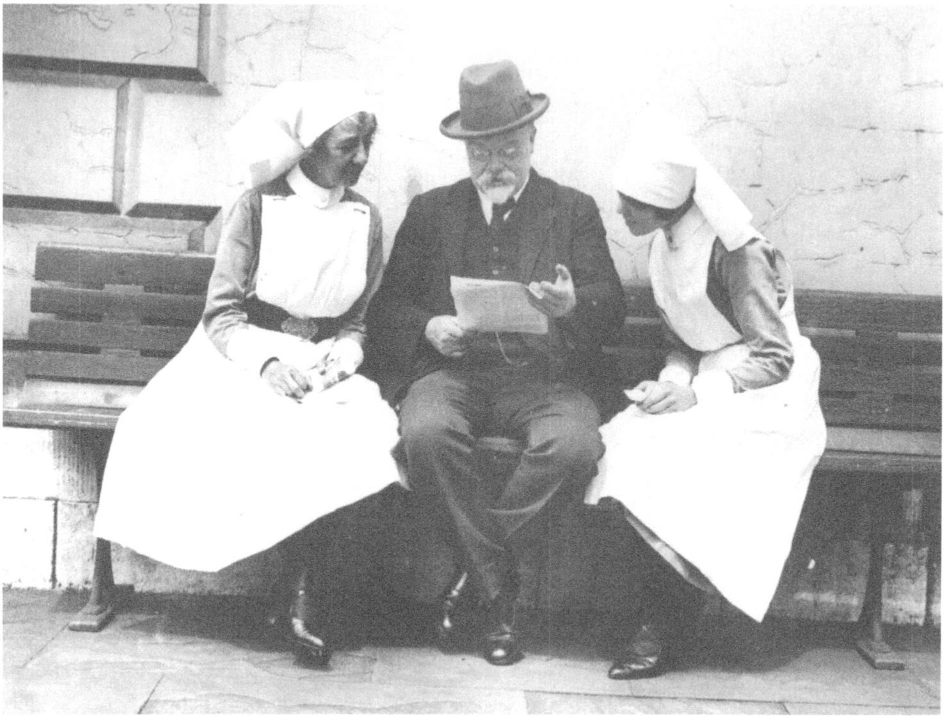

Figure 17.2: Two *Dreadnought* sisters talking to Sir George Hume in 1928. [SHS Archive].

ity of nurses employed by the Society at that time. Names of 53 Nurses and Sisters (15 had served *before* Collins was appointed) listed: four were dismissed for being 'drunk and disorderly', four were described as being 'incompetent', or 'dishonest', and several others had remained out after permitted hours (one 'till 10 p.m.'!); a mere 18 seem to have been able to carry out their duties responsibly![16] Clearly, a great deal of 'tightening up' in discipline was required, and in 1875 revised instructions for the *nurses* employed by the Society were therefore laid down (see Box 1).

Box 1

1. The Nurses will be selected by the Matron on trial for one month, at the expiration of which time, if approved of by the Surgeon, she will report them to the Secretary, and if approved by the Committee, a uniform will be provided for them.
2. They must be able to read and write. They will reside in the Hospital, be entirely under the control of the Matron, and always wear the uniform provided.

3. They shall take their meals in the room set apart for that purpose, and at the times appointed by Matron. They will rise in the morning at six o'clock; prayers and breakfast, 6-30; in wards, 7-0; dinner, 1-0; tea 5-0; supper 9-0; prayers 9-30; lights out at 10.30. The night nurses rise at 8-30 p.m.; in wards at 9-0 p.m.; dinner at 10.0 a.m.; bed at 1-0 p.m. They are to leave the wards by nine in the morning, and their rooms are to be tidy by ten o'clock.
4. All the patients are to be washed before their breakfast. The Night Nurses are to assist in washing them and making the wards ready for the visit of the Medical Officer at nine o'clock in the morning. The dining-hall, corridors, scullery, &c., are to be all in order by ten o'clock in the morning.
5. Any alteration that may appear in any patient before the Sister comes on duty is to be reported to the Medical Officer by the Night Nurse, and she is never to leave the wards until she has given her report to the Sister.
6. The Nurses shall take care that their wards, furniture, and utensils are cleaned, and in order, every day, by nine o'clock in the morning, at the latest.
7. They should have a list of all articles in their charge, and be held responsible for producing them.
8. They must positively prevent anything being brought into the wards by patients' friends or visitors. Any attempt to infringe this regulation must be reported by them immediately to the Steward.
9. They are to take especial care that no provisions of any kind, nor wine, spirits, beer, or anything not ordered by the Medical Officer, be supplied to any patient.
10. They are to be responsible for the general Instructions to the Patients being strictly complied with, and to report any misconduct to the Sister, who will immediately make known the same to Matron.
11. They are not to receive any present, acknowledgement, or gratuity, either in money or in any other way, from the patients or their friends.
12. They must be diligent in complying with the orders of the Medical Officers; and conduct themselves with tenderness to the patients, and with civility and respect to visitors.
13. At the times appointed for visitors, they are to see that not more than two persons at the same time visit any patient.
14. They are not to suffer any patient to sit upon his neighbour's bed, or on his own, without permission from the Matron.
15. They must be particularly attentive to the fires and lights in the ward; take particular care that the patients do not meddle with either; and that no patient smokes tobacco in the wards or in any part of the building, except in the place set apart for that purpose.
16. They will see that all patients, capable of doing so, attend the Daily Prayers, and Divine Service on Sundays.
17. They are to report immediately to the Sister should a wish be expressed by a patient to be visited by the Chaplain or Minister of his own persuasion.

18. They are to see that the patients go to bed at eight o'clock in the winter and nine in summer, and that there is no talking or noise among them afterwards.
19. They shall not carry out of the House any provisions, or other things, belonging to the Hospital, on pain of being immediately discharged and prosecuted.
20. They must be careful that there be no waste of provisions, medical comforts, coal, gas, water comforts, or other articles; nor any destruction of bedding or clothing.
21. They are to deliver to the Laundress all the dirty linen, and see that it is returned correctly.
22. They must not be absent from their wards, except on duty; nor go out of the Hospital, on any pretence whatever, without permission in writing from the Matron. When leave is granted, they must return not later than nine o'clock.
23. In the event of a Nurse being guilty of gross dereliction of duty, or disobedience to orders, the Matron (with the approval of the Surgeon) will have the power of dismissing her summarily without notice, or any claim either for wages or board, beyond the day of such dismissal.
24. No person to bring provisions of any kind, wines, spirits, or beer, into the Hospital, without leave from the Secretary. Any Nurses or Hospital Servants infringing this Rule will be dismissed.
25. They shall each give fourteen days' notice of their intention to resign their situation, and shall be subject to removal at any period upon a like notice.[17]

The Secretary's Report to a meeting held in December 1879 contains a disturbing revelation:

> *Ordered:* That one of the Nurses (Davis) be prosecuted for stealing money from one of the sisters as set forth in detail in the Secretary's Report. It was decided [however] not to put the above resolution into force if the Nurse made a written confession voluntarily, and threw herself upon the mercy of the Committee.

This matter seems to have been amicably resolved: 'The Secretary reported that Nurse Davis had confessed that she stole Sister M^{s} [?] money & so no further steps had been taken'.

It is of interest that problems such as these are 'glossed over' in the SHS *Annual Reports* of this era. It should be recognised however, that the *Annual Reports* were circulated to potential benefactors, and 'washing your linen in public' was not the best way forward with regard to fund-raising!

At a meeting of the Committee of Management held in 11 May 1888, the following criticism of Miss A G Cooke (Matron of the 'Dreadnought' since 1882 – *see* Chapter 15) was minuted:

> Your Sub Committee met at the Seamen's Hospital at Greenwich on Thursday the 3rd May 1888 to investigate a charge made by the Revd R.M. Spence of Fordoun [sic] N.13. against Miss Cooke … that the character of his daughter, who had been a nurse in the Hospital had been defamed by Miss Cooke in a conversation with Miss Westlake who had been a Head Nurse (Sister Somerset) in the Seamen's Hospital. After carefully considering the whole of the correspondence including a letter from Miss Westlake excusing herself from being present at the enquiry to which your Sub Committee had invited her but pointing out that all she had to say on the subject would be found in her letter to Mr Spence – a copy of which (dated 18th April 1888) was furnished by Mr Spence.
>
> Your Sub Committee put Miss Cooke through a searching examination and having taken also evidence of the [PMO] and the late Steward of the Hospital, are of opinion that the remark made by Miss Cooke to Miss Westlake on the occasion in question amounted to no more than that there had been a 'flirtation' between Miss Spence and the barber of the Hospital. This flirtation appears to be admitted by Mr Spence in his letter of the 13th of April to Miss Westlake in which he says that his daughter had 'engaged herself to him' (the Barber) 'in marriage'.
>
> Your Sub Committee therefore acquit Miss Cooke of the charge brought against her and are of opinion that no imputation injurious to character rests on Miss Spence. It was also suggested by Mr Spence that Miss Cooke had used her influence to damage Miss Spence's prospects of obtaining employment elsewhere as a nurse and especially that she had written in unfavourable terms of Miss Spence to Mrs Higginbotham of Glasgow. The Sub Committee learned from Miss Cooke that she had not written anything unfavourable of Miss Spence or calculated to injure her prospects of obtaining future employment. The charges made against Miss Cooke by Mr Spence were framed in language of excessive vehemence which only the concern of a parent at what had been represented to him as an attack on his daughter's fair game could excuse.
>
> S^{gnd} F Cleeve.
>
> It was resolved that the report now read be adopted and that a copy of it be sent to the Revd Mr Spence.

The minute books contain numerous other details of day-to-day activities at the *Dreadnought*. Thus a fire in the nurse's home did not escape attention. It was reported that a fire had occurred in a nurse's bedroom at Greenwich:

> A nurse had been reading in bed and having gone to sleep her bedclothes had taken fire, the nurse escaped uninjured the fire had been promptly put out and damage to the extent of about £9 had been done to the Society's property, the insurance office had been communicated with. It was resolved that it be an instruction to the Matron that all lights in bedrooms except gas be prohibited.

A nurse-training school

In 1877, the Committee Management at last gave the go-ahead for a 'Dreadnought School for Nurses' – largely for its own purposes; this pioneering move, presumably initiated by Mrs Brown, was probably ahead of its time. Previous emphasis on conditions of service and indeed the possibility of nurse-*training* is apparent from the Society's minutes shortly after removal to land. An early and recurring theme (by the Medical Officers to the Committee of Management) was a request for *more* nurses, e.g.:

> Read a letter from M^r^ [Harry] Leach [1836–79] [the Resident Physician on board the 'Dreadnought'] [*see* Chapter 15] on the recommendations of Dr Rooke urging the need of the appointment of an additional nurse on the Medical & one also on the Surgical Side of the Hospital. Granted.[18]

Appropriate conditions of service, including salaries for the nursing-staff were therefore matters for *urgent* consideration:

> Ordered that the "Instructions" received by the Committee ... be adopted with the alteration in the Case of Sisters and Head Nurses by requesting a Month's notice of resignation or dismissal in lieu of a fortnight and in the Case of Nurses the following addition, – "In the Event of a Nurse being guilty of gross dereliction of duty, or disobedience to orders, the Matron (with the approval of the House Governor) will have the power of dismissing her summarily without Notice, or any claim Either for wages or board, beyond the day of such dismissal."[19]

Beginning of nurse-training

From April 1878, the Society admitted *probationer* nurses; Mrs Raynard of the London Bible and Domestic Mission was responsible for organizing their interviews and selection. The number of probationers undergoing training varied from 11 to 12;[20] they underwent a three-month classroom induction, received board and lodging, and wore a recognized uniform; after three years' service with the Society they were considered fully qualified. By 1880, all SHS nursing vacancies had been filled – the majority by 'daughters of small tradesmen or farmers'.[21] During the 'Great War' (1914–18), Alice Hall was the *Dreadnought* matron; she was responsible for further improvements in the nurses' lot –providing both a tennis court, and more acceptable living accommodation.

Nurse training gets underway

Mr (later Sir Henry) Burdett[23] was extremely interested in nurse-training, and although probably suggested by Mrs Brown, it was undoubtedly largely due to his initiative that the *'nursing school'* actually got off the ground! The first clear documentation of training at the Society is to be found in a minute dated April 1878:

> Mr. Fred^{k} Cleeve, C.B., Deputy Chairman [of the SHS], *gave notice* that he should propose at the next meeting of the Committee *That Probationer Nurses be received* into the Hospital for training from Miss Ranyard's Bible & Domestic Mission.

This intention was duly fulfilled at that meeting:

> *On the Motion of Fred^{k} Cleeve, Esq., …* seconded by I. Holt Skinner, Esq., it was *Resolved*! That (a) [sic] it is desirable to train women in the duties & requirements of nursing, as *Probationers* for the term of three months; that they be provided with Board and Lodging; and that all such persons shall be exclusively subject to the Rules and Regulations of the Committee of management without reference or appeal to any outside authority whatever. That (β) until further notice the Probationers shall be recommended by Miss Ranyard [sic] of the London Bible & Domestic Mission, subject to the approval of the Surgeon and Matron.[24]

The training programme seems to have progressed well, for the Surgeon's Report at a meeting held in March 1879 records:

> *Ordered!* That the Surgeon be instructed to prepare a Return shewing the progress made under the new arrangements for training Nurses, &c,: 1. The number & names of Nurses and of Probationers on the Hospital Books on the 31 Dec 1878. 2. The names of Nurses entered on the Books of the Hospital during the Qr. end 31 March '79. 3. The names of Probationers d^{o} -------d^{o} -------- d^{o} ---------- 4. -----d^{o} -------- Nurses discharged -------d^{o} -------- d^{o} ---------- 5. -----d^{o} ---------- Probationers d^{o} -------d^{o} -------- d^{o} ---------- 6. The nature and duration of the instruction given by the Medical Officers & by the Matron to Nurses and Probationers. This Return to be continued until further notice.

A further Report at a meeting held the following month reads:

> *Ordered! …*The Surgeon submitted a report on the present conditions of *the Nursing Department* & also undertook to give the detailed Returns asked for by the next Committee.[25]

Welcome news regarding the nursing scenario generally, and *training* in particular was minuted at a meeting of the Committee of Management held in July 1880:

> The report …showed that for the first time since the formation of the Society the Matron would for the future be able to fill up all Vacancies in the Nursing Staff by probationers trained at the Hospital.[26]

Also minuted was the fact that that: 'A Dreadnought trained nurse has very little difficulty in obtaining employment in another Hospital should she desire a change'.

The 'probationer saga' continued; at a meeting held in June 1883:

> Some correspondence was read in which *M^{iss} M.A. Luard*, Lady Superintendent of the St Albans Diocesan Institution for trainee *Nurses* requested to be *allowed to keep over here* [i.e. at the *Dreadnought*] *as a proba-*

> *tioner* – Miss Luard suggested that her nurse should be for the first three months without wages, but after this period that she should be paid at the rate of £12 a year. It was *unanimously resolved* that *one* of Miss Luards Nurses should be *permitted* to be trained at the Seamens [sic] Hospital on the *same terms* and conditions *as the two* which *M*[iss] *Ranyard* sent, but the Committee could not entertain the proposal of payment in any way for her Services.

In May 1887, on the recommendation of the Principal Medical Officer (PMO) an additional Ranyard nurse (Miss Purvis) should, it was minuted, be specially trained in 'Hospital Nursing'; she was duly admitted as an unpaid probationer for twelve months 'on payment of a fee of twenty five guineas'. However, she had to undergo a 'one month [period] on Trial'. This nurse was obviously not alone in seeking training at the *Dreadnought*, which must by then (a decade after it was initiated) have become a very attractive proposition:

> A letter having been read from a Miss Sansone asking to be allowed to become a paying probationer it was resolved that [she] be allowed to enter the service of the Hospital as an *unpaid* probationer for twelve months on payment of a fee of twenty five guineas and that she is in all respects under the same discipline as the other probationers but that the second years service be dispensed with.

The same minute continued that it was essential, however, that Miss Ranyard's probationers should 'reside in the Hospital', and not 'attend the Hospital daily'.[27]

These developments were not *without* problems however, and the reason for the following course of action is not fully explained:

> A letter was read from the London Biblewomen Nurses' Mission stating that they intended in the future to arrange for their Nurses to be trained at a Hospital where they would obtain experience in the nursing of women. The Mission thanked the Committee for the privileges, which they had enjoyed at the Dreadnought Hospital for so many years. The Secretary was directed to acknowledge the receipt of the letter and to express the regret of the Committee at the severance of the connection between the two Charities.[28]

Nurses' lectures

Later, in June 1904, a Medical Council Minute records:

> The subject of lectures to Nurses was considered and it was resolved to recommend the Committee of Management to adopt the following scheme:

1. Instruction by Lectures to be carried on for six months every year – from October 1st to end of December: from beginning of year to Easter.

2. Two courses of lectures to be given, each course lasting three months.
   a) One course on Physiology and elements of practical medicine.
   b) The other on Anatomy and elements of practical surgery.
   The first two lectures of course 'a' to be devoted to Physiology, the first two lectures of course 'b' to Anatomy, the remaining . . . lectures in each course to deal with practical medicine and practical surgery respectively.
3. Each course to be followed by an examination.
4. The instruction by lectures to be supplemented by the present system of tutorial teaching or practical demonstration by the Sisters.
5. That a set of diagrams to illustrate the lectures be provided for both the Dreadnought Hospital and the [ADH].
6. That the grant to Lecturers be arranged on a scale of one Guinea per Lecture.
7. That the members of the full Staff at each Hospital be invited, in order of seniority, to deliver the lectures, but that no Physician or Surgeon having once given a course of lectures be asked a second time until each of his juniors has had the opportunity given him of undertaking the duty. The surgical courses shall begin in January and the medical course in October of each year.
8. That a Library for medical and special professional books, like that at Greenwich, be formed at the [ADH].[29]

The matter received ongoing attention, as is stated in the following minute: 'The Medical Council submitted new rules and regulations for lectures to Nurses. The regulations would involve an expenditure of over £40 per annum, but it was resolved to defer the consideration of the subject until the next meeting. In July 1904, a Minute records:

> The subject of lectures to Nurses, referred from the last meeting, was again under consideration. It was resolved to record that the recommendations of the Medical Council are favourably considered. The Secretary was instructed to obtain statistics as to the fees paid by Probationer Nurses at other Hospitals the two subjects to be then considered together.

Careful surveillance continued, and in October that same year:

> The Committee considered the revised regulations in reference to Lectures to Nurses at both Hospitals ... It was resolved to adopt the regulations and to suggest that two additional lectures be delivered at each Hospital on Tropical Nursing[30] [see below].

The Society's nurse's lectures were not merely of interest (and debate) by that body alone; there were much wider implications:

> A communication was read from the Central Hospital Council for London on the subject of the systematic training of the Nurses of the Society and suggesting that the period of training should not exceed three years. The Society however deems it essential that a Nurse shall have four years training; three at the Dreadnought Hospital and one at a Hospital for women, before the joint certificate from both Institutions

> is signed in her favour. The Committee approved of a letter being sent to the Secretary of the Central Hospital Council to this effect.[31]

Burdett later wrote a useful and practical guide to nursing training; this book summarises training throughout the UK, and abroad. The entry for the SHS summarises the situation at their 'flagship' hospital, the *Dreadnought*:

> Beds, 291. MATRON; 1 Home Sister; 1 Night Sister; 5 Ward Sisters; 1 Out-Patient Sister; 1 Theatre Sister; 18 Staff Nurses; 30 Probationers; 1 Male Dresser. Applications average 200, and vacancies 11 yearly. *Ordinary Probationers* are selected from among the daughters of professional or business men. After a personal interview and 2 months' trial, applicants are received for 4 years' training (including 1 year in a London hospital for women and children). Candidates should be between 23 and 30 years of age, and must produce satisfactory evidence as to character, education, health and physique, three certificates being necessary, health, dental, and re-vaccination. During their training nurses are instructed by systematic courses of lectures held during the winter and spring. LECTURES are given by the medical and surgical staff and include courses in medicine, surgery, gynaecology, diseases of children, and tropical diseases; nursing lectures are given by the matron. Examinations are held at the expiration of each course and each nurse is required to reach a certain standard of efficiency. Certificates are given upon satisfactory completion of engagement. RECREATION, 2 hours daily five days, and 4 hours on one day of the week; 3 hours on Sundays; 1 day monthly from 7 P.M. the night before; 2 weeks' holiday 1st year; 2nd year, 3 weeks; 3rd year, 4 weeks. PREMIUM, *nil*. SALARY, 1st year, £12; 2nd year, £15; 3rd year, £20; Nurses £25. Laundry and indoor uniform are provided. Nurses and probationers do not have separate bedrooms. Nurses are assisted to join the Royal National Pension Fund [see below], and pensions are also given on the merits of the case to old employees. *Paying probationers* are received for 1 year's training. At the end of the year they may continue as ordinary probationers if considered suitable. PREMIUM, 25 guineas per annum. They have no special privileges as regards work, but the ordinary regulations as to age are not so strictly observed.[32]

Insights into the duties of Sisters and Nurses at the *Dreadnought* Hospital at a later date are to be found in two anonymous articles in the *SHS Quarterly Magazine*.[33]

Renewed problems with nursing 'standards', and other matters

Although *training* seems to have been proceeding well by 1888, substandard practice – by no means a new theme (see above) – again came to the fore at a meeting in April of that year:

> Dr. Griffiths [Chapter 15] stated that the medical nursing of the Hospital was below the modern standard and recommended the superannuation of the sister of the Ground East Floor. The subject was referred to Dr. Macdonald, Inspector General of Hospitals and Fleets who kindly undertook to investigate the matter and report to the Committee.

This potential problem was subsequently resolved without too much trouble:

> Dr. Macdonald stated that he had visited the Hospital and thoroughly investigated the matter having seen the Principal Medical Officer and House Physician and he had come to the conclusion that Dr. Griffiths was mistaken in his conjecture, that the nursing of the Hospital was not below the modern standard and that in every particulars [sic], the orders of the Medical Officers are thoroughly carried out. The report was received and adopted.

A detailed copy of the Macdonald report was available at the meeting held in May 1888 (see Box 2).[34]

Box 2

I have the honour to report that in compliance with the request of the Managing Committee of the Seamen's Hospital Society I made the necessary enquiries as to the validity of certain statements made in reference to the Hospital Nursing by Dr. Herbert Griffiths on resigning his appointment as Visiting Physician to that Institution. The investigation was conducted on the 2nd inst in presence of Mr Cleeve C.B. the Chairman whose intimate acquaintance with the internal management and working of the Seamen's Hospital enabled him to afford me much valuable aid. I would say as a matter of preface that the letter containing the allegation in question was written by its author without having previously consulted his Medical Brethren who might very easily have set him right and deterred him from such an unwise proceeding. This fact alone would be quite enough to warrant the board to pass the document over in silence; but now that they have thought fit to put it to the test of a special inquiry, what I have further to say will I am sure be received with pleasure, as affording them satisfactory proof that the more the constitution, qualifications and the working of the superviewing [sic] and nursing staff is investigated the more it will be apparent that the medical and I will include the surgical nursing in the Seamen's Hospital is not one whit below the modern standard and that in every minute particulars [sic] the orders of the medical officers are thoroughly carried out. I would lay much stress upon the fact which seems to have escaped the consideration of Dr. Griffiths that the Seamen's Hospital unlike the other London Hospitals is really also a home for the poor sailor who after having derived benefit from treatment is permitted to remain in the Institution until suitable arrangement can be made for his disposal, thus, it will be seen that the total number of inmates can never give a fair estimate of the actual number of sick and hurt requiring daily treatment and nursing in the legitimate sense. Moreover, where it is known that the present Staff besides a most excellent Matron includes 4 Sisters, 10 Nurses, 10 Probationers and 2 Male Nurses for Venereal cases, the numerical strength is ample for the daily requirement. Thus, if we even take the number of men under treatment to be 150 the proportion of attendants to patients would be as 1 to 5.5. In our Naval Hospitals the proportion is seldom below 1 to 7. Now by evidence supplied from several sources I find that the nurses are not only duly qualified for their work but bestow the most scrupulous care on the patients committed to their charge. *The help of the Probationers is also most valuable, and while they are themselves deriving information under instruction it must be admitted that the exercise of the ordinary common sense of educated persons cannot fail to be of great service to the sick* [my italics]. Finally on enquiry I find that the Sister on Ground East, complained of by Dr. Griffiths, is possessor of large practical experience in nursing and those who have a better knowledge of her intrinsic merits than Dr. Griffiths appears to have gleaned in his weekly visits affirm that it would be difficult to fill her place so well, if she were superannuated as suggested. In support of this statement the testimony of Dr. Johnson Smith P.M.O. the Matron and Dr. Trevelyan who are resident and not merely visitors is quite satisfactory. I have only now to put in the accompanying reports of Dr. Johnson Smith and Dr. Curnow, made at my request and of which my own report I find is but an echo to smooth the troubled waters left by Dr. Griffiths and to be an additional source of gratification to the Board to know that the benevolent object they take so much to heart is so efficiently carried out whatever maybe said to the contrary. Signed: - John D. Macdonald.

Resignation of the matron

The resignation of Miss Cooke – third Matron of the land-based *Dreadnought* – in 1895 emphasises the insecurity of nursing as a profession at that time:

> Gentlemen, I beg to lay before you my resignation [letter dated 12 September] of the appointment of Matron. I am prepared to meet your convenience as to the date of my departure, any time next month, or early in November would equally suit me as I am not taking other duties, and am leaving with the feeling of having been many years at work and now requiring rest.
>
> It has been a matter of regret to me that I have not been able to join the Pension Fund [see below], but I could not put away my ready money in it, as I have hitherto had several members of my family to assist, as well as to keep an old Nurse.
>
> I am therefore constrained to throw myself on your generosity, in the hope that you may see your way towards according me some small

> annual grant. I am absolutely without any settled income, and shall be dependent upon what I can earn, and any allowance that you may give, will be a source of great comfort and assistance to me, now that I feel constrained to give up my appointment.
>
> Expressing my regret at having to leave the 'Dreadnought', thanking you for the many acts of kindness and consideration I have received at your hands in the past.
>
> I am, Gentlemen [–,] Your obedient servant [–,] A.G. Cooke [–,] Matron.

It was resolved that her resignation be accepted with regret, and that the subject of her application to the Committee for financial assistance be referred to the Finance Sub-Committee. At a subsequent meeting:

> ... it was moved by Capt Holdsworth and seconded by Col. Despard that a gratuity of £50 be given to the Matron on her leaving the Hospital, whereupon the following amendment was moved by Mr Burdett and seconded by the Rev'. Brooke Lambert [also a member of the Committee of Management] that a pension of £25 per annum be granted to Miss Cooke on her retirement from The Office of Matron. After some discussion this amendment on being put from the Chair was declared to be carried, it was then put as a substantive motion and carried.[35]

Increase in number of Dreadnought *nurses*

In April 1897 (Queen Victoria's diamond jubilee year) a minute states:

> D^r. Rogers having suggested an increase in the number of nurses at Greenwich it was ordered that a return of the number of special cases requiring extra nursing in the Hospital at Greenwich during the past twelve months be laid before the next meeting, and also a return of the number of infectious cases treated during the past twelve months, and a return of the comparative number of Nurses to Patients in this and other Hospitals.

This minute was followed by documentation, setting out the nurse:patient ratio at the *Dreadnought:*

> The figures showed that the number of Patients to Nurses was much larger at Greenwich than at any of the other [Metropolitan or Provincial] Hospitals mentioned and it was resolved that 4 additional Nurses be engaged. The Nursing Staff will therefore stand as follows:- 1 Matron, 1 Home Sister, 1 Night Sister, 4 Day Sisters, 15 Nurses, (including 2 Male Nurses), 9 Probationers, 4 Mission Nurses, 3 Paying Probationers = 38.

Male nurses at the Dreadnought*?*

The 'rules' for male nurses (who were not under the Matron's jurisdiction) were very different from those of their female counterparts, and were printed separately in the 1875 pamphlet (see above, and Box 3). Although the Society had employed male nurses on the Hospital-ships (see above), they had been largely replaced (certainly by the 1890s) by females. The question of whether to employ them, and more importantly where they should be *trained,* were clearly important contemporary issues.

Box 3

1. The Male Nurse will be selected by the Surgeon on trial for one month, at the expiration of which time, if approved, he will be recommended to the Committee, through the Secretary.
2. He must be able to read and write.
3. He will have charge of the wards in his department, and be responsible for their good order and cleanliness.
4. He will be held responsible that the lavatories and water-closets are kept clean and in good working order, and that daily use is made of a sufficient quantity of disinfectant fluid, which will be supplied by the Steward for that purpose.
5. He shall take especial care to keep the beds of the patients clean and decent and shall see that every patient be washed regularly in the morning before breakfast.
6. He shall also take especial care to prevent spirituous liquors, or provisions of any kind, being brought into the wards by the patients' friends or visitors, or by any other person. Any infringement of this Rule to be immediately reported to the Surgeon.
7. He shall see every morning that the card corresponding to the diet ordered for each patient is fixed over the bed, and that such diet and any extras as may be ordered, are regularly served.
8. He will see that all patients, capable of doing so, attend prayers regularly, and Divine Service on Sundays.
9. He must himself see that the orders of the Surgeon be strictly attended to. Any refusal on the part of the patient to take his medicine must be reported at once to the Surgeon.
10. He will receive from the Needle-woman the requisite quantity of clean linen, and he must see that no soiled linen be allowed to remain in the wards, but that it be at once taken to the Needle-woman.
11. He shall not carry out of the Hospital any provisions or other things belonging to the Institution, on pain of being immediately discharged and prosecuted.
12. He must be particularly attentive to the fires and lights in the wards. The patients are not allowed to meddle with either. He is not to allow smoking in the wards.

13. He must be careful that there be no waste of provisions, medical comforts, coals, gas, water, or other articles; nor any destruction of bedding or clothing.
14. He will never leave the wards at night without leaving them in charge of the Barber, Surgery-man, or Night Nurse.
15. He is to be responsible that the general instructions to the patients are strictly complied with, and should report immediately to the Surgeon any misconduct of patients.
16. He shall keep an inventory of every article in his wards.
17. He shall give fourteen days' notice previous to resigning his situation, and shall be subject to removal at any period upon a like notice.

An SHS minute dated April 1895 reads:

> [It was suggested that] the 'establishment' of a school for the training of *male* [my italics] nurses, [would be] a means of increasing the income of the Charity [and] …it was resolved to appoint a sub-committee to go into the matter and report. The following members were then formally elected to serve on the said sub-committee:-
>
> Mr. Burdett, Capt Ommamney [sic] and Dr. Rogers.[36]

A few weeks later: 'It was resolved to add the names of the members of the active medical staff to the sub-committee appointed on the 5th of April to consider the subject of a school for male nurses'. This subject was treated seriously by the Society's authorities; for example, at a meeting in November 1895:

> The Sub-Committee appointed to consider the proposal to introduce *male* [my italics] nursing into the Seamen's Hospital met on November the 5th when were present:- Dr. Rogers, Dr. Curnow, Dr. Anderson, Dr. Manson,[37] and Mr Johnson Smith.[38] Unfortunately Mr Burdett, who brought forward the proposal was absent, and the Sub-Committee had not therefore their advantage of hearing his views on the subject, as it must be assumed that before making the proposal he had thought it over fully and would have been prepared to advocate some definite scheme for carrying it out.
>
> In [Burdett's] absence the Sub-Committee endeavoured to regard the proposal from every point of view; 1stly Financially. 2ndly With regard to the peculiar and unfavourable architectural arrangements of the wards for such an experiment. 3rdly On the changes which must necessarily be made in the arrangements for nursing and supervision before such a plan could be introduced with any chance of success.
>
> After considering all these points the Sub-Committee were unanimously of opinion that such a scheme was impracticable. Financially, they considered that the scheme would entail a loss rather than a gain to the Hospital, even supposing that male candidates as probationers would be forthcoming, which the Sub-Committee did not think would

> be the case. They thought also that the peculiar construction of the hospital in a series of very small wards would be fatal to carrying out the experiment satisfactorily and the required changes in the supervising staff besides introducing confusion and expense would be futile in the event of the scheme being ultimately found unworkable, which the Sub-Committee anticipated it would prove to be.
>
> Some facts were mentioned in support of the view taken –. viz. D^r^. Curnow mentioned that the demand for male nurses in general was diminishing, and that therefore there was less probability of candidates willing to pay a premium for instruction coming forward. D^r^. Anderson stated that even in the army, women were taking the place of men as nurses. D^r^. Manson made the same report as to nursing in Hong Kong. Mr Johnson Smith stated that whereas on the old Hospital Ship "Dreadnought" nursing by both sexes was in force, one inducement to move the Hospital to dry land was to do away with this system [Chapter 13] and eliminate the male element except in the lock wards.[39] A resolution was proposed that in any changes made in the nursing staff, the nursing should be raised to the highest level of that existing in the large general hospitals, but the Chairman declined to receive this as being outside the reference to the Committee
>
> T.L. Rogers [---------] Chairman.[40]

A later Minute records:

> The School Committee had considered a letter from the Colonial Office dated 30th Novr. 1901 asking the [Society] to endeavour to make some arrangements for the training of Male Nurses and they recommended that this project be favourably entertained. The letter from the Colonial Office was read and it was resolved that it be referred to the Medical Council with the request that they will consider the subject, report and make such recommendations as they may see fit on the suggestion. It was further resolved that the Council be informed that the Committee are disposed to look favourably on the proposal if suitable arrangements for the training of Male nurses can be made without detriment to the discipline and administration of the Hospitals. The Council to be asked to report upon this matter at the meeting on January 10th.[41]

As a post-script to this saga, the following minute was written, in July 1897: 'It was resolved on the recommendation of the F.S.C. [Finance Sub-Committee] that the two Male Nurses at Greenwich (Jack & Taylor) receive an increase of 1/- per week each'.[42]

Conditions and nurse-training at the *Dreadnought* were therefore, in the latter days of the nineteenth century, well-advanced.[43] As in postgraduate medical education, and the 'new' clinical discipline *tropical medicine* – the Society was at the forefront of developments, and had a great deal to teach the majority of London's teaching hospitals![44]

Life of Dreadnought *nurses in the late nineteenth century*

In 1893, a committee was set up to investigate *pay* and *pensions* (see below) of nurses in the employ of the Society:

> The Special Committee [on wages] beg to report that:- They have had under consideration the rates of remuneration which the Sisters and Nurses receive, and they have prepared a table showing the wages paid by other London Hospitals. They are of the opinion that it is desirable to raise the maximum wages of the Sisters after 10 years' service from £35 to £40 per annum, and of the Nurses after 10 years' service from £25 to £30 per annum, in each case by annual increments of £1. Their attention has been directed to the importance of securing an adequate provision for each member of the Nursing Staff in case of incapacity from illness or from old age [see below].
>
> The increase of wages now recommended will give additional opportunity to Sisters and Nurses to secure such provision through the Royal National Pension Fund [RNPF] for Nurses [see below], which affords a ready means of securing this desirable result. At the present time the Committee pay half the premium of every Sister or Nurse, under 40 years of age, who joins the Pension Fund for a pension of £15 after the age of 60 years and sick pay up to that age. The conditions on which this payment is made include the transfer to the credit of the Nurse in the books of the Pension Fund, of the said half-premiums on her leaving the employ of the Society after two years' service.
>
> The Sub-Committee think that this arrangement should be modified:- (1.) They recommend that this regulation be rescinded so far as concerns any Sisters or Nurses to be hereafter engaged, or Sisters or Nurses in the service of the Society who have not availed themselves of its provisions, and that in lieu thereof the Society shall pay half the premium (for a pension of £15 per annum from the age of 60, and sick pay to that age at the rate of 10/- per week) of any Sister or Nurse who joins the Pension Fund before the expiration of her first three years of service, and that after such a Sister or Nurse has completed ten years of service, the Society shall pay the entire premiums for her pension and sick pay, and further increase the premium so that the pension shall be raised to £20 at the age of 60. (2.). That when a Sister or Nurse has completed ten years service, and has not availed herself of the foregoing regulations the Society shall insure for her in the Pension Fund a pension of £15 to commence at the age of 60 years, with sick pay at the rate of 10^{s}/- per week, up to that age.
>
> The Committee are of opinion that Sisters and Nurses on leaving the Society's service without having completed ten years' service should not be allowed to have any premiums paid in on their account transferred to their credit in the Books of the Pension Fund, unless the Committee shall determine otherwise for special reasons supplied to

> them in particular cases where Nurses have prematurely broken down in health in the Society's service... The Committee also recommend that Probationer Nurses be advanced to their maximum rate of pay in three years, instead of in four as at present.
>
> For the Special Committee [–,] (Signed) Perceval A. Nairne [–,] Chairman.[45]

At a meeting, also in 1893, the following minute regarding both nurses' and patients' *diet*, was written:

> The Special Committee [to take into consideration the following matters in connection with the staff of Nurses and Servants: - (1) The supply of milk and check on its consumption. (2) The Meals of the Nurses and where taken] beg to report [on 10 November] that: - They have examined the effect which the institution of beer money has had upon the expenditure of the Hospital.
>
> It appears that, whereas during the three years preceding its institution, the expenditure on beer, on an average was £1.3.1 for every occupied bed, it fell to 13/2 per occupied bed on an average of the next three years. To this $13^{s}/2^{d}$ must be added the amount of beer-money paid to the Staff during the latter three years in question, which, on an average, was $8^{s}/10^{d}$ per occupied bed giving a total of £1.2.0 per occupied bed spent upon beer and beer-money during the three years following the institution of the new system. This shews [sic] an apparent saving of $1^{s}/1^{d}$ per occupied bed per annum. The average cost for Milk per occupied bed rose however from £4-1-5 to £4.9.11., an increase of $8^{s}/6^{d}$ per occupied bed per annum. Deducting the average of the apparent gain of $1^{s}/1^{d}$ on the expenditure for beer, we have, concurrently with the institution of the beer-money, a net increase of expenditure of $7^{s}/5^{d}$ per occupied bed per annum.
>
> The Committee feel that the system of giving money in lieu of beer having once been introduced, it would be inexpedient to deprive the present Staff of their beer-money, and they therefore recommend that the pay of every Sister, Nurse, Petty Officer & Servant, already on the Establishment shall be increased by an equivalent in wages, say £3 for men & £2 for women. That all Sisters, Nurses, Petty Officers and, Servants be engaged at scale rate without allowance of beer-money. That [in future] all Sisters, Nurses, Petty Officers and Servants be entitled to draw the allowance of beer.
>
> The Committee consider it desirable that all Nurses Meals should be served in their own dining-rooms, and that all provisions, of whatever kind, issued from the Stores (1) for the Officers and Nurses, and (2) for the Patients, respectively, shall be served and kept in separate vessels, and remain wholly distinct one from the other. The Committee recommend that this scheme shall come into operation on the 1st January 1894.
>
> For the Special Committee [–,] (signed) Perceval A. Nairne [–,] Chairman.[46]

Controversy regarding nurses' registration

The timing of registration was at that time a highly contentious issue. Nightingale was opposed to registration; Burdett, on the other hand, was strongly in favour, and felt that one year's training was sufficient. The following minute regarding 'registration' was written at a Council of Management meeting in March 1891:

> A circular letter from the Treasurer of St Thomas' Hospital together with a memorandum of certain resolutions passed at a meeting of representatives of Nurses Training Schools protesting against granting of a license by the Board of Trade to the British Nurses Association for power to form a *Register of nurses* [my italics] was read. It was moved by Mr Burdett seconded by Adm^{l} R.Coote C.B., and carried unanimously that a memorial in the spirit of the resolution passed at the meeting of representatives of Hospitals and Nurses Training Schools held at St Thomas's Hospital on the 27th February 1891 be signed by the Chairman and [PMO], Matron and Lecturers to Nurses, and presented to the President of the Board of Trade. Mr Burdett and Adm^{l} R.Coote were subsequently elected to form a Committee of observation as Representatives of the [SHS].[47]

Nurses' Pensions and The (Royal) National Pension Fund for Nurses (RNPFN)

Burdett (see above), during his time as Secretary to the Society, was to set up a scheme – the (Royal) National Pension Fund for Nurses – which was to benefit not only SHS nurses but also nurses in general. The £20,000 required to initiate the Fund was provided (with no strings attached) by Junius S Morgan (1813-90), Baron Rothschild (1839–93), Sir Everard Hambro (1842–1925) and Henry Hucks Gibb (later Baron Aldenham) (1819–1907). By 1889, the fund had 1,000, and by 1899 7,000 members (i.e. 40 per cent of British nurses). At the *Dreadnought*, each nurse's subscription of £2 annually was matched by a £2 donation from the Society.

The Society (largely as a result of Burdett's initiative) was therefore a pioneer in nurses' pensions (see above). Although nurse-*training* at the 'Dreadnought' was by 1890 well established (and nursing was regarded as being more 'respectable' following Nightingale's example at St Thomas') a great deal of financial insecurity awaited a nurse in her latter years and this must have seriously hindered recruitment for nurse training. Burdett was thus a keen advocate of a Pension Fund for Nurses. Nightingale, on the other hand, was opposed to such a scheme as she felt that a Nurse's pay was so low that contributions to a Pension Fund were out of the question. On this matter, as well as registration, Burdett and Nightingale therefore disagreed.[48]

At a meeting held in February 1889, the following was minuted:

> It was moved by Mr Burdett, seconded by Mr Nairne [Chairman of the Committee of Management] and carried unanimously that with a view to encourage thrift and independence among the nursing staff it is desir-

able that this Society should become affiliated with the [(R)NPFN]. It was further moved by Mr Burdett, seconded by Rev^{d}. Brooke Lambert and carried unanimously, that an arrangement be made whereby the Seamen's Hospital will contribute £2 per annum per nurse [see above], for each member of the nursing staff who may pay at least an equal amount into the National Pension Fund out of her earnings as a nurse, and that the details be left to the Finance Sub Committee with power to act. (Box 4 describes these financial arrangements in more detail).[50]

Box 4

A 4-page pamphlet was circulated to all nurses in the employ of the SHS:

1. The Committee of the [SHS are prepared to assist all Sisters, and Nurses, under 40 years of age, who may desire to join the National Pension Fund for Nurses, by paying one half of the annual premium while they remain in the service of the Society.
2. These premiums shall be paid on the returnable scale [tables were appended]... to secure a pension of £15 per annum (minimum) to commence at the age of 50, 55 or 60 years of age.
3. Sisters and Nurses withdrawing their one half of the premium whilst in the service of the Hospital without the consent of the Committee or within twelve months of leaving, will forfeit the amount paid to their name by the Hospital, but otherwise the amount will be considered as belonging to them.
4. Sisters or Nurses who are discharged by the Hospital, or who leave within two years of their appointment on the permanent staff, will forfeit the amount paid by the Society to their names in the National Pension Fund.
5. In every instance money which has been paid in the National Pension Fund by the Seamen's Hospital Society and forfeited, shall remain in the Fund for the benefit of the Seamen's Hospital Sisters and Nurses.
6. Probationers in the service of the Seamen's Hospital Society Training School for Nurses who may join the National Pension Fund to secure a pension of £15 per annum (minimum) at 50, 55 or 60 years of age shall, if appointed on the permanent staff, on completion of their training, receive from the Committee one half of the premiums already paid by them to the National Pension Fund.
7. The Committee are prepared to consider what help shall be given to Sisters and Nurses over 40 years of age, with the view of making such arrangements as may seem best in each individual case.
8. Those who are desirous of joining the Pension Fund on these conditions should send in their names to the Matron.

NOTE...If a Nurse...should...become ill, and remain so, she will be provided for at the rate of 10s. per week until the age of 60, when she shall be entitled to her pension. As the donations to the Fund now exceed £35,000, and a Nurse is also entitled to share in the profits arising from surpluses, it may be confidently anticipated that her pension will be much increased. Premiums are paid monthly. The Secretary will be happy to see any Nurse and give her further information should she desire it.

GREENWICH, January, 1890.

P. MICHELLI.[49]
Secretary [of the SHS]

In a 'follow-up' at the next meeting, the following was minuted: 'The *Chairman* and the *Deputy Chairman* were *authorised to arrange* the *affiliation of the Hospital* with *the Nurses' Pension Fund* on the basis of *half premiums* instead of by *definite payments* as [previously] agreed.' Some six years later, the following report was read to the Committee of Management:

> The Sub-Committee appointed to consider the subject of Pensions to old Sisters and Nurses beg to report that they have investigated this matter and find that the two sisters – Ground East (Parker) and Middle East (Cook) the former of whom entered the service of the society in 1872, and the latter in 1873 – are now past work: the latter (Sister Cook) has already been obliged to give up work and left her duties on the 15th of October last.
>
> The Sub-Committee have referred to the minutes of the 8th December 1893 [see above], when the Committee adopted a scheme for pensioning the Sisters & Nurses of the Society. On that occasion it was pointed out that there were two Sisters in the service of the Society both over 60 years of age who could not in consequence of their age come under the operation of the scheme. These Sisters were already in some measure provided for through the R.N.P.F.N. but would require, when leaving the Hospital, some additional help to put them on an equally favourable footing with the younger members of the Nursing Staff. It is found that the above-mentioned Sisters have all their savings into the R.N.P.F.N. and so helped themselves. It is also found that in January 1892, the Committee granted to each of the Sisters a year's pay, which sum was placed to the credit of these Sisters with the R.N.P.F.N. and realised, in the case of Sister Parker £3:5:4 per annum.
>
> The Sub-Committee now beg to recommend that the Society pension these two Sisters at the rate of £20 per annum each, which is the amount that they would have received had they been able, when they entered the Hospital, to avail themselves of the scheme for Pensions authorised by the Society. To effect this it will be necessary to give to Sister Parker £16.15.2 per annum, and to Sister Cook £16.14.8 per annum. Sister Parker

is now 66 years and 3 months of age and has been in the service of the Society 24 years. Sister Cook was, at time of leaving the Hospital, 65 years and 8 months of age, and had been in the service of the Society 22 years.
(Signed) Perceval A. Nairne [–,] Chairman.

It was moved by Adm[l] Sir Walter Hunt-Grubbe, K.C.B., seconded by Cap[t] White and resolved that the Report ... be adopted... D[r] Rogers made an intensive verbal report from the Sub-Committee, appointed to consider the subject of additions to the Nursing Staff and on the recommendation of this Sub-Committee it was resolved that a Home Sister be engaged at a commencing salary of £35 per annum, and a Night Sister at the rate of £30 per annum.

Foundation of the London School of Tropical Medicine (LSTM) and the beginning of 'tropical' nursing at the ADH

Nursing at the ADH

The rigid routine (see below) and timetable expected of all nurses, including the Matron, at the ADH (shortly *before* it became the 'tropical centre') is revealed in a 'job description' dated 1895:

1: The Matron will be selected by the Committee, on probation for three months.
2: She will carry out such instructions as may be given her for the good order and well-being of the Hospital.
3: She will be empowered, subject to the approval of the Principal Medical Officer, to engage, and in case of misconduct or gross dereliction of duty to suspend all Sisters and Nurses. She will take care that the rules of the Hospital are strictly observed by them, and she will immediately report any instance of misbehaviour or neglect on their part.
4: She will be held responsible for the good order of Nurses and for the cleanliness of their apartments; and will see that their fires and lights are extinguished at the time appointed.
5: No Sister, Nurse or Servant shall absent herself from the Hospital without permission of the Matron, who will be held responsible for the good order, neatness and cleanliness of their apartments.
6: She will keep an account of the receipt and delivery of all articles in store under her charge. She will also keep an account of all the Hospital bedding, linen and clothing, of which, she will have the general charge and be responsible for its being properly marked, kept well mended, thoroughly aired and in good condition. When a further supply of any article is required, she will make a written application to the Secretary for an order for the same.

7: She will see that all articles committed to her charge are properly dispensed, and keep a separate account of the expenditure of each.
8: She will enforce the strictest attention to the personal cleanliness of the patients, and will see that the clean bed linen for each patient is issued at least once a week.
9: She will frequently visit the different Wards at night to see that the regulations about retiring to rest are duly observed.
10: She will at once report all such occurrences, in her departments, as she may deem of sufficient importance.
11: She will not on any day, except Sundays, absent herself from the Hospital between the hours of midnight and 3pm. In conjunction with the Resident Medical Officer, she will, on alternate days and Sundays after the regulation hours of duty, be the Orderly Officer for the day, and shall not be absent from the Hospital without permission from the Committee.
12: She will give a quarter's notice, in writing, previous to resigning her appointment, and be subject to removal upon receiving a notice from the Committee.

In view of her onerous duties, it is perhaps not surprising that by 1899, the incumbent had also applied for a salary increase: 'An application from the Matron for an increase of pay was referred to the Finance Sub-Committee'.

ORIGIN(S) OF TRAINING IN TROPICAL NURSING

As the following Minute (dated March 1899) makes abundantly clear, the training of nurses in this discipline (*tropical medicine*) was immediately given high priority – being mentioned by Joseph Chamberlain (Secretary of State for the Colonies) himself in the House of Commons:

> Communications have been received [by the SHS] from the Colonial Nursing Association [CNA] requesting that application may be made to this Board for permission for Trained Nurses to enter the service of the [SHS] for short periods so that they may obtain an insight into Tropical Nursing before proceeding to their destinations in the Tropics. The importance of Nurses obtaining this training before going abroad was emphasized by Mr. Chamberlain in his speech in the House of Commons on the 10th inst. And he foreshadowed that the Society would give facilities to obtain the necessary training.
>
> To meet the wishes of the Secretary of State for the Colonies and the Institution that is interested in sending the nurses to the Tropics it is suggested that four fully trained Nurses be admitted into the Hospital to go through a course of from six to 12 months training in Tropical Nursing. At the present time four Nurses are admitted to the Hospital for a period of one year only from the Raynard Mission for ordinary nursing training. These Nurses do not pay anything to the Hospital and the short course they go through is unsatisfactory.

> It is suggested that this number be reduced to two and that the two vacancies be filled by Nurses who desire training in *Tropical Medicine* [my italics] and furthermore that two additional Nurses who desire such training be added to the staff.
>
> This arrangement would enable four fully trained Nurses to go through a course of from six to 12 months in *Tropical Nursing* [my italics]. These Nurses would all be unpaid and the only additional cost to the Society would be the rations of two Nurses. It is believed that this arrangement would improve the efficiency of the nursing of the Hospital; it would give the services of four fully trained Nurses in the Wards in lieu of two of the Probationers sent by Raynard Mission who during the whole of the course of their training at the Hospital are of little service to the Society. It is believed that the Seamen's Hospital is the only one in London that receives Probationers from the Raynard Mission free of charge … it was resolved that the report now read be received and adopted and that the Secretary communicate with the Raynard Mission through the Revd Brooke Lambert.[51]

The importance of tropical nurse-training as another *new* Society initiative was also made clear at a committee meeting in May 1899:

> Sir Fredk Young having intimated that he had had an interview with Mr Chamberlain on the subject of the training of Nurses for Mrs Chamberlain's Association for supplying Trained Nurses to the colonies, it was resolved that Mr Chamberlain be informed that the Committee have made arrangements for four Colonial Nurses to receive training at the Dreadnought Hospital, and that the Matrons at [the Dreadnought] and the [ADH] will cordially co-operate.[52]

At the next meeting of the Committee, it was made clear that this line of action had already been implemented: 'It was reported that arrangements had been made for four nurses from the [CNA] to enter the service of the Society'. Later that year the matter was further aired:

> A letter was read from the [CNA] offering to send a Nurse to the Hospital for *training* in *Tropical Diseases* [my italics] in the middle of this month. Arrangements however having been made for a Nurse from the [CNA] to enter in January [1900] and there being no vacancy at present on the Hospital Staff the Secretary was instructed to inform the [CNA] that at the present time there is no vacancy for a Nurse.[53]

A report was read [at an SHS meeting in October 1899] with reference to Colonial Nurses, stating that as nearly all the cases of Tropical Diseases are now treated at the [ADH] it will be necessary for the Nurses from the [Colonial Nurses Association (CNA)] to attend at the [ADH]. It was resolved that a further report be submitted and that arrangements be made if possible for the *Colonial Nurses* to take the place of some members of the Nursing Staff at the [ADH].[54]

TROPICAL NURSING BECOMES ESTABLISHED

Despite minor problems, courses in *tropical nursing* were to become fully established and by 1909, a full programme of nurses' lectures, by then given by the distinguished medical staff of the LSTM – based at the ADH – was in full swing. The syllabus included lectures by Doctors Duncan, Sandwith, McLeod, Daniels and Leiper and Mr Cantlie (*see* Figure 17.3 and Chapter 18). Regarding remuneration for these lectures, a minute dated July 1909 records: 'The Committee also approved of the fee for Lectures to nurses on Tropical Subjects being fixed at One Guinea'.[55]

Care of patients with all manner of infectious illness was a major nursing activity. This was, however, an era in which 'tropical medicine' – the discipline *invented* to

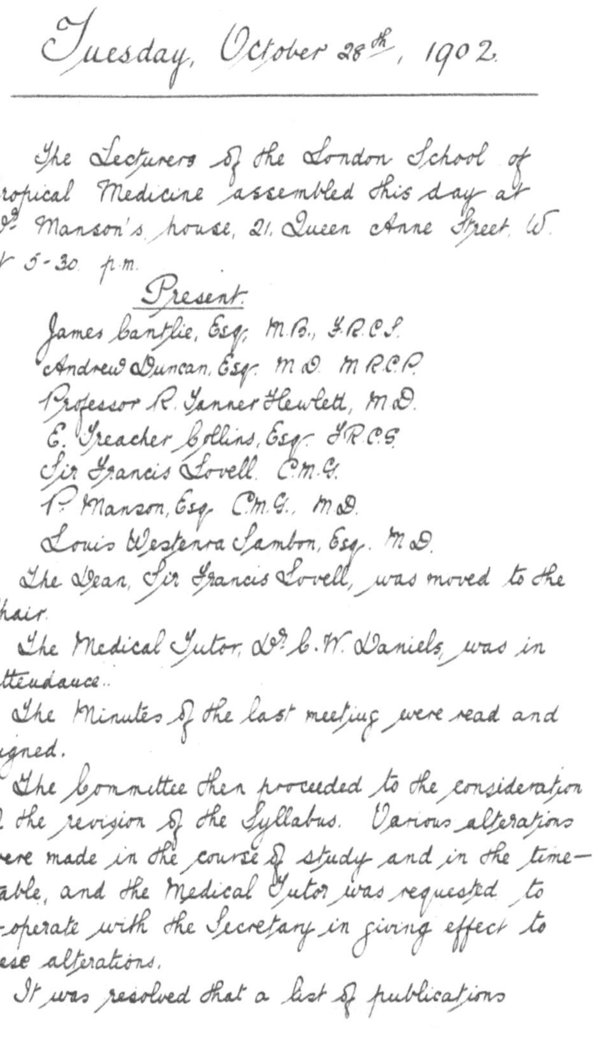

Tuesday, October 28th, 1902.

The Lecturers of the London School of Tropical Medicine assembled this day at Dr Manson's house, 21, Queen Anne Street, W. at 5-30. p.m.

Present.

James Cantlie, Esq. M.B., F.R.C.S.
Andrew Duncan, Esq. M.D. M.R.C.P.
Professor R. Tanner Hewlett, M.D.
E. Treacher Collins, Esq. F.R.C.S.
Sir Francis Lovell. C.M.G.
P. Manson, Esq. C.M.G., M.D.
Louis Westenra Sambon, Esq. M.D.

The Dean, Sir Francis Lovell, was moved to the Chair.

The Medical Tutor, Dr C.W. Daniels, was in attendance.

The Minutes of the last meeting were read and signed.

The Committee then proceeded to the consideration of the revision of the Syllabus. Various alterations were made in the course of study and in the time-table, and the Medical Tutor was requested to co-operate with the Secretary in giving effect to these alterations.

It was resolved that a list of publications

Figure 17.3: Part of a minute of a 'tropical lecturers' meeting in 1902. [SHS Archive].

care for disease involving the servants of the Empire and Raj – 'reigned supreme'. It was entirely appropriate therefore, that the training of nurses in this speciality was to become an important function of the Society.

Incidentally, if any nurse contracted an infectious disease – which many did – she (by permission of the Lewisham Local Board of Works) could be admitted to the 'Board's Hospital at Hither Green'.[56]

Difficulties with recruitment seem to have been a major ongoing concern. A later Matron highlighted some of the problems. Parents had difficulty in maintaining a daughter until she was old enough (19 or 20 years) to enter nurse-training. Between school and this age, she might learn short-hand and typing and become employable in another capacity. However, excellent opportunities existed with the Society: either a trained woman could serve in the colonies (with a certificate in *tropical nursing*) or else, go to sea![57]

A minute of March 1898 records:

> The subject of nursing at the [ADH] was discussed. It was resolved that a Nurse and Probationer be provided for the new [tropical] ward to be opened at the [ADH] next week. It was also resolved that so far as the nursing of patients at the [ADH] cannot be provided for by unpaid Probationers, paid Probationers be engaged to avert the necessity of calling in occasional assistance from Nursing Institutions, and that so far as may be possible nursing assistance be sent from Greenwich [i.e. the *Dreadnought*] to the [ADH] when required.[58]

Following the opening of the ADH, probationers had been trained there as well as at the *Dreadnought*.[59] The transfer of most 'tropical cases from the 'Dreadnought' to the [ADH] had already become a contentious issue amongst the SHS *Medical* Staff (Chapter 18). Although the LSTM had been founded at the ADH in October 1899 (Chapter 14), the hospital had been open since 1890. The major object, therefore, in recent years was to care for 'tropical' cases and to give formal instruction to Medical Officers who would be looking after British Subjects in Colonies throughout the Empire. But it was now clear that nurses should also be trained to care for those patients suffering from 'exotic' diseases.

A 1900 minute records:

> The Committee approved the following scheme for the future Staff of the [ADH where most 'tropical medicine' was by then centred]:- That 8 nurses, one maid and a boy be added making the total staff: 1 Matron, 2 Sisters, 12 nurses, 2 Out-patient Nurses, 5 Female Servants, 2 Porters and a boy.[60]

FUTURE OF TROPICAL NURSE-TRAINING

The SHS Nurses Training School, like the *Dreadnought* Hospital itself, closed on 31 March 1986. Training in the nursing of tropical diseases continued for a while at the Hospital for Tropical Diseases, St Pancras Way, NW1, and in 1996, the LSHTM (which had opened in 1929) rather belatedly assumed responsibility at the *Nurses' Training Centre in Tropical Medicine*.

A *new* nurses' home

Viscount Devonport[61] later raised a fund to erect a new Nurses' Home and Pathological Laboratory (*see* Chapter 20) – to the south of the *Dreadnought* Hospital. Figure 17.4 shows the presentation of a cheque to the SHS Chairman – Sir Arthur Clarke; the official opening of the *Devonport* buildings took place on 15 July 1929 (*see* Chapter 20).[62]

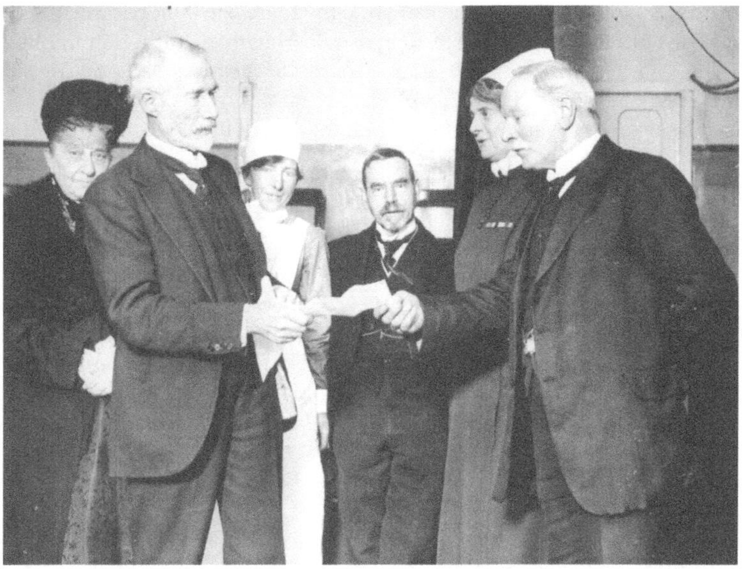

Figure 17.4: Presentation of a cheque to the Society's Chairman, Sir Arthur Clarke, in 1926 or 1927. [SHS Archive].

References and notes

1 Cook E T. *Life of Florence Nightingale.* Two vols. London: MacMillan 1914: 507 & 510; Woodham-Smith C. *Florence Nightingale 1820 – 1910.* London: Constable 1930; G C Cook, A J Webb. Reactions from the medical and nursing professions to Nightingale's 'reform(s)' of nurse training in the late 19th century. *Postgrad Med J* 2002; 78: 118–123; [*See also:* C Helmstadter. Early nursing reform in nineteenth century London: a doctor-driven phenomenon. *Med Hist* 2002; 46: 325–50; R G Huntsman, M Brain, D Holttam. Twixt candle and lamp: the contribution of Elizabeth Fry and the institution of nursing sisters to nursing reform. *Med Hist* 2002: 46: 351–80; M E Baly, H C G Matthew. Nightingale, Florence (1820–1910). In: H C G Matthew, B Harrison (eds). *Oxford Dictionary of National Biography.* Oxford: Oxford University Press 2004; 40: 904–12].

2 **Harry Calvert** (later Sir Harry Verney, Bt) (1801–94) was both brother-in-law (having married Parthenope Nightingale) and close confidante of Florence Nightingale. He was the son of General Sir Harry Calvert Bt, educated at Harrow and Cambridge, and later became MP for Buckinghamshire. After early experiences involving cholera, he promoted

the social reforms of the 7th Earl of Shaftersbury (1801–85) (and others), and played a leading role in providing aid to the sick and wounded during the Franco-German War (1870); *Op cit.* See note 1 above (Cook, Webb); [*See also*: M M Verney, H C G Matthew. Verney [*formerly* Calvert] Sir Harry, Second baronet (1801–1894). In: H C G Matthew, B Harrison (eds). *Oxford Dictionary of National Biography.* Oxford: Oxford University Press 2004; 56: 341–3].

3 **John Sutherland** (1808–91) was one of Britain's leading authorities on sanitation, and a prominent promoter of 'sanitary science'. He held an MD (Edinburgh) degree. After early experiences with cholera, he became head of a commission to the Crimea to inquire into the sanitary conditions in the British Army there. He later became Inspector General of the Board of Health. [*See also*: G C Boase, M Harrison. Sutherland, John (1808–1891). In: H C G Matthew, B Harrison (eds). *Oxford Dictionary of National Biography.* Oxford: Oxford University Press 2004; 53: 367–8].

4 F Nightingale to H Verney 1867; 7 March: 1 [Archives & Manuscripts Collection, Wellcome Library: MS 9002/114].

5 F Nightingale to H Verney. 1867: 15 March: 2 [Archives & Manuscripts Collection, Wellcome Library: MS 9002/128].

6 [PMH–P]. Travels of a Londoner. *General Steam Navigation Co. News Letter No. 73.* 1953; August 28: 4; Cook G C. *From the Greenwich Hulks to Old St Pancras: a history of tropical disease in London.* London: Athlone Press 1992: 338; *Op cit.* See note 1 above (Cook, Webb).

7 **Henry Rooke** (1824–1870) was the Principal Medical Officer (PMO) to the *Dreadnought* from 1858 until his death in 1870; H T L Rooke. In: *Seamen's Hospital Society: copy of three letters received by the Committee* 1864: 2–8 [SHS Archive]; Annual Report 21; [*See also*: Anonymous. Rooke, Henry T L. In: *Medical Directory.* London: John Churchill and Sons 1864: 553].

8 Committee of Management Minutes. 10: 142–3

9 *Ibid.* 10: 149–52.

10 *Op cit.* See note 7 above (Reports) 61: 13; 62: 12; 69: 10; 70: 14; 71: 13; 73: 13; 74: 13.

11 *Ibid.* 51: 20; G C Cook, A Webb. History of 'tropical nursing' in East London: the *Dreadnought* experience. *Int Hist Nursing J* 1996; 2 (2): 69–83.

12 *Op cit.* See note 8 above: 9: 240.

13 **Silas Kemball Cook** (1818–1874) (*See also* Chapter 12) had been appointed Secretary of the SHS in September 1849. One of his sons Sir Edward Cook KBE (1857–1919) became a well-known editor, and wrote a two-vol biography of Florence Nightingale (see ref 1 above). Kemball Cook's terminal illness began in 1873, and he died in the land-based '*Dreadnought*' Hospital which he had done so much to instigate.

14 *Op cit.* See note 8 above. 9.

15 *Ibid.* 9: 295.

16 Seamen's Hospital Society *'Names of Sisters & Nurses in the Hospital upon Appointment of Matron Decr 1 1870, with the names of those engaged and left since that date'.* 1870: December: 2 [SHS Archive].

17 *Instructions to Officers, Nurses, Servants, &c, employed in the service of the Seamen's Hospital Society (late Dreadnought) Greenwich*: 1875 [SHS Archive].

18 *Op cit.* See notes 1, 2 and 11 above.

19 *Op cit.* See note 8 above 9: 262.

20 *Op cit.* See note 7 above (Reports) 58: 13; 69: 14; 70: 13.

21 *Op cit.* See note 8 above 9: 210.

22 *Op cit.* See note 8 above.

23 **H C (later Sir Henry) Burdett** (1847–1920) KCB, KCVO had previously been Secretary of Queen's Hospital, Birmingham. On leaving the SHS (he served as Secretary from 1874

until 1880), he joined the London Stock Exchange but retained a keen interest in hospitals, nurses' education, and especially the National Pension Fund for Nurses – which he had initiated! [*See also*: G C Cook. Henry Charles Burdett (1847–1920): outstanding hospital administrator, successful Secretary of the Seamen's Hospital Society, and notable philanthropist. *J Med Biog* 2001; 9: 195–207; F Prochaska. Burdett, Sir Henry Charles (1847–1920). In: H C G Matthew, B Harrison (eds). *Oxford Dictionary of National Biography*. Oxford: Oxford University Press 2004; 8: 741–3].

24 *Op cit*. See note 8 above. 10: 112, 115–16 [*See also*: *Op cit*. See note 7 above (Reports) 59: 11, 13].

25 *Op cit*. See note 8 above. 10: 177–78, 180.

26 *Ibid*: 275. [*See also*: *Op cit*. See note 7 above (reports) 60: 13; 61.

27 *Op cit*. See note 8 above. 10: 491–2; 11: 335, 362, 372–3.

28 *Ibid*. 13: 177–8.

29 Medical Council Minutes 1904.

30 *Op cit*. See note 8 above. 14: 96, 100, 114–5.

31 *Ibid*. 14: 166.

32 Burdett H. *How to become a nurse. The nursing profession: how and when to train. Being a guide for trained nurses in their work and to training for the profession of a nurse, with particulars of nurse training schools in the United Kingdom and abroad and an outline of the principal laws affecting nurses, etc.* London: Scientific Press 1909.

33 Anonymous. *SHS Quart Mag* 1993; 5(1): 20; 1934; 6(1): 14.

34 *Op cit*. See note 8 above: 14: 393, 399–400, 402–3.

35 *Ibid*. 12: 352–3, 362.

36 *Op cit*. see note 18 above. G C Cook, A J Webb. Nurse-training at the *Dreadnought* Hospital, Greenwich in the late 19th century. *Int Hist Nursing J* 2002; 7: 12–22, 29–37.

37 **John Curnow**, **John Anderson** and **Patrick (later Sir Patrick) Manson** were Consultant Physicians to the SHS [*See also*: G C Cook. Doctor Patrick Manson's leading opposition in the establishment of the London School of Tropical Medicine: Curnow, Anderson, and Turner. *J.Med Biog* 1995; 3: 170–7].

38 **William Johnson Smith** FRCS (1940–1912) (see also Chapter 15) was the long serving Resident Surgeon to the SHS. [*See also*: Smith, Wm Johnson. *Medical Directory* London: J & A Churchill 1900: 363–4].

39 The *lock* wards were expressly devoted to male venereal diseases – syphilis and gonorrhoea, both of which were very common in seafarers. [*See also:* G C Cook. Disease in the nineteenth century merchant navy: The Seamen's Hospital Society's experience. *Mariners Mirror* 2001; 87: 460–71; D I Williams. *The London Lock: a charitable hospital for venereal disease 1746–1952*. London: RSM Press, 1995: 166].

40 *Op cit*. See note 8 above. 12: 329, 340, 362–4.

41 *Ibid*. 13: 388.

42 *Ibid*. 12: 500.

43 *Op cit*. See note 11 above. [See also Chapter 15.]

44 *Op cit*. See note 8 above. 12: 487–8, 490.

45 *Ibid*. 238–241.

46 *Ibid*. 236–8.

47 *Op cit*. See note 1 above (Cook). [*See also*: C Maggs. Ethel Manson and Henry Burdett: two great minds not thinking alike. *Hist Nurs Grp Roy Coll Bull* 1989; 2 (8): 1–5; *Op cit*. See also note 29 above: 47–8].

48 *Op cit*. See note 1 above (Cook); [*See also*: J Elliott. One Man's vision: Royal Pension Fund for Nurses; *Nursing Times* 1968; 26 July; C Maggs. Sir Henry Burdett and the RNPFN. *Lampada* 1987; 1(11): 12–14; C Maggs. Nursing's forgotten hero. *Nursing Times* 1987; 83 (36): 33–35; *Op cit*. See note 8 above. 12: 362–4].

49 **P J (later Sir James) Michelli,** CMG (1853–1935) was Secretary to the SHS from 1887 until 1927. He was also Secretary to the London School of Tropical Medicine from 1899–1924; *Op cit.* See note 29 above: 392–394.

50 *Op cit.* See note 26 above. 443; *Seamen's Hospital Society: National Pension Fund for Nurses: Regulations for distribution amongst the Nursing Staff.* [SHS Archive].

51 *Ibid.* 13:148–50, 208.

52 *Ibid.* 13: 166.

53 *Ibid.* 13: 174, 223.

54 *Op cit.* See note 8 above. 13: 158.

55 *Ibid.* 14: 446.

56 *Op cit.* See note 7 above (Reports).

57 Matron of the Dreadnought. The answer to a very big problem of today. *SHS Quart Mag* 1931; 3(2): 11–13.

58 *Op cit.* See note 8 above. 13: 40–41.

59 *Op cit.* See note 11 above (Cook, Webb); *Op cit.* See note 7 above (Reports): 74.

60 *Op cit.* See note 8 above. 13: 252–3.

61 **Viscount Devonport** (1856–1934) was a prominent politician and chairman of the Port of London Authority from 1909 until 1925. [*See*: R Davenport-Hines. Kearley, Hudson Ewbanke, first Viscount Devonport (1856–1934). In: H C G Matthew, B Harrison (eds). *Oxford Dictionary of National Biography.* Oxford: Oxford University Press 2004: 30: 960–1].

62 G C Cook. Transfer of hospitals and 'additional premises' to the state: questionable morality in the implementation of the National Health Service Act (1946) *Postgrad Med J* 2004; 80: 716–19.

Chapter 18

Genesis of the first school for *tropical* diseases at the ADH

Origins of the LSTM

The 1898 *Annual Report* recorded 'one of the most important [departures] in the annals of the Corporation: '... the establishment of the London School of Tropical Medicine [LSTM] ...'. The initial stimulus for creation of this school (under the aegis of the SHS) came in a letter from the Colonial Office (presumably triggered by Sir Patrick Manson (see Chapter 15) in early 1898; this was read at a Management Committee meeting – held at the Institute of Chartered Accountancy, Moorgate Place, EC – on 11 February:

> Downing Street
> 2 February 1898.
>
> Sir,
>
> The question of improving the medical service of the British Colonies in West Africa has been receiving Mr Secretary Chamberlain [the Rt. Hon. Joseph Chamberlain FRS (1836–1914)]'s serious consideration.
>
> At present the newly-appointed medical officers receive no special Training in the diagnosis and Treatment of tropical diseases before they proceed to West Africa; and, although an attempt is made to give them whenever possible some preliminary instruction at the Head Quarter's Hospital of the Colony, this course cannot be followed in every case and the arrangement is, on the whole, unsatisfactory.
>
> Mr Chamberlain feels confident that a marked advance would have been made, if some scheme could be devised by which all the newly-appointed officers should receive a sound and systematic training in this country before proceeding to take up their duties in West Africa.
>
> He is advised [again, presumably by Manson] that the experience and training to be obtained at the Seamen's Hospital would be the most suitable in the present instance, and he would be greatly obliged to the Managing Committee if they could give him their valuable assistance in the matter.
>
> Mr Chamberlain understands that the Committee are about to enlarge their Branch Hospital at the Albert Docks [the Albert Dock Hospital – ADH], and he would ask them to consider whether it might not be

possible to provide the necessary accommodation in the new building for the officers whom it is desired to instruct.

The Secretary of State for Foreign Affairs is being asked whether it is wished that the Protectorates in East and West Africa, at present administered by the Foreign Office, should be included in the proposed scheme; but in any case, it is not probable that more than six officers would be under instruction at any one time.

It is desired that the course of instruction should last for three or four months.

In the event of the Committee being willing to entertain these proposals favourably, Mr Chamberlain would be glad to know the terms and conditions on which they would be prepared to make the necessary arrangements.

I am,
Sir,
Your obedient servant,
H Bertram Cox.[1]

A minute of the same date stated:

> The Deputy Chairman [P A Nairne] was requested to prepare a reply to the effect that the matter will receive the careful and favourable consideration of the committee who hope to be able to see their way to propose a scheme which will carry out the views of the Colonial Secretary.[2]

The matter was further considered at the following meeting of the Committee, held at the same venue, on 11 March; it was '… resolved that the matter be referred to a Sub-Committee (which would 'consult with such members of the Senior Medical Staff of both Hospitals [the *Dreadnought* and the ADH] as they might think right') consisting of: - G Lidgett Esq., JP, Adml. E.S. Adeane, C.M.G. Rev[d] Brook Lambert M.A., B.Ch., TL Rogers Esq., M.D., Major the Hon. W Rowley, Silas Waymouth Esq., RN, Col. WE Despard, and Comm G Hodgkinson RN'. The first meeting was held at the Cannon Street Hotel on 15 March 1898. Having held four meetings and consulted with Manson who was at that time 55 years old, and at the height of his power(s) – being Medical Officer to the Colonial Office, in addition to his routine duties at the *ADH*. Clearly, to incorporate a tropical school necessitated a considerable extension of the existing buildings. Mr Johnson Smith, and 'the Architect', of the sub-committee reported (via P A Nairne) to the April meeting of the Committee of Management:

> … your Sub-Committee are of opinion that, should a School [of *tropical medicine*] be established, its teaching centre should be located at the [ADH]; this opinion is borne out by the Returns which shew that 78% of the cases of Tropical Diseases treated by the Society during the six months reviewed have either been treated at the [ADH] or have passed through the Docks immediately adjoining it.

> Your sub-Committee therefore recommend that in further reply to the letter from the Colonial Office the Government be informed of the lines on which the Committee consider that such a Medical School as the Secretary of State has suggested should be laid out, and worked.
>
> The present Branch Hospital [ADH] does not give sufficient accommodation for the treatment of all the cases of Tropical Disease that apply for admission and the extension to 30 beds had already been resolved on before the suggestion of the establishment of a School had been heard of. If the establishment of the School should be arranged the Sub-Committee would suggest that the accommodation should be still further increased to 45 beds which would avert the danger of sending on acute cases to Greenwich [i.e. the *Dreadnought* Hospital] and would at the same time give ample teaching material. It would also provide for cases of accident and emergency arising in the neighbourhood.
>
> They recommend that provision be made for the teaching of from 20 to 25 Students, with sleeping accommodation for about 10 persons. This would necessitate a fully equipped laboratory, pathological room, mess room, ante room, offices, etc.
>
> They further recommend that the Senior Medical Staff of the Society be invited to join the teaching Staff of the proposed School; those members of the Staff at Greenwich who accept to send their cases of Tropical Diseases to the teaching centre.
>
> That instruction be given to students on four days in the week for four hours each day by one or more members of the Senior Medical Staff.
>
> That a Medical Tutor (who should be also a bacteriologist) or other suitable instructor attend the school for six hours daily ...[3]

This report was accompanied by a draft letter (compiled by the Secretary – P J [later Sir James] Michelli [*see* Chapter 15]) to the Under Secretary of State at the Colonial Office, and was followed by an estimate of expenditure on the proposed School:

> Sir,
>
> In further reply to your communication of 2nd February, No. 16144/97, I am directed to inform you that my Committee have carefully considered the subject of the establishment of a School for the Study of Tropical Diseases which cannot be found elsewhere in the United Kingdom in the same amount and variety. There are on an average 190 cases of well marked typical Tropical Diseases coming under the care of the Society's Physicians and Surgeons annually. These are usually acute cases, such as are met with in actual practice in the Tropics and include a large percentage of Asiatics, Africans and West Indians, as well as Europeans of all nations and natives of British and other Colonies. Seventy-eight % of these patients land in the Royal Victoria and Albert Docks and are either treated at the [ADH] which adjoins the Dock Gates, or, if not too ill, are sent to the Dreadnought Hospital at Greenwich.
>
> The number of beds in the [ADH] is at present 18 and a large number of cases of Tropical Disease are sent to Greenwich, a distance of about

6 miles. The demand for additional accommodation has been so great that the Committee had lately arranged to increase the number of beds to 30. This increase, however, would not fully meet the demand and the Committee feel that if a School for the study of Tropical Diseases is to be formed the accommodation should be further enlarged to 45 beds which would usually be filled with cases affording excellent material for the purposes of the School.

It will be necessary that suitable school buildings and sleeping accommodation for students be erected, with appropriate laboratory, pathological room, mess room, ante room, offices, etc.

The distance of the [ADH] from London, the far greater opportunities enjoyed by students who are on the spot during the whole 24 hours, and the shortness of the period which most students will be able to give up for their course of study all combine to make it most desirable that provision for the residence of the Students in the Hospital should be made.

The Medical Staff of the [SHS] are by long experience exceptionally well qualified for the teaching of the treatment of Tropical Diseases and arrangements would be made for one or more Members of the Senior Medical Staff to attend and give instruction to students on four days in the week and on each occasion for four hours.

In addition a Medical Tutor (who would be also a bacteriologist) would be in residence to give daily instruction to students, not only in the study of Tropical Diseases but in Hospital administration and the treatment of patients generally.

Plans and specifications for the erection of a new wing and the School building have been submitted to the Committee by their Architect and will be laid before the Secretary of State if desired, and appended to this letter is an estimate of the capital and current expenditure shewing that the addition of the new wing will cost in construction approximately £10,000 and in maintenance £2,000 per annum, and that the School buildings will cost in construction approximately £3,500 and, with six students, in maintenance £1,100.

The Committee would propose to admit to the School Students, other than those sent by the Colonial Office, as it is believed that Missionary Societies and other bodies would wish to give their Medical Officers the advantage of training in the School.

The Committee of the [Society] will be happy to entertain any suggestions for the modification of the scheme that the Secretary of State may see fit to make.

I am, Sir

Your obedient servant.

P Michelli (Secretary)

April 14 1898

Estimate

Capital Expenditure

Estimated cost of establishing and working a School for the study of Tropical Diseases:-

Cost of New Wing:

Building	£7500	
Piling	1200	
Furniture, Fittings &c.	750	£9450
Cost of School Buildings		
One Laboratory		
One Pathological Room		
One Ante Room		
Sleeping accommodation		
Mess Room, Offices, &c	£3150	
Appliances for Laboratory	150	
Furniture, Fittings, &c.	250	3550
Total cost of new wing and School Buildings		13000

Current Expenditure

Cost of maintaining say 25 additional beds occupied (the total number added being 27) at £78 per annum	£1950	
Board of six students, one laboratory man and two Servants at £30 per annum each	£270	
Chemicals, repairs &c.	75	
Salary of Bacteriologist say	150	
Wages of laboratory man	30	
"of two Servants at £16 per annum each	32	
Sundries, clerical work, printing stationery &c &c	50	
Interest on capital (£13,000) at 3%	390	
Depreciation of School only – say	100	1097
Representing at 3% a capital sum of upwards of £100,000		£3047

Note

Maintenance of six students for 10 months in the year at 4 guineas per week approximately per annum	£1,100
Proposed fees for a course of not less than 4 weeks for Resident Students	£4:4:0 per week
"Non-Resident Students	£2:12:6 " "

It was resolved that the report now read be adopted and that the letter be written to the Under Secretary of State for the Colonies, enclosing an estimate of the Capital and Current Expenditure [see above].

A special Committee ('to provide for the efficient organisation and management of the new [LSTM]' was also formed); this consisted of the following:

PERCEVAL A. NAIRNE Esq. (*Chairman*)
Admiral Sir WALTER HUNT-GRUBBE GCB (*Deputy Chairman*)
Sir EDWIN ARNOLD KCIE CSI
Surg.-Col. OSWALD BAKER MD
ROBERT BARNES Esq. MD FRCP FRCS
Sir CHAS. GAGE BROWN KCMG MD FRCP
Sir THOMS. LAUDER BRUNTON MD FRS
JAMES CANTLIE Esq. MB CM FRCS
Surgeon-General JAMES CLEGHORN CSI MD
WILLIAM COLLINGRIDGE Esq. MD
The late S. LEONARD CRANE Esq. CMG MD
W H CROSSE, Esq. MRCS
H.H. THE THAKORE SAHIB OF GONDAL GCIE LLD DCL MD FRCP
Sir WILLIAM R KYNSEY CMG
Rev. BROOKE LAMBERT MA BCL
HERBERT H LANKESTER Esq. MD
ALLAN MACFADYEN Esq. MD
STEPHEN MACKENZIE Esq. MD FRCP
N C MACNAMARA Esq. FRCS
PATRICK MANSON Esq. CMG LLD MD FRCP FRS
JAMES LAIDLAW MAXWELL Esq. MD
JOHN WILLIAM OGLE Esq. MD FRCP
H J READ Esq.
T L ROGERS Esq. MD
Major the Hon. W ROWLEY
W JOHNSON SMITH Esq. FRCS
Sir H M STANLEY GCB DCL LLD MP
Admiral Sir RICHARD TRACEY KCB
Inspector-General ALEXANDER TURBULL RN MD
WILLIAM TURNER Esq. MS (LOND) FRCS[4]

At a July meeting, a reply from the Colonial Office was read:

Downing Street. 30th June 1898

Sir,

I am directed by Mr. Secretary Chamberlain to acknowledge the receipt of your letter of the 16th of April submitting the proposals of the Managing Committee of the Seamen's Hospital for the formation of a School of Tropical Medicine, at which the Medical Officers of the colonies and Protectorates administered by the Colonial Office and Foreign Office respectively may be given special instruction in the treatment of Tropical Diseases.

2. Mr Chamberlain desires me to ask you to convey to the Committee his thanks for their cordial co-operation in this matter and to inform

them that Her Majesty's Government are prepared to accept the scheme which they have put forward on the following terms:-

1) That a contribution of £3550 shall be made on behalf of the Colonies and Protectorates concerned towards the initial cost of School buildings, Laboratory, &c
2) That the fees for training students shall be as stated in your letter, namely £4:4:0 per week for Resident Students and £2.12.6 per week for non-Resident students.
3) That a representative of the Colonial Office shall be admitted to the Board of Management of the Hospital.

3. If these terms are acceptable to the Committee, Mr Chamberlain would ask that the necessary arrangements for the reception of the officers to be trained at the Hospital should be made with as little delay as possible, as he is anxious to bring the scheme into operation at an early date.

I am, Sir
Your obedient servant,
H. Bertram Cox

At the same meeting, the Chairman (P A Nairne) emphasised:

the liability that would be involved in the acceptance of the offer of the Colonial Office and pointed out that not only did the scheme involve an expenditure of capital and consequent diminution of income from invested property but that even if allowance were made for receipts from student fees an additional expenditure would be incurred of upward of £2000 per annum. On the other hand the establishment of such a school must of necessity advertise the Charity and be of benefit to the Institution and he saw no reason to apprehend that in time sufficient funds would be forthcoming from the public to meet the increased cost of maintenance, nevertheless the Committee should be alive to the fact that in all probability it would take some time to raise from annual subscriptions and donations sufficient funds to make the income equal to the expenditure. If on the other hand he was not correct in his surmise and it was found necessary to lessen the cost of maintaining the various establishments of the Charity it appeared to him that it would be found expedient to reduce the number of beds at Greenwich, rather than stop the active work which is being carried on at the [ADH]. He did not apprehend that such a course would ever have to be adopted and he felt that the committee might accept the offer of the Colonial Office and forthwith proceed with the work not only of the school buildings but also of the new wing to the [ADH].

This meeting:

unanimously resolved that the offer of the Colonial Office be accepted and that the erection of the School Buildings and new wing to the [ADH] be proceeded with forthwith.

The Secretary informed the Committee that the Editor of the Times had stated that he would give favourable consideration to a letter on the subject of the School for Tropical Diseases in view of a leading article in the Times. The Secretary was authorised to see Sir H Burdett [a Vice-President and former Secretary of the SHS] (Chapter 15), to lay the whole scheme before him, and to ask him to write a letter to the Times giving particulars of the proposed School.

The Architect (Mr Hall) was in attendance and was called before the Committee. He was instructed to proceed with the piling for the foundations of the School Buildings and new wing at once in the same manner as he had arranged for the piling for the Laundry, matters of detail in connection with the ground plan to be arranged with the Chairman & Secretary. The Architect was further instructed to prepare detailed plans of the School Buildings, Laboratory and New Wing, to have Bills of Quantities prepared and to obtain tenders &c for the consideration of the Committee at their meeting in October next.[5]

A serious controversy

Sir Henry Burdett (see Chapter 15) duly wrote to *The Times* outlining details of the proposed school. This letter (which was accompanied by a supportive leading article) was written in order to both give publicity to the proposed LSTM – as outlined in the previous correspondence – and to appeal for funding for the new venture. He also outlined the valuable role of the ADH in dealing with 'accident cases which occur with alarming frequency in the neighbouring Albert and Victoria Docks'. 'To emphasise this appeal [the 1898 *Annual Report* declared], Mr Chamberlain has consented to preside at a Festival Dinner [arranged by Sir Donald Currie, G.C.M.G., M.P., a Vice-President of the Society] to be held at the Hotel Cecil on the 10th of May next …'.[6] Burdett's letter brought forth a rapid but unwelcome response from the Senior Medical Staff (led by Doctors Curnow and Anderson, and Mr G R Turner) based at Greenwich. The reason(s) for their disgruntlement was essentially threefold: (i) they were being slighted in that it was being implied that they were unable to care (competently) for 'tropical cases', (ii) the scheme would move all 'tropical' cases away from the *Dreadnought* to the ADH, and (iii) there were in any case far more suitable venues for a School of Tropical Medicine (e.g. Netley[7] and Haslar[8]).

It was agreed at a meeting on 9 September that the following letter be sent to Turner 'in response to [his joint] communications to the Chairman' (for details of this correspondence see ref. 9 – below):

Dear Sir

Your letters to the Chairman of July 19th & 21st have been laid before my Board.

The Committee feel that their relations with the medical staff in the past are a sufficient answer to the suggestion that any discourtesy or want of consideration towards them in connection with the Society's reply to the Secretary of State's proposal for the establishment by the Society of a School for the Study of Tropical Diseases, was intended.

The Committee regret that any expression in Sir Hy Burdett's letter published in the 'Times' … should appear to you and to some of your colleagues to have represented that you and they had engaged to take part in the educational work of the school. Sir Henry Burdett (with the Committee) probably felt no doubt that the educational work would in the main be taken charge of by the Medical Staff of the Society's Hospitals, but the Committee do not read his letter as a pledge that each member of the staff would join in the educational work.

The Committee have read with much regret the joint letter of Dr. Curnow, Dr. Anderson, and yourself, published in the 'Times' of July 20th, and in some of the Medical papers a few days later, which they feel must tend to injure the success of the project into which the Committee have entered at the invitation of the Secretary of State. They will be glad to know whether they are to infer from it that the writers have renounced all connection with the proposed School and upon this point they ask for a definite reply at an early date.

Yours faithfully
P. Michelli
Secretary

Mr G Robertson Turner.

A reply was duly forthcoming, and was read to the following (October) meeting of the Management Committee:

9 Harley Street. W. October 10th 1898.

Dear Sir,

Referring to the proposed School for Tropical Medicine at the Royal Victoria & Albert Docks, and Mr Michelli's letter of the 14th July, we think our letter to the 'Times' of July 20th, was a plain statement of facts. We see nothing to regret on our part and if there is any meaning in plain English, Sir Henry Burdett's words can have but one interpretation, i.e.: that the Senior Staff of the Dreadnought were to be on the teaching staff of the proposed School.

On July 15th he wrote Dr. Anderson that his letter to the 'Times' was written under instructions from the Committee of the Dreadnought:- a Committee, we would remind you, who had not had the courtesy to let us know that such a scheme was on foot; still less to ask for our co-operation, until five days after the vice-President's letter appeared in the lay press, and he had been asked for explanation by Dr Anderson.

We beg to ask the Committee, as Dr Curnow has twice already asked the Secretary, whether they have decided to concentrate the cases of tropical diseases at the [ADH] and have done this without consulting the Visiting Physicians of the Parent Dreadnought Hospital?

It is impossible for us to give any answer to a request for co-operation until we have been put in full possession of the details of the scheme of the proposed school.

Believe us,

Yours faithfully,

John Curnow.

J. Anderson.

G.R. Turner.

The Chairman of the *Dreadnought* Hospital Committee.[9]

At the same meeting the Committee resolved to send the following reply to this joint letter:

14th October 1898

Dear Sirs,

I am instructed to acknowledge the receipt of your letter of 10th inst. which was laid before the General Committee at their meeting this day.

The Committee regret that you still feel aggrieved by Sir Henry Burdett's letter …

They also much regret that you do not feel able to signify your wish to co-operate with them in carrying out the scheme of H.M. Secretary of State for the Colonies for the establishment, in connection with the Society's Branch Hospital, of a School for the study of tropical diseases.

The details of the scheme must necessarily remain open for consideration by the Committee which will be appointed to manage the School.

I am, Dear Sirs, Yours faithfully

P Michelli (Secretary).[10]

RESIGNATIONS OF FOUR MEMBERS OF THE HONORARY MEDICAL STAFF OF THE DREADNOUGHT

A great deal of acrimonious correspondence followed, in which many leading figures in the medical profession, including Sir William Broadbent Bt FRS (1835–1907) (see Chapter 19) joined in. Sir William, although he had been defeated in the RCP's presidential election of 1889, was Physician-Extraordinary to Queen Victoria (1896) and was to become Physician-in-Ordinary to the Prince of Wales (1901). Curnow was, however, not only the senior physician at the Dreadnought Hospital, but also on the staff of the *Lancet*, a journal which clearly sided with him and his colleagues. The thoughts and feelings of the Society's Committee of Management were summarised in a *Memorandum* 'adopted' at a meeting held on 9 December 1898:

It appears from the article published in the [*BMJ* 1898; ii: 1716] … that the two points of which the Visiting Staff complain are:-

a) A paragraph in Sir Henry Burdett's letter … which stated – 'the teaching staff will consist of the Senior Medical Staff of the Dreadnought Hospital at Greenwich as well as of the [ADH], together with a number of teachers specially selected and attached to the new School'.
b) The statement that the Committee propose to 'concentrate cases of tropical disease' at the [ADH]. The [*BMJ*] expressed the opinion that an apology and explanation are due to the visiting Staff, and a hope that this may be frankly given and as frankly accepted.

The Committee of the [SHS] have already in the correspondence expressed regret that any statement in … Burdett's letter should have caused the Visiting Staff to feel aggrieved. The Committee regret also that the statement relating to the proposed constitution of the Teaching Staff was capable of bearing the interpretation that the Greenwich Visiting Staff had pledged themselves to take part in the teaching work of the School. The Committee wish to make an honourable apology to the visiting Staff for any injury or indignity that has unconsciously been caused to them through the statement.

The Visiting Staff in their letter of October 29th say 'We are still more aggrieved by the Committee's want of courtesy in not asking the opinion of the Senior Medical Staff of the Dreadnought Hospital at any time during the inception of the scheme'.

On this point the Committee would explain that the enquiry of the Secretary of State for the Colonies was 'whether it might not be possible to provide the necessary accommodation in the new building' about to be erected for the enlargement of the [ADH] for the officers whom it is desired to instruct. No enquiry as to the possibility of providing accommodation at the Dreadnought Hospital at Greenwich was made.

The two Hospitals are worked as separate establishments with separate Visiting Staffs and separate Resident Staffs, the only Medical Officers having duty at both Hospitals being the Society's Principal Medical Officer [Johnson Smith] and the Ophthalmic Surgeon [Donald Gunn FRCS] who visits each Hospital.

In 1892, on the recommendation of a Sub Committee of which the Greenwich Visiting Staff were members, a Visiting Physician [Manson] to the [ADH] was appointed and the Greenwich Visiting Physicians were relieved of duties at the [ADH]. They subsequently objected to the Visiting Physician being described as an officer of the 'Seamen's Hospital, Greenwich', thereby emphasising the disconnection of the two Hospitals.

The establishment of a School at the [ADH] in which the Visiting Staff of the Dreadnought Hospital, with the exception of the Ophthalmic Surgeon, have no duties will thus not affect them and no want of courtesy to that Staff was intended by the Committee in not asking their opinion on a matter which did not relate to the Hospital to which they were attached.

With reference to the concentration of cases of Tropical Disease at the [ADH] it may be explained that previous to the establishment of the [ADH] a large proportion of the cases of Tropical Disease landed in the Port of London were treated at the [Royal] London Hospital. A smaller percentage applied for admission and were treated at the Dreadnought Hospital at Greenwich. Since the establishment of the [ADH] the number of cases of Tropical Disease treated at the Dreadnought Hospital at Greenwich has been decreased through the transfer from the [ADH] of convalescent patients originally admitted and treated there. The necessity of enlarging the [ADH] to avert the removal of convalescent patients at too early a stage had been so strongly felt by the Committee that plans had been prepared and arrangements made for an enlargement of that Hospital before the suggestion of the Secretary of State for the Colonies for the establishment of a Tropical School was received.

As the majority of patients coming to the Society's Hospitals suffering from Tropical Diseases are usually landed in the Docks on the north side of the Thames it is manifest that a large percentage of such cases will be treated at the [ADH], which was built there with the express object of treating patients landing at, or sustaining injuries in those Docks. But there is no reason to suppose that the patients suffering from tropical diseases who have hitherto applied for admission and been treated at the Dreadnought Hospital will be fewer than heretofore and the Committee do not contemplate the transfer of such patients to the [ADH].

D^r. Curnow, the Senior Visiting Physician of the Dreadnought Hospital, in a letter published in the 'Daily Chronicle' [1898: 26 November] advanced reasons for the establishment of the School at the Dreadnought Hospital in preference to the [ADH]. His letter was forcibly answered by 'a Colonial Physician' in a [later] letter [1898: 29 November] the arguments in which need not be here repeated.

Amongst the reasons which moved the Committee to decide on the [ADH] as the more suitable place were the following:-

The Society hold the Dreadnought Hospital, formerly the Infirmary of Greenwich Hospital, from the Lords of the Admiralty on a tenancy determinable by either party by six months' notice. They have no additional land at Greenwich, and they have no reason to think that the Lords of the Admiralty would either grant additional land or sanction the erection of additional buildings within the precincts of Greenwich Hospital.

They hold the land on which the [ADH] stands on lease for about 90 years from the London and India Docks Joint Committee, and the Joint Committee have both offered additional land for the extension of the Hospital and the building of the School and have approved the plans of the new buildings.

Above all other considerations it is manifest that the Hospital must be placed where it will best serve the needs of patients and that the School must be attached to the Hospital at which tropical diseases can best be studied.

It is not open to question that the Society's … Hospital at the Victoria & Albert Docks [ADH] is the Hospital which affords the best opportunities in London for the study of Tropical Diseases and the Society have throughout the negotiation for the establishment of the London School of Tropical Medicine been in full and constant consultation with the Visiting Staff of that Hospital.[11]

It is clear therefore, that a vehement and acrimonious controversy followed the announcement of the Manson/Chamberlain plan! G R Turner (one of the key 'opponents' was to summarise his views many years later (Chapter 15). The controversy was to escalate, and culminated in a letter to *The Times* (supportive of Curnow and his colleagues) signed by no less than 15 distinguished members of the professions, including: Sir Joseph Fayrer (doyen of the Indian Medical Service), Sir Dyce Duckworth (who was, interestingly, later appointed to the SHS – Chapter 15) and Sir William Selby Church (President of the Royal College of Physicians from 1899 until 1905). The distinguished *Dreadnought* trio had by this time had enough, and they, together with the ophthalmic surgeon (Gunn) sent their letters of resignation (which were immediately 'accepted with regret'). The resignations were recorded at a Management Committee meeting on 24 March 1899:

The following letter was read:-

9, Wimpole Street, W. 12th March 1899

To the Board of Management, Dreadnought Hospital
Greenwich
Gentlemen,

We beg to tender our resignation of the posts we hold as physicians and surgeons of the Seamen's Hospital Society.

We shall be happy to continue to perform the duties of our office until our successors are selected, who, we venture to hope, will be appointed with as little delay as may be convenient to you.

We are, Gentlemen
Your obedient servants,

John Curnow
John Anderson } Physicians, Dreadnought Hospital

G.R. Turner Surgeon, do

A separate letter was also read from Donald S Gunn resigning his appointment as Ophthalmic Surgeon.

At the same meeting a Sub-Committee was set up to meet at Cannon Street Hotel on 28 March; their brief was 'to consider and report what regulations it is desirable to make with regard to the duties and status of the Senior Medical Staff of the Society'. The 1898 Annual Report recorded that 'in connection with the subsidy from Her Majesty's Government [from the Colonial and Foreign Offices both of which would be nominating a representative] to serve on the Committee of Management …'.[12]

Formation of an LSTM Committee

An LSTM Committee had by this time been formed. This consisted of P A Nairne (Chairman), Commander D Hodgkinson RN, G Lidgett Esq JP, Stephen Mackenzie Esq MD FRCP, R Tanner Hewlett Esq MD MRCP, James Cantlie MB FRCS and P Manson Esq LLD MD FRCP; the first meeting had been held on 5 July 1899. These minutes, ending in July 1924 are preserved at the SHS in nine volumes.[13]

RELATIONSHIP BETWEEN THE SHS AND THE LSTM

Not everyone was persuaded that this Society – formed principally to care for Merchant Seamen – should undertake an academic (teaching) role as well; in April 1905, for example, a letter was read at the Management Committee meeting from Mr Silas Waymouth RN (a member of the Sub-Committee which had been set up in early 1898 to advise on the feasibility of a *tropical school)*. He complained that the LSTM should not be 'worked as an integral part of the [SHS]' (see above).

Early years of the LSTM

The 79th *Annual Report* (1899) recorded that after completion of the extension, the LSTM was opened (with 28 post-graduate students) on 2 October 1899 when Dr Manson was due to deliver an inaugural address. 'Mr Perceval A. Nairne occupied the Chair, and many members of the Medical profession and supporters of the Charity were present …'. Figure 18.1 shows the interior of the 'tropical' ward at the ADH.

However, events had not been as straightforward as documented: Dr Alphonse Laveran (1845–1922) or William Osler FRS (1849–1919) had initially been invited to give the opening address but both were unable to attend. Guido Baccelli (1832–1916) was then invited, but he too declined! The reason(s) for these decisions were not stated. Manson was unwell on the day of the address (possibly suffering from gout) and his words were in fact read by James Cantlie.[14]

Expansion

The following Report (1900) recorded a highly successful first year – 100 post-graduate students (42 from the Colonial Service, four the Foreign Office, two the Navy, five the Army, 16 from Missionary Societies and 31 private students [five of them women]) had 'passed through a course of study'. Indeed, so successful was this new venture that increased facilities (i.e. 'extension of the Laboratory, Museum, and domestic buildings') were soon required, and the Hon Sir Francis Lovell CMG, formerly Surgeon-General of Trinidad (and from 1902, Dean of the LSTM) travelled to many of the Colonies in order to raise funds; this he did to the tune of £8,000! Subsequent Reports recorded further successes. It was intended that Lovell was to undertake a further fund-raising tour, but unfortunately his health failed and did not allow it; fortunately he was able to go to 'the East' from February to June 1904. Also, a further fund-raising Banquet was arranged, again with Chamberlain present (but chaired on this occasion by His Grace the Duke of Marlborough) on 10 May 1904.[15]

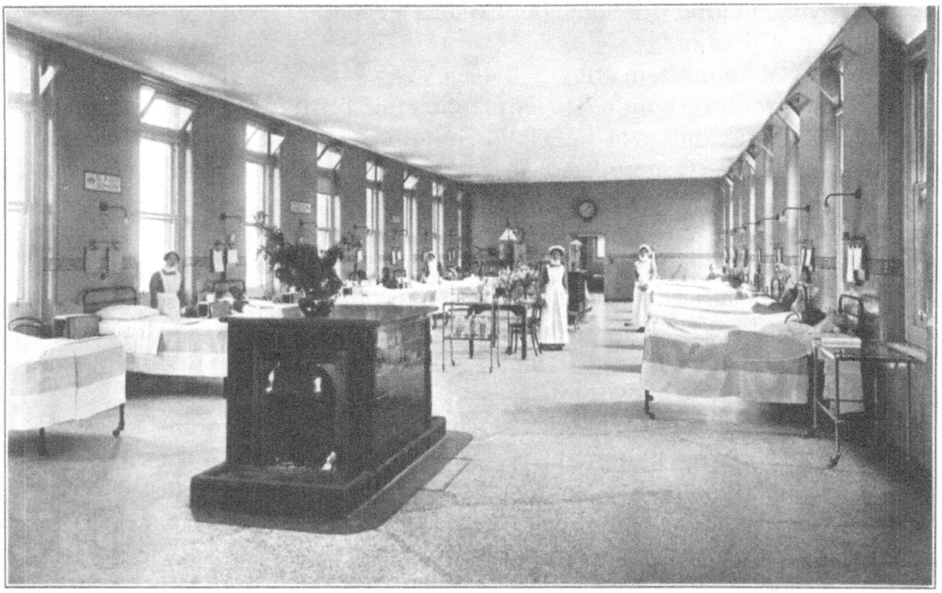

Figure 18.1: Interior of the 'tropical' ward at the Albert Dock Hospital. (Undated, but probably early 20th century).

The 1906 Report recorded that 'over 600 Students [had by then] passed through the School … now scattered throughout the Tropical Regions of the World'. On 28 February 1911, with the Lord Mayor presiding, a meeting at Mansion House was addressed by Mr (later the 1st Viscount) Lewis Harcourt (1863–1922), Secretary of State for the Colonies (1910–15).[16]

In 1909, another extension of the ADH had been required by the expanding LSTM, and this was made possible by a gift of £500 from Mr P Blessig. This expansion required additional land – from the Port of London Authority; however, only a small plot of land was offered, and it was declined, with thanks.[17] A further extension of the LSTM, and also the ADH was required in 1912; this would 'bring the laboratory accommodation for ordinary students up to about 100 and sleeping accommodation for about 25'. The King (George V, 1865–1936) accepted an invitation to lay the foundation stone of this new Wing on 17 July 1912, but he later declined.[18]

Internal matters

RULES FOR THE LSTM MEDICAL STAFF

The rules for the teaching staff of the LSTM were clearly stated at a meeting held on 11 December 1913:

1. That the director, Lecturers, Heads of Departments and other Members of the Teaching Staff be appointed by the Board of Management on the

recommendation of the School Committee after consultation with the committee of Teachers.

2. They shall retire from office at the age of 65.
3. They can only be required to retire from office by the Board of Management on the recommendation of the School Committee after the said School Committee has offered the Committee of Teachers an opportunity to report thereon – the School Committee to be specially convened, two-thirds of its members to be present and its recommendations made on a majority of two-thirds.
4. Three months' notice of termination of office to be given on either side, such notice to be terminable at the end of a session.
5. The Directors, Heads of Departments and Demonstrators shall devote their whole time to the service of the School unless permission to do otherwise be granted by the School Committee.
6. The Director, Heads of Department and Senior Members of the Teaching Staff shall be eligible for election to the School Committee.
7. The Director shall attend all Meetings of the School Committee.
8. The Teaching Staff shall recognise the Director as their Principal in all matters relating to the arrangements for Teaching, and the general management of the School.
9. The Director, Heads of Department and Senior Members of the Teaching Staff will constitute the Committee of Teachers.[19]

MANSON'S RESIGNATION

In August 1912, Sir Patrick Manson (then approaching 69 years) resigned:

50, Welbeck Street,
Cavendish Square
2nd August 1912
The Secretary of the Seamen's Hospital Society

Dear Sir

I greatly regret to have to request you to place my resignation of my appointment as a Physician to the [SHS] in the hands of the Management. My health is such that I feel I can no longer discharge my duties satisfactorily. I should like my resignation to take effect from the 15th inst. when I propose to retire from active practice.

In resigning my office I would ask you to express to the Chairman and Committee of Management my appreciation of the courtesy and consideration I have invariably experienced at their hands, and this more especially in connection with the [LSTM] which they have so successfully fostered.

Needless to say, although thus severing myself from the active staff of the Hospital at the Albert Docks, my interest in the work of the Hospitals and Schools [this included the LSCM – Chapter 19] will continue unabated.

Believe me. Yours faithfully,
Patrick Manson

Although then a relatively old man, Manson had been the instigator of the plan to establish both the LSTM and also the LSCM. This news must therefore have been a considerable blow to the Management Committee and his resignation was received 'with very great regret'.[20]

THE CHAMBERLAIN WARD

The 1912 Annual Report referred to 'the splendid and successful efforts of the Rt Hon (Sir) Austen Chamberlain, MP (1863–1937) [who had been elected a Vice-President of the Corporation] to complete the noble monument to the Imperial ideal begun by his father'. Sir Austen Chamberlain had launched an appeal for renewed funding for the LSTM; this ultimately reached a total of £63,000. The SHS Committee decided to name a ward – 'Chamberlain Ward' – in recognition of the efforts and interest shown by both of the Chamberlains to the LSTM. The opening ceremony and unveiling of 'bronze portrait reliefs' of both of these senior statesmen was carried out by the Rt Hon Lewis Harcourt (see above) on 23 June 1914. Figure 18.2 shows these images – preserved to this day at the Hospital for Tropical Diseases, London.[21]

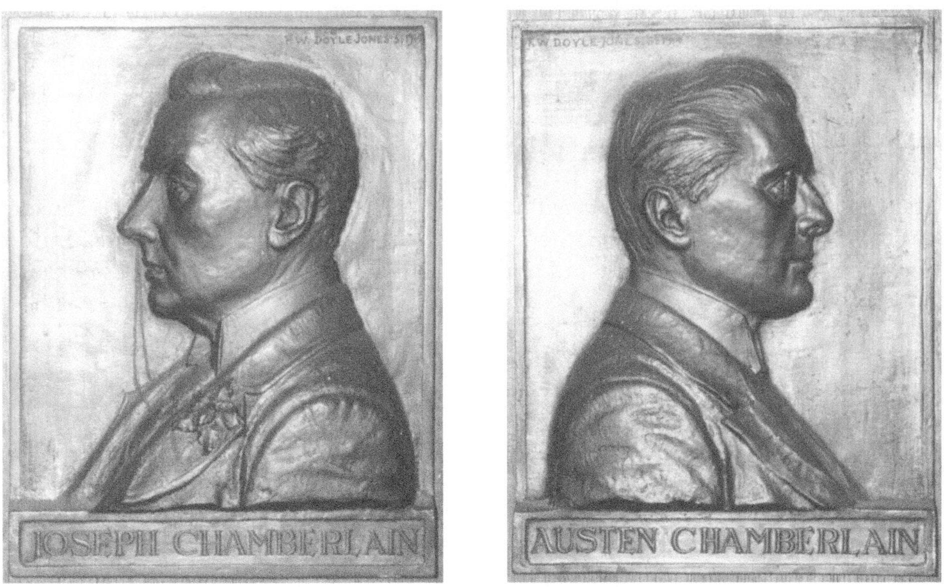

(a) (b)

Figure 18.2: Images of the Rt Hon Joseph Chamberlain FRS (1836–1914) (a) and his son Sir (Joseph) Austen Chamberlain (1863–1937) (b) on bronze plaques unveiled at the ADH on 23 June 1914. These are presently displayed at the Hospital for Tropical Diseases, University College Hospital, London.

ADDRESSES TO THE LSTM

During the period under review, a number of addresses were delivered at the LSTM – most by eminent figures in medicine; amongst those delivered, some have survived.[22] An inaugural address was in fact given at the start of each session.

Outside recognition

In October 1899 a minute records that the Royal Geographic Society 'had placed their Library and map collection at the disposal of Students attending the School'. The library of the Royal Colonial Institute was also put at the 'disposal' of the School.

A minute in March 1900 records that the LSTM had been 'admitted as a School of the reconstituted University of London ...'. However, this did *not* apparently mean that the School was *recognised* by the University; Sir Michael Foster FRS (1836–1907) had 'advised [in June 1903] that a formal application should be made to the Senate ...'. At a later meeting that year it was announced 'that the Senate of the University of Cambridge had decided to grant a diploma in Tropical Medicine'. Ultimately, the University of London resolved '... that Tropical Medicine should be added to the list of branches in which the M.D. degree may be taken' and in March 1905, the LSTM was admitted as a School of the University [of London] in the Faculty of Medicine. The Royal Colleges of Physicians and Surgeons, however, had no intention of establishing diplomas in Tropical Medicine. The question of dissociation of the LSTM from the London Post Graduate Association and the Polyclinic (Chapter 19) was raised in 1919.[23]

Future of tropical medicine in London

The discipline of *tropical medicine* had thus been successfully launched. Manson-Bahr (1956) has termed the SHS, the 'Foster Mother' of tropical medicine in London. For the future of this specialty in London, the reader is referred to Cook (1992 and 2007) and Chapter 25.[24]

References and Notes

1 P H Manson-Bahr, A Alcock. *The life and work of Sir Patrick Manson* London: Cassell & Co Ltd 1927: 273; Anonymous. The father of tropical medicine. *SHS Quart Mag* 1929; 1: 35-38; R Ross. *Memories of Sir Patrick Manson*. London: Harrison and Sons Ltd 1930: 26; P Manson-Bahr. Founders of the School. In: *History of the School of Tropical Medicine in London (1899–1949)*. London: H K Lewis & Co Ltd. 1956: 113–25; P Manson-Bahr. *Patrick Manson: the father of tropical medicine*. London: Thomas Nelson and Sons Ltd 1962: 192; G C Cook. *From the Greenwich Hulks to Old St Pancras: a history of tropical medicine in London*. London: Athlone Press 1992: 68–79. [See also Chapter 15].

2 **Joseph Chamberlain** MP FRS (1836–1914) was the British Secretary of State for the Colonies from 1895 until 1903. [See also: P T Marsh. Chamberlain, Joseph (Joe) (1836–

1914). In: H C G Matthew, B Harrison (eds). *Oxford Dictionary of National Biography.* Oxford: Oxford University Press 2004; 10: 923–34]; 78 Annual Report: 18, 22–26; SHS Committee of Management Minutes 13: 34–37; Anonymous. Modern treatment of tropical disease: the great work of Endsleigh Gardens. *SHS Quart Mag* 1935; 7(1): 13–24; Famous film actress seeks help from Endsleigh Gardens. *SHS Quart Mag* 1935; 7(2): 14–16; G C Cook, A J Webb. The Albert Dock Hospital, London: the original site (in 1899) of Tropical Medicine as a new discipline. *Acta Tropica* 2001; 79: 249–255.

3 *Op cit.* See note 2 above (Minutes) 13: 38–44, 50–9.

4 *Op cit.* See note 2 above (Reports) 79: 21–4; *Op cit.* See note 2 above (Minutes) 13: 143–4; G C Cook. 'Tropical' cases admitted to the Albert Dock Hospital in the early years of the London School of Tropical Medicine. *Trans R Soc trop Med Hyg* 1999; 93: 675–7.

5 *Ibid* (Minutes) 13: 77–86.

6 H C Burdett. A school for tropical diseases in London. *Times, Lond* 1898: 11 July: 12; Leading article *Times, Lond* 1898; 11 July; 11; *Op cit.* See note 1 above (Manson-Bahr [1956], Cook).

7 P Hoare. *Spike Island: the memory of a Military Hospital.* London: Fourth Estate 2001: 417.

8 A L Revell. *Haslar: The Royal Hospital.* 2nd ed. Gosport: The Gosport Society 1984: 50.

9 G C Cook. Doctor Patrick Manson's leading opposition in the establishment of the London School of Tropical Medicine: Curnow, Anderson, and Turner. *J Med Biog* 1995; 3: 170–7 [*See also Op cit.* See note 2 above (Minutes) 13: 88–90, 92–6, 110–11, 114–5, 120–21].

10 *Op cit.* See note 2 above (Minutes) 13: 97–103. [*See also*: *Op cit.* See note 1 above (Cook)].

11 *Ibid* (Minutes) 13: 121–2, 123–8, 140.

12 G R Turner. *Unorthodox reminiscences.* London John Murray 1931: 90; *Op cit.* See note 10 above: 123–6; *Op cit.* See note 2 above (Minutes) 13: 147–8; *Op cit.* See note 1 above (Cook).

13 *Minutes of the London School of Tropical Medicine* (nine vols. July 1899 to July 1924); these minutes contain a great deal of information about the day-to-day workings of the LSTM; however, all *major* events were recorded in the SHS Committee of Management minutes – see note 2 above [Minutes]).

14 P Manson. *The London School of Tropical Medicine (under the auspices of Her Majesty's Government) in connection with the Royal Victoria and Albert Docks Branch of the Society. Some observations in reference to this new school, together with the Introductory Address for the session commencing 2nd October 1899.* London: E G Berryman & Sons 1899: 22; *Op cit.* See note 2 above (Minutes) 13: 180–81, 191, 197, 200; See note 2 above; (Reports).

15 *Op cit.* See note 2 above (Reports) 80: 22; 81: 22–24; 82: 24–6; 83: 22; 84: 22–3. *Op cit.* See note 2 above (Minutes) 13: 257, 265–6, 379–80, 495–6. *Op cit.*

16 **Lewis Harcourt** MP (1863–1922) was a prominent British politician who was Secretary of State for the Colonies from 1910 until 1915. *Op cit.* See note 2 above (Reports):86 (1906); 15–16; 91 (1911): 17. [See also: P Jackson. Harcourt, Lewis Vernon, first Viscount Harcourt (1863–1922). In: H C G Matthew, B Harrison (eds). *Oxford Dictionary of National Biography.* Oxford: Oxford University Press 2004; 25: 125–8].

17 *Op cit.* See note 2 above (Minutes) 14: 438–9, 456–7; 480, 484.

18 *Ibid.* 15: 96–7, 113–4, 117–8.

19 *Ibid.* 15: 214.

20 *Ibid.* 15: 121–2, 124.

21 **Sir Austen Chamberlain** MP (1863–1937) was a prominent English politician, who became British Foreign Secretary. *Op cit.* See note 2 above (Reports): 92; [*See also*: *Op cit.* See note 2 above (Minutes) 15: 189–90, 192–3, 205–6, 251; Anonymous. Sir Austen Chamberlain *SHS Quart Mag* 1937; 9 (2): 15; D J Dutton. Chamberlain, Sir (Joseph) Austen (1863–1937) In: H C G Matthew, B Harrison (eds). *Oxford Dictionary of National Biography.* Oxford: Oxford University Press 2004; 10: 906–14].

22 W MacGregor. *An address on some problems of Tropical Medicine, delivered at the London School of Tropical Medicine, on October 3rd 1900.* Blackheath: E G Berryman & Sons 1901: 25; [SHS]. *The London School of Tropical Medicine: report of proceedings at the Royal United Service Institution on Wednesday 16th October 1901*; Opening of the third winter session, and departure of the Hon Sir Francis Lovell, CMG to the tropics on behalf of the School. Blackheath: E G Berryman & Sons 1901: 16; C Bruce. Colonial Sanitary Administration and Tropical Diseases. *Introductory Address delivered by St Charles Bruce GCMG at the Opening of the 16th Session on Friday, 7th October, 1904. BMJ* 1904: ii: 1105–8; G H F Nuttall. Scientific Research in Medicine. *Introductory Address at the Opening of the 19th Session on Wednesday the 11th of October 1905.* London: E G Berryman & Sons 1905: 20; J Catto. *Schistosoma cattoi*: a new blood fluke of man (Craggs Prize Essay 1904). *BMJ* 1905: i: 11–13; K MacLeod. *Introductory Address delivered at the Opening of the 22nd Session on Monday October 8th 1906.* London: John Bale, Sons & Danielsson Ltd. 1906: 21; P W Bassett-Smith. An investigation into the value of the serum diagnosis of Mediterranean or Undulant Fever, and the Treatment of the Disease by means of Vaccines (Craggs Prize Essay 1906) *J Trop Med Hyg* 1907; L Brunton. *Fleas as a national danger. Introductory Address delivered at the Opening of the 25th Session on Monday Oct. 21st, 1907; R L Antrobus, Esq., C.B. (Assistant Under Secretary of State for the Colonies, in the Chair.* London: E G Berryman & Sons 1907: 12; *Report of Proceedings at the unveiling of a portrait of the Hon. Bomaji Dinshaw Petit (a munificent benefactor of the School) on Friday July 19th 1907.* London: E G Berryman 1907: 16; R Howard. *Malaria prophylaxis in small communities in British central Africa.* London: John Bale, Sons and Danielsson Ltd 1908: 47.

23 *Op cit.* See note 2 above (Minutes) 13: 205, 215, 243–4; 14: 5, 54, 63, 145, 149–51, 233, 446; G C Cook. *John MacAllister's other vision: a history of the Fellowship of Postgraduate Medicine.* Oxford: Radcliffe Publishing 2005: 186.

24 *Op cit.* See note 1 above (Cook). [*See also*: G C Cook. Tropical Medicine: an illustrated history of the Pioneers. London: Academic Press 2007 (in press)].

Chapter 19

The London School of Clinical Medicine (1906–14), and structural changes to the *Dreadnought* Hospital

Undergraduate medical training in London has a very long history, but organised postgraduate education did not commence until the latter years of the nineteenth century. At the time of the foundation of the *London School of Clinical Medicine* (LSCM) in 1906, although there were four schemes in operation, there was very little *clinical* input into any of them. At the West London Hospital, the surgeons Charles Keetley (1848–1909) and L A Bidwell (1865–1912) had started a Post-graduate College in 1894. Meanwhile, Sir Jonathan Hutchinson FRS (1828–1913) had initiated the Medical Graduate College and Polytechnic. The London Postgraduate Association had already been started by Sir Raymond Crawfurd (1865–1938), and the North East London Postgraduate College had been founded at the Prince of Wales Hospital, Tottenham. Therefore, London (and in fact England) badly needed a *clinical* school (a 'Mecca') for postgraduate study.[1]

By 1900, the Society had successfully launched a Nurse-training School (in 1877) and also the LSTM at the ADH (in 1899). By 1905, the time was considered ripe for pursuit into *Postgraduate Training* in *General Medicine*. Therefore, the Management Committee of the SHS decided to go ahead with the formation of the LSCM – which was to be based at the *Dreadnought* Hospital, Greenwich. Creation of this school necessitated a number of important architectural alterations to the *Dreadnought* Hospital (see below). Sadly, this pioneering venture was never well financed and was forced to close at the outbreak of the Great War (1914–18); it was never resuscitated – largely for financial reasons. It thus survived for a mere eight to nine years.

A *new* clinical school

In early 1906, the *British Medical Journal* summarised details of the newly formed *School of Clinical Medicine* which, the writer claimed, marked 'the dawn of a new era in the history of the [SHS]':

> [It] was founded in response to the ever-increasing demand for post-graduate teaching in London. Although the function of supplying such teaching is well discharged by the London Post-graduate Association,

> the Polyclinic, the West London Post-graduate College, and the North-East London Post-graduate College connected with the Tottenham Hospital – see above [the anonymous writer recorded], it was felt to be a pity that the large opportunities for *clinical* [my italics] study offered by a hospital containing such an abundance and variety of cases of exceptional interest should be lost to medical education. Another consideration which had weight [with the Society] was the fact, proved by universal experience, that the usefulness of a hospital in regard to the successful treatment of patients is vastly increased when the work is done under the eyes of critical observers.
>
> The presence of ordinary students is found to be a check against inefficiency and negligence, and quickens the energies of the medical and surgical staff to the highest pitch. Obviously the presence of qualified medical practitioners must be a still more powerful incentive. Moreover, the accommodation was often inadequate to the demands made upon the hospital by the class of sufferers [mostly seafarers] whom the Society exists to relieve, and it was recognized that the establishment of a *clinical* [my italics] school would necessitate an increase in the number of beds and a development of the out-patient department, and afford an opportunity for a general reorganization of the institution.
>
> It may be mentioned [the writer concluded] that before [the SHS] came to a definitive decision the opinion of the medical profession as represented by many of its leading members was asked for, and found to be favourable to the scheme. Several of the foremost men in the various provinces of practice gave a practical proof of their approval by consenting to take an active part in carrying it into effect.

This article (which had been preceded by three shorter ones[2]), then listed the existing staff (see below and Chapter 15) of the new school, which was intended 'not to supersede but to complement the [LSTM] carried on in connexion with the [ADH]'. The staff consisted of both permanent and 'extramural' members:

> *Physicians:* Sir Dyce Duckworth MD LLD FRCP; Fredk Taylor MD FRCP; J Rose Bradford MD FRCP FRS; R Tanner Hewlett MD MRCP; Guthrie Rankin MD MRCP. *Surgeons:* Sir William H Bennett KCVO FRCS; A W Mayo Robson DSc FRCS; Albert Carless MB MS FRCS, William Turner MB MS FRCS; Lawrie H McGavin FRCS. *Ophthalmic Surgeon:* L Vernon Cargill FRCS. *Surgeon for Diseases of the Skin:* Malcolm Morris FRCS Edin. *Physician for Diseases of the Throat, Nose, and Ear*: St Clair Thomson MD FRCP FRCS. *Physician in Charge of the Electrical Department:* James Mackenzie Davidson MB CM. *Dental Surgeon:* Kenneth W Goadby MRCS LDS. *Assistant Physicians:* S Russell Wells MD MRCP; A Ernest Jones MD MRCP. *Assistant Surgeons:* Harold Burrows MB BS FRCS; E Rock Carling MB BS FRCS. *Assistant Ophthalmic Surgeon:* Stephen Mayou FRCS. *Assistant Surgeon for Diseases of the Skin:* Wilfrid S Fox MA MD FRCP. *Assistant Surgeon for Diseases of the Throat, Nose, and Ear*: S A Lawrence FRCS.

> EXTRAMURAL LECTURERS.
>
> … Diseases of the Nervous System: James Taylor MD FRCP. Mental Diseases: W H B Stoddart MD MRCP. Hygiene and Public Health: W J R Simpson MD FRCP DPH. Applied Anatomy: James Cantlie MB FRCS. Gynaecology: William J Gow MD FRCP; Herbert Williamson MA MB MRCP. Surgical Diseases of Women: John Russell Howard MB MS FRCS. Medical Diseases of Women: Alexander Haig MA MD FRCP; Robert O Moon MD MRCP. Medical Diseases of Children: Charles O Hawthorne MD MRCP; Thomas D Lister MD FRCS MRCP. Surgical Diseases of Children: Herbert S Pendlebury MA MB FRCS. Midwifery: Wm. Radford Dakin MD FRCP; Robert Boxall MD MRCP. Operative Surgery (additional): W Johnson Smith FRCS. A lecturer on anaesthetics has still to be appointed.

Several special hospitals (in addition to the *Dreadnought)* became 'affiliated' for teaching purposes; these were:

> The General Lying-in Hospital, York Road, for midwifery; the Royal Waterloo Hospital for Diseases of Children and Women, and the Bethlem Royal Hospital for mental diseases. The large opportunities for observation and practical study offered by these institutions make [the writer continued] the teaching equipment of the [LSCM] unusually complete. Although the [LSTM] is a distinct institution, students at the [LSCM] can avail themselves at a reduced fee of the educational advantages which it offers.

Details of the course(s) of instruction also received attention:

> There will be three sessions in the year, each of ten weeks' duration. Practical courses will be given in the following subjects: the practice of medicine; the practice of surgery; diseases of the eye; diseases of the throat, nose, and ear; diseases of the skin; diseases of the nervous system; operative surgery; clinical pathology; microscopy and bacteriology; mental diseases; radiography; dental surgery; the administration of anaesthetics; hygiene and public health; gynaecology; surgical diseases of women; surgical diseases of children; medical diseases of women; medical diseases of children; applied anatomy; and midwifery. Arrangements will also be made for a short vacation course of instruction in September, if a sufficient number of students present themselves.
>
> Besides the clinical demonstrations given in the wards and out-patient rooms, and the practical classes just enumerated, tutorial classes are conducted in medicine by the Medical Registrar, in surgery by the Surgical Registrar, and in pathology by the Pathologist. Owing to the relatively large number of unclaimed bodies, there are exceptional facilities for acquiring skill in operative surgery.

The article then gave details of the laboratories and museum attached to the *Dreadnought* Hospital:

> There are two pathological laboratories, each of which is fully equipped with the instruments and apparatus requisite for pathological work. It may be mentioned that the laboratory staff undertakes clinical investigations and supplies reports on urine, sputum, blood, faeces, and morbid specimens sent by practitioners for examination. The Museum, though small, contains specimens illustrating a considerable variety of diseases. An especially interesting feature is a collection of specimens of malposition of the fragments in fracture, showing the results of the rough-and-ready surgery which sailors have to endure at sea in ships which do not carry a surgeon. [This descriptive piece ended:] ... The contents of the Museum also include a collection of skulls, interesting from an ethnological point of view, made by Mr Busk[3] [*see* Chapters 8 and 12], who was at one time surgeon to the *Dreadnought*.

Certificates of attendance (given at the end of each session) were: 'accepted for study leave by the Admiralty and, for special subjects, by the War Office. The Dreadnought Hospital is also recognized [the writer continued] by the University of London as an institution from which certificates of post-graduation study for the higher degrees are accepted.' The prospectus, the article concluded, was readily obtained from Mr P Michelli, the SHS Secretary.[4]

Several years later (probably in 1914 – the final year of the enterprise), the syllabus for the School had been perfected; the two sessions (winter and summer) ran from 1 October to 28 February and from 1 April to 31 July. It contained details (with tuition fees) for the various courses together with lists of the lecturers and venues (see above and below); the Miller General Hospital was 'at a distance of ten minutes walk, or halfpenny tram ride from the Dreadnought'. Also included were the Post-graduate Members of the School (presumably those medical practitioners who had availed themselves of the various courses – numbering between 700 and 800 post-graduates) since March 1906. The aspiring post-graduate student was advised that 'A list of good and comfortable lodgings is kept in the Dean's Office, for the convenience of those who desire to live in Greenwich, Blackheath, or Lewisham', and that the 'Annual Dinner of the Past and Present Members of the School is held at the beginning of the Winter Session'. 'The Hospital and School [the Syllabus assured potential applicants] are provided with a complete telephone installation (Greenwich 968)'.[5]

Moves to create the LSCM

The project (which subsequently involved sweeping changes – both architecturally and staff-wise – had been inaugurated at a meeting at Rankin's House on 12 December 1904; others present at that meeting were: Cargill, Hewlett and Turner (see above and Chapter 15). The following 'suggestions' were made: The establishment of a post graduate school at Greenwich. (i) An increase in the Medical Staff, and (ii) The establishment of a Nurses' Home, and the removal of the Nurses from the *Dreadnought* Hospital itself. The latter alteration would enable the tuberculosis wards to be increased in size, as well as extension of the Lock wards (for men with sexually transmitted diseases). Other suggestions were: Establishment of a Club for Post-graduates, an emergency ward for women and children (on the medical side) and appointments of a Pathologist, an extra House Surgeon, and a Superintendent – who should have medical administrative jurisdiction over the Junior Medical Officers and the School. The meeting also considered that: one or two Out-Patient Physicians and Surgeons should be appointed, and provision made for special departments 'so far as such are necessary for a full post-graduate curriculum.[6]

In January the following year, a Sub-Committee appointed by the Medical Council of the SHS met at 13A Cockspur Street, SW. In addition to those present at the previous meeting, Sir Patrick Manson[7] (who was to become Chairman) attended. The meeting came 'unanimously to the conclusion that the present is an opportune time to found a *post-graduate* [my italics] School in connection with [the SHS]'. At that meeting, various projects were finalised, including the following: (i) an increase in the number of Physicians and Surgeons (at Greenwich) to three or four; (ii) extension of the 'Dreadnought Hospital' by sleeping the Nurses outside the Hospital – thus increasing the number of beds; and (iii) affiliation of the [SHS] with the Royal Waterloo Hospital for children & Women; the Royal Eye Hospital; the Blackfriars Skin Hospital and the Bethlem Hospital.

The Sub-Committee considered that if the scheme (i.e. the *Post-graduate School*) were a sufficiently prominent one, it would be likely to attract 'some of the leading members of the medical profession and it was resolved that as a first step some of these should be approached and sounded [out] as to whether, if invited, they would be willing to join the Medical Staff [of the SHS] and take part in the founding and teaching of the School'. The following names were suggested: *On the Medical side*: Dr Mitchell Bruce, Dr Fredk. Taylor, Dr David Ferrier and Dr G A Heron; and *On the Surgical side*: Mr A W Mayo Robson, Mr Edmund Owen, Mr A Marmaduke Sheild and Sir Wm. H Bennett KCVO.[8] *For the Rõntgen Ray department:* Dr Jas. Mackenzie Davidson.[9]

The following additional names were later suggested: *On the Medical Side:* Sir Dyce Duckworth MD,[10] Sir Lauder Brunton MD[11] (Figure 19.1) and David Ferrier; *On the Surgical Side:* Mr G H Makins CB, Mr H T Butlin FRCS and Mr A Carless MS FRCS. The sub-committee also 'suggested that the Junior Resident Medical Staff be increased by one ... with a Senior Resident Medical Officer appointed for a year – who should have jurisdiction over the Junior Resident Medical Officers and take part in the teaching of the new School'. It was considered 'that the most suitable title for the new School would be – *The London School of Clinical Medicine.*[12]

A fortnight later, the Sub-Committee met again, at Manson's House, 21 Queen Anne Street, London W, when it was announced that Bruce, Carless, R Godlee, Pendlebury, and Davidson were willing to co-operate; Bennett (see above), Dr Radcliffe Crocker and Mr Colcott Fox were also 'lined up', as were W H Allchin, J Kingston Fowler, J F Payne, Sir Wm. H Broadbent[13] (*see* Figure 19.2), C P Field and St Clair Thomson.[14]

The early March meeting was an important one, for in addition to the members of the Sub-Committee, the following were 'also present by invitation': Duckworth, Bruce, Taylor, Allchin, Robson, Godlee, Pendlebury and Crocker, as were: Sheild, Field and Mackenzie Davidson (see above). This meeting was addressed by Manson (who was by this time, although in his early 60s, extremely enthusiastic about this new venture); he pointed out the advantages that were likely to accrue by the proposed augmentation of the staff and the establishment of a *new* [post-graduate] School.

With the exception of Bruce and Godlee, all those invited 'spoke in favour of the proposition and intimated their willingness to assist it'. The meeting resolved 'That there is opening and need in London for a Post-Graduate School founded on a broad and influential basis, in connection with a Hospital'. It was also decided 'That the facilities possessed by the Dreadnought Hospital so far as clinical material, and educational opportunities are concerned, are such as might form the nucleus for ensuring the success of such a scheme as that proposed'.

Three other resolutions were also carried at that meeting: (i) 'That the members of the medical profession who have been invited to meet the Sub-Committee [of the SHS] to consider a scheme proposed by them for such a School, express their willingness to assist the Sub-Committee's endeavour', (ii) 'That it is desirable that a report thereof should be presented without delay to the Medical Council [of the SHS] and suggesting that a full report thereof should be made to the Committee of Management [of the SHS] with a request that the body may appoint a Sub-Committee

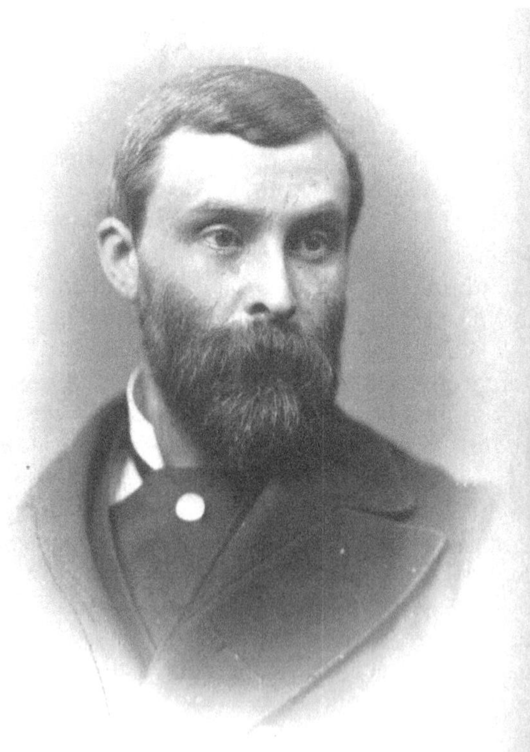

Figure 19.1: Sir (Thomas) Lauder Brunton Bt FRCP FRS (1844–1916). [Courtesy: The Wellcome Library, London].

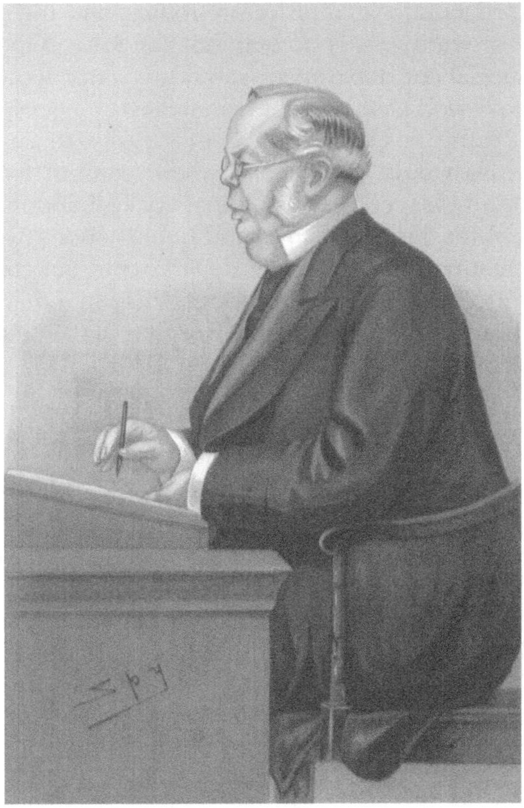

Figure 19.2: Sir William Henry Broadbent KCVO FRCP FRS (1835–1907) depicted in a 'Spy' cartoon. [Courtesy: The Wellcome Library, London].

to co-operate with the Sub-Committee of the Council, for the consideration of this scheme' and (iii) 'That a future conference of these gentlemen whose names it is proposed to place upon the full staff with members of the Sub-Committee should be summoned for the purpose of criticism and discussion of the scheme in extensio, before it is finally presented to the Medical Council [of the SHS].[15]

Later that month 'the Sub-Committee agreed to a detailed Report outlining proposals for setting up the LSCM which was to be 'circulated amongst members of the Medical Council [and would be] considered at a Special meeting of the Council' to be convened in April. Provided the Medical Council agreed with the Sub-Committee, it should be sent to the Board of Governors. The report considered that a *clinical* school (which should be founded along similar lines to the *tropical* school) would be established in the wake of Johnson Smith's[16] imminent retirement. The top floor of the Hospital (then occupied by nurses' accommodation) should be utilised to house additional patients (thus creating a total of 285 beds); the nurses meanwhile should be accommodated in 'an outside Home in Greenwich'. Smith's present house [at the southern extreme of the *Dreadnought* Hospital] would furthermore be utilised for laboratories and lecture-rooms, and the post-mortem rooms increased so as to 'provide greater accommodation for … Operative Surgery and Pathology'. The out-patient department should be extended, and the East India Dock Road and Gravesend Dispensaries reorganised.

Negotiations with other hospitals (see above) were also discussed. The Admiralty and Army authorities would be approached for consent to send their officers to the School for study-leave; and the University of London would (hopefully) recognise the School for 'higher degrees and qualifications'. Other recommendations referred to creation of several new departments, set courses, appointment of a School-Committee, establishment of lectureships in gynaecology, and mental and public health, and expansion of the Hospital staff, details of which were provided.[17]

INVOLVEMENT OF THE SHS'S COMMITTEE OF MANAGEMENT

The Medical Council at this stage reported to the Society's Management Committee. The fact that the 'efficiency and energy [of an institution] are most satisfactorily fulfilled when the cases are investigated and treated under the critical observation of students who are qualified medical men' was again stressed.

In May, the Committee of Management considered a synopsis of the report by the Medical Council; it was resolved that a Sub-Committee (consisting of the Chairman [Mr P A Nairne], Deputy Chairman [Admiral Sir R Tracey KCB], Sir Stephen Mackenzie MD FRCP, Mr C T Orford and Sir Frederick Young KCMG) be appointed to confer with a Sub-Committee of the Medical Council (see above).[18] Representatives of the two Sub-Committees duly met at 13A Cockspur Street, SW the following month. It was resolved that '… this joint Sub-Committee consider that the establishment of a Post-Graduate School at the Dreadnought Hospital is likely to promote the general efficiency of the Hospital for the service of seamen in the Port of London, provided that it can be shewn [sic] that such a School is likely to be *self supporting* [my italics] and not a burden on the endowments or income of the [SHS].[19]

A Sub-Committee of the Medical Council appointed by this Joint Sub-Committee met in July and drafted a report – which was intended to be a discussion document for a meeting of the Joint Sub-Committees three days later. This meeting endorsed earlier decisions, and insisted on the architectural alterations previously mentioned (see below). It was resolved that the report be 'laid before the meeting of the Board of Management on August the 11th'; in actual fact it was deferred until the October meeting. It also recommended the following appointments: McGavin as surgeon to in-patients (replacing Smith – who was retiring) and Evans as surgeon to in-patients – with duties at the [ADH].[20] These appointments were ratified by Council later that month. Meanwhile, members of the Sub-Committee visited the *Dreadnought* Hospital 'with a view to submitting an estimate, and the Architect having been consulted …'. At another Sub-Committee meeting of Council, chaired by Manson, in July, structural changes required to accommodate 'almost 40 students' were considered; the cost of these (including the Architect's estimates) were:

Conversion of the Principal Medical Officers (Johnson Smith's) House	£313.00
Addition to Nurses' quarters	£60.00
Addition to Post Mortem Room (to provide additional teaching space)	£145.00
New Out-Patients Department (between Somerset and Ground West wards)	£1500.00
	£2018.00

When the cost of erecting '[open air] accommodation for phthisical patients on the East roof[21] and equipment added', the total would probably be covered by an initial outlay of £3000' which, it was suggested the Board 'might be willing to advance ... as they did for the establishment of the [LSTM]'. These changes were also expected to provide an additional 33 beds (12 on Somerset, 15 Middle East, and six Ground East wards) producing a grand total of 258. 'In the event of the School prospering [the meeting concluded] it would be possible at a future date to consider the subject of the Nurses living out ...'.

At the October meeting, a provisional School Committee (Hewlett, McGavin, Rankin and Turner – 'with power to add to their number') was appointed. Their report was duly considered by the Management Committee three days later, and it was concluded that:

> It might be reasonably anticipated that very shortly the School would become a source of important revenue to the [SHS], it would prove a helpful adjunct to the [LSTM], the patients would benefit by the greater efficiency and care with which their treatment would be conducted; and the usefulness of the Charity would be enhanced by the contribution which the Hospital would afford to the progress of scientific medicine and the conquest of disease.

The Management Committee agreed with the various recommendations in the report, with the exception of the proposed changes to the Out-Patients' Department. It was also agreed that Dr T L Rogers be appointed to the Joint Sub-Committee (as a representative of the Committee of Management in place of Mackenzie – whose health was declining).[22] Rogers immediately produced a detailed 'critique' of the Joint Committee's report. His (undated) report recommended that the matter of structural changes be referred back to the Sub-Committee for further consideration; one detail would *not* however be acceptable today: 'If the smoker's room is removed [where are] the men to smoke in wet weather – I suggest that one of the numerous rooms in the basement ... might be fitted up for their use.[23]

The 'London School of Clinical Medicine' becomes a reality

The composition of the *new* Joint Sub-Committee (hereafter entitled the 'Committee of the [LSCM]') was finalised: P A Nairne (Chairman), Adml Sir Richard Tracey KCB, Orford, Rogers (see above) and Sir Frederick Young KCMG. Representatives from the Medical Council were to be: Hewlett, McGavin,

Rankin and Turner (Vice-Chairman). At a subsequent meeting, Commander G Hodgkinson RN was invited to join as an 'additional representative of the Board of Management'. It is clear therefore that the Sub-Committee (of the LSCM) by no means dominated the scenario.

STAFFING AND OTHER MATTERS

At the first meeting of the LSCM Committee, the following were 'invited to join the Extraordinary Teaching Staff' of the School: Duckworth, Allchin, Taylor, Robson, Carless, Sheild, Thomson, Crocker, and Davidson (of these, Allchin, Sheild and Crocker subsequently declined). Captain A E Hayward Pinch (Medical Graduate College and Polyclinic) was to be approached regarding the post of 'Medical Superintendent at the Hospital and new School; pending his reply, Smith would be asked to 'undertake the duties of Superintendent until Christmas [1905] or until such time as the permanent Superintendent [had] been appointed'. Hayward Pinch subsequently declined – because the salary was less than his present one.[24]

At the following meeting, it was resolved to invite 'Mr Malcolm Morris ... as Dermatologist [in place of Crocker] and either Sir Douglas Powell [he subsequently declined], or Dr Head as a Physician in place of Allchin'. The subject of a surgeon 'in place of Sheild was deferred'. Sir Thos. Barlow later declined on account of the 'state of his health'. At the following meeting it was reported that Bennett (see above) 'had consented to join as a member of the Extraordinary Staff', and that Prof W J Simpson ('Hygiene'), Dr Stoddard ('Mental Diseases') and Mr Cantlie ('Applied Surgery') would accept the posts of Extra-mural Lecturers.

The Architect (Keith D Young FRIBA) was present at that meeting and submitted plans for: (i) alterations to the Principal Medical Officer's house, (ii) modified nurses' quarters, and (iii) reconstruction of the post-mortem room. Also, the Sub-Committee (consisting of the two physicians and two surgeons at Greenwich) previously appointed, reported on their recommendations:

- i) a syllabus, fees and payments to teachers;
- ii) the Billiard room (Ground West floor), rooms occupied by the 'Working Gang' (Upper West) and Porters' Rooms (Ground West), which they suggested be removed to the basement;
- iii) 'Venereal Cases', which should be distributed throughout the wards ('ordinary gonorrhoea' was considered surgical, and 'gonorrhoeal rheumatism' medical); furthermore, on each floor 'on both sides [medical and surgical] there should be a small Lock Ward – for men suffering from syphilis – on the medical side (for the infectious stage) and on the surgical (for "foul sores")';
- iv) the whole of Upper West floor should be reserved for tuberculosis;
- v) the Gravesend Dispensary should be closed, and the money saved could be used to increase the salary of a Medical Officer at the East India Dock Dispensary (EIDD), and also provide a salary for a Pathologist;
- vi) Mr Steele be offered the post of Surgeon to the EIDD (at £100=00 per annum) whilst the agreement with Oxley (Dispensary Surgeon) be terminated;

vii) the posts of two Honorary Anaesthetists be advertised, and
viii) a Clinical Pathologist and curator be appointed (at £100=00 per annum).

(v), (vi) and (viii) were immediately rejected by the Management Committee; the last of these was however, ratified in principle at a subsequent meeting on 14 December[25] but they considered that they could grant only £50=00, and the School Committee should contribute 'a like amount'. This minute presumably reflects a growing anxiety that the 'new scheme' would absorb too much of the Charity's funds.

Other recommendations were:

ix) appointment of a Specialist in Nerve Diseases (who should be a member of the Extra-Mural Staff) – Dr James Taylor and/or Dr Purves Stewart would be approached;
x) Dr Stoddart (Bethlem Royal Hospital) and Cantlie should be invited to be the Extra-Mural lecturers;
xi) Medical and Surgical Registrars should be appointed – to attend Out-patients on 'two days in the week'; and
xii) apportionment of beds should be: 10 to each member of the Extraordinary Staff (later designated Honorary Medical Staff), 10 to the Ophthalmic Surgeon, five to the Dermatologist, five to the ENT Specialist, and the remainder to be divided amongst the Ordinary Staff – who were to have the entire control of the tuberculosis wards.[26]

The following meeting held in late November approved, with only minor alterations, the architect's plans for reconstruction of the Mortuary and rooms for Operative Surgery, as well as plans for the 'formation of a new Out-Patients Department adjoining Somerset Ward'. Approval for these alterations was later received from Mr Perfect (Civil Engineer at the Royal Naval College) declaring that he saw 'no reason why permission should not be granted by the Admiralty for the Out-Patient Department to be erected outside the building on the north side and in such a position that it would harmonise with the Policy Barracks across the way'. The meeting also approved of Professor Rose Bradford (or failing him, Dr Sharkey) being invited to serve as an Extra Physician. At the following meeting, Bradford (who had accepted) and Morris (see above) were invited to join the Committee of the LSCM – as 'representatives of the elected Medical Staff'. It was also resolved that the Society apply for 'recognition of the School to London University, the Royal College of Physicians and the Royal College of Surgeons ...' (see below). Meanwhile, a letter received from the Admiralty indicated that the School would be recognised for post-graduate courses of instruction for Naval Medical Officers.

A meeting of the LSCM Committee in December resolved both to accept the recommendations of the Medical Committee, and to recommend that the list of the following Officers be placed before the Board of Management:

i) Medical Superintendent of the Hospital and School: C C Choyce MD FRCS;
ii) Assistant Surgeons: H Burrows FRCS; E Rock Carling FRCS;
iii) Assistant Ophthalmic Surgeon: S Mayou FRCS;
iv) Assistant Surgeon of Diseases of the Skin: W S Fox MD MRCP.

The November meeting also emphasised the need for *isolation* wards at the *Dreadnought*: '...if the Admiralty agree to the Outpatient Department being built *outside* [my italics] the Hospital ... it might be possible to place [isolation wards] on top of the Department'. These structural alterations were approved two days later by the Management Committee.

At a subsequent meeting, a letter from Tracey was read intimating that he had had an interview with Mr Stansfield (Director of Greenwich Hospital) who 'expressed his willingness to meet the views of the [SHS] as regards the new Out-Patient Department, &c as far as lay in his power'. At that meeting, Turner explained the arrangements which had been made for 'Operative Surgery': 'the Licence hitherto granted to Smith be transferred to Choyce ... and that the classes be taught by Turner and McGavin ... Smith should take part in the teaching of Operative Surgery [but from then on] as an Extra-Mural Lecturer'. It was also 'resolved to recommend to the Board [of Management] that the wives and children of Seamen, Watermen, and others be admitted for treatment in the Out-Patient Department under the new scheme'; this was ratified by the Board at the December meeting.

Regarding the Gravesend Dispensary, the Committee resolved to arrange a meeting between Captain Clarke, a member of the Honorary Medical Staff, the Secretary, and the Surgeon at the Dispensary 'with a view to improving the service [there]'. Meanwhile, Steele declined to 'accept the post of Dispensary Surgeon at £80 per annum. It was reported that Dr S Russell Wells and Dr A Ernest Jones had been elected Assistant Physicians and Mr L A Lawrence Surgeon to the ENT Department. Also, the BMA was permitted to hold a meeting (followed by tea in the School) at the *Dreadnought* Hospital in February, and that Dr [C W] Daniels be invited to bring his class over [from the LSTM]'.

It was also recorded that 'two students were [already] attending the School'. General practitioners 'in the immediate vicinity of the School' who had been in practice there for 'not less than two years' were authorised to be admitted to the 'clinical practice of the Hospital at Three Guineas [per] Session'.[27]

Regarding the Museum (*see* Figure 19.3), it was recommended that 'the curator of the Museum at Guy's Hospital ... provide specimens at an all-round cost of 5/= each, subject to the approval of the Pathologist'. It was also resolved 'that application be made to the Royal College of Surgeons for a grant of specimens, of which they have duplicates, for ... use of the school Museum'.

FINANCE MATTERS

Expenditure remained at the forefront of deliberations; the sum chargeable to the Charity for establishment of the [LSCM] (including enlargement to 250 beds, and employment of an additional House Surgeon, Nurses, Maids, Scrubbers, etc. amounted to £599=6=0; with the addition of 'cost of food, washing, etc for the extra patients'; this amount would 'bring the additional annual expenditure to over £1000'.[28]

ADVERTISEMENT OF THE SCHOOL

Discussion on the best means of advertising the new School took place at a meeting on 30 January; however, a decision was postponed until the following meeting! The

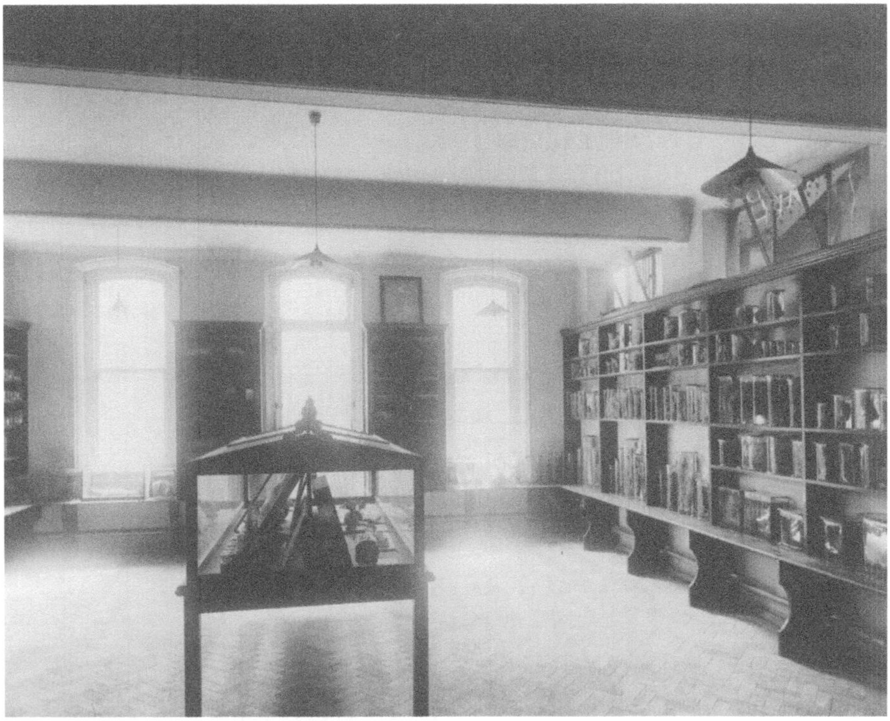

Figure 19.3: The interior of the *Dreadnought* Hospital Museum. [SHS Archive].

Committee also agreed to order 1000 copies of a new Syllabus – to be distributed amongst 'Universities at home, ... America and the Colonies, and among General Practitioners in and near London'. One thousand copies would cost £6=16=9 (from Berryman & Sons); but 2,000 were in fact acquired at £10=2=6.[29]

Structural alterations

Figure 19.4 shows the ground-floor plan of the *Dreadnought* Hospital in 1906 (i.e. when the LSCM was launched). It was felt by the joint Sub-Committee that new buildings 'should be constructed for In-Patients and *not* Out-Patients', and that the 'present Somerset Ward [should be] converted into an Out-Patient Department'. It was therefore decided to recommend to the Board: 'the building of a wing to the Hospital instead of a new Out-Patient department, previously recommended, provided of course funds were available. However, at the following meeting a letter from the architect was read indicating that the cost of building a new wing (with three storeys) to the east of the Hospital, would cost 'at least £35,000 exclusive of furniture and fittings'. Furthermore, a letter from the Admiralty to the Board of Management which was read to the LSCM Committee in April 'indicated that [in any case] sanction could not be given for buildings to be erected on the north or

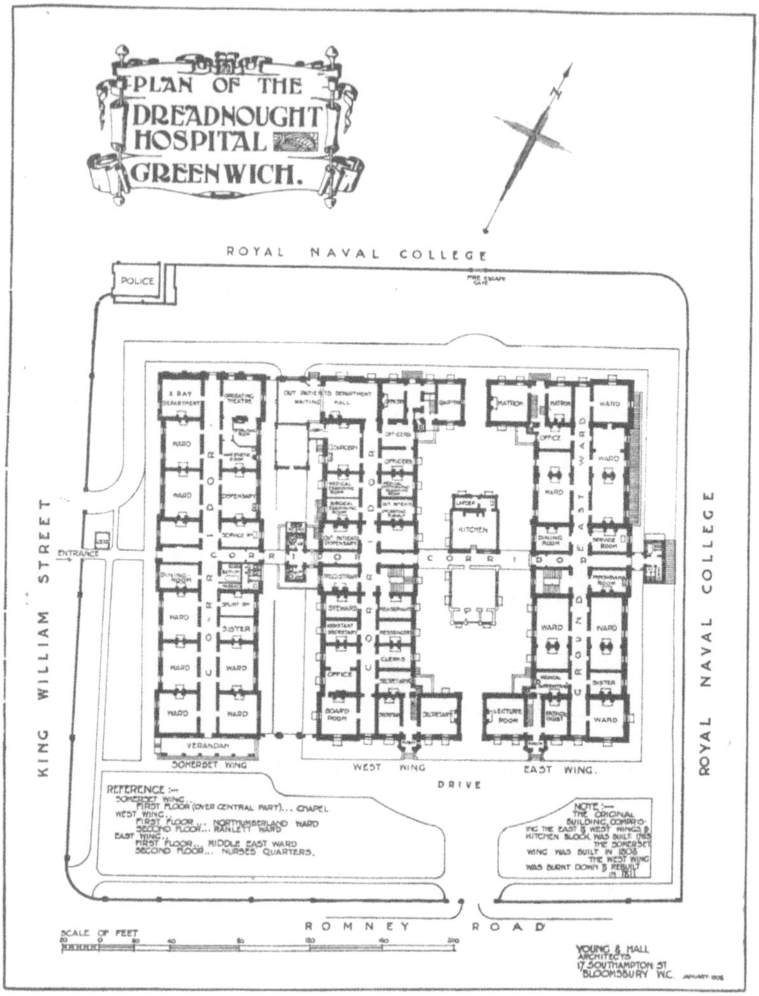

Figure 19.4: Groundfloor plan of the *Dreadnought* Hospital in 1906. [SHS Archive].

east side of the *Dreadnought* Hospital'. On receiving this letter, the Board apparently instructed the Secretary to enquire about 'the possibility of obtaining suitable premises for a Nurses' Home either in Haddington Terrace or elsewhere in the neighbourhood of the Hospital'.

The next meeting considered a plan for *improving* the Out-Patient Department: 'provision of an additional waiting room at the back of the Smoke Shed, two Water Closets in the West Tower, the removal of the Dispensary into the present Casualty room, [and] conversion of the present Dispensary into an Anaesthetising … and a sterilising room'. At a meeting in February 1906, the LSCM Committee was informed that the SHS Board was asking for an estimate for conversion of 'the Smoke Shed into a Billiard Room'.[30]

Regarding these structured alterations (see above), the Architect was asked, in September 1906, to provide 'further details in regard to certain plans for a Mortuary, Sterilizing and Anaesthetising Room, Out-Patient Department, etc'; his estimates were:

Post Mortem Room	£550
New Out-Patient Department	£500
W.C.s in connection therewith	£100
	£1150

This meeting also resolved to 'urge the Board to proceed with the whole of the work without delay'; the cost 'might be equally divided between the Charity and the School'.

The Board of Management stalled at this request, and failed to give a rapid reply. A minute records '... since the resignation of Mr Johnson Smith, and concurrently with the establishment of the [LSCM], the [SHS] had expended upon the Hospital a sum of about £456 on structural alterations etc [so that the] ordinary expenditure had been raised by £600 per annum'. When everything (including students' fees) were taken into account, this left 'a sum of £747 due to the Hospital'.

At the November meeting, a Board of Management minute indicates that they were:

> ... not prepared at present to extend the Mortuary accommodation, nor to remove the Dispenser from his quarters in the Hospital, but they [would] put in hand the enlargement of the Out-Patient Department and alter the lavatories in connection therewith.

And at the following meeting, it was reported that the plans for enlargement of the Out-Patient Department had been returned by the Civil Engineer of the Royal Naval College and sent to the Admiralty for approval, which was duly obtained in February 1907.[31]

Later alterations

At a meeting some five years later, in December 1912, the Committee further considered erecting 'additional accommodation for the School, etc, *outside* [my italics] the Hospital'. It was suggested that plans should provide accommodation for: A Pathological Department, Lecture Rooms, an Out-Patient Department, and a Nurses' Home (*see* Chapters 14 and 20). A memorandum of a School Finance Sub-Committee meeting held in February 1913 again considered the possibility of acquiring a site in Haddington Terrace (to the west of the Hospital) from the Admiralty to allow extension of the work of the School. The Sub-Committee concluded:

> i) ... it is advisable to obtain a definite statement from the commissioner of Greenwich Hospital as to the amount of land they would dispose of and the terms upon which it would be either let or sold,
> ii) That as soon as the particulars are to hand this Sub-Committee be again called to consider the matter,

iii) That the Architect be requested to get out a route plan and estimate for a steel framed building suitable to the requirements, and
iv) That a detailed estimate of the cost of upkeep be prepared.

Sir Malcolm Morris (he had been knighted in1908) offered to 'approach Prince Louis of Battenberg and ask him to lay the scheme before the King'.[32]

Offical opening

At the May 1906 meeting, it was decided to 'invite Professor Osler [who subsequently declined because he was to give the Harveian Lecture to the Royal College of Physicians at about that time] ... to deliver the opening address of the School during the second week in October [1906]'; it was resolved at the next meeting therefore, to 'adjourn the official opening of the School until the following March'. A later meeting suggested that an address be delivered by Sir Herbert Ellis, Director General of the Medical Department of the Navy on 4 October (i.e. at the beginning of the winter session) and failing him, Sir Douglas Powell (who did in fact deliver the Inaugural Address on 8 October 1907) or 'some other prominent member of the profession'.

For the opening address of the 1908–9 Winter Session the following names were suggested: 'Professor W H Welch, of Baltimore, Dr Wm. White, of Philadelphia, Mr Wm. May, or his brother, of Rochester, USA, Mr Howard Kelly, of Baltimore, and Mon. Lucas Championierre, of Paris'. None of these accepted however, and at a later meeting, it was minuted that the Sub-Committee 'had failed to get anyone to deliver an Address at the opening of the Winter Session'. It was therefore recommended that the idea of a dinner be abandoned, but that they would 'endeavour to make arrangements for a Dinner in March [hopefully with Sir Frederick Treves in the Chair]'. Treves was unable to be present, however, and the December meeting suggested Lord Robert Cecil. He did accept and was willing to preside at a dinner on 19 February; however, he was indisposed on the day, and P A Nairne chaired the occasion – 125 were present and the dinner was apparently a success.[33]

Teaching and students

At a meeting in early May 1906, it was stated that four students had entered for the complete course, three for pathology, three practical surgery and 'about 10' for operative surgery, since the opening of the school, and that a total of £100-00 had been received in fees. By June, the Medical Superintendent was able to report that: '25 students had joined the School and ... a sum of £152. 15. 6. had been received for Tuition Fees, etc.'. In December 1907, the Dean (C C Choyce) gave details of fees which 'were due to Teachers in The School'; these ranged from three (Bickerton) to 10 (Johnson Smith) guineas and the total amounted to £44=2=0. Smith was evidently suffering the effect(s) of advancing years: 'in consequence of [his] infirmities Students [were refusing] to attend his classes'; it was thus considered inviting him to resign and he 'should be replaced on account of his advancing years and inability to perform his [teaching] duties'. It was resolved that Choyce and Lawrence Jones be appointed teachers in Operative Surgery.

A request that 'holders of the Conjoint Postgraduate Association and Polyclinic [see above] might attend courses at the LSCM for lower fees' was rejected! The Committee noted that the LSTM permitted its name to appear as one of the constituent hospitals of the London Postgraduate Association; it was resolved that as students of the LSCM have no right to attend cliniques at the LSTM, the latter should consider disassociating themselves from the London Postgraduate Association and Polyclinic. It was also resolved that the Medical Council (of the SHS) should consider 'the desirability of members of the Dreadnought Hospital and [LSCM] delivering lectures or taking part in teaching at the Polyclinic'.

In October 1909, the Dean was able to report that 20 students had entered for the present session, and by the November meeting this number had risen to 26. In January 1910, he reported that 17 students and eight Naval Surgeons were 'on the books' for the session. In June, the total was 32. By October 1911, he was able to state that 22 students had started that session, and of those eight were Naval Surgeons. By October 1912, 38 students (including 23 Naval Surgeons) had joined. At a meeting at 31 Wimpole Street on 3 April 1913, Choyce reported that 24 Naval Students and six ordinary students had entered for the present session.

In January 1914, it was resolved that the pathological work of the Borough of Deptford should be carried out in the School's laboratory, and at the following meeting a similar resolution was passed concerning similar work for another Borough, i.e. that of Greenwich. It was estimated that the additional income from the work of these boroughs would amount to £330 for that year, and £450 for subsequent years. The salary of Dr Arthur Davies, the pathologist was raised by £100 to £350=00.[34]

Outside organisations also used the facilities of the new school: thus, the West Kent Medico-Chirurgical Society held a meeting at the *Dreadnought* Hospital on 8 March 1912.

Some day-to-day events at the new school

Owing to a sharp increase in numbers of out-patients (which was at that time causing considerable concern), the Dispenser at the *Dreadnought* asked for a separate Out-Patient colleague; a meeting of the LSCM Committee therefore recommended to the Board that such an appointment be made. Similarly, Mr Goadby indicated that due to the escalation of out-patients, he could not undertake dental management without the assistance of an Assistant; this matter was referred to the Medical Council. At a meeting in 1909, the Dean drew attention to the fact that, due to very few attendances by the anaesthetists, it was very difficult for students of the School to obtain instruction in this subject![35]

At the October 1911 meeting, the Dean reported that he had been in correspondence with Dr Pritchard and Mr Keogh Murphy, members of the staff of Miller Hospital who had expressed themselves willing to take part in teaching at the LSCM and to make 'cases in the Miller Hospital under their care' available; this soon became a reality. It was also reported (at the same meeting) that 'there was a possibility of amalgamation between the Pathological Departments of the *Dreadnought* Hospital [see below] and the Miller Hospital', this was also rapidly accomplished.[36]

In February 1912, Choyce reported that he had attended 'meetings of the Licensed Teachers of Anatomy ... and submitted a confidential report of the proceedings of their proposed action, shewing [sic] that they hoped to procure new legislation making compulsory the handing over of all unclaimed cadavers for distribution under the instruction of a Government Official as yet un-named'.

Resignation of Bennett in March 1912 necessitated significant changes to the surgical beds, and the following changes were recommended to the Medical Council:

Turner:	16 in 'North'; 4 in 'Ranlett'
McGavin:	26 in 'Somerset'
Rock Carling:	24 in 'North'
Choyce:	4 in 'North' and 9 Venereal
[Locum]	4 in 'Ranlett' and 6 Venereal[37]

The possibility of changing the timing of School sessions was considered by a Sub-Committee set up at the May 1912 meeting, and the following meeting recommended: 'That the School year be divided into two sessions of five and four months each, October-February and April-July. It was also recommended that the General lying-in Hospital be deleted from the list of affiliated Hospitals, and the Miller Hospital be added'. Another recommendation was that '... a specially selected number of men of the highest professional repute (e.g. Sir William Osler, etc) be invited to lecture once a session ...'. At the second July 1912 meeting, it was decided to invite Sir Thomas Barlow PRCP and Sir Rickman J Godlee Bt PRCS to deliver special lectures for the session opening in October 1912. At the same meeting, the following were made Emeritus Teachers of the School: Robson, Mackenzie Davidson, Carless, Bennett and Thompson.[38]

The following meeting of the Committee (October 1912) was held not at the Medical Society of London, but at 31 Wimpole Street (Choyce's house). It was considered that the next Annual Dinner should be held the following February (the organising Sub-Committee to consist of Rankin, Biggs and Hooper), and that Lord Haldane be invited to preside. It was also resolved 'that Professor Osler be requested to deliver an oration on the day of the dinner or near thereto'. The Dean also recorded that Mr A[ndrew] Balfour had been invited [but he later declined] to preside at the School Dinner. It was later reported that as none of those invited had agreed, Surgeon/General A W May CB (the new Director General of the Navy) should be invited, and failing him, Adml. Sir Frederick Fisher, KCVO; the former accepted.[39]

In December 1912, the Committee resolved that Sir John Rose Bradford be invited to speak at the International Congress the following year 'on the subject of Postgraduate Medical study'. They also considered 'provision of better laboratory accommodation [with new buildings between the Somerset and West Wings of the Hospital] with a view to meeting the requirements of the University of London and thus becoming a recognised School in the University'. It was felt, however, that 'much better accommodation' could be provided by the 'erection of suitable buildings outside the Hospital grounds' (*see* Chapter 20). A further suggestion was that to obtain University recognition as soon as possible (a subject of continuing urgency) smaller laboratories might be built above Somerset Ward.[40]

The subject of special lectures on *Hospital Administration* had been broached at the previous meeting but the Dean reported that 'he had been in communication with the Director General who refused to allow the Naval Surgeons to attend any other course on [that subject] than that already established at the North West London Fever Hospital'. Memoranda were written of two meetings held in January 1913, the first at the Medical Society of London and the second at 31 Wimpole Street. At the first, the Committee unanimously resolved to recommend to the Medical Council the offer by the Borough of Woolwich to 'place the laboratory work of the district in the Laboratory of the [LSCM]'. At the second, they considered a letter from the Army Council with regard to postgraduate tuition to 'about 50 Captains of the Royal Army Medical Corps'; the plan was to'divide the Students into classes distributed among five of the 11 London Hospitals which possessed Medical Schools, each receiving £100 with an additional £10 10 0 for a Tutor to direct studies …'. The meeting felt that the proposed fees were inadequate! It was decided at the following meeting that the local Medical Officers of Health should become Associates of the School.[41]

As early as October 1906, the question of *women* graduates attending the LSCM courses had been raised; the meeting resolved to '… ask [the Medical Council] to reconsider the question of admitting women either to the clinical work or to the classes in the School, or to both'. In February 1913, a letter was read from the Colonial Office suggesting that a *woman* graduate appointed to the Straits Settlements (Malaysia) should be offered facilities for Operative Surgery in the School; the Committee reiterated its view that women graduates were *not* acceptable as students!

Dr Bernard G Klein was appointed Assistant Pathologist in 1913. It was also resolved to invite Professor Arthur Keith to lecture at the School at a time convenient to him.[42] A special meeting of the Committee was called for January 1914, when it was resolved to offer Gordon Holmes three beds (later increased to four, previously used for venereology), to allow him to set up a neurology out-patient session, and to appoint him 'Neurologist to the Hospital'. The whole question of teaching, especially 'on the medical side', was to be considered by a Sub-Committee consisting of Rankin, Turner, Rock Carling, Singer, the Dean and Assistant Dean.

A 'memorandum' attached to the minutes of a meeting on 22 January 1914 states that 'informal' consideration be given to a letter from Dr Sydney Davies, Medical Officer of Health for the Borough of Woolwich 'suggesting that phthisical patients be sent from the Borough Tuberculosis Dispensary for consultation with the Medical Staff and for treatment'; he was aware, he wrote, that 'only sailors could be treated as In-patients'. The meeting resolved to do everything in their power to implement these suggestions; furthermore '… on occasions arrangements may be made for the admission of a special case not of the seafaring class'.[43]

The Secretary of State for the Colonies had intimated that in the event of the School running a course in Venereal Diseases, he would 'from time to time' send Colonial Medical Officers to attend; as a consequence a four-week course was established. It was suggested at that time also that Out-patient treatment of syphilis (by

Salvarsen injections) should be considered by the Medical Council with a view to 'every such patient paying for his treatment ...'; this was agreed.[44]

In February 1913 the Board of Management approved of the Billiard Room being placed at the disposal of the Pathological Department (see above) of the Hospital and School.

FEES AND ATTEMPTS TO RAISE THE PROFILE OF THE NEW SCHOOL

The question of finance was always to the forefront; it was resolved that a student attending the LSTM should be 'allowed an abatement of 10%' and it was further recommended that the LSTM should 'reciprocate in this matter'. In an attempt to repay its debt to the Society, 'it was resolved to ask the Board to approve ... a Banquet for the charity and the Clinical School next Session, and that of the Prince of Wales should be invited to take the Chair'. The Board of Management were, however, less than enthusiastic on the grounds that (i) this was too soon after the last Banquet, and (ii) the Committee 'desired to see the Clinical School in a more advanced and thriving state before bringing the claims of the Society again before the public'. However, the Committee later suggested a Banquet (also to be chaired by the Prince of Wales) in the Spring of 1908; this too failed to receive support from the Board on the grounds that the period since the last Banquet was still rather short. An alternative plan was a Garden Party, but this too was shelved until they could get 'a prominent man, possibly from abroad, to deliver the opening address ...'.

At the January 1911 meeting, arrangements for the Annual Dinner of the School (to be held in the last week of March) were considered: Lord Chas. Beresford was to be invited to preside, and the Sub-Committee to make arrangements would consist of Mr Biggs, Choyce and Mr McGavin. Later that year, it was reported that Lord Ilkeston 'had consented to preside at the next School Dinner', to which ladies would *not* be invited. However, at the January 1912 meeting it was recorded that '... Ilkeston had ... withdrawn his promise to preside; in his place, Prince Louis of Battenberg would take the Chair, on Friday 1 March'.

ATTEMPTS AT OUTSIDE RECOGNITION OF THE NEW SCHOOL

On 29 October 1911, a deputation (consisting of Sir Henry Miers [Principal of the University], Professor [Ernest] Starling, Professor Hill and Mr Waring visited the School, but 'declined to recognise the [LSCM] as a School of the University of London' on the grounds that the improvements in the laboratories were insufficient, that there was inadequate accommodation for post-mortems, and the Out-Patient Department was 'inefficient in some points'. The Report concluded that 'while the question of medical teaching in the University ... is being discussed it would be inadvisable to complicate matters by the admission of new Schools, especially when there is doubt about their adequacy'.

The subject of University of London recognition of the LSCM was however repeatedly raised; provided that Rose Bradford and Russell Wells (both members of the Senate) felt the time was opportune, a formal application was to be made. At the next meeting, however, both of these members of Senate expressed doubts as to whether the School would be recognised; Wells 'intimated that there were certain members of the Senate who had scruples to a School, which was not a complete medical School …', but this issue continued to be discussed and in December 1907 a Sub-Committee consisting of Tanner, Hewlett, Russell Wells and Choyce, was set up to approach (unsuccessfully) both the University of London and Royal College of Surgeons (RCS). The RCS regretted their inability recognise the LSCM, but felt that the School fell short of 'the clinical instruction in Medicine and Surgery required as of the curriculum of candidates who desire to take the Diplomas of the Royal Colleges'. A later letter from the RCS intimated however that they were able to 'recognise the Dreadnought Hospital for the additional year of Hospital practice required in the case of Candidates for the Fellowship who are not members of the College'. In October 1908 it was recorded that the Conjoint Board 'had decided to recognise the course of Operative Surgery … as fulfilling the conditions of paragraph XXI, clause I, section II of the Regulations of the Board'.[45]

In April 1908, 'The Secretary was requested to ascertain from the Admiral President [of the Royal Naval College], Sir Arthur Fanshawe, whether surgeons from the Royal Navy might be permitted to reside in the Royal Naval College and become members of their Mess while attending the [LSCM]'; it was recorded at the following meeting that he had no objection to the idea, but the School should first obtain clearance from the Director General of the Medical Department of the Navy. At the July meeting, a letter from the Mess Secretary of the Royal Naval College was read to the Committee; in it, he intimated that 'the Officers of the College will be pleased to make Naval Surgeons attending the [LSCM] Honorary members of their Mess'. At the July 1912 meeting, the Dean also reported that 'he had had an interview with the Director of the Royal Army Medical Corps [regarding] clinical teaching at the [LSCM]. [He] expressed the hope that Officers would be sent for instruction to Greenwich'.[46]

The India Office apparently refused to acknowledge the certificate of the LSCM as sufficient evidence of Ophthalmic work in 'an Ophthalmic Hospital of the Ophthalmic Department of a General Hospital'.[47]

Progress of the School

The Medical Superintendent indicated in January 1907, that 14 students were now 'attending the various classes at the School'. It was also reported that another BMA meeting (the Norwood Division of the South-eastern Branch) would be held at the *Dreadnought* in February. The Sydenham Society had offered most of their publications at a price of £5=5=00; this offer was accepted. The minutes of the February meeting contain a notice that 'Thos. Lewis, Esq., M.B., B.S., [later to become a distinguished cardiologist] had been appointed Medical Registrar …'. Later that year, it was agreed that Choyce's title be changed from 'Medical Superintendent' to 'Dean' of the LSCM.

Encouraging news was reported at the December 1907 meeting. 'The Dean reported that during the [previous] session 24 students, in addition to 17 Associates, had been in attendance. This is the largest number since the School was established', he added. Rankin, Choyce and Lake were appointed to make arrangements for the Annual Student's Dinner to be held the following February.[48]

In June 1909, the following fees to staff members were approved; these ranged from 2½ guineas (Jones and Lewis) to 27½ guineas (Choyce); the total amounted to £82=18=6. At the November meeting that year, fees were again approved; they ranged from 2½ guineas (Lewis) to £32=12=0 (Choyce); the total amounted to £107=12=0. Totals at the April and June 1910 meetings were £91=17=6 and £75=12=0, respectively.

The possibility of a School *journal* was raised in 1910; Mr Lake offered his services as editor. The matter was again aired at the October 1911 meeting, when a Sub-Committee was set up consisting of C C Choyce FRCS, A Davies MB BS, Hewlett, Gordon Holmes MD, R Lake FRCS and Sir Malcolm Morris KCVO. However, it was ultimately decided that the time was inopportune to establish such a publication.[49]

At the April 1910 meeting (the first, apart from Committee Meeting to be held at the Medical Society of London) encouraging news was reported that 'the Colonial Office had arranged for Medical Officers in the WAMS [West African Medical Service] to be seconded for study after five years service and that the [LSCM] had been adopted as one of the approved places [for] study'.[50]

Overall financial position of the enterprise

The precarious state of the finances (a complete statement was due in January 1908) was reported to the meeting in December 1907:

Income	**Tuition fees**			**Pathological fees**		
1st Session	£58	16	0			
2nd Session	£100	0	6	£1	19	6
Vacation Classes	£81	9	6		5	0
October Session	£159	0	2	£3	3	0
Total	£399	6	2	£5	7	6

The financial position, however, continued to be extremely unsound; in fact, 'at the end of 1907 the School was indebted to the SHS to the tune of £1047.13.6'. In order to increase income, Choyce was asked 'to make arrangements for the Saturday classes to visit the [ADH] and for the students [at the LSTM] to visit the Dreadnought'. In early 1908 the Committee 'approved of the [SHS] charging the School 4% interest on its overdraft'.[51]

By December 1908, finances had marginally improved: receipts 'amounted to £703 as against £499 in the previous year'. It was resolved to recommend to the Board of Management that an 'Appeal Dinner … for the [LSCM] be held in May 1910 and that Lord Rosebery should be invited to preside. The Sub-Committee also recommended that Lords Howard de Walden and Ridley, and Mr Gordon be invited to be Chairmen and Hon Secretary of the dinner Committee, respectively. However, the Board again rejected this idea (see above), and ruled that the 'ordinary Annual Social Dinner' [with Sir James Crichton-Browne presiding) should be held on 15 March; when about 140 were present.

'It was unanimously resolved in November 1910 that the financial position of the School is considered by this Committee as satisfactory and sufficient to justify the School in looking forward to future prosperity'. This transpired, however, to be an over optimistic viewpoint! Subsequent accounts of the School indicate that in the year 1913, for example, income had again exceeded expenditure, by £114=5=9.[52]

A course for Naval Officers – an opponent to the LSCM

In March 1909 it was reported that the Admiralty intended establishing a School for Naval Officers in London – probably at the Royal Naval College, Greenwich; 'in these circumstances [the meeting heard] it was likely to affect the [LSCM]'. It was resolved, therefore, that this subject be referred to a Sub-Committee (which met on 7 May 1909) consisting of Bennett, Rankin, Manson, the Chairman of the SHS Committee of Management (P A Nairne) – or, if he should be unavailable, Orford – and the Dean as an Ex-Officio member. At a subsequent meeting, Choyce reported that 'the naval Surgeons seconded for study-leave were now resident at the Royal Naval College, [and] by order of the Director General they had been sent to attend the curriculum at the *West London Hospital* [my italics]'.

By 1912, relationships with the RN had improved, somewhat. A letter was received by the Committee of the LSCM 'from the Admiralty ... in which various suggestions were made for the Students of the new Naval School at Greenwich to receive instruction at the *Dreadnought* Hospital'. The Admiralty 'also asked for six beds to be placed at the disposal of the Naval Professor of Clinical Pathology for the treatment of Naval ratings suffering from tropical diseases'. Both requests were acceded to.[53]

Associated Hospitals

The April 1911 meeting resolved that 'a Sub-Committee consisting of Rock Carling, Choyce and Harlett be appointed to consider the expediency of associating other hospitals with the Seamen's Hospital and the [LSCM]'. The following meeting minuted the fact that the following hospitals were being invited to become affiliated: The Soho Hospital for Women, Queen Charlotte's, City Road Hospital for Diseases of the Chest, and Plaistow Fever Hospital. It was also 'resolved to ascertain whether there [was] a definite system of teaching now carried on at the York Road Hospital, and if there is not this Hospital [should be] deleted from the list of affiliated Hospitals'.[54]

The Pathology Department; the sole financially viable component of the LSCM

The budget of the Pathological services of the *Dreadnought* was considered at the May 1913 meeting. Total annual expenditure was £350 (£245 was paid by the hospital and £105 by the School). This meeting resolved to ask the Hospital authorities to pay £350 as a contribution to the £670 cost of running the Pathological Laboratory (receipts from Woolwich and the Royal Naval surgeons amounted to £170 and £20 respectively, leaving the School £130 to pay annually). At the July meeting of the Committee, the advisability of 'improving the Pathological Department [various structural alterations were envisaged] in order to meet the requirements of the University of London' was considered; the work (and also the increase in contributions to the fees) was sanctioned by the Board of Management and subsequently implemented. At the May meeting, 'The Medical Superintendent suggested the propriety of making the *Dreadnought* Hospital a *centre for pathology* [my italics] of the group of hospitals associated with the [LSCM]'. The Countess von Pappenheim had apparently been assisting (unpaid) in the Pathological Laboratory; the December meeting recommended an honorarium of 25 guineas a year for her invaluable services.

The future of the Pathological Department (see above), which seems to have been the only component of the LSCM which was financially viable, was further discussed in 1913; it was agreed that the pathological work of the Borough of Woolwich be done in the School's laboratory at a rate similar to that charged by the Lister Institute. This, of course, meant that the Pathologist (Davies) should receive a higher salary and be helped by a medically qualified assistant as well as an additional laboratory technician. He was also granted the right to act as Pathologist to the Miller Hospital. With minor amendments made in a letter to Michelli, Davies accepted these conditions.[55]

The Great War (1914–18) and after

The involvement of the Society during the 1914–18 war will be described in Chapter 20, but this event had a devastating effect on the LSCM. The final meeting of the LSCM Committee prior to the Great War was held on 3 September 1914. The Director-General of the Navy had intimated that there would be no more students from the RN until 'hostilities cease', and the Dean also felt that 'very few (if any) other Students would thenceforth present themselves, and in particular there would be no students from the Indian Medical Service, the Royal Army Medical Corps, Colonial Service and other Government Departments'.

The Committee reviewed the general financial position at that time; if the Classes in *Operative Surgery* were to be maintained [they claimed] there may be a profit on this branch of the School's work of about £80 per annum, and a profit on the *Pathological Department* of approximately £150. It was resolved to recommend that a sum of £50 be appropriated to 'improving the Museum' during the period of closure. Both the Dean and Assistant-Dean agreed to forego their honoraria for the duration of the war and that the 'collection of skulls [assembled by George Busk] be lent to the Royal College of Surgeons for exhibition there'. It was also resolved that a notice that the School was closing be circulated to 'every Member of the Honorary Medical Staff and Teachers in the School, including the extra mural Teachers' and that 'the Annual School Dinner be abandoned this year'.[56]

Cessation of hostilities and continuation of the Pathological laboratory

At the conclusion of the war, the Medical Council had to give serious consideration to the viability (or otherwise) of the LSCM. Its prognosis was gloomy, and it felt that in view of the original objectives of the SHS 'the suggestions for the admission of women and children with a view to the better treatment of sick Seamen is not met with approval and support and that in consequence it is deemed by their Council impossible to continue to carry on the [LSCM] in its present form'. It was further resolved that 'an inventory of School Property be prepared with a view to its value being put as a set off against the debt of the School to the Hospital'. It was resolved that £33=16=10 [i.e. 20% of 'monies received from the Ministry of Pensions for the treatment of pensioners in this Hospital'] be handed to the Hospital as a further set off towards defraying the debt.[57]

At the following meeting in November 1919, resignation of several members of staff who had joined in the days when the LSCM appeared promising, were announced; these included: Rose Bradford, MacCormac, Cargill and Rock Carling; Bradford, Cargill and Carling were thenceforth appointed to the *Consulting* Staff. At the following meeting the Dean (Choyce) too resigned 'in consequence of his being appointed Director of Surgery at University College Hospital, and he also was appointed to the *Consulting* Staff.[58] The Pathological Services, however, went from strength to strength and undertook to work for Queen Mary's Hospital East Ham (for £400), and the Miller Hospital (for £225) annually.

The LSCM was at this time in debt to the Society to the extent of £502. 'This School [a minute recorded] is kept in being in order that funds may be available to repay the loan made … and during the last few years all surplus profits … have been devoted to that purpose'. 'It was stated that the equipment of the Pathological laboratories was the property of the School and it was again suggested that this might be utilised as a set-off against the debt'. '… the matter of the employment of women graduates was again considered, but no decision was [made]'. Regarding House Surgeons, it was approved of 'their being advertised for at the rate of £150 per annum in order to secure the services of graduates of *British* [my italics] origin'.

The next meeting of the LSCM did not take place until January 1921; there were more resignations, and *no* applications for the vacant position of Physician to the Out-Patients Department.[59]

Postscript

The LSCM had been launched in good faith to make good a deficiency in post-graduate training in London and to strengthen the *clinical* dimension of the *Dreadnought*'s activities. However, it was never financially viable – despite the fact that several distinguished physicians and surgeons had been invited to serve on its teaching staff. The SHS was, after all, a Charity, which could not allow its donated funds to be drained in order to create another School of Medicine – however good the teaching material was! After less than a decade, therefore (and hastened by the outbreak of the Great War) the venture came to an abrupt (and premature) end. Thereafter, the Dreadnought Hospital Medical Committee continued meeting, usually monthly (at the LSTM, at Endsleigh Gardens, WC1) – but without the LSCM.

The LSCM however, again entered the SHS minute books on 30 May 1922; 'the [Society had provided] generous grants to the School and a sum of money on loan for the use of certain premises'. 'Up to 1914, although the other Departments at the [LSCM] had a [substantial] income, their expenses were … heavy [and] the pathological department was the only one to show a profit'; after 1914, almost the entire income of the [LSCM] had in fact been earned by the Pathological Department. Year by year portions of the loan from the [SHS] had been repaid until, at the close of the last financial year, the whole financial indebtedness of the [LSCM] to the [SHS] had been wiped out.

The *Pathological Department* had thus shouldered the burden of the entire school debt and succeeded in paying it off. Until 1914 (the last minute book declared) 'the benefits accruing to the Hospital were fully as great as had been hoped; how great can only be appreciated now when the deplorable effect of the failure to re-establish the School *after* the war can be seen everywhere in the working of the Institution'. The minute concluded by summarising the 1922 situation:

1. The [LSCM] is defunct except for the Pathological and Operative Surgery Departments.
2. The Operative Surgery classes are intermittent and each class is so arranged that when all expenses are paid there remains a small surplus.
3. The debt to the [SHS] has been paid off [and]
4. The Pathological Department is making a profit of some £400 per annum.

Owing to the viability of the Pathological Services, it was resolved at that meeting to appoint 'a sub-committee [consisting of Davies, Fisher, Hewlett, Prentice and Russell-Wells] to consider the extension and scope of [that] department.[60]

References and notes

1 C Newman. *The evolution of Medical Education in the Nineteenth Century*. Oxford: Oxford University Press 1957: 341; G Rivett. Postgraduate Study. In: *The Development of the London Hospital system 1823–1982*. London: King Edward's Hospital Fund for London 1986; 159–60; G C Cook. *John MacAlister's other vision: a history of the Fellowship of Postgraduate Medicine* Oxford: Radcliffe Publishing 2005: 178.

2 Anonymous. A new clinical post-graduate school for London. *BMJ* 1905; ii: 1306–7; Anonymous. London School of Clinical Medicine. *BMJ* 1905; ii: 1472, 1608.

3 **George Busk** FRS (1807–1886); (*see* Chapter 12).

4 The Seamen's Hospital, Greenwich. The new school of clinical medicine. *BMJ* 1906; i: 211–5.

5 *The London School of Clinical Medicine (Postgraduate): In connection with the Dreadnought Hospital, Greenwich (250 Beds): with which are affiliated for teaching purposes the following hospitals: - 1. – Royal Waterloo Hospital for Children and Women. 2. – Bethlem Royal Hospital. 3 - Miller General Hospital for South-east London:* 1914: 51 [SHS Archive].

6 London School of Clinical Medicine: *Preliminary Meeting 1904: 12 December*, 1.

7 **Sir Patrick Manson** GCMG FRCP (1844–1922) (*see also* Chapters 15 and 18) is often referred to as the '*father* of tropical medicine'.

8 **Sir William Henry Bennett** KCVO FRCS (1852–1931); *see also* Chapter 15.
9 *LSCM Sub-Committee Meeting*, 1905: 1: 2–3.
10 **Sir Dyce Duckworth** Bt FRCP (1840–1928); *see also* Chapter 15.
11 **Sir (Thomas) Lauder Brunton** Bt FRCP FRS (1844–1916) was a Consultant Physician to St Bartholomew's Hospital. He was also the author of several texts on medicine and therapeutics. [*See also:* J A Gunn, M P Earles. Brunton, Sir Thomas Lauder, first baronet (1844–1916). In: H C G Matthew, B Harrison (eds). *Oxford Dictionary of National Biography.* Oxford: Oxford University Press 2004; 8: 369–70].
12 *Op cit.* See note 9 above. 1905: 4–7.
13 **Sir William Henry Broadbent** FRCP KCVO FRS (1835–1907) was Physician in ordinary to King Edward VII, and the Prince of Wales (subsequently King George V). He was also Physician Extraordinary to Queen Victoria. He was a Consultant Physician at St Mary's Hospital, London. Broadbent was President of the Medical Society of London, the Clinical Society, and the Neurological Society. [*See also*: K Brown. Broadbent, Sir William Henry, first baronet (1835–1907). In: H C G Matthew, B Harrison (eds). *Oxford Dictionary of National Biography.* Oxford: Oxford University Press 2004; 7: 725–7].
14 *Op cit.* See note 9 above. 1905: 8–10.
15 *Ibid.* 1905: 11–14.
16 **William Johnson Smith** FRCS (1840–1912); *see also* Chapters 12 and 15.
17 *Op cit.* See note 9 above: 1905: 15–32.
18 *Ibid.* Board of Management consideration of synopsis submitted by the Medical Council 1905: 2 May 44–8.
19 *Ibid. Joint Sub-Committee meeting* 1905: 14 June: 49–51.
20 *Ibid.* Memorandum of Medical Council and Board of Management. Meetings 1905: 6 July and 17 July: 53; *Joint Sub-Committee Meeting* 1905: 20 July: 54–64.
21 G C Cook. Early use of 'open-air treatment for 'pulmonary phthisis' at the Dreadnought Hospital, Greenwich, 1900-1905. *Postgrad Med J* 1999; 75: 326–7.
22 *Op cit.* See note 9 above. Note on Medical Council Meeting 1905: 10 October: 65; Committee of Management Minutes 1905: 14: 66–79.
23 Dr T L Rogers. *Suggestions … on the Report of the Joint-Sub-Committee relating to the proposed establishment of a Post Graduate School and concurrent alterations in the arrangements of the Dreadnought Hospital; Op cit.* See note 5 above: 81–9.
24 London School of Clinical Medicine (LSCM): Minute Book 1; *Joint-Sub-Committee Report* 1905: 3–5; *Op cit.* See note 1 above (Cook).
25 *Op cit.* See note 22 above (Minutes): 1905; 14: 220–224.
26 *Op cit.* See note 24 above. 1905: 1: 6–8; 9–13.
27 *Ibid.* 1905; 1: 14–12; 34–6; 25–30; **Sir John Rose Bradford** Bt KCMG FRCP FRS (1863–1935) was Professor of Medicine at University College London, and President of the Royal College of Physicians (1926–31); *see also* Chapter 15.
28 *Op cit.* See note 9 above: 1; 37–9, 40–3.
29 *Ibid.* 1; 44–6, 47–51.
30 *Ibid.* 1; 52–4, 55–6, 57–60, 61–3.
31 *Ibid*: 1; 83–6: 87–90.
32 *Ibid*: 1912: 20 December: 77–80; 1913: 29 May: 99–102; 1913: 24 July: 103–6; 30 October: 108–11.
33 *Ibid.* 1906: 22 May: 67–9; 19 June: 73–7; 1907: 9 July: 116–8; 15 October: 119–20; 1908: 31 March 130–1; 1908: 9 December: 138–40; 1909: 5 January: 141; 1913: 29 May: 99–102; 24 July: 103–6.
34 *Ibid.* 1906: 22 May 67–9; 1908: 9 December 83–6; 1913: 30 October 108–11; 1913: 29 May: 99–102; 24 July: 103–6; 1914: 30 April 125–9.

35 *Ibid.* 1: 61–3, 121–4; 2: 5–8.
36 *Ibid.* 2: 38–40, 42–5.
37 *Ibid.* 2: 46–8.
38 *Ibid.* 2: 51–6, 63–5.
39 *Ibid.* 2: 65–9, 77–80, 103–6.
40 *Ibid.* 2: 71–6, 77–80.
41 Memorandum of the Clinical School Committee. 1913: 81, 82–3, 84–8; *Op cit. See* note 1 above (Cook).
42 *Op cit.* See note 9 above. 1913: 91–5; 108–111.
43 Special meeting of the Committee of Management. 1914: 115–7; Sub-Committee of the LSCM Committee: 118–22.
44 *Op cit. See* note 9 above. 1914: 123–4; 125–9.
45 *Ibid.* 1906: 83–6, 107–8; 1911: 3: 29–30, 38–40, 42–5.
46 *Ibid.* 91-4; 95–9, 121–4: 104–6, 132–4, 135–7, 4: 5–8, 15–18, 19–21, 51–6.
47 *Ibid.* 95–9, 125–6, 127–9, 15–18; 1910: 30 November: 25–8.
48 *Ibid.* 5–8; 1909: 30 November 11–14; 1910: 25 January: 15–18, 19–21; 22–4, 38–40.
49 *Ibid.* 15–18, 38–40.
50 *Ibid.* 100–3, 119–20, 19–21.
51 *Ibid.* 125–6.
52 *Ibid.* 138–40, 215–18, 25–8.
53 *Ibid.* 2: 1–3, 49–50; *Op cit.* See note 1 above (Cook).
54 *Ibid.* 31–2, 34–7.
55 *Ibid.* 91–5.
56 *Ibid.* 132–4.
57 *Dreadnought* Medical Council. Book 3: 1–5.
58 *Op cit.* See note 9 above. 1919: 6–11, 12–14, 17–20.
59 *Ibid.* 21–25, 26–30.
60 *Ibid.* 69–77; *Op cit.* See note 1 above (Cook).

PART IV

Two World Wars, introduction of the National Health Service, and insidious decline of the Society (1914–2006)

'Change and decay in all around I see; O Thou, who changest not, abide with me.'

H F Lyte (1793–1847)

Chapter 20

The Great War (1914–18); the inter-war years; and several new facilities

The 1914–18 War

The 1915 Annual Report (i.e. shortly after the beginning of the Great War) commented: 'The trumpet call to action has been sounding throughout the Empire for the past year, and its message has been just that upon which the Voluntary Hospitals of this country have for so long depended – willing sacrifice'. The Society, during this worldwide conflict, played a major rôle in care, not only of merchant seamen, but also Naval Ratings (and to a lesser extent soldiers also) – most of whom 'arrived by ambulance train at Greenwich Station'; the 1918 Report stated that during that year alone 1,720 Naval Ratings had been treated by the Society – bringing the total since the outbreak of war to 4,717 (a number which was to increase to 5,282 by the time the 1920 Annual Report was written). To give some idea of the immense burden on the SHS, the 1915 Report (see above) continued:

> In the early part of the year comparatively few Admiralty patients were in the Wards, but as the casualties from the Dardanelles* began to return in growing numbers, more and more beds were required. During the last three months of the year the accommodation was taxed to the utmost, the record number of 320 patients being at one time in the Wards.

The closer association in time of war between the Royal Navy (RN) and the Mercantile Marine (MM) is outlined in the 1918 Report:

> One of the results of the War has been that a very large proportion of the men of the MM were drafted into the [RN]. As a consequence of this an arrangement has been entered into with the Admiralty by which many thousands of Naval Ratings from the Fleet have been succoured and tended in the Wards of the two Hospitals [the *Dreadnought* and ADH] since the year 1914, as well as large numbers of their equally gallant brothers of the [MM], and Mine Layers, Mine Sweepers, and the men

* This campaign (also known as Gallipoli) took place between March 1915 and January 1916. It was an Anglo-French war against Turkey, but failed to produce a clear-cut result and produced an enormous number of Allied casualties.

> of the small Patrol Boats – men from every Naval engagement that has taken place, from the Jutland* fight, from Zeebrugge and Ostend.†[1]

Morale at the SHS was to a certain extent kept up by several Royal visits; on 21 September 1915, HM the King (George V) and Queen (Mary) visited the wards of the *Dreadnought*:

> Their Majesties paid tribute to the brotherhood of the sea and placed the Merchant Seaman as worthy to stand side by side with his comrade of the [RN] in the community of service, sacrifice, courage and endurance: even as at that moment they were lying side by side in the Wards of the Dreadnought in the common bond of illness and suffering.

On 20 November 1917, His Majesty also visited the ADH, and on 27 February the following year, the Queen accompanied by the 'Prince of Wales and Princess Mary' did likewise.

Increased public recognition of the crucial role of the Sailor in the war effort is emphasised in the 1917 Report: 'There is evidence that the part played by the Sailor in this War is receiving much larger recognition than heretofore, and very generous support has been forthcoming for his treatment and maintenance.'[2]

As with all Institutions, it was difficult to maintain satisfactory service in time of war, because so many of the staff from both hospitals (including the physicians and surgeons) were fighting for their country; however 'many Officers of the Colonial Medical Service [contributed] a large part of their leave to the service of the Society' and 'Officers of the West African Medical Staff' and a 'number of V.A.D. Nurses [gave] their services to the Hospital'.[3]

The *Dreadnought* facilities expand

Figure 20.1 shows an aerial view of the Hospital in 1926. The need for 'additional premises' in Greenwich, not least a dedicated nurses' home, had been aired long ago. Although the war precluded any 'improvements' in the *Dreadnought* Hospital, the Devonport Special Appeal (see below) which, according to the 1921 Annual Report then stood at >£200,000 continued apace; in recognition of this, a floor of the hospital was named *'The Devonport Floor'*. The Report for 1923 documented the removal of the;

> Royal Hospital School boys to new premises in Suffolk; the Admiralty [had] generously granted the Society a new and extended lease for 99 years, comprising the buildings and grounds of the Dreadnought

* A major battle (31 May – 1 June 1916) between the British and German fleets, off the coast of Denmark.

† The harbour of Zeebrugge (Belgium) was raided by the British in 1918, sinking blockships, and thus denying use of the port by German submarines. Ostend (also in Belgium) was a German submarine base until the British fleet sealed the port in 1918.

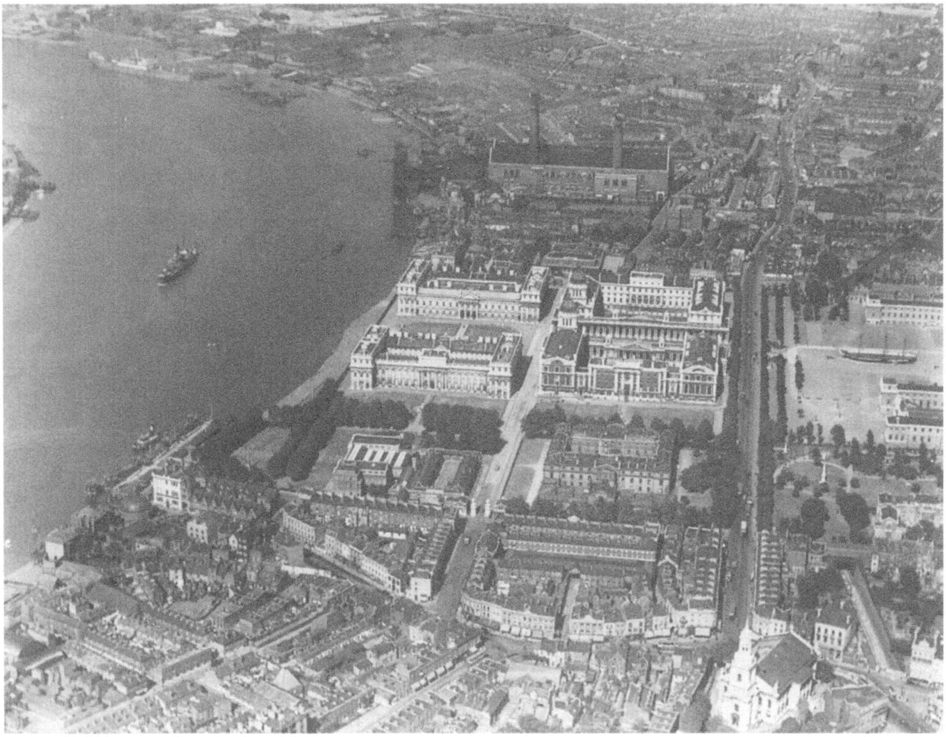

Figure 20.1: Aerial view of the *Dreadnought* Hospital and surrounding buildings in 1926. [SHS archive].

> Hospital, and, in addition, the Infirmary of the Royal Hospital School, Greenwich, and the grounds surrounding it, on the south side of the Romney Road [thus paving the way for the Devonport buildings – see below]. This extension of site [was expected to] provide facilities for the erection of a Nurse's Home and other departments, for which Lord Devonport's fund . . . will afford opportunity for the extensive improvements in the old building which are urgently needed. Plans are now being prepared [the Report continued] for the erection of the Nurses' Home and other improvements, and these [it is anticipated] will be carried out in the immediate future.

Work on the 'improvements' was not in fact to begin until 1925; the first Viscount Devonport (1856–1934)[4] chaired a Sub-committee to which plans by the architect Sir Edwin Cooper FRIBA (1874–1942)[5] were submitted; the idea was to erect a *new* Nurses' Home (incorporating 130 bedrooms, sitting, recreation, and classrooms), and a 'pathological unit' to provide for 'the growing needs of science and the well-being of the patients in the care of the Society'. In order to erect these new buildings, an Act of Parliament had to be passed. Figure 20.2 shows the interior of the Chapel in 1930.

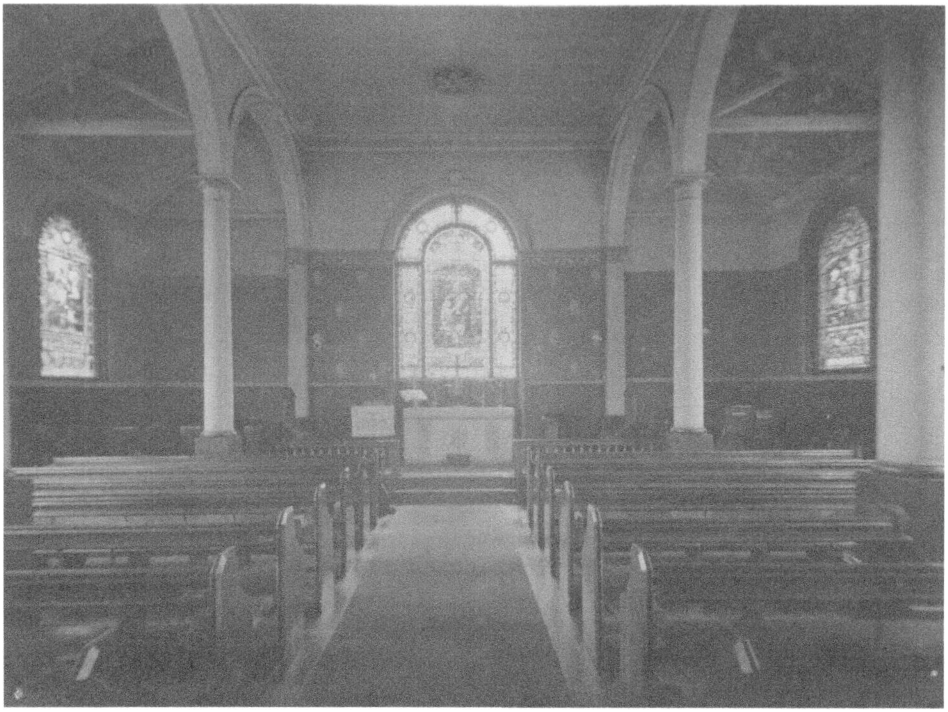

Figure 20.2: Interior of the *Dreadnought* Hospital Chapel (1930). [SHS archive].

The Devonport buildings

Devonport had therefore headed a most successful fund-raising campaign, initiated in 1916. The 1926 Report began:

> A very successful year, fraught with good omens for the future, in that the foundation stone of the new Nurses' Home was laid on the 23rd June. The Home is on the site provided by the Admiralty [to the south of the *Dreadnought* Hospital] and the ceremony was performed by the Rt. Hon. Viscount Devonport. A large number of Governors and supporters of the Society were present, and a delightful day lent hope and brightness to the occasion.

This Report continued:

> The Pathological block lying to the south-west of the site, being smaller, has made more rapid progress, and is nearing completion. Until the Nurses' Home is available it is not possible to proceed with the Officers' unit, which will be in the part of the old building vacated by the Nurses, but it is the desire of the Society to see that improved accommodation for Officers of the Merchant Service is provided, affording the amenities of sitting room, etc., for these men who, by their efforts when at sea, help to interest the public in the well-being of the

> mariner, and so augment the funds of the Society. Where possible the remodelling of the old Hospital is being proceeded with; the Architect is preparing plans for this work, which has been so long needed.

The 1929 Report was able to record details of completion and the official opening of the *Devonport* buildings:

> The outstanding feature of the year was the completion of the Devonport Nurses' Home [see Figure 20.3] and the Pathological Laboratories, both built to the designs of Sir Edwin Cooper, F.R.I.B.A. The Pathologists moved into their new quarters in February, and the Nurses into their new Home in May. Both buildings were formally declared open by T.R.H the Duke [later King George VI (1895–1952), President of the SHS] and Duchess of York on Monday, the 15th of July [see Figure 20.4] ... about 1,500 were present in the quadrangle to greet T.R.H. the President and the Duchess of York. The erection and equipment of these two buildings are the first-fruits of the fund which Lord Devonport raised during the [1914–18] war for the improvement and extension of the Dreadnought Hospital, and as a memorial to the work of the men of the Merchant Service in war and peace. In the evening a dinner at the Langham Hotel was given to Lord Devonport by the Honorary Medical Staff of the Hospital.

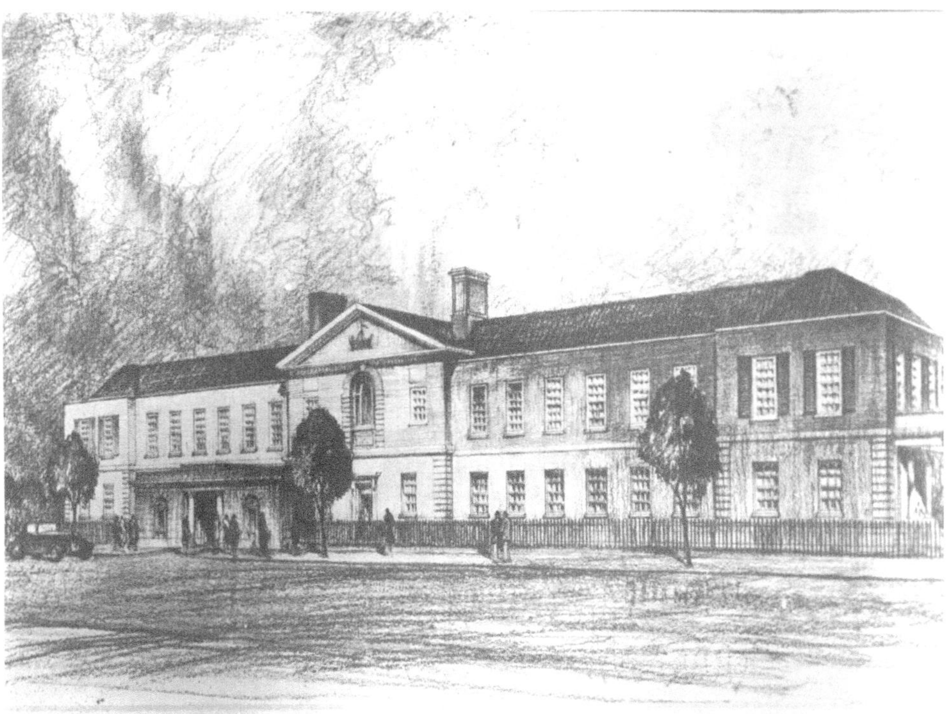

Figure 20.3: The completed Devonport nurses' home in 1929. [SHS archive].

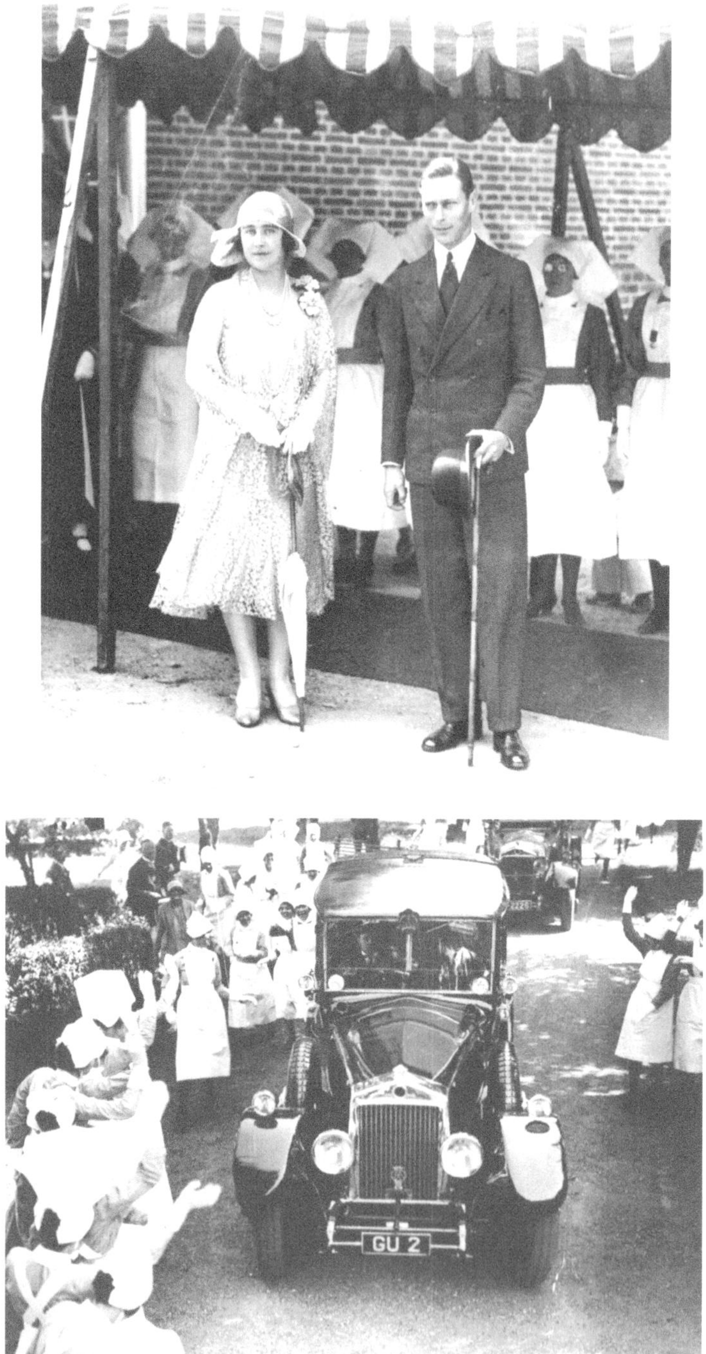

(a)

(b)

Figure 20.4 (a, b): (a) The Duke (later King George VI) and Duchess of York at the official opening of the Devonport building on 15 July 1929; (b) the 'motor-cade' at their departure.

An SHS Committee of Management minute records:

> On Monday the 15th July [1929] the new Nurses' Home and Pathological Department [now residential accommodation and the conference centre of the University of Greenwich] were formally opened by T.R.H., The Duke [President of the Society & the future King George VI] and Duchess of York. Their Royal Highnesses arrived at the entrance to the Pathological Department at 3 o'clock where they were welcomed ... by his Worship the Mayor of Greenwich. [They] were then received by Viscount Deopport [sic] and other Vice Presidents of the Society: Captain Sir Arthur Clarke, Captain Sir Ion Hamilton Benn, members of the Board, and Sir Edwin Cooper, the Architect. They were then conducted to the Library where the Directors of Pathology and the Dean of the London School of Clinical Medicine were presented…
>
> After a tour of the Laboratories [which were opened by the Duke] Their Royal Highnesses proceeded to the dais erected in the quadrangle of the Nurses' Home where an address of welcome was made by Lord Devonport, H.R.H.; The Duke of York then addressed the assembled gompany [sic] and the Rt. Rev. the Lord Bishop of Fulham dedicated the new buildings. [They] then entered the Nurses' Home by the main entrance and H.R.H. The Duchess declared open the Devonport Nurses' Home. After a tour of the Home the royal party left at 4 o'clock. About 1,500 people were present including Lady Devonport, Sir John [President of the Royal College of Physicians] and Lady Rose Bradford, Adml. Mansell, Commdr. G. Hodgkinson, Captain and Mrs. A.M. Hughes, Adml. W.H.D. and Lady Florence Boyle, Adml. and the Hon. Mrs Oliphant, Mr. A. L. l. Sturge, Mrs. Spencer Stidolph, Adml. and Mrs. Hopwood, Captain H.C. Birnie, Mr. R.T. Garrett, Mr. and Mrs. A.W. Smallwood, Mr. and the Hon. Mrs. McAlister, Mr. and Mrs. C.F. Leach, Lord and Lady Southborough, Mr. F.S.A. Baker and Adml. Sir George and Lady Webb, etc., etc. Music was provided by the Kneller Hall Band. It was resolved that the thanks of the Board be expressed to Their Royal Highnesses for their gracious act in performing the opening ceremony.

Simultaneously with this notable achievement, the Committee had approved plans (also by Cooper):

> …for the provision of a new Out-Patient Department and … a complete theatre unit at the Dreadnought Hospital. These urgently needed improvements will be effected by adding a storey to the present 'Somerset' wing and by roofing in the quadrangle between north-east 'Somerset' and 'Ground West'. The Lords Commissioners of the Admiralty have given their approval to this scheme, and it is proposed to make a start in the early spring. The cost will amount to about £35,000.

Progress with these much needed alterations was outlined the following year:

> The added storey to the 'Somerset' wing is roofed in, and it is hoped that the new surgical wards, new theatres, and Out-Patient department may be available for use towards the end of this year. There will then remain the new kitchen and dining-room block, which is to be built inside the quadrangle, and this work will be taken in hand very shortly. All these improvements and rebuilding schemes are absolutely essential in order to fit the Hospital for its work, and the Board felt that they could not delay matters any longer, although a very large capital expenditure is involved. … the Board feel it incumbent upon them to launch a special appeal to meet this expenditure.

Nurse-training

Caring for 'landsmen', women and children had always been a highly contentious issue; the 1930 Report contained the following:

> The Board have taken the important step of approving the provision of a ward of twenty-five beds for the treatment of women, and twenty beds for children, in the Dreadnought Hospital, Greenwich … This will enable the Hospital to be recognised by the General Nursing Council as a self-contained Training School for Nurses, and obviate Nurses having to take part of their training in a hospital for women and children, and will also reduce the period of their training from 3½ to 3 years.

With further emphasis on nurse-training, the 1934 Report recorded another important development:

> The Board of Management has, during the year, undertaken a new phase of activity in effecting a change over from an Affiliated Training School to a self-contained Training School for the Nursing Staff in the confidence that such a step could not but benefit its Nursing Staff and consequently the patients cared for in its wards. It is their earnest hope that nurses will now be able to leave the 'Dreadnought', having completed their training without the burden of attending special Hospitals for part of the curriculum, with as complete and efficient a training as can be obtained elsewhere.

Of more general interest is an extract from the 1937 Report:

> A number of changes and improvements have taken place in the grounds and buildings. Immediately between the Devonport Nurses' Home & Devonport Pathological Laboratories and Greenwich Park, the disused Church of St. Mary has been demolished and the site, having been conveyed to the Society by the Ecclesiastical Commissioners, has been handed over to H.M. Office of Works for maintenance in perpetuity under a deed of guardianship. A commemorative tablet and rosemary hedge mark the vaults of the old Church and in the centre of the lawn now stands the Statue of King William IVth, transferred by the

Corporation of the City of London from its former position near London Bridge.[6]

Work on the 'Old' Building

Following the launch of the new Devonport buildings, 'the much-needed re-modelling of the old buildings' could begin (see above). Unfortunately, rebuilding of the 'kitchen and dining room block' had to be abandoned for financial reasons, although the new Somerset Wing (incorporating 'The Viscountess Devonport Ward', had been completed. These extensions comprised: an out-patient department, three surgical wards, an operating theatre unit (see below) and a chapel, the latter (after restoration and redecoration, incorporating the John Lydekker memorial stained glass window) having been re-opened on 2 November 1931.

Towards the end of the Great War, an appeal for a *new* ward – the *Silver Thimble Ward* – was launched. This had been founded by Miss Hope Clarke on behalf of women worldwide, to commemorate the services of men of the MM during that War. A plaque was unveiled by Queen Alexandra (then a Patron of the Society), accompanied by HRH Princess Victoria, on 5 June 1919.

These extensions had been officially opened by the Duke of York after the Annual Court (at the *Dreadnought* Hospital) on 8 June 1932:

> After the Court His Royal Highness declared open the new Out-Patient Department, the new Operating Theatres, and the three new Surgical Wards – the 'Viscountess Devonport Ward,' the 'Arthur Clarke Ward', and 'King George's Fund for Sailors' Ward. About 600 to 700 governors and friends of the Society were present, including Admiral of the Fleet Sir Roger Keyes.

In fact, so acute was the financial position following this building programme (the Society had clearly overstretched itself) that the Chairman (Sir Arthur Clarke [1857–1932]) – who incidentally died a mere two months later – felt obliged to write to *The Times* on 24 November 1931 appealing for further donations.[7] Clarke had succeeded Nairne as SHS Chairman in 1922, having served on the Board of Management since 1905. He had inaugurated the King George's Fund for Sailors in 1917, and served on the Board of Management of: the Marine Society, the Royal Alfred Merchant Seamen's Institution, the Royal Merchant Seamen's Orphanage, the Sailors' Home and Red Ensign Club.

Numerous subsequent 'improvements' are recorded in later Reports; in 1937, for example:

> The whole Upper East Floor of the Hospital [had] been reconstructed and redecorated, the patients [then] being accommodated in larger wards at the north end, while the remainder [provided] suitable accommodation for the male staff who [had] hitherto been ill provided for. A new Lift [was also] installed giving direct service to all Floors of the East Wing. The improvements to the main and ward kitchens, [were] made possible by special donations from King George's Fund for Sailors ....[8]

The Angas Convalescent Home, Cudham

Not all was doom and gloom during the Great War. The 1918 Report referred to one of 'the great features of the year':

> The opening of a new branch of the Society – the Angas Convalescent Home [*see* Figure 20.5], of which Mrs Gilbert the widow of the Chaplain of the ADH – the Rev. T.H. Gilbert – who had died the year before, was appointed Matron. [The Home had been] a gift to the Sailor from Mrs. Angas, of Stoke Poges, in response to the appeal made by Sir Rosslyn Wemyss and Sir Henry Jackson at the [1917] Annual Meeting. This is the first occasion [the Report continued] upon which the Sailor has had provided for him a Home in which he can rest awhile to complete recovery after treatment in the wards of the Seamen's Hospital at Greenwich, or at the [ADH]. It is hard to compute the value of this gift, for the Sailor needs such a place of rest perhaps more than any other member of the community, as he is generally far from his home and friends when ill, and has no one to go to for that care and succour so very necessary in the trying days of convalescence. The Angas Home is at Cudham, on the North Kentish Downs. It stands on a freehold estate comprising about eighteen acres of ground, well wooded, and admirably situated. The Home provides [the Report concluded] accommodation for thirty patients, and was opened on 8th July.

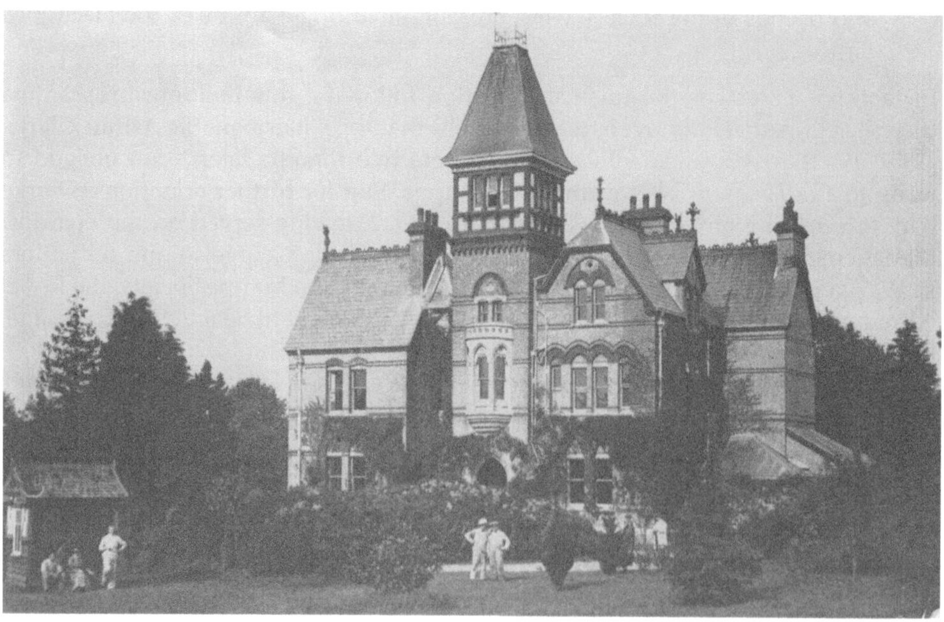

Figure 20.5: The Angas Convalescent Home at Cudham, Kent – in 1918. [SHS Archive].

An increase in accommodation was, however, soon required and on 11 September 1925, 'Mrs Angas … declared open the *new* buildings'. The Report for 1919 praised these new facilities, which in addition to the Sailor (who is 'frequently far away from his native port or place') was of value to 'sick Nurses'. Following the Great War, British schoolgirls and boys endowed a 'Schools bed' as a memorial to the bravery of seamen during the war.[9]

The *new* Hospital for Tropical Diseases

Two years after the armistice was signed (on 11 November 1918) the SHS's 'tropical' component moved from the ADH to Endsleigh Gardens, WC1 – becoming the Hospital for Tropical Diseases (HTD). The 1919 Report stated:

> [This year] will ever be memorable in the annals of the [SHS] as the year in which premises were acquired in London for a Hospital to be wholly devoted to the care and treatment of persons suffering from Tropical Diseases. The British Red Cross [BRC – who were generous benefactors to the SHS] and [the] Order of St. John of Jerusalem made possible the acquisition of premises situated at the west end of Endsleigh Gardens [*see* Figure 20.6]. The building had been used during the [Great] war as a Hospital for Officers, and is admirably suited [the Report continued] for the purpose for which it is intended. The establishment is a large one, and there is accommodation for 60 beds. The gift provides for the partial endowment of a moiety of these, and ten other beds are also endowed by the Mesopotamia Comforts Fund in memory of the late General Sir FREDERICK STANLEY MAUDE.

The Report gave details of the inscriptions on two plaques:

> Tablets are being erected in the new Hospital bearing the following inscriptions:-
>
> £100,000
> WAS GIVEN TO THE SEAMEN'S HOSPITAL SOCIETY, GREENWICH,
> For the Purchase of these Premises and
> Endowment of Beds therein by the
> JOINT WAR COMMITTEE OF THE BRITISH RED CROSS
> AND ORDER OF ST. JOHN OF JERUSALEM,
> in recognition of the SERVICES RENDERED to the EMPIRE
> By SAILORS IN THE GREAT WAR,
> and in order to provide immediate Medical Treatment for
> those Sailors and Soldiers who have contracted Tropical
> Diseases while on Active Service;
> And ultimately for the Benefit of Sailors.

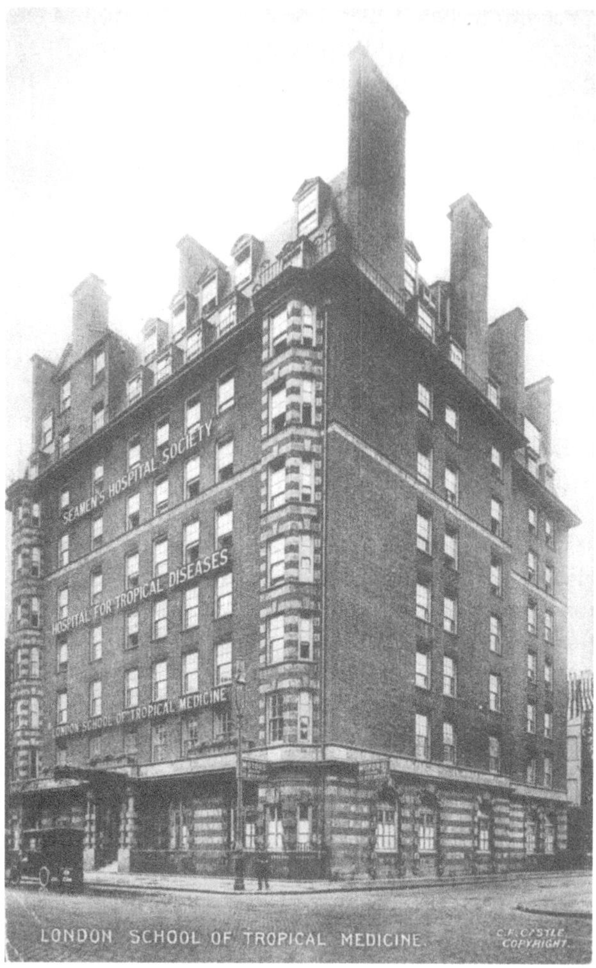

Figure 20.6: The Hospital for Tropical Diseases at Endsleigh Gardens, WC1 – officially opened on 11 November 1920. [Courtesy: The Wellcome Library, London].

THE STANLEY MAUDE WARD.
On this floor is Endowed by the
MESOPOTAMIA COMFORTS FUND
A Ward in Memory of the gallant deeds and noble death
OF THE LATE
LIEUTENANT-GENERAL
SIR FREDERICK STANLEY MAUDE,
K.C.B., C.M.G., D.S.O.,
who gave his life for his country in Mesopotamia in 1917.

So ample [the Report continued] is the accommodation that it has been found possible to provide space in the lower floors for the London School

> of Tropical Medicine [LSTM]. It has been deemed advisable to remove the School from its present position in association with the [ADH], and no more suitable situation could be found than in the same building as the [HTD] with Miss C Graham Knight, MBE as Matron, JC Gilbert as Steward, and the Vicar of St Pancras (the Rev EL Metcalfe) as Chaplain.

Further details were provided in the following Report:

> The year under review witnessed the beginning of the work of the [HTD], Endsleigh Gardens. The first patient, C.E. Long, suffering from Bilharzia [schistosomiasis], [had been] admitted on the 9th February. Very soon all the beds were occupied, and during the latter part of the year 50 beds were in daily occupation. The facilities which the munificent gift of the [BRC] has enabled this Hospital to afford have been of the very greatest service. All patients treated there were suffering from some form of Tropical Disease. On the 11th November [1920], H.R.H. The Duke of York [see above] formally declared the buildings open. … On the same occasion His Royal Highness unveiled [the] Memorial Tablet [see above] … in memory of the late General Sir Stanley Maude.

Other endowments were to follow; for example, the St Michael and St George bed.[10]

The following fatality involving a member of staff at the HTD is recorded in the 1930 Report:

> The Board regret to record that Mr. H.P. Lilles, one of the Laboratory Assistants at the [HTD], died from yellow fever contracted in the performance of routine laboratory duties. Mr. Lilles was a most promising and able young man of fine character, who for the past five years had been associated with the laboratories, first of the London School of Tropical Medicine [LSTM], and later of the Hospital for Tropical Diseases. A tablet [*see* Figure 20.7] to his memory is being erected in the laboratory in which he worked.

The following Report recorded that this tablet was unveiled on 27 May (1931) 'before a gathering of his relatives'.[11]

A competitor?

There was, soon after the opening of the newly located hospital, an 'opponent' to the Society's HTD. *The Ross Institute & Hospital for Tropical diseases* (RIHTD) was officially opened at Putney by the Prince of Wales (later King Edward VIII, 1894–1972) on 15 July 1926 (i.e. nearly six years after the 'tropical' component had moved from the ADH site to Endsleigh Gardens, WC1 [the HTD]). This institution had been founded to commemorate the discovery in India, by Sir Ronald Ross (1857–1932),[12] of mosquito involvement in the transmission of malaria. To most observers, it was obvious that London did *not* require *two* tropical hospitals. When, in 1932 (i.e. some six years after its foundation) the RIHTD was

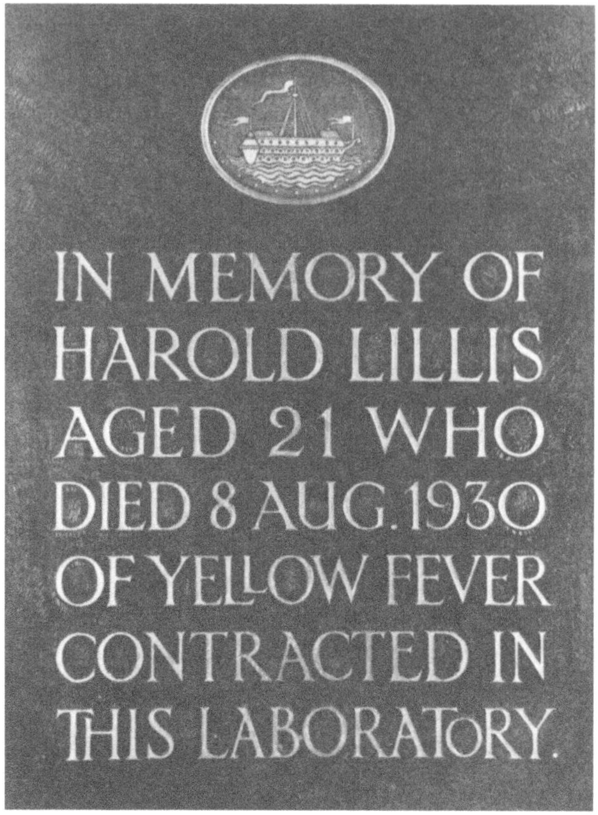

Figure 20.7: Plaque commemorating Harold Lillis who died of yellow fever contracted at the HTD in 1930. [SHS Archive].

compelled to close for financial reasons, and facilities were transferred to the London School of Hygiene and Tropical Medicine (LSHTM) as the Ross Institute; there was a need for *clinical* facilities for a member of its staff who was a physician – which the LSHTM could not provide. After lengthy negotiations, three beds (in the Ross Ward) were provided at the HTD (which was still under the control of the SHS), and A Castellani (the Director of Tropical Medicine and Dermatology at the RIHTD) was given a post at the HTD on the Associated Staff. Meanwhile, new wards, laboratories, and the 'Manson' *clinical* lecture theatre were added to the HTD, following the departure of the non-clinical departments to the newly opened LSHTM. On 20 November 1930, the HTD was formally re-opened by the Under Secretary of State for the Dominions (William Lunn MP) and the Secretary of the MRC (Sir Walter Fletcher). The HTD fund had by that date raised £13,000 – headed by a donation from Sir Leslie Wilson.[13]

Tropical nursing seems to have blossomed during these inter-war years; the 1936 Report, for example, refers to the fact that no less than '55 Nurses attended the winter courses in tropical nursing'.[14]

Opening of The London School of Hygiene and Tropical Medicine (LSHTM)

Since its inauguration at the ADH in 1899, the LSTM had remained under the auspices of the SHS. The 1924 Report referred to another important event:

> … in 1923, the Rockefeller Foundation offered a sum of £450,000 to the Ministry of Health, with a view to establishing a School of Hygiene [LSHTM], in which diseases peculiar to hot climates were also to be dealt with, and the Government also promised a substantial subsidy towards maintenance. It was felt by the [SHS] that it would be to the advantage of the medical profession, of the Tropical Colonies, and of all concerned, that these activities should be grouped under a single administration, it being at the same time agreed that the name of the [LSTM] be retained or continued in the new building, and that the teaching staff and other employees should be secure in the continuation of their interests. Two members of the Board of Management of the [SHS] are members of the Court of Governors, and one a member of the Board of Management of the [LSHTM]. These changes do not affect the [HTD] which remains one of the establishments of the Seamen's Hospital Society. …
>
> This highly-successful and thriving School will carry on both the research work and the instruction of medical graduates with increased facilities and a more extended sphere of action.

Progress was rapid, and the 1929 Report referred to the transfer of the *LSTM* to the newly built *LSHTM* building in Keppel Street. This thus gave:

> an opportunity … to effect the much-needed extension of accommodation for in-patients at that branch of the Society, and to carry out other improvements in the Hospital. In order to be ready for the leave season of 1930, the Board resolved to carry out the alterations inmediately [sic]; by the end of April, 1930, therefore, the number of beds at the [HTD] will be increased to 80. The new Pathological Department will not only fulfil the requirements of the Hospital, but will act as a centre for consultation by members of the medical profession in cases of diseases peculiar to the tropics. The new clinical lecture theatre – to be known as the 'Manson Memorial Theatre' [Mansion had died in 1922] – will be evidence of the continued close alliance between the Hospital and the School. The cost of these extensions and alterations is estimated at £20,000.

The first (and only) Director of the LSHTM was (Sir) Andrew Balfour (1873–1931), who suffered from a manic depressive psychosis, committed suicide in 1931. A plaque erected to his memory, was unveiled on 6 October 1932 by The Earl of Athlone [1974–1957].

There was, however, disquieting news from the HTD; in the 1932 Report 'a sad felling off in the number of paying patients' is recorded, and this was deemed:

> due to the world depression, which kept away undoubtedly a certain number of patients, and also prevented others from paying full maintenance charges. There has also been a much smaller flow of persons home from the East than usual. Steps have, however, now been taken which will, it is hoped, bring the [HTD] into touch with a larger number of tropical cases needing treatment in London than has hitherto been the case, and it is hoped that this branch of the Society will be able to show a better record in the coming year.

On a more optimistic note, the 1933 Report announced:

> The Board record with satisfaction the successful cooperation between [the HTD] and the [LSHTM]. The School relies for its *clinical* [my italics] teaching upon that Hospital, and members of the Hospital Staff are also members of the School Council. During the year the Ross Institute was amalgamated with the [LSHTM] and the Hospital at Putney closed [see above]. The [HTD] is now the only institution of its kind in London. In this connection the Ross Institute very kindly made over a gift of £1,000 to the [HTD] to commemorate the name of Sir Ronald Ross, and a ward has been named the 'Ronald Ross' Ward. The Hospital received also from the same donors some most useful Hospital equipment and furniture [through the kind offices of Major Lockwood Stevens].

Refurbishment of the HTD was also aired in the following Report:

> … the extensive internal rebuilding and alterations [to the HTD], which were begun in the autumn of 1929, were completed during the past year. Twenty-five beds have been added, extra accommodation … provided for the Nursing Staff, the Theatre unit and X-ray department have been entirely remodelled, and a large Clinical Demonstration Theatre (known as the "Manson" Clinical Lecture Theatre), and new Pathological Laboratories, have been provided.
>
> An oil-burning boiler plant has been installed, and the whole Hospital has been redecorated. The reconstruction and redecoration were carried out by Messrs. Higgs & Hill, from designs by, and under the supervision of, Mr. Stanley Hamp (Messrs. Collcutt & Hamp).[15]

The Albert Dock Hospital

The 1919 Report pointed out that, despite removal of the tropical component, the ADH (*see* Chapter 14) would remain open as a 'Hospital for Seamen', Miss E E Wheeler was appointed Matron in place of Miss C G Knight, and it was anticipated that all 'tropical' cases admitted there would be transferred to the HTD.

In May 1927, the new chapel at the ADH was dedicated by the Bishop of Barking. Furthermore:

> The Port of London Authority [PLA] have [the 1930 Report recorded] very kindly granted the Society some additional land, which ... enabled it to provide a tennis court for the use of the resident staff of the Hospital. This is a great acquisition, which is particularly acceptable in that district, where there are no amenities for sport and recreation.

The 1930 Report, however, also contained worrying news about the ADH:

> At the [ADH] the Society is faced in the near future ... with considerable capital expenditure. For many years no alterations or improvements have been effected there, as it was thought that the site might be required by the [PLA] for the new thoroughfare. This is now definitely ruled out, and the Board have instructed Mr. Stanley Hamp to prepare a plan for the urgent alterations required to bring the Hospital up to date.

The news was to become increasingly alarming – as the Report for 1933 illustrates:

> For several years grave anxiety has been felt in regard to the [ADH] owing to the serious movements which have taken place in the foundations. In the last few weeks it has been necessary to pull down and rebuild a portion of one of the main walls of the Hospital. It is, therefore, with much pleasure that the Board are able to announce that they have been able to come to an agreement with their landlords, the [PLA], who have met them in a most sympathetic spirit. It has been arranged that the Society's lease, which has another 36 years to run, shall be terminated at the end of five years and that in consideration, the [PLA] will make payment of £25,000 to the Society and also provide a new site [at Alnwick Road] of 1½ acres for the erection of a new Hospital. It will cost approximately £45,000 to build a new Hospital of 60 beds, and funds are urgently needed to enable the Society to begin building with as little delay as possible ...

By the following year the situation had become dire:

> Anxiety concerning the present [ADH] has greatly increased during the past year and it has been necessary on two occasions to shore up different parts of the Hospital. The building was therefore condemned and the [PLA] have most generously assisted the Society by providing a new site not far from the present one (*see* Figure 20.8), and by promising £25,000 towards the cost of the building. The total cost of the new Hospital will be approximately £65,000, so that there is still £40,000 to find, and the Board of Management most earnestly appeals to all who can help in any way to raise this sum.[16]

The new ADH

In order to raise funds for this huge project, the President launched an appeal for the 'doomed hospital':

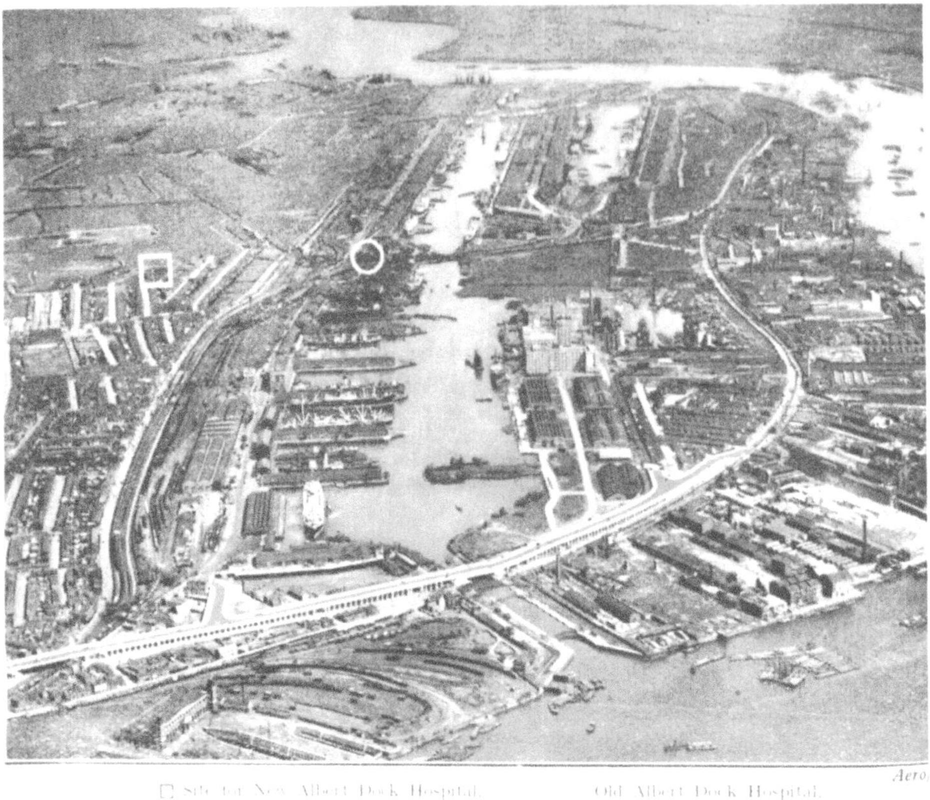

Figure 20.8: Aerial photograph (c1936) showing the sites of the *original* and 'new' ADH. [SHS Archive].

> The appeal issued by H.R.H. The Duke of York [see above] for rebuilding the [ADH] which will cost £75,000, has already met with much generous response, and there has been published a first list of donations amounting of £45,355. The [PLA] have throughout the year greatly assisted the Society in complicated negotiations concerning the new site. The condition of the old Hospital is such that the new building must be started immediately, and the Board earnestly hope that the total amount for which His Royal Highness has appealed will be contributed during the current year.

At a meeting at Trinity House on 22 October of that year in order to raise £50,000 'over and above the gift from the [PLA]' the Duke of York had this to say:

> There is no one who can disclaim his debt to the men of the Merchant Navy. The Commerce and Industry not only of the United Kingdom but of the whole Empire, depend upon the safe transport overseas of both raw materials and manufactured goods. Indeed the health and

welfare of merchant seamen are important factors in the revival of trade throughout the world.[17]

The *'new'* ADH (which was by then under construction) (*see* Figure 20.9) received extensive coverage in the 1936 Report:

> [It] will continue to offer all those services which have been available during the past 45 years in the old establishment, the principal feature of the buildings which are now rising close by will be a Model Fracture Clinic [run by Mr H Ernest Griffiths MS FRCS, and rehabilitation centre] for the treatment of the seafaring community and all those who may be injured during the loading and unloading of vessels in the Port of London. It is the aim of the Board to provide a complete service from the moment when one of the Society's motor ambulances picks up an injured

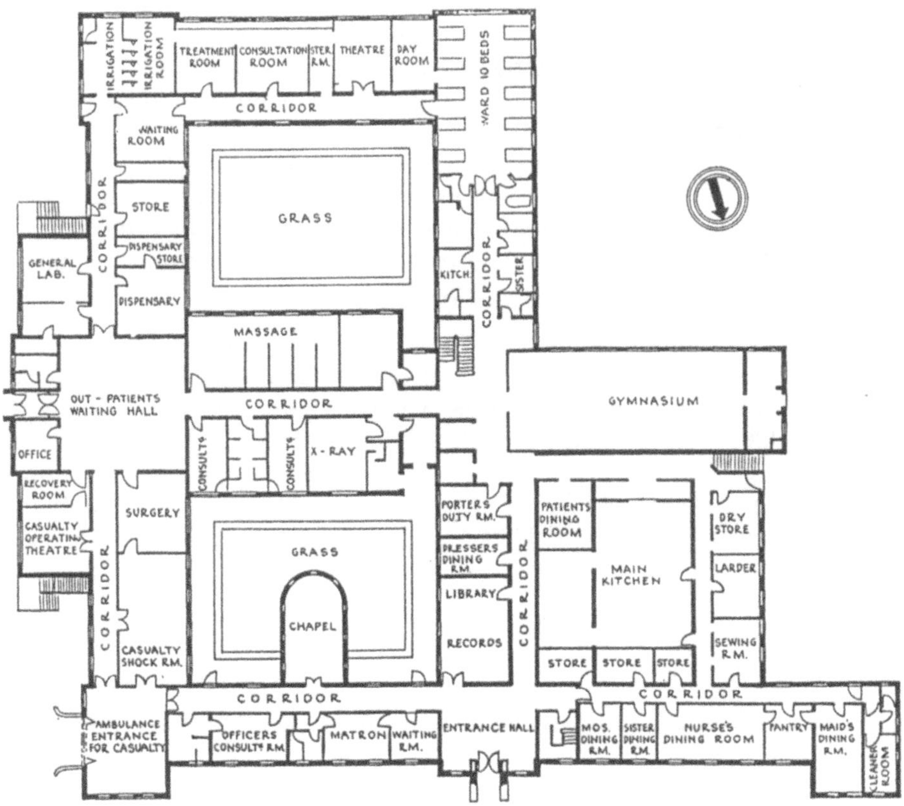

NEW ALBERT DOCK HOSPITAL—Plan of Ground Floor.

Figure 20.9: Plan of the ground-floor of the newly built ADH. [SHS archive].

> man at the scene of the accident, to the time when he is able to return to work, or the best possible physical end-result has been obtained.

But, the building programme was *not* without hitches, as the 1937 Report summarised:

> The erection of the new [ADH] ... has proceeded steadily throughout the year and it is hoped that patients and staff may be able to move over from the old buildings towards the end of the summer. The Committee are however deeply concerned over the financial position. The intervention of the Ministry of Transport, which induced the Society to relinquish for the purposes of a new highway the site granted by the [PLA] rendered useless the plans and quantity statistics which had been prepared. Fresh drawings and figures had to be made for the buildings upon another site – made available by the further help of the Port Authority – portions of which had to be subject to Closing Orders.
>
> In the new situation [Alnwick Road] it was found that instead of being on the ground level only, the necessary accommodation could only be provided in a two-storey building and this necessitated the driving into the soil of over 800 piles to support the reinforced raft carrying the buildings. In the intervening period before the building operations could be begun, there had been a marked rise in the cost of both labour and materials. These circumstances, which were entirely beyond the control of the Committee of Management, have resulted in a considerable increase in the total cost of the new Hospital and it is estimated that £11,000 is still required.

When laying the Foundation Stone of the New [Hospital] on 13 July, 1937, Lord Ritchie of Dundee, proclaimed: 'As a maritime Nation with our wealthy banking, commercial and industrial interests, we owe a great deal to the sailors who are responsible for the safe transport of goods and passengers across the seas. I hope that the greater measure of prosperity being enjoyed by those with commercial interests and those in dock areas will result in increased support so that that Hospital can be opened free of debt.'[18]

OPENING THE 'NEW' ADH

The 'new' hospital was opened in 1938:

> The In-Patients were safely transferred to the new Hospital on the morning of Thursday, the 22nd September, and the old Hospital closed its doors after 49 years of work which had made its name famous not only among sailors, but in all parts of the tropics as the home of the [LSTM].
>
> Her Majesty Queen Mary, Patroness of the Society, visited and formally declared open the new [ADH] ... on Trafalgar Day, the 21st October. At that ceremony, 'Lord Lloyd [now President of the SHS] offered an address of welcome to Her Majesty and presented to her

> a paper knife made from some wood from the laboratory bench used by the late Sir Patrick Manson in his work in tropical medicine at the old [ADH].

Therefore, the rebuilt hospital had reached completion in late 1938, a year which, according to the Report for that year:

> ... will take its place as a red-letter year, notable [not only] for the completion of the new ... Hospital [but] for the gracious marks of personal favour bestowed upon the Society's work by Her Majesty Queen Mary and His Royal Highness the Duke of Kent. Although the new [ADH] is now in full working order – and is achieving results in both medical and surgical cases as remarkable as were ever obtained formerly at the old [ADH] – the sum of £6,000 is still required to complete the Rebuilding Fund. The Committee assure the Governors that all possible steps are being taken to keep alive the Society's claim for compensation arising from the change in the site of the new Hospital at the request of the Ministry of Transport to facilitate their plans for a new arterial highway to improve road transport in the dock area.[19]

King George's sanatorium at Bramshott Place, Liphook, Hampshire

In 1919 the first steps were taken to establish a sanatorium:

> ... Seamen suffer from consumption (*see* Chapter 23) almost more than any other class of the community, and the Society is establishing an Institution in the country where they may treat and care for those who may recover, and comfort and succour others whose health may never be restored. Mrs. Angas, of Dirry Mor, Stoke Poges, the founder of the Convalescent Home, was the first to come forward with an offer of a substantial sum towards the foundation of this Sanatorium and this was quickly followed by a grant from King George's Fund for Sailors. With this encouragement the Committee of Management have found a site in Hampshire and have entered into negotiations for Bramshott Place [to be called the 'King George's Sanatorium for Sailors' (*see* Figure 20.10) – with the Rector of Bramshott (the Rev. A F Polehampton) as Chaplain], a suitable building with an estate of about 100 acres. This has been approved by Dr [Christopher] Addison [1869–1951, *see* Figure 20.11],[20] the Minister of Health, who will make the usual Government grant towards initial expenses, and Lord Inchcape[21] is inviting contributions to a Subscription List which he has headed with £10,000 [this Appeal had reached £100,000 by the end of 1921]. It is to endow and partly to equip this branch of the Society's work that the Committee earnestly appeal to all supporters of the Charity and all others who recognise what we owe to the Sailor.[22]

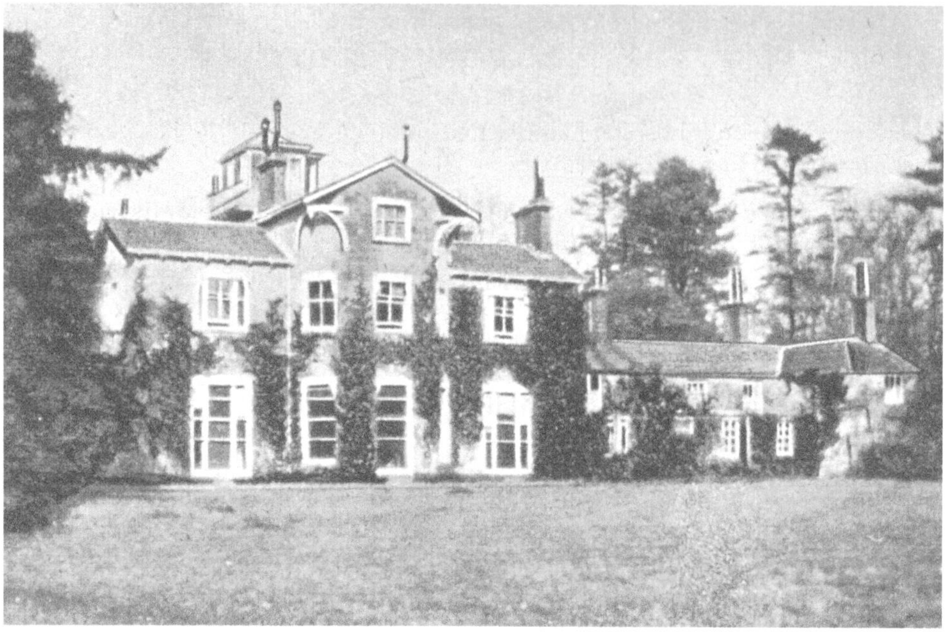

Figure 20.10: The King George's Sanatorium for Sailors at Bramshott, Hampshire – opened in 1921. [SHS Archive].

Opening the Sanatorium

The sanatorium consisted of a pavilion 'containing 80 beds and standing in 100 acres of grounds amid wooded walks and old gardens'. In addition to merchant seamen, a good many naval ratings and marines were treated there.

The 1920 Annual Report recorded:

> H.R.H. The Duke of York [President of the SHS] declared open the Sanatorium on the 12th of July [the first patients had been admitted on 8 July, and the Matron was Miss J Williams – formerly a sister at the *Dreadnought*], and so for the first time in the long history of this Corporation special and adequate accommodation has been provided for the Sailor suffering from the dire disease of consumption, where he may receive the most approved modern methods of treatment. For this great boon the Sailor is indebted to Lord Inchcape, who raised the Fund that enabled the Sanatorium to be provided. Prior to this establishment being open the Sailor suffering from consumption was treated on the roof [the Ranlett ward – named after two SHS physicians Rankin and Hewlett – *see* Chapter 21] of the old Hospital at Greenwich, but the proximity of this building to the river, and its lack of modern appurtenances, did not give the patients the best chance of recovery.

The Sanatorium Chapel was dedicated on 27 September 1922 by Bishop Crossley. A distinguished visitor in 1919 was Queen Alexandra (see above) who on 5 June

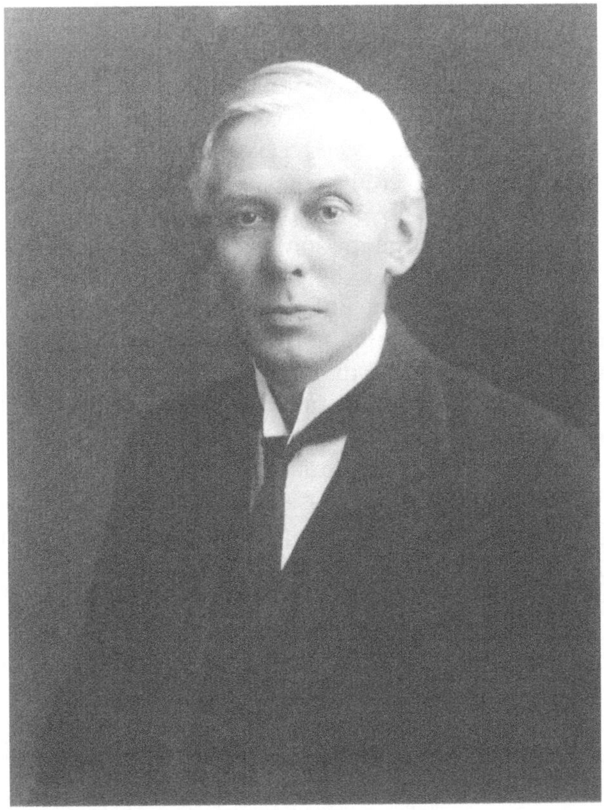

Figure 20.11: Christopher Addison (later first Viscount Addison) (1869–1951) the first Minister of Health. [Courtesy, the Wellcome Library, London].

unveiled a Tablet 'commemorating the gift of £10,000 from the Sliver Thimble Fund'.

During the first full year (1922), it is recorded that the sanatorium 'fully justified its existence', and the cost of running worked out at £2=18=9 per bed per week. It was not long, however, before extensions were required, and the 1925 Report informed its readership that a new kitchen and lift were required, as well as ultra-violet rays for the 'treatment of tuberculosis patients'. Details of the functioning of the Sanatorium (including staff lists and a 'breakdown' of disease encountered (Chapter 23) were presented in subsequent Annual Reports.[23]

A hospital for the Tilbury docks

The Report for 1923 documented developments at Tilbury, by now a booming dock town, about 25 miles down river:

There has … been fulfilled a scheme which was first under consideration in the year 1888, that is, the establishment of a Branch of the Society in the Tilbury Docks. At that time the Committee did not feel justified in undertaking the care and responsibility of another establishment, and although the matter has been receiving attention on more than one occasion during the intervening years, it has not been possible to bring it to fruition. In the year 1896 a small Hospital was established at the Tilbury Docks, with accommodation for 15 in-patients. This Institution, known as the 'Passmore Edwards' District Cottage Hospital' [PEDCH*] has done excellent work; but, in the view of the extension of the docks, the Committee of that Hospital felt that it was time the establishment was enlarged and brought up to date, to enable it to meet the increased demands which will be made upon it. Accordingly the [SHS] was approached with the request that they should take over the management of the [PEDCH]. This additional responsibility the Committee has accepted, and the Hospital passed into their administration as from January 1st, 1924. In future, this Hospital will be known as the 'Tilbury Hospital [*see* Figure 20.12],' the name 'Passmore Edwards' being retained in connection with the present building, which will form one of the wings of the Hospital when enlarged. Dr. J.J.S. Rowe, an old official of the Society, who has served for some years at the Hospital at Greenwich, has been appointed Resident Medical Officer at Tilbury, and took up his duties on the 1st January, and the Committee have every confidence in feeling that the traditions of the Dreadnought will be maintained in this new branch of their activities. It is hoped to extend the Hospital, so as to afford proper accommodation for the Out-Patient Department and to bring up to 30 the number of beds for in-patients. Before handing over to the [Society] the former Tilbury Hospital Committee had made arrangements for the provision and housing of an X-Ray installation of the latest pattern, and had also completely re-equipped the operating theatre.

An important feature of this Hospital [the Report continued] is that, by the generosity of Mr. P.J. Singhanee, of Bombay, separate accommodation is provided for Indian patients. Mr. Singhanee presented a sum of One Lakh of Rupees (£6,732) for the construction and equipment of the ward and for its endowment. This ward is now in the course of erection.

The acquisition of the Tilbury Hospital rounds off the Society's work, making them responsible for sick and injured Seamen in the whole of the Port of London.[24]

* This hospital had been founded by the philanthropist John Passmore Edwards (1823–1911) in 1896 and enlarged in 1900. It is first listed as Tilbury Hospital (one of the SHS's establishments) in the *Medical Directory* for 1926.

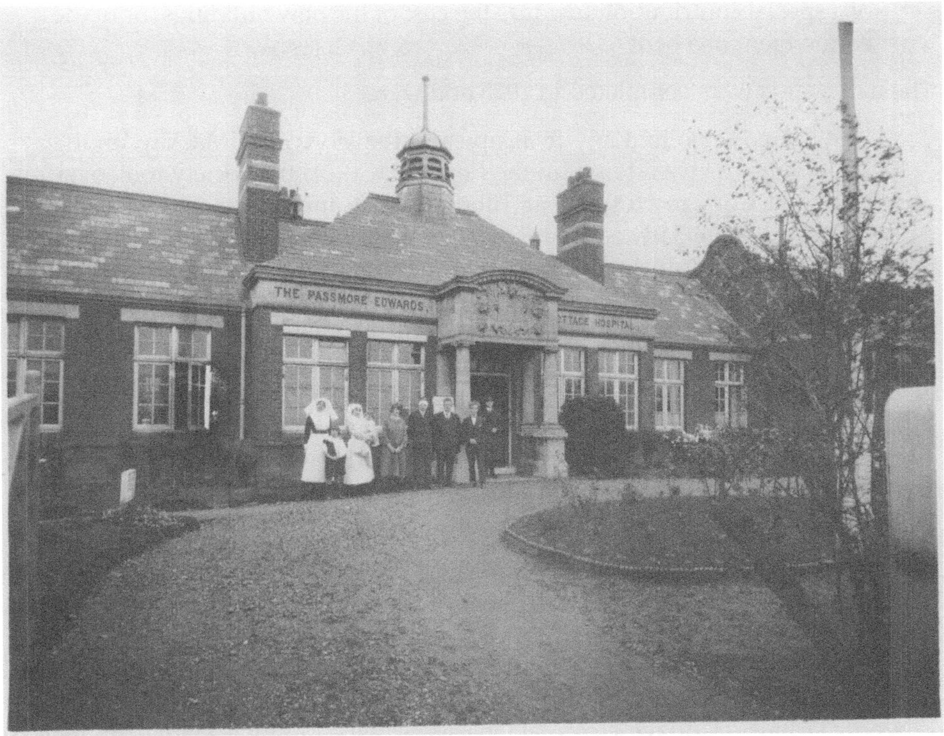

Figure 20.12: The Tilbury Hospital (which incorporated part of the old 'Passmore Edwards' District Cottage Hospital') in 1925; it was opened in 1924. This building was situated at the Dock Gate(s). [SHS Archive].

Opening the Tilbury Wards

The following report referred to the laying of the foundation stone of the *new* building:

> On the 27th June, the President ... visited the Society's Hospital at Tilbury, in order to declare open the Singhanee Ward [for Lascar patients, and which was enlarged to 16 beds in 1928], and at the same time to lay the foundation stone of the new buildings. These comprise a Nurses' Home and two new Wards of 22 beds each. Mr. Stanley Hamp, F.R.I.B.A., of Messrs. Colcutt & Hamp, who designed the Sanatorium Pavilion at Bramshott for the Society [see above], is the Architect. The Tilbury buildings are single-storied pavilions [which] may be taken to be the most up-to-date example of hospital construction. Such good progress is being made that it is hoped to open the new Hospital [the Chaplain was to be the Vicar of St. John's, Tilbury (the Rev. W.C. Bown)] during the course of the summer. It will cost upwards of £30,000 to enlarge and equip this branch of the Society, and the Committee invite the assistance and support of every well-wisher of the Sailor, in the form either

> of a special contribution towards the cost of the new buildings, or of the endowment of a bed.

The new wards were completed in 1925 and were:

> … declared open by Lady Inchcape and the Hon. Elsie Mackay, on the 24th of June. As was stated [in the Report for 1924] the Society took over the small Cottage Hospital at Tilbury, which then contained 17 beds, with an average daily occupation of 7 patients. Now it has been enlarged to 65 beds, and during the last two months of the year there was an average daily occupation of 55. … Here, at the threshold of the Port of London, patients who have become ill or who have met with accident upon the high seas, can obtain immediate attention on the arrival of the ship. The quayside is in close proximity to the Hospital and therefore patients can be landed and tended without delay. By the opening of this Branch, another important development of the work of the [SHS] has been accomplished, and it is proving of the greatest advantage to the shipping community and others.

After the surrender of the Tilbury Hospital to the NHS in 1948 (Chapter 22), the SHS Secretary sent a number of documents relating to that hospital to the Secretary, South East Essex Hospital Management Committee; these included: (i) the agreement to transfer the Passmore Edwards Hospital to the SHS (12 December 1923), (ii) three agreements between the SHS and PLA (1925), (iii) copies of the Passmore Edwards (Tilbury) Cottage Hospital Charity Scheme (30 June 1928), (iv) the lease of the Hospital and adjoining premises for the PLA to the SHS, for 80 years from 25 December 1926, (v) the Charity Commissioners scheme (20 October 1925), and (vi) a schedule of dilapidations to the Children's Ward (21 February 1945).[25]

The Marseilles' venture

The 1927 Report stated that:

> During the summer the Committee of the Queen Alexandra Memorial Hospital at Marseilles [southern France] opened negotiations with a view to entrusting the administration and management of their Hospital to the [SHS] … A Scheme for providing a British Hospital at Marseilles [had been] started in January, 1918. The work of … raising the necessary funds and carrying out the building and equipping of the Hospital has been done [the Report continued] by a Committee in Marseilles under the chairmanship of H.M. Consul-General, and by a Finance Committee in London. It was not until September, 1927, however, that the Hospital was finished and equipped, and ready to receive patients.
>
> [The SHS] Board decided to undertake the maintenance of the Hospital as from 1st January, 1928. They felt the more justified in doing so as the Hospital was always mainly intended for sailor patients, and was originally called 'The British Merchant Seamen's Hospital'. After

> the death of Queen Alexandra [in 1925], H.M. the King [had] graciously permitted the Hospital to be known as the 'Queen Alexandra Memorial Hospital'. By happy coincidence, our Royal President was already Patron, and H.R.H. the Duchess of York, Patroness of the Hospital.

And this Report continued with a description of the Hospital and its administration:

> [It] stands in its own grounds, and is situated in the higher part of the town overlooking the docks [*see* Figure 20.13]. In addition to the general wards it provides accommodation for Officers of the [MM] and a certain number of private patients. An important feature is a separate section for infectious or contagious cases. The total number of beds is 60. A British Medical Officer is resident in the Hospital, and the Nursing Staff is composed of fully-trained British Nurses. The Board have appointed the old Executive Committee in Marseilles *en bloc* as Local Advisory Committee; this body, with a resident Secretary, will be responsible to the Board for the details of administration. ... This is the first time that the Society has undertaken the work of caring for sick seamen outside the shores of Great Britain, and it is hoped that the Hospital may also be a boon to many travellers east or west on the highways of the sea.

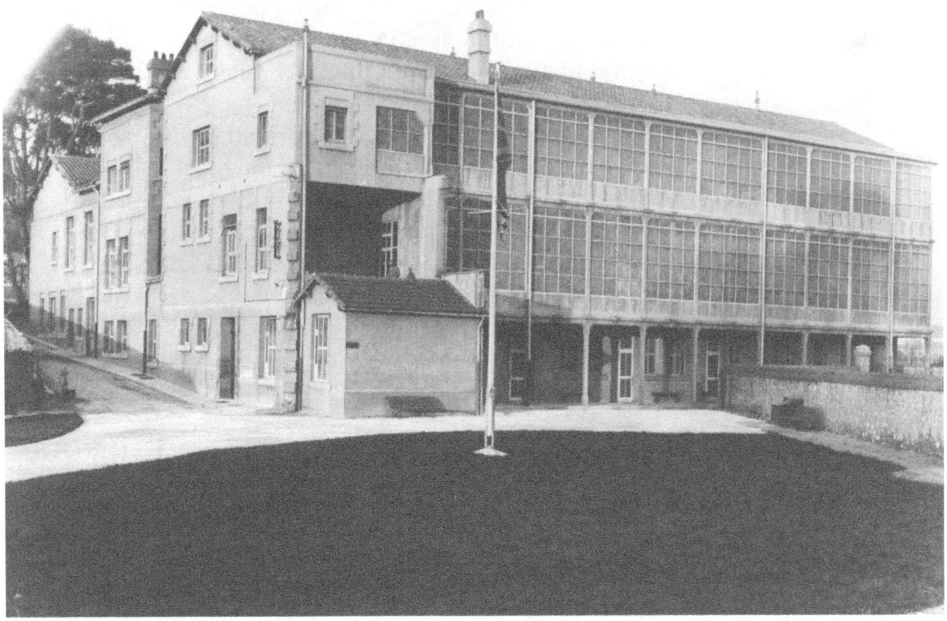

Figure 20.13: Queen Alexandra Memorial Hospital, Marseilles, in 1928. [SHS archive].

The following year (1928), the Report recorded:

> [This hospital has now] been successfully taken over and is now being administered by the Society. As is natural during the first year of administration, there have been difficulties to overcome, but, thanks to the guidance of the local Advisory Committee ..., the goodwill of the French authorities, and the good service of ... the Resident Secretary, this new branch has now found its footing. During the year there has been an average daily occupation of 20.5 patients.
>
> The Board report with much gratification that Their Royal Highnesses the Prince of Wales [later King Edward VIII] and the Duke of Gloucester paid a visit to the Hospital on their way to Africa last September. They were received by Sir Arthur Clarke, the Chairman of the Society, and a large number of members of the British colony of Marseilles were gathered within the Hospital grounds to welcome the royal visitors. ... The Hospital ... has more than justified its existence, and has earned the gratitude of many patients who have had occasion to seek in the Port of Marseilles the aid of a Hospital run on British lines.

Closure of the Queen Alexandra Memorial Hospital

Sadly the Marseilles enterprise did not last long (less than five years); the 1932 Report recorded:

> The Queen Alexandra Memorial Hospital, Marseilles, was closed in July. The Board were forced to this decision with much regret, but the Hospital had always been a costly one to administer and maintain and the percentage of beds occupied remained very low, and since the serious decline in the value of the pound sterling in France, the burden became intolerable.
>
> The Board wish to thank all those who have supported the Marseilles Hospital. They also owe a deep debt of gratitude to the local Advisory Committee with whom they have always worked in the greatest harmony during the 4½ years that the Hospital was in the care of the [SHS]. The members of the Honorary Medical Staff (all French Doctors) gave most loyal and whole-hearted service and the Hospital is particularly indebted to Dr. Hawthorn (French, despite his name) for his devoted work in the interests of the Institution.[26]

Closure of the East India Dock Dispensary, and the opening of one at Southampton

Expansion of the SHS 'Empire' was a prominent feature during the inter-war years, but clearly a close watch on facilities was paramount. The 1929 Report, for example, outlined the history of what had been an important development (i.e. the first SHS dispensary [*see* Chapter 14]) almost 50 years previously:

> This Dispensary, which first started at Well Street, London Docks, in 1880, was transferred to East India Dock Road in 1891, but of late years the number of patients attending has sunk to such a comparatively low figure that it was felt that the time had come to close this branch of the Corporation.
>
> At the same time there have been indications that a dispensary at Southampton would meet a need amongst the seafaring folk of that port, and steps were taken to acquire a suitable building and to open a new dispensary there. The old East India Dock Dispensary [EIDRD] closed its doors on 31st December, 1929, and the new institution at Southampton opened on 3rd December, 1929. Immediate first-aid treatment will be given there by the Society's Medical Officer, who may, if necessary, draft suitable cases for admission to one of the Society's hospitals [see above]. The Board hope that by the end of the year [1929] they will be able to submit a report which will justify the action taken in extending the work of the Society to that large and growing port. … Dr. Bernard Bourke, who some years ago was a House Surgeon at the Dreadnought Hospital, and who is now in practice in Southampton, has been appointed Medical Officer to this new branch.

The following Report stated:

> Dr. W.H.F. Oxley, who held the post of Medical Officer to the [EIDRD] for nearly thirty years, has been appointed Consulting Medical Officer to [the Southampton] Dispensary. Dr. Bernard Bourke continues as Medical Officer in charge of the Dispensary.

But this institution was also a victim of financial constraints, and the 1932 Report recorded: 'The closing of the Dispensary at Southampton, was a further step in saving expense. It was felt that the number of patients attending there hardly justified the maintenance of the establishment'.[27]

Other SHS matters

Venues for Society meetings

The Report for 1933 recorded: 'During the year the Chamber of Shipping of the United Kingdom has again generously placed its Board Room at the disposal of the [SHS] for its Monthly Board Meetings, and the Tilbury Contracting & Dredging Co., and the Orient Steam Navigation Company for the Meetings of Sub-Committees. The Board gratefully acknowledge this most valuable help'.[28]

Dreadnought Hospital

In July 1930, the old operating theatre at the *Dreadnought* Hospital was demolished and replaced with a new one (*see* Figure 20.14).

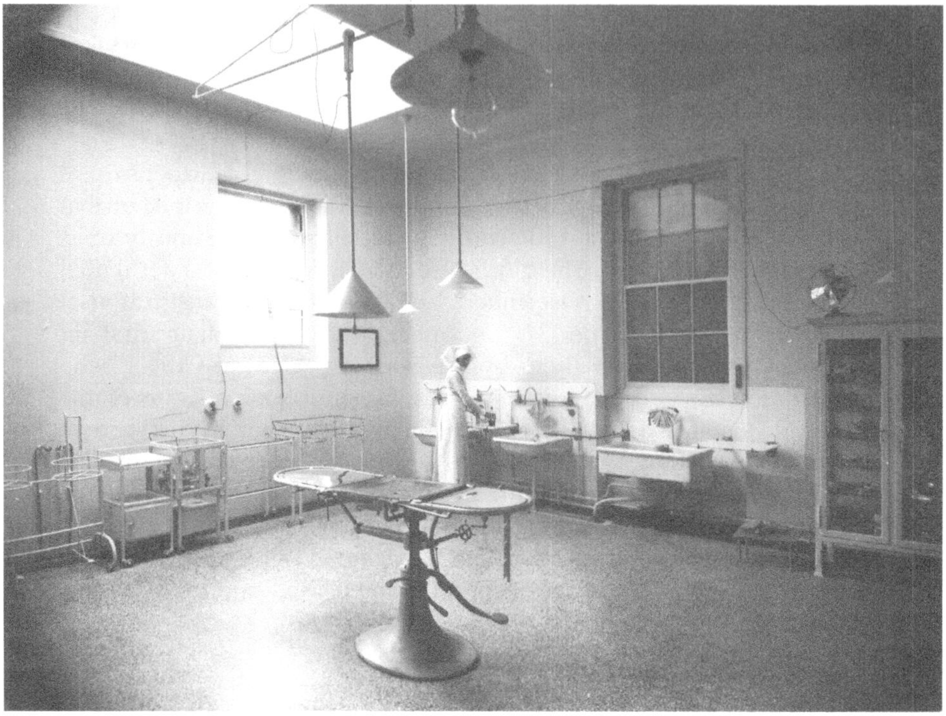

Figure 20.14: The new *Dreadnought* Hospital operating theatre, circa 1920s.

Ambulance facilities

The 1924 Report referred to the fact that captains of ships could now send 'a wireless message, to have one of the Society's Ambulances (*see* Figure 20.15) waiting at the quay-side when his vessel births'. 'By this means [the report continued] it is now possible ... by preventing sepsis from becoming fatal, to save the limb, or even the life, of a Sailor'. The Society was apparently, in 1931, the only organisation to maintain its own fleet of *motor* ambulances; there were four vehicles; three 'Guy chassis fitted respectively with an ambulance body, a converted ambulance body and a laundry van body ... and one 12hp Austin runabout van ...'

The 1932 Report recorded: 'On Wednesday, 27th April, Sir Malcolm Campbell kindly attended a ceremony at the Dreadnought Hospital when the fleet of two motor ambulances and a laundry van, the gift of the Seamen's Hospital Aid Committee, were formally handed over to the Society. Sir Malcolm ... named these Ambulances: "Grampus" and "Dreadnought".'.[29]

Outbreak of the Second World War (1939–45)

The Report for 1939 declared:

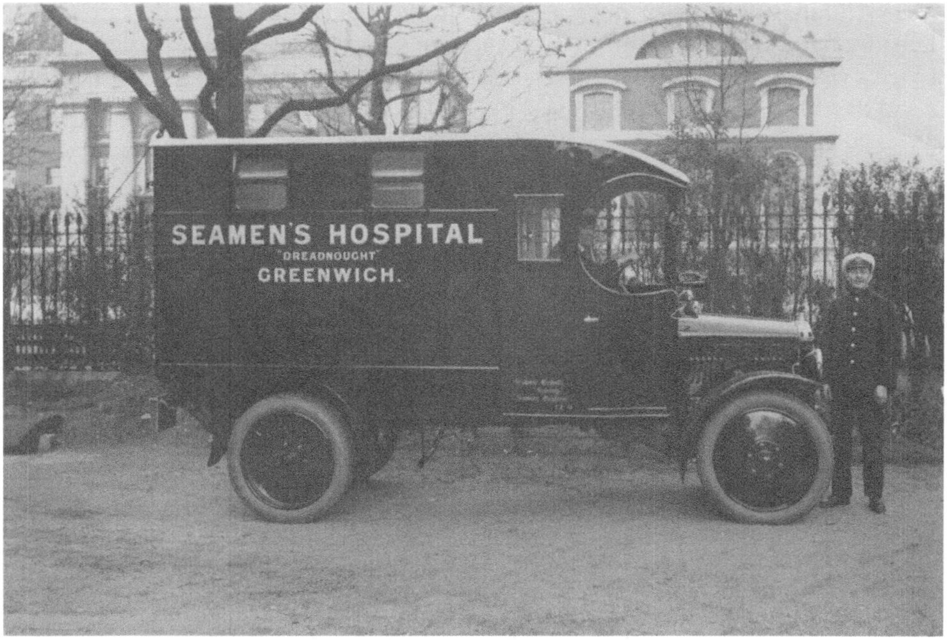

Figure 20.15: The Society's first *motor* ambulance. [SHS archive].

> On the outbreak of War [on 3 September 1939] three of our Hospitals were called upon to play their part as Casualty Clearing Hospitals in the Minister of Health's Emergency Hospital Service [EMS], which had been designed to meet the needs of air raid casualties, and consequently a considerable number of beds have remained reserved by the Minister for this purpose. Nevertheless, no seriously sick, injured or wounded officer or man of the British Merchant Navy, or from vessels of allied or friendly countries, has been denied the treatment he requires...
>
> [This report continued] The sailors now in the Society's Hospitals are those who have been injured directly by the enemy's mines, torpedoes or bombs, or whose health has been impaired by the great hardships of their ceaseless vigil while maintaining the seaborne trade of the nation. The Society's work in War is therefore identified with the relief of distress among sailors whose gallantry on active service is the admiration of the British Empire, of our Allies and of all friendly Nations.

Furthermore, the report pointed out: the *Angas Convalescent Home* was 'equipped and staffed as a Recovery Hospital', and the *King George's Sanatorium* was 'now receiving Royal Naval Ratings suffering from tubercle'. Meanwhile the *HTD* (an 8-storey building at Endsleigh Gardens, WC1) had been evacuated, being deemed 'unsuitable for the retention of In-patients in the event of enemy attack from the air'; arrangements were therefore made 'to give In-Patient treatment to a very limited number of *tropical* [my italics] cases in the Officers' Wards of the Dreadnought Hospital', and a 'Consultative Out-Patient Clinic' was to be held twice a week at the LSHTM. This was, as Manson-Bahr subsequently related, thus a sad day for *clinical* tropical disease in London.[30]

References and notes

1. Annual Report 95: 11–12; 98: 10; 100: 18.
2 *Ibid.* 97: 11.
3 *Ibid.* 95.
4 **Hudson Ewbanke Kearley** (1856–1934), who was a grocer and politician (who became in 1905 Parliamental Secretary to the Board of Trade); he was appointed Chairman of the newly created Port of London Authority (PLA) in 1909, a position which he held until 1925. Kearley's first experience of the *Dreadnought* Hospital dates back to 1916. He was created Baron Devonport in 1912. [*See also:* J Michelli. Lord Devonport: one of the Society's greatest benefactors. *SHS Quart Mag* 1934; 6 (4): 8–9; R Devonport-Hines. Kearley, Hudson Ewbanke, first Viscount Devonport (1856–1934) In: H C G Matthew, B Harrison (eds). *Oxford Dictionary of National Biography.* Oxford: Oxford University Press 2004; 30: 960–1].
5 **Sir (Thomas) Edwin Cooper** FRIBA (1874–1942) was a distinguished British architect. Amongst many buildings designed by him were the Port of London Authority (PLA) building, and the SHS buildings at Greenwich. He was knighted in 1923. [*See also*: A Powers. Cooper, Sir (Thomas) Edwin (1874–1942) In: H C G Matthew, B Harrison (eds). *Oxford Dictionary of National Biography.* Oxford: Oxford University Press 2004; 13: 246–8].
6 *Op cit.* See note 1 above: 106: 13–14; 109: 14–15; 110: 14–15; 114: 15; 117: 13–14; Anonymous. An Act to authorise buildings to be erected on a disused burial ground forming part of Greenwich Hospital – 7 August 1925. 15 & 16 Geo. 5. cap 58.
7 *Op cit.* See note 1 above: 101: 13; 103: 14–15; 105: 14–15; 111: 14–15; 112: 18; Anonymous. Wards in the Hospitals of the Seamen's Hospital Society: (i) The Silver Thimble Ward. *SHS Quart Mag* 1931; 3 (4): 12–13; Anonymous. Captain Sir Arthur Clarke: a friend of all seamen. *Ibid.* 1932; 4 (1): 9–10; Anonymous. The work of the 'Silver Thimble': an incident of the Great War. *Ibid.* 1938; 10 (2): 14–15; A Clarke. *Times, Lond* 1931: 24 November.
8 *Op cit.* See note 1 above: 117: 14.
9 *Op cit.* See note 1 above: 98: 11; 99: 13; 105: 15; [*See also*: J Michelli. What the schools are doing for the sick sailor: the first Schools' bed at the Angus Home, Cudham. *SHS Quart Mag* 1932; 4 (l): 14–16].
10 *Op cit.* See note 1 above: 98: 11–12; 100: 11; Anonymous. "St George for England!": the Order of St Michael and St George. Proposed endowment of a bed. *SHS Quart Mag* 1932; 4 (1): 14–16.
11 *Op cit.* See note 1 above. 110: 25; 111: 26; G C Cook. Fatal yellow fever contracted at the Hospital for Tropical Diseases, London, UK, in 1930. *Trans Roy Soc Trop Med Hyg* 1994; 88: 712–713.
12 **Sir Ronald Ross** KCMG (1857–1932) was born in India to Scottish parents. He served in the Indian Medical Service (1881–99) and in 1897 demonstrated at Secunderabad a rôle for the mosquito in human malaria transmission. The following year, at Calcutta, he delineated the complete life cycle of *avian* malaria (*Proteosoma*). Ross was awarded the Nobel prize for Physiology or Medicine in 1902. He spent the latter years of his life at the *Ross*

Institute & Hospital for Tropical Diseases at Putney, which had been founded in his honour. [*See also*: W F Bynum. Ross, Sir Ronald (1857–1932) In: H C G Matthew, B Harrison (eds). *Oxford Dictionary of National Biography.* Oxford: Oxford University Press 2004; 47: 842–6].

13 Anonymous. Hospital for Tropical Diseases: opening of wards, laboratories and 'Manson' clinical lecture theatre. *SHS Quart Mag* 1930; 2 (4): 7–8; G C Cook. The Ross Institute and Hospital for Tropical Disease. In: *From the Greenwich Hulks to Old St Pancras: a history of Tropical Disease in London.* London: Athlone Press: 1992: 259–266; G C Cook. Aldo Castellani FRCP (1877–1971) and the founding of the Ross Institute & Hospital for Tropical Diseases at Putney. *J Med Biog* 2000; 8: 198–205; G C Cook. A difficult metamorphosis: the incorporation of the Ross Institute & Hospital for Tropical Diseases into the London School of Hygiene and Tropical Medicine. *Med Hist* 2001; 45: 483–506.

14 *Op cit.* See note 1 above: 116: 20.

15 *Ibid.* 104: 14–16; 109: 14–16; 112: 15; 113: 15–16; *Op cit.* See note 13 above; [*See also*: Anonymous. Memorial to Sir Andrew Balfour: his work for tropical medicine. *SHS Quart Mag* 1932; 4 (4): 11; G C Cook. Evolution: the art of survival. *Trans R Soc Trop Med Hyg* 1994; A S MacNalty, M E Gibson. Balfour, Sir Andrew (1873-1931). In: H C G Matthew, B Harrison (eds). *Oxford Dictionary of National Biography.* Oxford: Oxford University Press 2004; 3: 493–4].

16 *Op cit.* See note 1 above: 107: 24; 110: 16; 113: 14–15; 114: 15; G C Cook, A J Webb. The Albert Dock Hospital, London: the original site (in 1899) of tropical medicine as a new discipline. *Acta Trop* 2001; 79: 249–255.

17 *Op cit.* See note 1 above: 115: 14.

18 *Ibid.* 116: 13; 117: 13–14.

19 *Ibid.* 118: 13.

20 **Christopher Addison** KG MD FRCS, first Viscount Addison (1869–1951) received his medical training St Bartholomew's Hospital, and became a lecturer in anatomy there. Amongst numerous senior government appointments, he was the first Minister of Health (1919–21). [*See also*: K O Morgan. Addison, Christopher, first Viscount Addison (1869–1951) In: H C G Matthew, B Harrison (eds). *Oxford Dictionary of National Biography.* Oxford: Oxford University Press 2004; 1: 315–9].

21 **James Lyle Mackay** (1852–1932), who became the first Earl of Inchcape, was throughout his life involved with shipping. Having served in India, he returned to England in 1893 to take charge of the British India Company. He was to become the Government's authority on commercial relations between Britain and India. Inchcape was in fact to become 'the most prominent figure in British shipping'. He was also the founder of the KGSS and was elected a Vice-President of the SHS in 1921. [*See also*: Anonymous. Capt. The Rt. Hon. Earl of Inchcape, G.C.S.I, G.C.M.G., K.C.I.E., R.N.R. *SHS Quart Mag* 1932; 4 (2): 10–11; K Grieves. Mackay, James Lyle, first earl of Inchcape (1852–1932) In: H C G Matthew, B Harrison (eds). *Oxford Dictionary of National Biography.* Oxford: Oxford University Press 2004; 35: 515–8].

22 *Op cit.* See note 1 above: 99: 15; 100: 12; 101: 14. [*See also*: Anonymous. The foundation of King George's sanatorium: what the Seamen's Hospital Society owes to Lord Inchcape. *SHS Quart Mag* 1932; 4 (3): 15].

23 *Op cit.* See note 1 above: 100: 13; 102: 13–14. 105: 13; Seamen's Hospital Society. King George's Sanatorium for Sailors, Bramshott Place, Liphook, Hants. Medical Superintendents' Report for the year 1938. London: E G Berryman. *Ibid* 1943, 1944.

24 *Op cit.* See note 1 above: 103: 14–15; Seamen's Hospital Society: *Tilbury District Cottage Hospital – 1896–1910* [SHS Archive]; *Ibid* 1911–1923.

25 *Op cit.* See note 1 above: 104: 13–14; 115: 13–14; F A Lyon to E E Taylor. *Tilbury Hospital* 1949; 13 June: 2.

26 *Op cit.* See note 1 above: 107: 16–17; 108: 14–15; 112: 16.
27 *Ibid*: 109: 15–16; 110: 17, 112, 16.
28 *Ibid*: 113, 17.
29 *Ibid*: 104: 13; 112: 23; [*See also:* Anonymous. A Hospital's own fleet. *SHS Quart Mag* 1931; 3 (2): 13–15; Anonymous. New ambulances for Seamen's Hospital: named by Sir Malcolm Campbell. *SHS Quart Mag* 1932; 4 (2): 20–21].
30 *Op cit.* See notes 1: 119: 4–5; and 13 above (Cook, 1992: 267–96); P Manson-Bahr. *History of the School of Tropical Medicine in London (1899–1949)* London: H K Lewis 1956: 75; G C Cook. History of tropical medicine – William Ernest Cooke FRCSI (1879–1967) and his Asian tour of 1929–1930. *Acta Tropica* 2006; 100: 1–10.

Chapter 21

Staffing during the Great War and inter-war years

During the two decades prior to the Great War (1914–18), many additions were made to the medical staff (*see* Chapters 15 and 19). This had had a great deal to do with the foundation of the two schools under the auspices of the Society – the *LSTM* in 1899, and the *LSCM* in 1906 (*see* Chapters 18 and 19). With the exception of the war years, when most of the medical and also administrative staff served the country in the armed services, this chapter dwells on a period of temporary stability for the Society. Short biographies of many of the more influential, or colourful, office-holders in the Society between 1914 and 1939 are given.

Non-medical staff

Table 21.1 summarises the senior non-medical staff from the beginning of the Great War and during the inter-war years.

Table 21.1: The Society's Honorary and administrative staff (1914–39).

Patron:	
19[14]–36	King George V (1865–1936) and Queen Mary (1867–1953)*
1936–37	King Edward VIII (1894–1972)
1937–[39]	King George VI (1895–1952)
President:	
19[14]–21	Admiral HSH Prince Louis of Battenberg (later Admiral the Most Hon. The Marquess of Milford Haven) GCB GCVO KCMG (1854–1921)*
1921–37	HRH (later Vice-Admiral, RN) The Duke of York KG KT GCMG GCVO [later King George VI] (1895–1952)
1938–[39]	The Rt Hon. Baron Lloyd of Dolobran PC GCS GCIE (1879–1941)
Chairman, Committee of Management:	
19[14]–21	(Sir) P A Nairne (1841–1921)*
1922–32	Captain Sir Arthur W Clarke KCVO KBE (1857–1932)
1932–37	The Rt Hon. Baron Lloyd of Dolobran PC GCSI GCIE (1879–1941)
1937–[39]	Captain Sir Ion Hamilton Benn Bt CB (1863–1961)

Table 21.1 – *continued*

Secretary:	
19[14]–27	P J (later Sir James) Michelli CMG (1853–1935)*
1927–35	R E V Bax (?–1970)
1935–[39]	F A Lyon (?–?) OBE
Treasurer:	
19[14]–[39]	Colonel (Sir) Robert Williams Bt MP (1848–1943)*
1927–36	Sir James Michelli, CMG (1853–1935)
Dreadnought	
Medical Superintendent:	
19[14]–19	R S Lawson
1919–25	H Ridley Prentice
1926–28	Richmond McIntosh
1928–33	L H Savin
1929–30	J W Illius
1930–[39]	J Walker Wilson
1933–[39]	W Ogilvy Reid
1935–38	B J Dunn
1938–[39]	H J Ross
Matron:	
19[14]–25	Miss A M Hall MBE*
1925–27	Miss E J Williams
1927–34	Miss C E Hayden
1934–[39]	Miss K L Bone
ADH	
Director:	
19[14]–[39]	H B Newham
Matron:	
19[14]–19	Miss C Graham Knight
1919–21	Miss E E Wheeler
1921–24	Miss E N Price
1924	Miss E Alderman
1924– [39]	Miss H S Sheard
Tilbury	
Matron:	
1920–24	Miss A M Fairbairn
1924–[39]	Miss M Ireland
Resident Secretary:	
1926–28	C E H Lloyd
1930–[39]	D A C Price
Hospital for Tropical Diseases	
Matron:	
1919–26	Miss C Graham Knight
1926–27	Miss C E Hayden
1927–30	Miss E Lloyd
1930–34	Miss K Bone

Table 21.1 – *continued*

1934–36	Mrs J C Sinnatt
1936–[39]	Mrs M Hill
KGSS	
Resident Secretary:	
1922–25	F H Gerty
1925–35	H J D Spriggs
1937–[39]	C F Loveless
Matron:	
1921–22	Miss J Williams
1925–26	Miss A M Hobling
1926–28	Miss M Ruck
1929– [39]	Miss A M Wootton
Angas Home	
Matron:	
1918–37	Mrs T H Gilbert
1937–[39]	Miss D Lewis

*See also Chapter 15.

Chairman, Committee of Management

Sir Perceval Nairne (1841–1921) (*see* Chapter 15) received a knighthood in 1915, and continued as Chairman of the Committee until his death in 1921. Following this long 'reign', came Captain Sir Arthur Clarke (1857–1932) (Figure 21.1), an elder Brother of Trinity House, who occupied that office for a decade until his death in 1932; he had had a distinguished naval career and served in numerous administrative posts. Previously a member of the Port of London Authority (PLA) and Deputy Chairman of King George's Fund for Sailors, he was to be a member of the Court of Governors of the London School of Hygiene and Tropical Medicine (LSHTM).[1]

For the following five years (1932-37), Baron Lloyd of Dolobran (1879–1941) (Figure 21.2) chaired the Board. During this time, a dominant theme involved the future of *tropical medicine* as a 'formal' discipline (*see* Chapters 18 and 25). It had become clear that the Ross Institute & Hospital for Tropical Diseases (RIHTD) at Putney (never a viable institution) was heading for disaster. Thus, when Ross died in 1932, i.e. shortly after Lloyd had taken up the mantle, negotiations led to the Society instituting a Ross Ward (containing a mere three beds) in the Hospital for Tropical Diseases (HTD) at Endsleigh Gardens, while the remainder of the Putney institution was absorbed into the LSHTM, which was of course never under the Society's control. Lloyd (who had been enobled in 1924) was educated at Eton and Cambridge, after which he travelled extensively and had had a distinguished career in the Great War – serving in Egypt, Gallipoli, Mesopotamia and the Hedjaz. Following the war he became successively: Governor of Bombay, Conservative MP for Eastbourne, High Commissioner for Egypt and the Sudan, President of the Navy League, and Chairman of the British Council. After his period of service with the Society (five years as Chairman of the Committee of Management, and two as

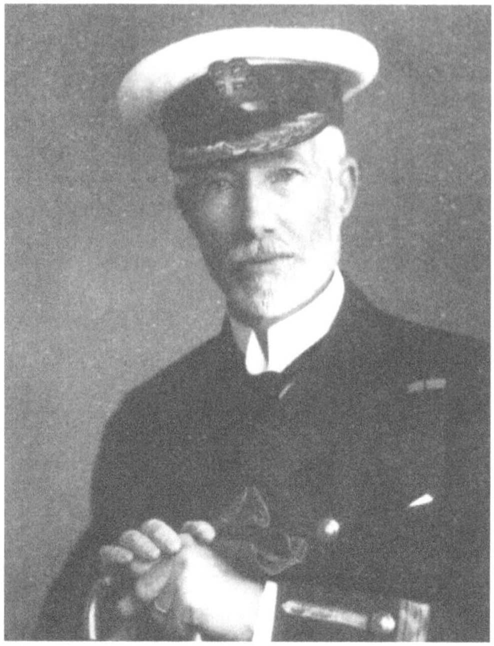

Figure 21.1: Captain Sir Arthur Clarke (1857–1932), Chairman of the Committee of Management (1922–32). [SHS Archive].

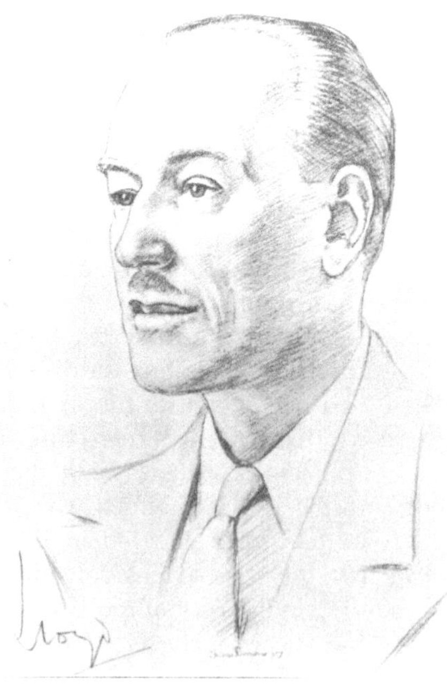

Figure 21.2: Baron Lloyd of Dolobran (1879–1941), Chairman of the Committee of Management (1932–37) and President (1938–41). [SHS Archive].

President), he became in 1940, Secretary of State for the Colonies until his death from myeloma a year later.[2]

Following Lloyd, Captain Sir Ion Hamilton Benn Bt (1863–1961) (Figure 21.3) – later to also become President of the SHS – took over the chairmanship of the Committee of Management. He had already served for long periods with the PLA and the Thames Conservancy, was a former Mayor of Greenwich, had served as a member of the London County Council (LCC) for Greenwich, and had been elected Unionist MP for Greenwich 1910–22. During the Great War, Benn served on the Belgian Coast.[3]

Secretaries

The previous era (*see* Chapter 12) had seen two outstanding and highly influential secretaries – following Kemball Cook (who had died in 1874 – i.e. shortly after removal to land). The first of these was Sir Henry Burdett (1847–1920) (*see* Chapter 15); the second was Sir James Michelli (1864–1939) who was firmly in command during the Great War. In the latter part of the period under review in this chapter (1927–39), the Secretaries were successively R E V Bax – a Barrister-at-Law – and FA Lyon (Figure 21.4).[4] Doubtless, both of these men pursued a steady course for the now well established society, but both seem to have lacked the charisma of their immediate predecessors.

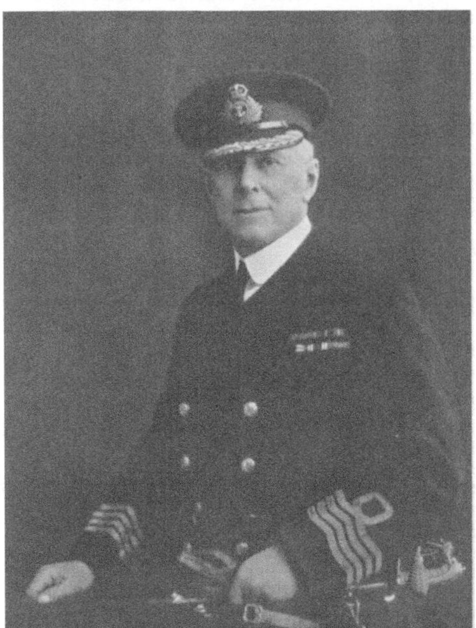

Figure 21.3: Sir Ion Hamilton Benn (1863–1961), Chairman of the Committee of Management (1937–46). [SHS Archive].

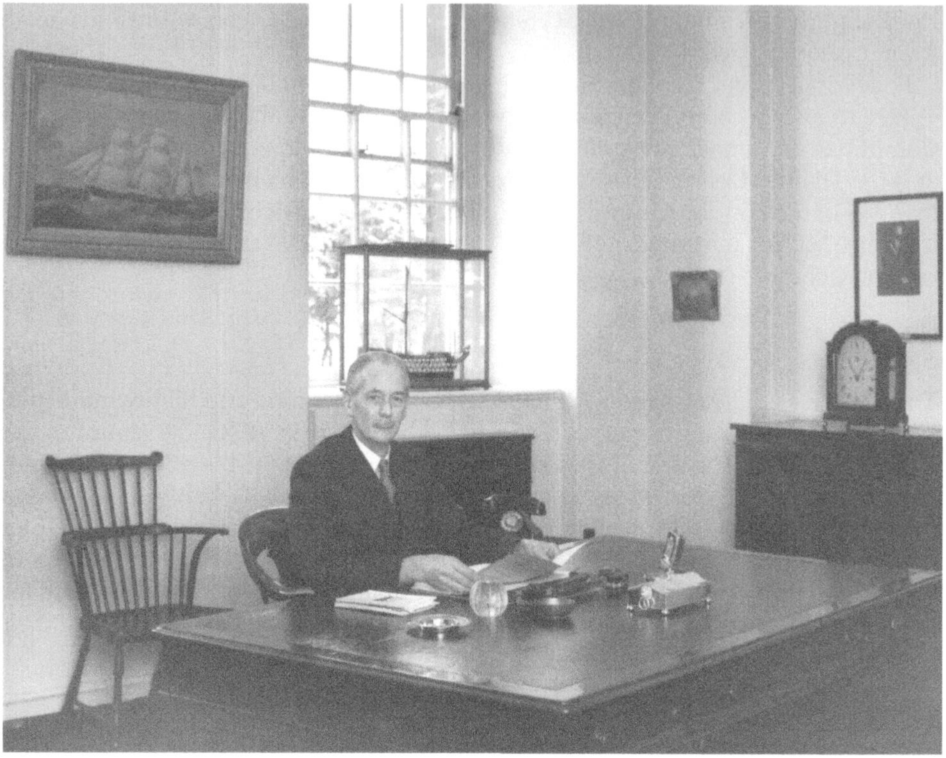

Figure 21.4: F A Lyon, Secretary (1935–69). [SHS Archive].

Medical Staff of the *Dreadnought* Hospital 1914–39

Table 21.2 summarises senior medical personnel who were employed at the *Dreadnought* at Greenwich, during the inter-war years. Many of their biographies have been outlined in Chapter 15.

Physicians

Amongst the 'new recruits' were the following:

HOLMES

(Sir) Gordon Holmes CMG CBE FRCP FRS (1876–1965) (Figure 21.5) was neurologist at the *Dreadnought* from 1914 until 1937. He was born in Dublin; his father had Yorkshire origins. He read natural sciences and medicine at Trinity College, Dublin, and pursued anatomical training in Frankfurt. On return to London he entered the National Hospital Queen Square (where he followed in the footsteps of: Hughlings Jackson, Brown-Séquard, David Ferrier, William Gowers, Charles Bastian and Victor Horsley), and with which he was closely associated until 1941. During the Great War, Holmes had become a consultant to the British Expeditionary

Table 21.2: Medical staff of the *Dreadnought* (1914–39).

Consulting Physicians:	
1917–19	Guthrie Rankin*
1917–28	Sir Dyce Duckworth*
1919–35	Sir John Rose Bradford FRS*
1937–[39]	(Sir) Gordon M Holmes FRS
Consulting Surgeons:	
19[14]–31	Sir William Bennett*
1919–[39]	W Turner*
1919–[39]	E (later Sir Ernest) Rock Carling*
1919–35	C C Choyce*
1921–33	L H McGavin*
Consulting Ophthalmic Surgeon:	
1919–[39]	L V Cargill*
Consulting Dermatologists:	
1919–24	Sir Malcolm Morris*
1924–[39]	Henry MacCormac
Consulting Surgeon for Diseases of the Throat, Nose and Ear:	
1920–[39]	Richard Lake
Consulting Pathologist:	
1935– [39]	Prof R Tanner Hewlett*
Physicians:	
19[14]–19	Sir Dyce Duckworth*
19[14]–21	(Sir) Frederick Taylor
19[14]–19	Sir John Rose Bradford*
19[14]–17	Guthrie Rankin*
19[14]–25	S (later Sir Sydney) Russell-Wells MP*
1917–[39]	C E Sundell
1920–25	H Ridley Prentice
1925–30	J Conway Davies
1926–30	J Purdon Martin
1930–[39]	A C Hampson
Surgeons:	
19[14]–19	W Turner*
19[14]–21	L H McGavin*
19[14]–19	E Rock Carling*
19[14]–19	C C Choyce*
1919–[39]	P P Cole
1919–27	Cecil Rountree
1921–[39]	E T C Milligan
1928–[39]	T G D Bonar
Surgeon(s) with Charge of Out-Patients:	
1920–21	E T C Milligan
1921–25	A G Timbell Fisher
1925–28	R Ogier Ward

Table 21.2 – continued

1928–37T	G D Bonar
1928–[39]	R Lester Williams
Physician(s) with Charge of Out-Patients:	
1929–30	A C Hampson
1930–[39]	R G Ranyard West
1930–32	E C Warner
1932–38	D Krestin
1938–[39]	W G Oakley
1939–[39]	A Wingfield
Ophthalmic Surgeons:	
19[14]–19	L V Cargill
1919–[39]	R E Bickerton
Surgeon for Diseases of the Skin:	
19[14]–19	Sir Malcolm Morris*
ENT Surgeons:	
19[14]–20	Richard Lake
1923–[39]	F Courtenay Mason
Honorary Dermatologist (Diseases of the Skin):	
1932–[39]	J Franklin
Gynaecologist:	
1935–[39]	K M K Duff
Neurologist:	
1914–37	(Sir) Gordon M Holmes FRS
Directors of the Venereal Diseases Clinic:	
1917–19	H M Mogridge Woodward
1933–[39]	P P Cole
Physician-in-charge of the Electrical Department:	
19[14]–20	T D Collis Barry
1920–[39]	Martin Berry
Physician for Diseases of the Skin:	
1939–[39]	D Erskine
Director-in-Charge of Department of Physical Medicine:	
1931–[39]	J Sainsbury
Physician-in-Charge of Psycho-Therapeutic Department:	
1937–[39]	C Allen
Directors of Pathology:	
19[14]–35	Prof R Tanner Hewlett FRCP*
1926–35	[co-director] Arthur Davies
1935–[39]	Arthur Davies

*See also Chapter 15.

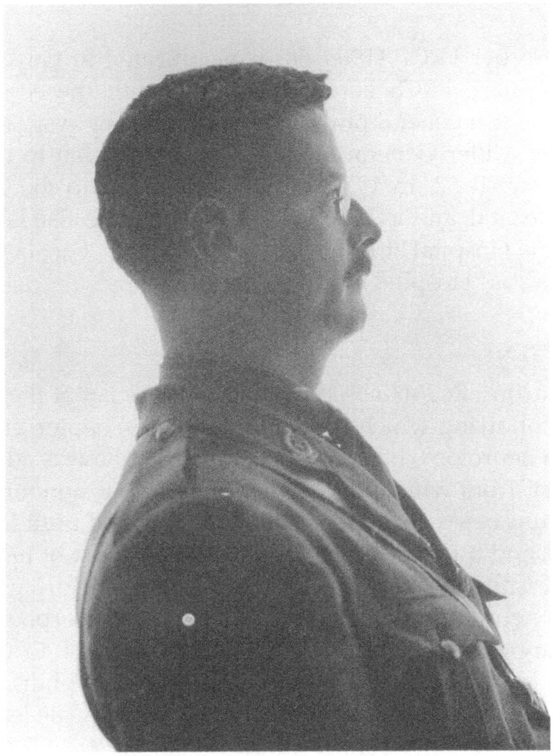

Figure 21.5: Sir Gordon Holmes FRCP FRS, neurologist to the *Dreadnought* Hospital (1914–1937). [Courtesy of Wellcome Library, London].

Force (BEF) and made important observations on the effect of gun-shot wounds of the spinal cord and brain. At the RCP, he was Goulstonian and Croonian lecturer, Councillor, Censor and Conway Evans prizeman; Holmes was knighted in 1951. He had three daughters.[5]

SUNDELL

Charles Ernest Sundell MRCP (1883–1964) qualified from the (Royal) London Hospital in 1907 with the MB, BS degrees, and passed the MRCP in 1910. During the Great War, he served as a Major in the RAMC, and researched trench fever in France. Sundell subsequently became Senior Physician to the *Dreadnought*, physician to the Evelina Hospital for Children, visiting physician in charge of the children's department at the Prince of Wales Hospital, and visiting physician to King George's Sanatorium, Enfield Hospital and Tilbury Hospital (*see* Chapter 24). Sundell was a general physician who 'was equally at home in every field of medicine, including tuberculosis, and tropical medicine of which he saw his full share at the Seamen's Hospital, Greenwich and Tilbury'. Sundell was never elected FRCP; the reason remains unclear.[6]

WARNER

Edwin Charles Warner FRCP (1900–68) was educated at Guy's Hospital, where he passed the primary FRCS before qualifying with the conjoint diplomas in 1925. He later became a general physician. Warner was physician to the children's department of the Miller General Hospital, and physician to out-patients at the *Dreadnought* from 1930–32. In 1931, he was appointed to the consultant staff of Charing Cross Hospital, and in 1936 Putney Hospital; he also later joined the staff of the New Victoria Hospital at Kingston-upon-Thames. For six years, Warner was Dean of Charing Cross Hospital Medical School.[7]

PURDON MARTIN

James Purdon Martin FRCP (1893–1984) was a physician at the *Dreadnought* from 1926 until 1930, following which (like Holmes – *see* Chapter 21) he had a distinguished career in neurology. Born in County Antrim, he was educated at Queen's University, Belfast, from which he obtained a first-class honours degree in mathematics. On account of severe psoriasis, he was declared unfit for military service in the Great War; and qualified in medicine in 1920. Most of his career was spent at the National Hospital for Nervous Diseases, although during the Second World War, he served as neurologist to Eastern Command. At Liverpool, he suffered from encephalitis lethargica, and henceforth devoted his research to studies of the basal ganglia. He was also a pioneer in the treatment of neurosyphilis with penicillin. At the RCP, Martin was Lumleian, and at the RCS Aris and Gale lecturer. Martin was twice married; there were two sons from the first of these.[8]

HAMPSON

Arthur Cecil Hampson FRCP (1894–1972). Born near Wigan, Lancashire, Hampson had a distinguished career with the Royal Field Artillery during the Great War, following which he studied medicine at Cambridge, qualifying with the conjoint diplomas in 1924, and the MB, BChir degrees in 1927. In 1930, he was elected Assistant Physician and in 1947 Full Physician, to Guy's Hospital, and also Physician to the children's department. In 1930 Hampson was elected to the staff of the *Dreadnought*. When the Second World War started in 1939, he was appointed Deputy Group Medical Officer to Sector 10.[9]

Surgeons

ROUNTREE

Cecil Rountree FRCS (1880–1943) was educated at Islington High School, University College London, and the Middlesex Hospital; he qualified in 1902. He lectured and published several papers on malignant disease, and was aware of its connection to radiation. At the Royal Cancer (now Royal Marsden) Hospital he was: surgeon, senior surgeon and consulting surgeon respectively. He was elected surgeon to the *Dreadnought* (1919–29), Woolwich and District War Memorial Hospital, and the Caterham, Erith, and East Grinstead Cottage Hospitals. During the Great War,

Rountree served as medical officer to the 16th Battalion the Queen's Westminster Rifles, having been commissioned as a Captain in the RAMC territorial force in 1911. He was also consulting surgeon to the American Red Cross. Rountree became internationally known for his cancer research. There were two sons and a daughter of his marriage; for the last four years of his life, he 'suffered from [a] severe [form of] cardiac illness'.[10]

Specialist medical/surgical staff

The inter-war years were ones of increasing specialisation. The SHS, not to be outdone by this trend, appointed several staff members who were specialists in their respective fields. The following notes embrace a gynaecologist, two dermatologists, two ENT surgeons and an ophthalmic surgeon.

DUFF

Keith Mitchell Keitley Duff FRCS FRCOG (1893–1980) qualified from Guy's Hospital in 1919 and became a gynaecologist. After practicing in England (at the *Dreadnought* [1935–48]), he served in Kenya, and the Transvaal, South Africa.[11]

MacCORMACK

Henry MacCormack CBE FRCP (1879–1950) was the grandson of a physician with an identical name, who was an early exponent of open-air treatment of 'phthisis' (see Chapter 16). MacCormack graduated MB ChB (Edinburgh) in 1903, and afterwards studied in London and Paris; he held several junior appointments, mostly in London, and specialised in *dermatology* – a discipline for which he was appointed to the SHS. During the Great War he had been consulting dermatologist to the BEF in France (where scabies was a great problem) and was in medical charge of the 25th General Hospital. At the RCP MacCormack gave the Lumlian lectures in 1945. There was one son of his marriage.[12]

FRANKLIN

John Lewis Franklin FRCP (1904–72). Born in London, Franklin qualified at St George's Hospital, and specialised in *dermatology* and *venereology*. He was one of the last physicians to combine these two specialities. Franklin was consultant dermatologist to the *Dreadnought* from 1932–39. In 1934, he became Head of the Skin Department at Westminster Hospital. He was thrice married; there was a son and daughter of the first.[13]

LAKE

Richard Lake FRCS (1861–1949) was educated at Trent College, Bonn (Germany), and St Thomas's Hospital, qualifying in 1885. He joined the National Aid Society (the forerunner of the British Red Cross) and served in the Sudan; the following year he served in the Servo-Bulgar War. On return to England, Lake became a Captain in the RAMC in the 2nd Middlesex Volunteer Artillery. He specialised in disease of the ear, nose and throat and became surgeon-laryngolgist to Mount Vernon Hospital for Consumption and to the *Dreadnought*; he also lectured to the LSCM (Chapter 19). During the Great War, Lake was surgeon to the Royal Flying Corps Hospital, and Princess Christian's and Robert Lindsay's hospitals for officers. Between 1898 and 1926, he was consulting surgeon to the Royal Ear Hospital. Lake was twice married; a daughter resulted from the first.[14]

MASON

Francis Courtenay Mason FRCS (1891–1953). Educated at Haberdasher Aske's Hampstead School and the Middlesex Hospital, Mason qualified in 1916. He served with the RAMC during the Great War, and passed the FRCS and MS (London) examinations in 1920. After junior appointments at the Middlesex and the Hospital for Sick Children, he specialised in laryngology. Mason was subsequently: surgeon to the ear nose and throat department of the *Dreadnought* (from 1923), the King George Hospital, Ilford, and West Middlesex Hospital; he was also oto-rhino laryngology consultant to the LCC. There was a son and daughter from his marriage.[15]

COLE

Percival Pasley Cole FRCS (1878–1948) qualified first as a dental surgeon at Guy's Hospital in 1899; he obtained the conjoint diplomas in 1904, and served as house surgeon at Guy's. In 1906 he obtained the FRCS, and in 1909 MB ChB (Birmingham). After several junior appointments, Cole was elected assistant surgeon to Queen Mary's Hospital for the East End in 1911, and the following year to the *Dreadnought* (where he became surgeon in 1919, and consulting surgeon in 1947; Cole was also Director of the VD department there). He also held appointments at the (Royal) Cancer Hospital (where he worked with: Charles Ryall, Ernest Miles, Jocelyn Swan, Cecil Rountree [*see* Chapter 24] and Cecil Joll), Bethnall Green, and Tilbury Hospitals (from 1930). During the Great War, Cole was surgeon to King George Hospital, Waterloo Road and the Brook War Hospital. He succeeded C C Choyce (Chapter 19) as Dean of the LSCM in 1919. Towards the end of his life, he up-dated Leach's *Ship-captain's medical guide* (*see* Chapter 11). Cole also 'perfected [McGavin's] filigree operation for inguinal hernia'. Twice married, there was a son and daughter from the first.[16]

Medical staff of the Albert Dock Hospital (ADH) 1914–39

This hospital had been founded in 1890 (Chapter 14) and from 1899–1920 housed the *clinical* base of the LSTM (Chapter 18). In order to *strengthen* the tropical expertise, Manson was responsible for several appointments of junior colleagues (physicians) with a special interest in this discipline. Amongst the earliest appointments were those of Sandwith and Daniels (Chapter 18). Two other relatively early appointments were those of G C Low and P H Bahr (later Sir Philip Manson-Bahr) (see below); the latter had married Manson's daughter, and became Manson's principal biographer. Table 21.3 summarises the medical staff during the inter-war years.

Table 21.3: Medical staff of the Albert Dock Hospital (1914–39).

Consulting Physicians:	
19[14]–22	Sir Patrick Manson*
1920–26	C W Daniels*
1937–[39]	G C Low
Consulting Surgeons:	
1921–26	Sir James Cantlie*
1921–37	J J Pratt
1929–[39]	T Pomfret Kilner
Physicians:	
19[14]–18	F M Sandwith*
19[14]–20	C W Daniels*
1918–37	G C Low
1921–[39]	P H (later Sir Philip) Manson-Bahr
Surgeons:	
19[14]–21	J (later Sir James) Cantlie*
1914–21	J J Pratt
1921–[39]	H E (later Sir Hugh) Griffiths
1921–29	T Pomfret Kilner
1929–[39]	C Hope Carlton
Ophthalmic Surgeons:	
19[14]–27	L V Cargill*
1927–[39]	E Wolff
Radiologists:	
1927–29	J V Sparks
1930–[39]	F G Wood
Directors of the Venereal Diseases Clinic:	
1917–19	R P Cockin
1919–21	H M Hanschell
1933–[39]	H M Hanschell
Physician for Diseases of the Skin:	
1934–[39]	N F C Burgess
Pathologist (and Honorary [Medical] Superintendent):	
1920–[39]	H M Hanschell

*See also Chapter 15.

Physicians

LOW

George Carmichael Low FRCP (1872–1953) (*see* Figure 21.6) was born at Monifieth, Forfarshire, Scotland and educated at Madras College (St Andrews) and St Andrew's University. Following qualification (with the MB, CM [Edinburgh] degrees), he held house appointments at Edinburgh Royal Infirmary. Low had joined Manson's staff at the ADH in 1899, and subsequently studied at Heidelberg and Vienna; on return to London, he established the mosquito-man component of the life-cycle of *Wuchereria bancofti* (a helminth responsible for lymphatic filariasis). He then undertook (as a Craggs Research scholar) a study of the filariases in the Caribbean. In 1902, he led the first (unsuccessful) Royal Society (RS) expedition to Uganda in an attempt to determine the cause of the 'negro lethargy' (African trypanosomiasis).

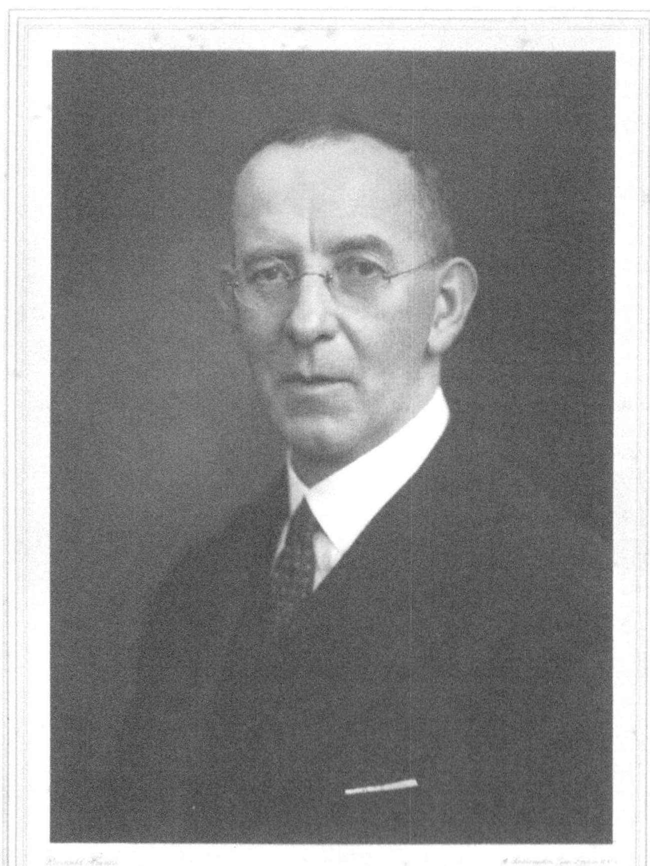

Figure 21.6: George Carmichael Low FRCP (1872–1953), physician at the ADH. [Courtesy of Royal Society of Tropical Medicine and Hygiene].

Despite these early achievements abroad, Low's major contribution was to the newly-founded discipline – where he became: superintendent, lecturer, consulting pathologist, and director of the division of *clinical* tropical medicine at the LSHTM; he also lectured at several London hospitals. During the Great War, Low held the rank of Major (IMS), and in 1918 he was appointed physician to the ADH, and subsequently physician to the HTD and Tilbury Hospital (see below) both of which were at that time administered by the SHS. He was largely instrumental in the founding of the (Royal) Society of Tropical Medicine and Hygiene – which he served as Secretary (1912–20) and President (1929–33). There were no children of his marriage.[17]

MANSON-BAHR

(Sir) Philip Henry Manson-Bahr CMG FRCP (1881–1966) (see Figure 21.7) as P H Bahr was born in Liverpool, and educated at Rugby School and Trinity College,

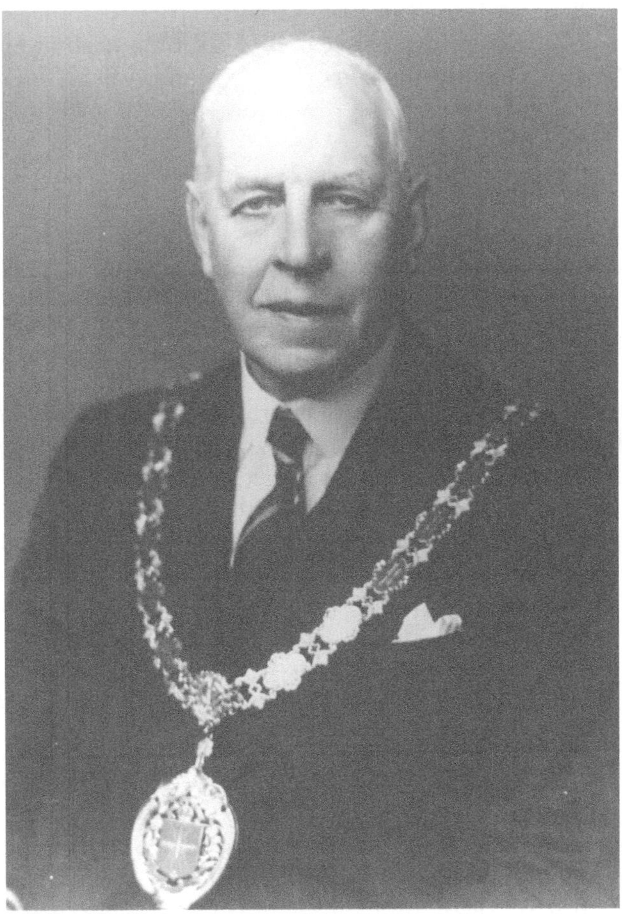

Figure 21.7: (Sir) Philip Manson-Bahr FRCP (1881–1906), physician at the HTD. [Courtesy of Wellcome Library, London].

Cambridge – qualifying from the (Royal) London Hospital in 1907. From early in his career he was an accomplished zoologist and ornithologist. His first overseas work was in Fiji, where he worked on dysenteric diseases and lymphatic filariasis. He later (1914) studied sprue in Ceylon (now Sri Lanka). During the Great War, Bahr served in Egypt, Palestine and the Dardanelles, where he studied 925 cases of pellagra among Middle East prisoners. Manson-Bahr was appointed to the staff of the ADH in 1921, and became a lecturer at the LSTM; from 1937–47 he was director of the LSHTM's Department of *Clinical* Tropical Medicine. From 1927 he was (together with Low) consulting physician in tropical diseases to Tilbury Hospital (see below), and from 1927 until 1947, consultant physician to the Colonial Office and the Crown Agents. He was President of the RSTMH from 1946 until 1948, and the Medical Society of London (1946–7). Manson-Bahr became editor of Manson's *'Tropical diseases: a manual of diseases of warm climates'* from 1921 until 1960. Manson-Bahr was a prolific author; several of his publications exist in the Society's archive. His marriage to Manson's daughter in 1909 ended with her death in 1948; he remarried in 1950 – Edith Mary Crossmith. Bahr altered his name to Manson-Bahr (according to *Munk's Roll* 'at the wish of his father-in-law, Sir Patrick Manson'). One of his sons (P E C Manson-Bahr) followed him into tropical medicine.[18]

Surgeons

At the ADH it was essential to have surgeons 'on board' – especially one with a 'tropical' background. James Cantlie (a colleague of Manson in his China days) had already been appointed (see also Chapter 18).

PRATT

James John Pratt FRCS (1860–1937) was born at Valene, France; his father was a surgeon and his mother (Maria Louisa Harvey) 'claimed descent from … William Harvey …'. Following medical education at Westminster Hospital, he entered Netley Hospital, and was gazetted IMS in September 1883; the following year, he took part in the Zhob Valley expedition. Pratt retired (on pension) in December 1912, when he became a student at the LSTM. He served as surgeon to the ADH and subsequently the HTD from 1914 until 1921; following this he became consulting surgeon until his death. Pratt was also a lecturer at Westminster Hospital from 1913. In December 1914, he was appointed officer-in-charge of the Hospital for Indian Wounded at Brighton. There was a son and a daughter of his marriage.[19]

CARLTON

Charles Hope Carlton FRCS (1889–1951) was born at Grantham, and educated at Doncaster Grammar School, St John's College, Oxford, and St Mary's Hospital; he qualified (MB, ChB) in 1914. During the Great War, Carlton served with the RAMC and saw active service in France and West Africa. Following cessation of hostilities, he pursued a career in surgery at St Mary's, Harvard, the Mayo Clinic and

Toronto. He became surgical registrar at the Royal National Orthopaedic Hospital and Surgeon to the ADH; he was also: surgeon (and curator of the museum) of the National Temperance Hospital, and the South-eastern Hospital for Children. At the outbreak of war in 1939 he was appointed ADMS 1st Anti-Aircraft Division; he was also in command of the 7th and 3rd General Hospitals, and the 34th West African General Hospital. Carlton was present at the invasion of Crete in 1941. After the introduction of the NHS in 1948 (Chapter 22), he became consultant surgeon to the North-West (Paddington) and South-east (Bromley) metropolitan regional hospital group; he also served on the council of the Regional Hospital Consultants and Specialists Association. There were two sons and a daughter of his marriage.[20]

Specialist medical/surgical staff

A particular requirement was for surgeons with *specialist* knowledge, both at the ADH, and also the *Dreadnought* – a plastic surgeon and one in 'orthopaedics and rehabilitation':

KILNER

Thomas Pomfret Kilner CBE FRCS (1890–1964) was educated at Queen Elizabeth Grammar School, Blackburn and Manchester University; he qualified from the latter in 1912 (MB, ChB). After appointments at the University of Manchester and Manchester Royal Infirmary, he served during the Great War as a captain in the RAMC – surgeon to No 64 Casualty Clearing Station, and surgical specialist to No 4 General Hospital. Following hostilities he was appointed plastic surgeon to Queen Mary's Hospital for Face and Jaw Injuries, Sidcup; with (Sir) Harold Gillies he took a key rôle in the establishment of plastic surgery as a separate specialty in the UK.

In 1921, Kilner was also appointed surgeon to the *Dreadnought*; he resigned in 1929 and was made a consulting surgeon. He was appointed associate plastic surgeon at St Thomas's Hospital in 1934. Kilner took a leading role in creation of the plastic surgery unit at Stoke Mandeville Hospital, and took charge of the plastic surgery division of the Ministry of Pensions. During the Second World War, Kilner was to become consultant to the pensioners at Roehampton, and in 1944 he was appointed Nuffield Professor of Plastic Surgery at Oxford, a post from which he retired in 1957. Kilner was twice married; he had one son by his first marriage, and two sons by the second.[21]

GRIFFITHS

(Sir) Hugh Ernest Griffiths CBE, FRCS (1891–1961) studied medicine at the University of Wales and St Bartholomew's Hospital – qualifying (with the conjoint diplomas) in 1916. He served as surgeon-probationer in the RNVR (1914–15) and between 1916–18, he was surgeon to the 1st London General Hospital. From 1916–26, Griffiths was a demonstrator in anatomy; in 1918, he was Research Scholar in surgery, and from 1919–22 Chief Surgical Assistant. At the RCS, he was

Hunterian Professor in 1923, and Arris and Gale lecturer in 1924. In 1920, Griffiths was appointed surgeon to the ADH (he also served on the staff of the Hertford County, Potters Bar Cottage, the Wimbledon and All Saint's Hospitals).

At the ADH, he made 'an intensive study of the work of seamen and dock-workers'. With his profound knowledge of anatomy and physiology, Griffiths was able to assess the physiological requirements of handicapped men. Therefore, his advice was greatly sought after by insurance companies, solicitors and trade unions. When the '*new*' ADH was being planned (in 1936) he studied (together with the Society's Secretary) 'the construction and administration of many hospitals abroad'. As Director of the hospital's Accident and Rehabilitation Centre, he advocated remedial intensive exercises in the gymnasium. Griffiths played a major role in rehabilitation of the disabled resulting from injury in the MM and docklands. He played a major part in establishing the Cripples' Training College at Leatherhead, and assisted Dame Georgina Bullet in setting up the British Council for Rehabilitation for the Disabled in 1944. During the Second World War, he became consulting surgeon to the Ministry of Supply, and in 1945 was responsible for the establishment of an *industrial rehabilitation service* in newly liberated Poland. There was a son and daughter of his marriage. Several of Griffiths' publications have been preserved in the SHS archive.[22]

Dispensaries and the Convalescent Home

These institutions were manned by relatively junior staff and in the majority details of their careers have not survived; Tables 21.4 and 21.5 summarise the medical and senior nursing staff.

Table 21.4: Medical staff of the Dispensaries (1914–39).

East and West India Docks Dispensary	
Consulting Surgeon:	
19[14]–17	Walter Fowler
Medical Officer:	
19[14]–30	W H F Oxley
Gravesend Dispensary	
Surgeon:	
19[14]–[39]	C E Robbs
Southampton Docks Dispensary	
Consulting Medical Officer:	
1930– [39]	W H F Oxley
Medical Officer:	
1929– [39]	B Bourke

Table 21.5: Medical staff of the Angas Convalescent Home, Cudham (1914–39).

Medical Officers:	
1918–25	H H Dummere
1925–30	W J Symes
1932–37	H J Hendley
1937–[39]	R G Dingwall
Matrons:	
1928–29	Miss A M Higgs
1929–30	Miss M Wootton
1930–31	Miss C Warner
1931–32	Mrs Scott Scott
1932–?	Miss Edith Jones

Medical staff of the Hospital for Tropical Diseases (HTD) 1920–39

This hospital opened in central London in 1920 (Chapter 20); all *tropical* cases were transferred there from the ADH (the original 'home' of tropical medicine in London).[23] Some of the leading administrative and medical staff have already been mentioned in connection with the ADH. Most, but not all, had had experience of medicine in a *tropical* environment – usually India.[24] The medical staffing in the inter-war period is shown in Table 21.6. The HTD remained under the administration of the Society until the introduction of the NHS.

Physicians and pathologists

WALSHE

(Sir) Francis Martin Rouse Walshe FRCP FRS (1885–1973) was born in Ireland; his father had served as a Colonial Surgeon in the West Indies. He was educated at Bath, University College School, and UCL, and qualified (MB, BS) from UCH in 1910. Walshe's whole career was devoted to neurology and neurophysiology. He later became President of the Association of British Neurologists, and the Royal Society of Medicine; for 16 years, he was editor of *Brain*. At UCH, Walshe was a house-surgeon to Sir Victor Horsley, and a colleague of T R Elliot (who founded the department of neurology there); another colleague was Wilfred Trotter. Walshe served in the RAMC during the Great War. He was consulting neurologist to the HTD from 1933 until his retirement at the age of 70. There were two sons of his marriage.[25]

Table 21.6: Medical staff of the Hospital for Tropical Diseases, Endsleigh Gardens (1920–39).

Consulting Physicians:	
1919–21	Sir Patrick Manson*
1020–25	C W Daniels
1937–[39]	G C Low
Consulting Surgeons:	
1921–24	Sir James Cantlie*
1924–[39]	J J Pratt
1935–[39]	T Pomfret Kilner
Consulting Ophthalmic Surgeon:	
1925–[39]	R H Elliot FRS
Consulting Neurologist:	
1933–39	F M R Walshe FRS
Consulting Gynaecologist:	
1928–[39]	V B Green-Armytage
Consulting Cardiologist:	
1929–[39]	D Evan Bedford
Consulting Physician for Diseases of the Chest:	
1939–[39]	F G Chandler
Physicians:	
1919–37	G C Low
1921–[39]	P H (later Sir Philip) Manson-Bahr
1937–[39]	N (later Sir Neil) Hamilton Fairley, FRS
Extra Physician (for Clinical Research):	
1921–[39]	Sir Leonard Rogers FRS
Hon Physician Representing the Colonial Office:	
1921–33	W T (later Sir William) Prout
Surgeons:	
1919–21	Sir James Cantlie
1919–24	J J Pratt
1924–32	(Sir) Thomas Carey Evans
1924–35	T Pomfret Kilner
1932–[39]	A H McIndoe
1935–[39]	C Naunton Morgan
ENT Surgeon:	
1930–[39]	W M Morris
Cardiologist:	
1935–[39]	D E Bedford
Respiratory Physician:	
1939–[39]	Mr F C Chandler
Physician in Charge of Electrical Department:	
1921–[39]	Martin Berry

Table 21.6 – *continued*

Ophthalmic Surgeons:	
1919–25	R H Elliot
1927–36	H Kirkpatrick
1937–[39]	R E Wright
Physician for Diseases of the Skin:	
1919–34	J M H MacLeod
1934–[39]	N F C Burgess
Gynaecologist:	
1928–38	V B Green-Armytage
Honorary Helminthologist:	
1929–[39]	Professor R T Leiper FRS
Honorary Protozoologist:	
1929–37	J G Thomson
Director of Pathological Department:	
1919–[39]	N H (later Sir Neil Hamilton) Fairley FRS
Pathologist:	
1933–37	Col F P MacKie
1937–[39]	P H Martin
Honorary Bacteriologist:	
1934–[39]	W W C Topley FRS
Ophthalmic Surgeons:	
1919–25	R H Elliot
1927–37	H Kirkpatrick
Radiologist:	
1931–[39]	G R M Cordiner
Medical Superintendents:	
1920–25	A L Gregg
1925–36	W E Cooke
1935–[39]	J S McNair

*See also Chapter 15.

FAIRLEY

(Sir) Neil Hamilton Fairley FRCP FRS (1891–1966) (*see* Figure 21.8) was born in Melbourne, Australia and educated at the Scotch College and Melbourne University, qualifying (MB, BS Melb) in 1915. During the Great War, Fairley joined the Australian Army Medical Corps, and between 1916–18 served in Egypt (where he carried out research on schistosomiasis – especially its immuniological aspects) and Palestine; he also investigated malaria-associated anaemia. In the 1920s he was Professor of Tropical Medicine in the University of Bombay – where he carried out research on 'tropical sprue'. In 1929, Fairley was appointed Director of Pathology at the HTD; there, his major research interest continued to be malaria-

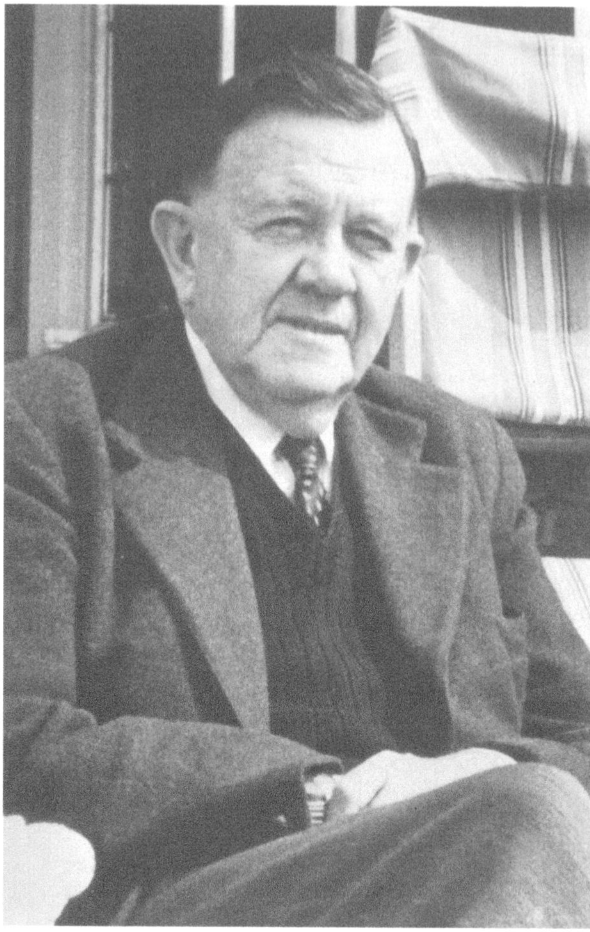

Figure 21.8: (Sir) Neil Hamilton Fairley FRCP FRS (1891–1966), physician at the HTD. [Courtesy of Wellcome Library, London].

associated anaemia, although he also carried out work on leptospirosis. At the outbreak of war in 1939 Fairley enlisted in the Australian Army Medical Force, and carried out important work at Cairns on the chemoprophylaxis and chemotherapy of malaria; this work led to mepacrine and proguanil being widely used by soldiers in the Pacific, India and Burma. He also demonstrated the cure of shigellosis with sulphaguanidine.

Following the war, he returned to the HTD, and in 1946 was appointed first Wellcome Professor of Clinical Tropical Medicine at the LSHTM; three years later he suffered a stroke which led to his resignation from the Chair, but he continued with hospital work. He served as President of the Royal Society of Tropical Medicine and Hygiene (1951–53). Fairley was twice married; there was one son of his first and two of the second. One son, who was a clinical oncologist at St Bartholomew's Hospital was murdered by the IRA on 23 October 1975.[26]

ROGERS

Sir Leonard Rogers FRCP FRS (1868–1962) (*see* Figure 21.9) was born near Plymouth, and educated at Tavistock Grammar School, Plymouth College, and St Mary's Hospital London; he qualified (MB, BS Lond) in 1892. The following year he enlisted in the IMS and initially investigated kala-azar in Assam – where the disease was epidemic. Although he soon demonstrated that the infection had a predilection for certain localities (and removal from these prevented infection), he was unable to disassociate it from chronic malaria; he demonstrated that antimony compounds were effective in its management.

In 1900, he was appointed Professor of Pathology in Calcutta – where his research work was dominated by *Entamoeba histolytica* infection, and liver 'abscess'; he demonstrated that emetine is effective in treatment. In India, Rogers developed a modified regimen for intravenous rehydration in cholera; he used the active ingredient of chaulmoogra oil (replaced by the sulphones in the early 1940s) in leprosy, and

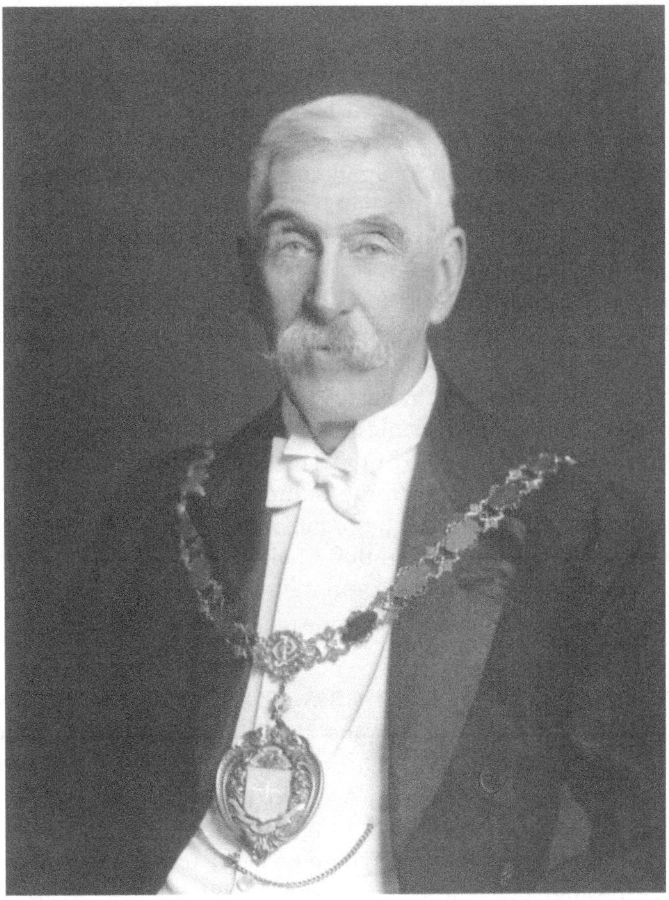

Figure 21.9: Sir Leonard Rogers FRCP FRS (1868–1962), extra physician to the HTD. [Courtesy of the Royal Society of Tropical Medicine and Hygiene].

carried out research on snake venoms, and the trypanosomiasis of horses. His overwhelming interest lay in the epidemiology of many of the diseases of Bengal.

Rogers also took a leading rôle in the establishment the School of Tropical Medicine at Calcutta – which opened in 1920. In 1920, he retired to England, and became medical adviser to the Secretary of State for India, physician to the HTD, and lecturer at the LSTM. He devoted a great deal of time to the British Empire Leprosy Relief Association. Rogers was later President of the Royal Society of Tropical Medicine and Hygiene (1933–35). At the RCP, he was Milroy and Croonian lecturer. There were three sons of his marriage, one of whom became a Professor of Mathematics at University College, London.[27]

MacKIE

Frederick Percival Mackie CSI OBE FRCS FRCP (1875–1944) was educated at Dean Close School in Cheltenham, Bristol University and St Bartholomew's Hospital, qualifying in 1897. After house appointments at the Bristol General and Fever Hospitals, and the County Asylum, Shrewsbury, he obtained the FRCS in 1902. In the same year he joined the IMS and was appointed medical officer with the Younghusband expedition to Tibet. Moving to Bombay in 1905, he became assistant director of the Plague Research Laboratory and demonstrated that relapsing fever was transmitted by body lice. Between 1908 and 1910 Mackie served on an RS sleeping sickness expedition to Uganda. However, the following year he returned to India in order to undertake research on kala-azar in Assam (see above). He saw active service in Baluchistan, and France and Mesopotamia during the Great War. In 1920 Mackie became Professor of Pathology at Calcutta, and in 1921 Director of the Pasteur Institute at Shillong. In 1923, he was appointed Director of the Haffkine Institute, Bombay (where he carried out research on 'tropical sprue' with Fairley, see above). In 1928, Mackie was appointed officiating public health commissioner to the Government of India, and chairman of the League of Nations Plague Committee; a year later he became surgeon-general with the Bombay Government. Before retirement from the IMS in 1932, he had briefly resumed his post at Shillong. After return to England, he became pathologist to the HTD (1933–38), and then chief medical officer of BOAC; he organised preventive measures against yellow fever on airfields, and the fumigation of aircraft. Mackie was twice married; there was one son of the first, and two from the second.[28]

EVAN BEDFORD

Davis Evan Bedford CBE FRCP (1898–1978) was born at Boston, Lincolnshire and educated at Epsom College and the Middlesex Hospital Medical School – qualifying MRCS LRCP in 1921. During the Great War, he had served as Surgeon-sub-lieutenant RNVR. Following a series of junior appointments at the Middlesex Hospital, he was appointed officer in charge of the cardiac wards at the Ministry of Pensions Hospital at Orpington, where he came under the influence of the distinguished cardiologist (Sir) John Parkinson. Following a short period in France, he carried out pioneering work (with Parkinson) on electrocardiographic changes in myocardial infarction. In 1926, Bedford was appointed assistant physician to the

Middlesex, and in 1933 physician to outpatients at the National Heart Hospital. In 1935 he was appointed consultant cardiologist to the HTD. During the Second World War he assumed the rank of Brigadier, RAMC, and was consulting physician to the Middle East Forces. After demobilisation, Bedford pursued his career in cardiology, rapidly gaining an international reputation. There were two sons of his marriage in 1935.[29]

CHANDLER

Frederick George Chandler FRCP (1885–1942) was born at Sutton in Surrey, and was educated at the Leys School, Jesus College, Cambridge, and St Bartholomew's Hospital from which he qualified in 1911. Following junior appointments at Bart's, the Hospital for Sick Children, and the Brompton Hospital, he became a medical registrar at the (Royal) London Hospital. During the Great War he served as a medical officer (RAMC) to the 2nd Argyll and Sutherland Highlanders. Following the war, Chandler was elected to the staff of the London Hospital for Diseases of the Chest, and in 1922 to Charing Cross Hospital; in 1930 he resigned the latter appointment, and became assistant physician to St Bartholomew's Hospital. Chandler became an authority on respiratory diseases, and was also briefly on the staff of the HTD and King Edward VII Sanatorium, Midhurst. There was a son and two daughters of his marriage.[30]

MacLEOD

John Macleod Hendrie MacLeod FRCP (1870–1954) was born at Galston, Ayrshire, and graduated at the University of Aberdeen. Deciding to embark on a career in *dermatology* (he was initially devoted to physiology), he studied at Vienna, Berlin, Hamburg and Paris. From 1903–30, MacLeod was on the staff of Charing Cross Hospital; he was also appointed to the LSHTM and the Victoria Hospital for Children, Chelsea. In 1923, he succeeded Sir Malcolm Morris (the founder) as medical officer to the Homes of St Giles for British Lepers. During the Great War, MacLeod was consultant in skin diseases to the Royal Flying Corps. There were a son and daughter of his marriage.[31]

MARTIN

Peter Henry Martin FRCP (1896–1963) was born in London; his father was a general practitioner at Southwick Place and several of his ancestors were also doctors. After schooling at Radley, he entered the Royal Naval Air Service – transferring for three years in 1916 to the RAF. He then studied medicine at New College, Oxford and St Bartholomew's Hospital, qualifying BM (Oxon) in 1924. After three years of junior appointments at his teaching hospital, he was appointed (in 1927) assistant pathologist at the HTD. Following this he served in Malaya as pathologist and later bacteriologist at the Institute for Medical Research at Kuala Lumpur; much of his work there was on typhoid and typhus fevers, and melioidosis.

In 1934, Martin returned to England as assistant pathologist at the British Postgraduate Medical School; shortly afterwards he was appointed to the LSHTM and, in 1937, accepted the post of *pathologist* to the HTD. When the war began in 1939 he joined the Emergency Public Health Laboratory Service and worked at Colchester, Ipswich (at the East Suffolk County Laboratory) and ultimately the newly built public Health Laboratory at Borough General Hospital. Martin retired due to ill-health (myocardial ischaemia) in 1948. His published work included contributions on paratyphoid fever and food-poisoning, and cultivation of *Mycobacterium tuberculosis*. There were no children of his marriage.[32]

Surgeons

EVANS

(Sir) Thomas John Carey Evans (Carey-Evans from 1921) KB FRCS (1884–1947). Born at Festiniog, Merionethshire, and educated at University College Cardiff – from which he qualified in 1905 – his medical career was pursued at Glasgow, St Bartholomew's Hospital, Brussels, and Vienna. Following qualification, he served in the 7th Battalion, Royal Welsh Fusiliers from 1908–9. In 1909, Evans was commissioned in the IMS, and in 1910 appointed surgical specialist in the Lucknow division; he saw active service 'against the head-hunters at Abor on the North-East frontier in 1911–12'. He also served as medical officer to the Mishin expedition which 'explored the Tibetan frontier and mapped the upper course of the river Brahmaputra'. During the Great War, Evans served with the Indian Army at Gallipoli, Egypt and Mesopotamia and in 1917, he became civil medical officer for Baghdad. In 1920 he was appointed resident medical officer of the State of Mysore.

Carey-Evans was a surgeon to the HTD from 1924 until 1932; he retired from the IMS in 1926. He was elected consulting surgeon to St Paul's Hospital for Genito-Urinary Diseases following return to England, and in 1933 appointed (first) Medical Superintendent of the Hammersmith Hospital 'when the [Royal] Postgraduate Medical School was established there' – a position which he held for ten years. During the Second World War, he 'organized the hospital under war-time and air-raid conditions', taking '[a] full personal share in the activities of the hospital's Home Guard detachment'. He retired in 1944 in order 'to cultivate his lifelong interest in [the] Welsh language, literature, and history'. His wife was the elder daughter of David Lloyd-George (1863–1945), prime-minister from 1916 until 1922; there were four children of the marriage.[33]

Specialist medical/surgical staff

As at the *Dreadnought*, the era of specialists was considered to have arrived; hence a plastic, colo-rectal, an ophthalmic surgeon, and a gynaecologist were appointed; in addition, a helminthologist was taken 'on-board', presumably at the request of Manson himself!

McINDOE

(Sir) Archibald Hector McIndoe FRCS (1900–60) was born at Dunedin, New Zealand, and educated at Otago High School and University. He qualified (MB,

ChB, *NZ*) in 1923, and after a house surgeon's post (at Waikato Hospital), was awarded a Fellowship to the Mayo Clinic, USA; he worked there from 1925–27, and published several papers on hepatic pathology. A post as first assistant in surgery followed. In 1931, he proceeded to England and was appointed clinical assistant in the Department of Plastic Surgery at St Bartholomew's Hospital, at the suggestion of his cousin, Sir Harold Gillies. In 1932, he was appointed surgeon and lecturer in *tropical surgery* at the HTD and LSHTM, and in 1939, was elected as consulting surgeon to: St Bartholomew's, the Chelsea Hospital for Women, St Andrew's Hospital, and the Hampstead Children's Hospital; he was also consulting plastic surgeon to the Royal North Stafford Infirmary and Croydon General Hospital.

In 1938, McIndoe was appointed consultant in plastic surgery to the RAF, and when war was declared in 1939 he chose the (newly rebuilt) Queen Victoria Hospital, East Grinstead as his preferred site for the plastic and jaw surgery centre; there, he rehabilitated badly burned air crew, and founded the notorious 'Guinea Pig Club'. McIndoe also accomplished a great deal for the RCS, where he was a major fund-raiser. He was twice married; there were two daughters of the first. A memorial service, at which an address was given by the PRCS – Sir James Patterson Ross, was held on 12 May 1960 at St Clement Danes, London.[34]

NAUNTON MORGAN

(Sir) Clifford Naunton Morgan FRCS (1901–86) was born at Penygraig, Glamorgan and educated at the Royal Masonic School (Bushey), University College, Cardiff, and St Bartholomew's Hospital; he qualified in 1923 and held junior appointments at the Metropolitan, London and St Mark's Hospitals. In 1927, Naunton Morgan became an anatomy demonstrator at St Bartholomew's, and the following year was appointed assistant surgeon to the Metropolitan Hospital. In 1936 he was appointed surgeon to St Mark's, and assistant director of the surgical unit at St Bartholomew's. During the Second World War, Morgan served in the RAMC and was initially posted to Egypt; he later became: consultant surgeon to the Persia-Iraq Force, and afterwards East Africa Command. Following the war, he returned to St Bartholomew's and St Mark's. He was also appointed to the HTD and the King Edward VII Hospital for Officers; he also became consultant surgeon to the Navy, Army and RAF. At the RCS, he was a member of Council, and Bradshaw and Vicary lecturer. Naunton Morgan was to become the doyen of *proctological surgeons* of Britain.[35]

ELLIOT

Robert Henry Elliot FRCS (1864–1936). Educated at Bedford School and St Bartholomew's Hospital, Elliot qualified MRCS in 1889, MB (Lond) in 1890, and BS in 1891. In 1892, he entered the IMS and had a distinguished period at Netley. From 1892–4 Elliot was on sanitary duty in India, and served on the NE frontier in the Chin Hills campaign of 1892–3. For a decade – beginning in 1904 – he was Superintendent of the Government Ophthalmic Hospital, Madras (now Chennai), and Professor of Ophthalmology at the Medical College there. For a time, he was secretary to the Surgeon-General of Madras. He became an authority on snake-bite.

In 1915, Elliot retired from the IMS and settled in London. In 1919 he was appointed lecturer on *ophthalmology* at the LSTM, and until 1925 was on the staff of the HTD; he was also ophthalmic surgeon to the Prince of Wales Hospital. Elliot was an expert on the surgical management of glaucoma. He wrote a great deal about Indian magic, being a member of 'The Magic Circle'. There were three sons of his marriage.[36]

GREEN-ARMYTAGE

Vivian Bartley Green-Armytage FRCP FRCS (1882–1961) was a *gynaecologist*. He was born at Clifton, and from Clifton College studied at the University and the Royal Infirmary, Bristol. In 1907, he joined the IMS (in which he served for seven years) having already completed a house-post, post-graduate studies at Paris, and a short time at the RAMC College, Millbank. Following distinguished service in the Great War, he spent a further 11 years in India, occupying the chair of midwifery and gynaecology at the University and Medical College of Calcutta. In 1933, he was appointed gynaecological and obstetric surgeon to the Bristol Post-Graduate, and West London Medical Schools, honorary gynaecological surgeon to the HTD and Italian Hospital, and obstetric surgeon to the Jewish Maternity Hospital. Green-Armytage was a foundation fellow of the British (later Royal) College of Obstetricians and Gynaecologists.[37]

LEIPER

Robert Thomson Leiper FRCP FRS (1881–1969) was born in Kilmarnock, Ayrshire and educated at Warwick (to where his parents had moved soon after his birth) School, Mason College in Birmingham and the University of Glasgow (where he studied medicine). Leiper graduated in medicine in 1904, and the following year was successfully 'head-hunted' by Manson as helminthologist to the newly-formed LSTM; he remained there or the LSHTM (which opened in 1929) until 1946. In 1929, he was made Honorary *helminthologist* to the HTD. He played a key role in persuading the Rockefeller Foundation to donate $2 million to establish the LSHTM.

Leiper undertook numerous expeditions to tropical countries, including the Far East, East and West Africa, Egypt, the Caribbean and South America, where his researches involved helminths of humans, and domestic and big game animals. He elucidated the full life-cycles of *Dracunculus medinensis* and *Loa-loa*. During the Great War, Leiper was posted by the RAMC to Egypt (where he had previously worked with Loos) and established the full life-cycles of *Schistosoma haematobium* and *S. mansoni*. He later established the *Journal of Helminthology* (1923) and *Helminthological Abstracts* (1932). There was a son and two daughters of his marriage.[38]

Surgical staff of King George's Sanatorium for Sailors (KGSS) 1914–39

Table 21.7 summarises the medical/surgical staff of the SHS sanatorium during the inter-war years. The two surgeons appointed at this establishment were,

Table 21.7: Medical/surgical staff of King George's Sanatorium for Sailors (1914-39).

Physician:	
1922–[39]	C E Sundell
Surgeons:	
1921–[39]	Gilbert Smith
1922–[39]	Sir Henry Gauvain
Chest Surgeon:	
1938–[39]	A Tudor Edwards
Laryngologist:	
1927–[39]	F Courtenay-Mason
Medical Superintendent (and Director):	
1921–23	H Sharpe
1923–[39]	J E Wood (*see* Chapter 24)

respectively – a local general practitioner/surgeon, and a leading authority (in this country) on the management of tuberculosis (phthisis). Sundell (the physician) was of course already on the staff of the *Dreadnought* hospital.

SMITH

Gilbert Smith FRCS (1874–1950) was the second son of Sir Thomas Smith Bt, a consulting surgeon to St Bartholomew's Hospital. He received his education at Marlborough School and St Bartholomew's Hospital, graduating MRCS, LRCS in 1896. He became clinical assistant in the throat department there, and also at the children's department at the Middlesex Hospital. Smith entered general practice at Hindhead, Surrey in 1900; In the Great War, he served in France a base hospital at Rouen with the British Red Cross, as a surgical specialist with the RAMC. In 1921, he was appointed surgeon to the KGSS at Bramshott. There were four sons and two daughters of his marriage.[39]

GAUVAIN

(Sir) Henry John Gauvain FRCS (1878–1945) was born at Aldernay and, having survived a severe attack of scarlet fever ('scarlatina') whilst at a preparatory school in England, undertook further education at Aldernay, St John's College, Cambridge and St Bartholomew's Hospital. He developed an interest in bone and joint tuberculosis, which he believed could be cured by 'fresh air and sunlight', whilst first medical superintendent of Lord Mayor Treloar's Cripples Hospital and College at Alton, Hampshire – to which he had been appointed in 1908. In 1920, he started a 'seaside branch' at Hayling Island and was a pioneer of occupational therapy and rehabilitation. Gauvain was also an 'excellent speaker and administrator'. He was an authority on hospital planning. Gauvain was also consulting surgeon to the King Edward VII Welsh National Memorial Association for treatment of tuberculosis, the London and Essex County Councils, Hampshire County Council, and KGSS (between 1922 and 1943) – where he established an 'open-air' ward. Gauvain was a pioneer in sea-bathing in the management of tuberculosis, and in 1938 was making plans for a hydrotherapeutic centre for the treatment of poliomyelitis at Hayling Island. There was a son and daughter of his marriage.[40]

TUDOR EDWARDS

A later appointment (shortly before the outbreak of World War II) was that of Arthur Tudor Edwards FRCS (1890–1946). Born at Langlands, Glamorgan, Tudor Edwards was educated at Mill Hill School, St John's College, Cambridge and the Middlesex Hospital Medical School. Having served as a surgical registrar, he was commissioned at the outbreak of war in 1914, to the RAMC, serving in France with No. 6 Casualty Clearing Station. Following the war, he became assistant surgeon to the Westminster and Brompton Hospitals, and researched (with collaboration of R A Young and Ivan Magill) surgical management of pulmonary tuberculosis, bronchiectasis, tumours of the mediastinum, tumours of the lung and was instrumental in establishing the *new* speciality of thoracic surgery. In 1936, Tudor Edwards was appointed first Director of the Department of Thoracic Surgery at the (Royal) London Hospital. He was also consultant thoracic surgeon to King Edward VII Sanatorium, Midhurst, and Queen Alexandra Hospital, Millbank. He was also a surgeon under the Ministry of Pensions to Queen Mary's Hospital, Roehampton, and supervised the LCC Thoracic Unit at St Mary Abbott's Hospital, Kensington. During the Second World War, he was civilian consultant to the RAF, adviser for thoracic casualties to the Ministry of Health, and civilian adviser to the War Office. He also organised reception centres for thoracic casualties under the EMS. Edwards was a prolific author. There were no children of his marriage in 1920.[41]

Medical staff of the Tilbury Hospital, and the Queen Alexandra Memorial Hospital, Marseilles

Table 21.8 summarises the physicians and surgeons who were responsible for patient-care at the Tilbury Hospital in the inter-war years. Most medical/surgical cover at the Tilbury Hospital was carried out by members of the staff of the *Dreadnought* Hospital and ADH, or by local general practitioner/surgeons. The remainder of the staff were relatively junior, and details of most of their careers have *not* survived. The Queen Alexandra Memorial Hospital at Marseilles was staffed entirely by French practitioners, and was merely administered by the Society.

Table 21.8: Medical staff of the Tilbury Hospital (1914–39)

Consulting Physicians in Tropical Diseases:		
1927–28	G C Low	(see above)
1927–[39]	P Manson-Bahr	(see above)
1937–[39]	N Hamilton Fairley	(see above)
Consulting Surgeons:		
[1896]–1930	T Openshaw	
1926–[39]	C J Pinching	
1930–[39]	C G E Plumstead	
1930–[39]	P P Cole (see above)	
Consulting Physician(s):		
19[14]–27	T Openshaw	
1921–25	A J Couzens	
1932–[39]	C E Sundell (see above)	
Ophthalmic Surgeon:		
1924–[39]	R H Balfour-Barrow	
Radiologist:		
1937–[39]	G W Phillips	
Visiting Tuberculosis Officer:		
1927–[39]	W T G Boul	

References and notes

1 Annual Report 112; *Who Was Who 1929–40:* 257.
2 *Op cit.* See note 1 above. (Reports); *Who Was Who 1941–50*: 691; G C Cook. A difficult metamorphosis: the incorporation of the Ross Institute & Hospital for Tropical Diseases into the London School of Hygiene and Tropical Medicine. *Med Hist* 2001; 45: 483–506; [*See also:* Anonymous. The Rt Hon Lord Lloyd of Dolobran, PC, GCSI, GCIE, DSO. *SHS Quart Mag* 1932; 4(2): 9; J Tomes. Lloyd, George Ambrose, first Baron Lloyd (1879–1941) In: H C G Matthew, B Harrison (eds). *Oxford Dictionary of National Biography.* Oxford: Oxford University Press 2004; 34: 124–7].
3 *Op cit.* See note 1 above (Reports) 141; *Who Was Who 1961–70*: 86.
4 Anonymous. The new Secretary: Mr [FA] Lyon takes up his duties at Greenwich. *SHS Quart Mag* 1935; 7(2): 7.
5 Anonymous. *Times, Lond* 1965; 30 December: 10: F M R Walshe. Gordon Morgan Holmes *Biog Mem Roy Soc* 1966; 12: 311–9; F M R Walsh. Sir Gordon Morgan Holmes *Nature* 1966; 209: 853–4; Anonymous. Gordon Morgan Holmes *Lancet* 1966; i: 101; Anonymous. Sir Gordon Holmes *BMJ* 1966; i: 111–2; Anonymous. Holmes, Sir Gordon Morgan *Munk's Roll* 5: 195–7; W Penfield. Holmes, Sir Gordon Morgan (1876–1965) In: H C G Matthew, B Harrison (eds). *Oxford Dictionary of National Biography.* Oxford: Oxford University Press 2004; 27: 788–90.
6 Anonymous. Charles Ernest Sundell *Lancet* 1964; ii: 1247.

7 Anonymous. *Times, Lond* 1968; 9 January: 8; Anonymous. Edwin Charles Warner. *Lancet* 1968; i: 152; [SJRR]. E C Warner. *Br Med J* 1968; i: 187; PBS Fowler. Warner, Edwin Charles. *Munk's Roll* 6: 450–1.
8 [JAVB]: James Purdon Martin: *Lancet* 1984; i: 1135–6; [AS]. J P Martin. *BMJ* 1984; 288: 1698; R E Kelly. Martin, James Purdon *Munk's Roll* 8: 323–5.
9 W N Mann. Hampson, Arthur Cecil. *Munk's Roll* 6: 216–7; *Guy's Hosp Gaz* 1972; 86: 570–1.
10 Anonymous. *Times, Lond* 1943; 15 October: 7; *Lancet* 1943; ii: 558; *BMJ* 1943; ii: 528 & 561; *Plarr's Lives 1930–51*: 692–4. [*See also* C W Rountree. Hunterian lecture on X-ray carcinoma, and an experimental inquiry into the conditions which precede its onset. *Lancet* 1909; i: 821–4].
11 Anonymous. *Plarr's Lives 1974–1982*: 115.
12 Anonymous. *Lancet* 1950; ii: 937–8; *BMJ* 1950: ii: 1449, 1500; *Munk's Roll 4:* 552.
13 Anonymous. *Times, Lond* 1972; 22 May: 16; *Lancet* 1972; i: 1295; *BMJ* 1972; ii: 535; *Munk's Roll* 6: 183–4.
14 Anonymous. *Times, Lond* 1949; 38 5 November: 47; Anonymous. Richard Lake. *Lancet* 1949; ii: 921–2; Anonymous. Richard Lake. *BMJ* 1949; ii: 1118; Anonymous. Lake, Richard. *Plarr's Lives 1930–51*: 461–2.
15 Anonymous. *BMJ* 1953; ii: 294; Anonymous. Mason, Francis Courtenay. *Plarr's Lives 1952–64*: 279–80.
16 Anonymous. *Times, Lond* 1948; 28 October: 7; Anonymous. Percival Pasley Cole. *Lancet* 1948; ii: 710; Anonymous. Percival P Cole. *BMJ* 1948; ii: 801, 962; Anonymous. Cole, Percival Pasley *Plarr's Lives 1930–51:* 155–6. [*See also:* P P Cole: Three cases showing late results of pedicle bone-graft for fractured mandible. *Proc Roy Soc Med* 1938; 31: 1131–4; Pathological fracture of the mandible. *Lancet* 1940: i: 1044–5; War injuries of jaws and face. *Postgrad Med* J 1940 16: 233–44; Experiences in reparative surgery of the upper limb. *Br J Surg* 1941: 28; The filigree operation for inguinal hernia. *Br J Surg* 1941: 29; Inguinal swellings. *Med Press Circ* 1942; 207: 91–6].
17 Anonymous. *Times, Lond* 1952; 1 August: 8; *Lancet* 1952; ii: 296–7; *BMJ* 1952; ii: 341–2; *Munk's Roll* 4: 594–5. [*See also:* [D A C Price] G Carmichael Low MD FRCP *SHS Quart Mag* 1937; 9(3): 15–16; G C Cook. George Carmichael Low FRCP: twelfth President of the Society and underrated pioneer of tropical medicine. *Trans R Soc Trop Med Hyg* 1993; 87: 355–60; G C Cook. Correspondence from Dr George Carmichael Low to Dr Patrick Manson during the first Ugandan sleeping sickness expedition. *J Med Biog* 1993; 1: 215–29; M Worboys. Low, George Carmichael (1872–1952) In: H C G Matthew, B Harrison (eds). *Oxford Dictionary of National Biography.* Oxford: Oxford University Press 2004; 34: 550–1].
18 Anonymous. *Times, Lond* 1966; 21 November: 12; Anonymous. Philip Henry Manson-Bahr *Lancet* 1966; ii: 1198–9; Anonymous. Sir Philip Manson-Bahr. *BMJ* 1966; ii: 1332; *Munk's Roll* 6: 328–30; [*See also:* P H Manson-Bahr, A Alcock. *The life and work of Sir Patrick Manson.* London: Cassell & Co Ltd 1927: 273; *P Manson-Bahr:* The jubilee of Sir Patrick Manson (1878–1925): a tribute to his work on the malaria problem. *Postgrad Med J* 1938; 14: 345–57; Treatment of dysentery. *Med Press Circ* 1941; 206: 64–8; Diarrhoea, with some notes on treatment. *Med Press Circ* 1942; 208: 100–2; The nature and treatment of war-time malaria relapses in England. *Med Press Circ* 1944; 212: 342–7; *Ibid.* The post-graduate teaching of clinical tropical medicine. 361–73].
19 D G Crawford (ed). Pratt, James John. *Roll of the Indian Medical Service 1615–1930* Calcutta: Thacker & Co 1930: 205.
20 Anonymous. *Times, Lond* 1951: 4 October: 8; Anonymous. Charles Hope Carlton. *Lancet* 1951: ii: 740; *Anonymous.* C Hope Carlton. *BMJ* 1951; ii: 976–7; Anonymous. *J Roy Army*

Med Corps 1951; 47: 508; Anonymous. Carlton, Charles Hope. *Plarr's Lives 1930–51*: 132–3.

21 Anonymous. *Times, Lond* 1964; 3 July: 14; Anonymous. Thomas Pomfret Kilner. *Lancet* 1964; ii: 103–4; Anonymous. Thomas Pomfret Kilner. *BMJ* 1964; ii: 127–8; *Brit J Surg* 1964; 51: 945; *Br J Plast Surg* 1964; 17: 330–4; Kilner, Thomas Pomfret *Plarr's Lives 1952–64*: 227–9.

22 Anonymous. Hugh Ernest Griffiths Lancet 1961; i: 1176–7; Anonymous. Sir Hugh Griffiths *BMJ* 1961: i: 1545; Anonymous *Plarr's Lives*. Griffiths, Sir Hugh Ernest 1952–64: 173–4; [*See also: H E Griffiths: Injury and incapacity with special reference to industrial insurance.* London: Jordan & Sons Ltd 1935: 270; The organisation of fracture clinics in Europe and America. *Postgrad Med J* 1938; 14: 167–175; Observations on the treatment of air raid casualties in Barcelona. *Postgrad Med J* 1939; 15: 371–5; Modern fracture treatment. *J Indust Welfare Soc* 1940: 55; Medical aspects of workmen's compensation. *BMJ* 1940; i:1060–1; Treatment of the injured workman. *Lancet* 1943; i: 729–33; The experimental approach – 4. Rehabilitation – the Albert Dock Hospital of the Seamen's Hospital Society. *Nat News-Letter* 1944; [H E Griffiths] Medical problems of workmen's compensation. *BMJ(suppl)* 1940; i: 103–107; Rehabilitation of the disabled in Poland – a UNRRA Report: 98 [SHS Archive].

23 G C Cook, A J Webb. The Albert Dock Hospital, London: the original site (in 1899) of Tropical Medicine and a new discipline. *Acta Trop* 2001; 79: 249–55.

24 G C Cook. *From the Greenwich hulks to Old St Pancras: a history of tropical disease in London.* London: Athlone Press 1992: 163–241.

25 Anonymous. *Times, Lond* 1973; 23 February: 19; [W G]. Francis Martin Rouse Walsh *Lancet* 1973; i: 496–7; Anonymous. Sir Francis Walshe. *BMJ* 1973; i: 555; C G Phillips. Francis Martin Rouse Walshe. *Biog Mem Roy Soc* 1974; 20: 457–81; W Gooddy. Walshe, Sir Francis (Martin Rouse). *Munk's Roll* 6: 448–9; W Gooddy. Walshe, Sir Francis Martin Rouse (1885–1973). In: H C G Matthew, B Harrison (eds). *Oxford Dictionary of National Biography.* Oxford: Oxford University Press 2004; 57: 126–7.

26 Anonymous. *Times, Lond* 1966; 21 April: 18; Sir Neil Hamilton Fairley. *Nature, Lond* 1966; 210: 1205; Neil Hamilton Fairley. *Lancet* 1966; i: 987–8; Neil Hamilton Fairley *BMJ* 1966; i: 1117–8; J Boyd. Neil Hamilton Fairley 1891–1966. *Biog Mem Roy Soc* 1966; 12: 123–45; Anonymous. *J Trop Med Hyg* 1973; Anonymous. *Med J Aust* 1969; ii: 991; J Boyd. Fairley, Sir Neil Hamilton (1891–1966). In: H C G Matthew, B Harrison (eds). *Oxford Dictionary of National Biography.* Oxford: Oxford University Press 2004; 18: 948–9.

27 Anonymous. *Times, Lond* 1962; 20, 22, 26 September: 18, 12, 15; Anonymous. Leonard Rogers. *Lancet* 1962; ii: 666–7; Anonymous. Sir Leonard Rogers. *BMJ* 1962: ii: 862–3; Anonymous. *Bull Calcutta Sch Trop Med* 1962; 10: 174–5; Anonymous. *St Mary's Hosp Gaz* 1962; 68: 268–9; C Wilcocks. Sir Leonard Rogers *Nature, Lond* 1962; 196: 517–8; J S K Boyd. Leonard Rogers *Biog Mem Roy Soc* 1963: 9: 261–85; *Munk's Roll* 5: 353–5. G McRobert, H J Power. Rogers, Sir Leonard (1868–1962) In: H C G Matthew, B Harrison (eds). *Oxford Dictionary of National Biography.* Oxford: Oxford University Press 2004; 47: 572–4; G C Cook. Leonard Rogers KCSI, FRCP, FRS (1868–1962) and the founding of the Calcutta School of Tropical Medicine. *Notes* Rec R Soc 2006; 60: 171–81. [*See also*: L Rogers. *Happy toil: fifty-five years of tropical medicine.* London: Frederick Muller 1950: 271].

28 D G Crawford (ed.). Mackie, Frederick Percival. *Roll of the Indian Medical Service 1615–1930*: Calcutta: W Thacker & Co 1930 524; F Percival Mackie *Lancet* 1944; ii: 263–4; Col. Frederick Percival Mackie. *Br Med J* 1944; ii: 164–5; Anonymous. Mackie, Frederick Percival. *Munk's Roll* 4: 566–7; Anonymous. Mackie, Frederick Percival. *Plarr's Lives 1930–51*: 510–3.

29 W Somerville. Bedford, Davis Evan. *Munk's Roll* 7: 28–30.

30 Anonymous. Chandler, Frederick George. *Munk's Roll* 4: 598.
31 Anonymous. MacLeod, John MacLeod Hendrie. *Munk's Roll* 5: 260–1.
32 Anonymous. Martin, Peter Henry. *Munk's Roll* 5: 270–1. [*See also*: Martin P H. *Monthly Bull Min Hlth Lab Service* 1947; 6: 148–51; 1949; 8: 38–47; 1952; 11: 187–206; 1953; 12: 232–41; 1957; 16: 103–22].
33 D G Crawford (ed.). Evans, Thomas John Carey. *Roll of the Indian Medical Service 1615–1930*: Calcutta: W Thacker & Co. 1938; 551; Anonymous. *Times, Lond* 1947; 26 August: 6; Anonymous. Thomas John Carey Evans *Lancet* 1947; ii: 373, 409; Anonymous. Sir Thomas Carey Evans. *Br Med J* 1947; ii: 352, 399; 1948; i: 180. Anonymous. Evans, Sir Thomas John Carey. *Plarr's Lives 1930–51*: 270.
34 Anonymous. *Times, Lond* 1960; 13 April: 15; 19 April; 13 & 13 May: 16; Anonymous. Archibald Hector McIndoe. *Lancet* 1960: i: 929–30; Sir Archibald McIndoe. *Br Med J* 1960; i: 1280–1; Anonymous. *Ann R Coll surg Engl* 1960; 26: 333 & 27: 62; Anonymous. McIndoe, Sir Archibald Hector. *Plarr's Lives 1952–64*: 266–8. R Battle, H C G Matthew. McIndoe, Sir Archibald Hector. (1900–1960) In: H C G Matthew, B Harrison (eds). *Oxford Dictionary of National Biography.* Oxford: Oxford University Press 2004; 35: 474–5. [*See also*: H M[c]Leave. *M[c]Indoe: plastic surgeon* 1961: 231; L Mosley. *Faces from the fire: the biography of Sir Archibald M[c]Indoe.* 1962: 269; Shaw J. Recognition of a special civilian on Battle of Britain Day. *Times, Lond* 2000; 15 September: 24].
35 Anonymous. *Times, Lond* 1986; 26 February: 16; *Daily Telegraph* 1986; 22 February; Anonymous. Clifford Naunton Morgan. *Lancet* 1986; i: 692; Anonymous. Sir Clifford Naunton Morgan. *BMJ* 1986; 292: 772; Morgan, Sir Clifford Naunton. *Plarr's Lives 1983–1990*; 261–2.
36 Anonymous. *Times, Lond* 1936; 10 November: 18; Anonymous. Robert Henry Elliot. *Lancet* 1936; ii: 1240; Anonymous. R H Elliot. *BMJ* 1936; ii: 1061–2; Anonymous. Lieut-Colonel R H Elliot. *Nature, Lond* 1936; 138: 913–4; Elliot, Robert Henry. *Plarr's Lives 1930–51*: 257–8.
37 Anonymous. Green-Armytage, Vivian Bartley. *Munk's Roll* 5: 163–4; Anonymous. Green-Armytage, Vivian Bartley (1882–1961). *Plarr's Lives 1952–1964*: 169–70.
38 Anonymous. *Times, Lond* 1969; 23 May: 12; Anonymous. Robert Thomson Leiper. *Lancet* 1969; i: 1103–4; *BMJ* 1969; ii: 579–80; P C C Garnham. Robert Thomson Leiper 1881–1969. *Biog Mem Roy Soc* 1970; 16: 385–404; J Farley. Leiper, Robert Thomson (1881–1969). In: H C G Matthew, B Harrison (eds). *Oxford Dictionary of National Biography.* Oxford: Oxford University Press 2004; 33: 280–1.
39 Anonymous. *Times, Lond* 1950; 24 June: 1; Anonymous. Gilbert Smith. *Lancet* 1950; ii: 461; Gilbert Smith (1874–1950). *Plarr's Lives 1930–51*: 721.
40 Anonymous. *Times, Lond* 1945; 20 January: 7; Anonymous. Henry Gauvain *Lancet* 1945: i: 162–3; Anonymous. Sir Henry Gauvain. *BMJ* 1945; i: 167; *Public Hth* 1945; 58: 60; Anonymous. *Med Press* 1945; 213: 96; Anonymous. *J Roy Inst Public Hlth* 1945; 8: 78; Anonymous. *J Bone Jt Surg* 1945; 27: 342; Anonymous. *Br J Phys Med* 1945; 8: 55; Gauvain, Sir Henry John (1878–1945). *Plarr's Lives 1930–1951*: 317–9; W J Bishop, L Bryder. Gauvain, Sir Henry John (1878–1945). In: H C G Matthew, B Harrison (eds). *Oxford Dictionary of National Biography.* Oxford: Oxford University Press 2004; 21: 653–4.
41 Anonymous. *Times, Lond* 1946: 27 August 1, 6; 28 August: 7; 29 August: 6; Edwards, Arthur Tudor. *Plarr's Lives 1930–1951*: 253–5.

Chapter 22

The Second World War (1939–45): introduction of the National Health Service (1948) and decline in the Society's activities

Little more than a year after the outbreak of War on 3 September 1939, the mood of the Society was 'darkened by the [sudden] death on February 5th [1941] of the President after [only] 2 years in office'. The Chairman of the Society (Benn) wrote in the Annual Report for 1940: '... [Lloyd had] devoted himself with passionate energy and singleness of purpose – to enrich the prestige of the British Empire and to increase its sea power'.

An aura of gloom surrounding the war had rapidly swept through the land, and all and sundry were prepared for air-raids, accompanied by fire, injury and death. The SHS archive contains several documents (1940–42) which highlight this increasingly disturbing situation. By late 1940, the SHS's bed complement was:

Dreadnought Hospital, Greenwich	53
Albert Dock Hospital, Custom House, E16*	55
Tilbury Seamen's Hospital	116
Angas Home, Cudham, Kent	42
King George's Sanatorium for Sailors, Bramshott, Liphook, Hampshire	80
	346

A diminution to 'little more than one-fifth of its normal size' of the *Dreadnought's* capacity was occasioned by destruction of the North West Wing – opened in 1932; the Chapel was also totally destroyed by a German bomb in 'the early morning [2.30am] of 10th September 1940' (Figure 22.1); 'By God's mercy there were [however] no casualties'. Shortly afterwards, the hospital received visits from 'the Prime Minister [Winston Churchill (1874–1965)] – on the 25th September, and HRH The Duke of Kent [1902–42] – on 30th September'. A 'Dreadnought Restoration Fund' was immediately set up, and help came from the British War Relief Society of New

* This hospital (the site of the first School of Tropical Medicine) played an enormously important part in the 'Blitz' of 1940.[1]

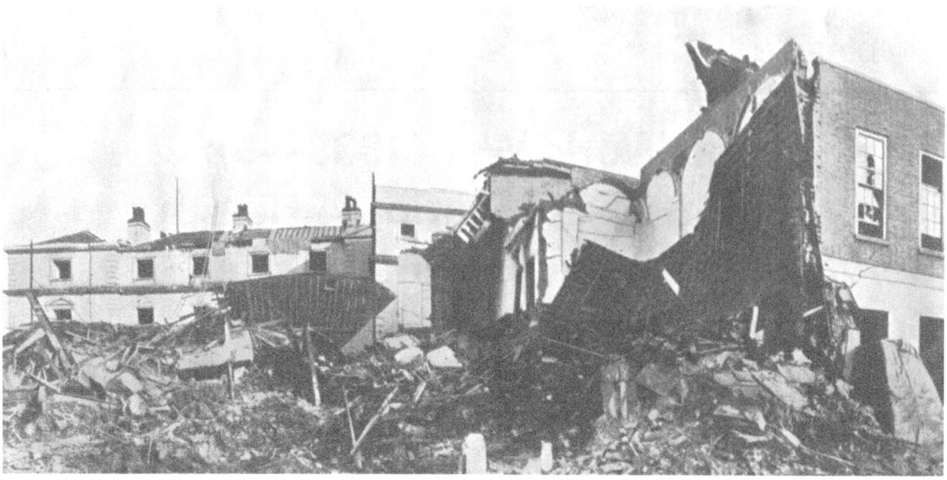

Figure 22.1: Destruction by enemy bombs of the *Dreadnought* Hospital in 1940. [SHS Archive].

York. Both the ADH and Tilbury Hospital were also damaged that year as a result of enemy action; the HTD had of course been closed since 1939 (and the patients transferred to the *Dreadnought* Hospital) on Ministry of Health orders. The 1940 report concluded by reminding its readership that 'no State aid is received for sailors of the Merchant Navy … whose gallant service is a vital, perhaps the paramount, factor in the Empire's war effort'.[1]

The 1941 Report contained further gloomy news:

> Further damage has been suffered by enemy action. The major part of the top storey [the roof of the *Eastern* Wing] of the Dreadnought Hospital was destroyed by the last of three showers of incendiaries on the night of the 19th April [1941], and the damage by water to the emergency hospital, reconstructed after [the] destruction wrought in September, 1940, interrupted its work for some weeks and has made working conditions difficult throughout the rest of the year.[2]

On two other occasions that year, the *Dreadnought* was damaged by enemy action. The 1942 Report recorded: 'A section of Middle East Floor, damaged on two occasions by enemy action, has been reconditioned to serve as a Scabies Unit working in conjunction with the scheme operated by Dr M.T. Morgan [Chapter 23], Medical Officer of the Port of London'.[3]

When the War entered its fourth year, it became increasingly difficult to maintain staffing at the five SHS establishments. The Report for 1943 also commented on entitlement to Emergency Medical Scheme [EMS] treatment:

> Arising from representations made by the Society, the rights of officers and men of the Merchant Navy to free treatment under the [EMS] have been clarified by the following definition 'officers and seamen of all

> nationalities who are injured in the course of duty or who are suffering as the result of exposure on duty are entitled to hospital treatment free of charge under the Scheme'. Those members of the Merchant Navy who do not fall within these categories are required to contribute towards the cost of their maintenance in E.M.S. Hospitals ...[4]

The former HTD building at Endsleigh Gardens had meanwhile been seriously damaged by 'a land mine which fell close to it on 10th May' 1944. Further bomb damage to the *Dreadnought* Hospital, and also the Devonport Nurses Home was recorded in the 1944 Report. 1945 was, however, the final year of the War, and the Report for that year recorded that, since VE day* 'some of the damaged wards [the hospital had received 'only superficial damage from V1 or V2 rocket bombs'] at Greenwich [had] been reconditioned [bringing the number of beds up to] 126'.[5] Figure 22.2 shows the ground-floor plan of the newly designed *Dreadnought* Hospital, and Figure 22.3 shows a corridor in the rebuilt hospital.

Other matters during the war years

A continuing discrepancy between the treatment of RN and Merchant Navy sailors had been highlighted by the 12th Earl of Cork and Orrery (1873–1967), Deputy Chairman of the SHS, during a debate in the House of Lords in 1941:

> ... Merchant Navy sailors in hospital are classed as 'Civilian Sick or Casualties', and therefore receive less ample rations than the [RN] ratings in R.N. Hospitals. This discrimination between sailors who are sick or injured after facing the same dangers and hardships has been remedied only insofar as R.N. ratings treated in Civil hospitals are in future to receive only civilian rations.

His Lordship again supported the Merchant sailors in a House of Lords debate the following year; as a result tuberculosis (Chapter 23) was specifically included as a 'war injury' and made eligible for compensation under the 'Pensions (MM) Act'.[6]

The 1944 Report began by paying tribute to the Society's late President, Lord Moyne (1880–1944)[7] (Secretary of State for the Colonies [1941–2], and subsequently Minister of State in the Middle East [1942–4]) who had been assassinated in Cairo on 6 November of that year.[8] The Society had thus lost two of its more distinguished Presidents during the War Years.

Together with interruptions in most of the Society's activities, the nurse-training programme also suffered. However, this was rapidly resumed as the following minute, also written in late 1944, makes clear:

> With the approval of the General Nursing Council, The Associated Training School for Student Nurses of the Dreadnought and Royal Waterloo Hospitals [teaching was soon] re-established. The training [the minute continued] will be over a period of 3½ years.

---

* Victory in Europe (VE) was celebrated on 8 May 1945.

THE BUILDINGS OF THE SEAMEN'S HOSPITAL SOCIETY

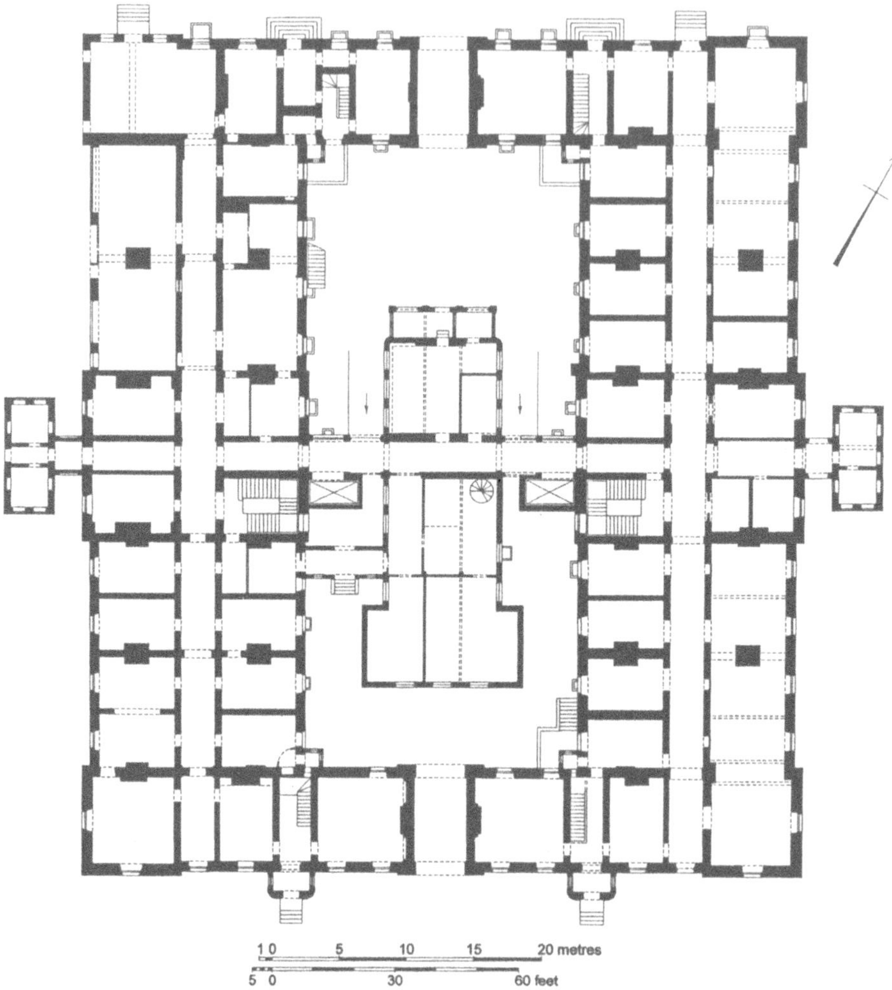

Figure 22.2: Plan of the ground-floor of *Dreadnought* Hospital in 1986, i.e. at closure of the establishment. [After J Bold. *Greenwich: an architectural history of the Royal Hospital for Seamen and the Queen's House*. London: English Heritage, 2000: 219.]

The National Health Service Act (1946)

Advanced notice of the setting-up of the National Health Service (NHS) in July 1948 had been publicised in 1942:

> In connection with the Survey of London Hospitals which is being undertaken by the Minister of Health in connection with his declared policy to co-ordinate all hospital services, a Memorandum was pre-

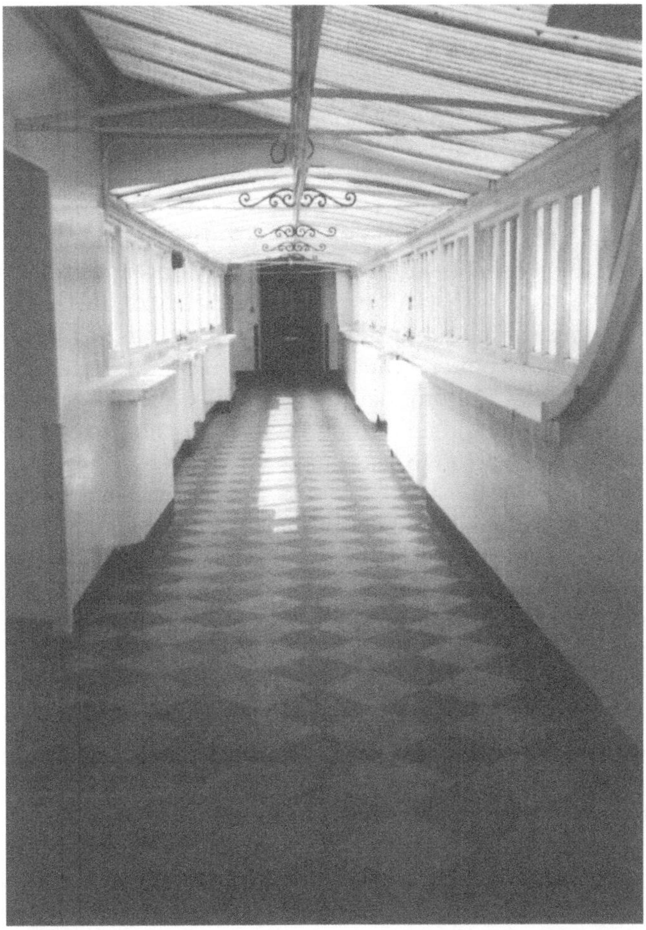

Figure 22.3: Corridor in the rebuilt *Dreadnought* Hospital prior to 1986. [SHS archive].

> pared describing the unique character and organisation of the group of Seamen's Hospitals and its identity with the Shipping Industry. This was approved by the Shipping Federation [SF] and the National Union of Seamen [NUS] and was then forwarded to the Co-ordination Committee for the Voluntary Hospitals of London and also handed to the Ministry of Health Surveyors.[9]

By 1944 the date for introduction of the NHS was fast approaching, and the Report for that year commented:

> In the view of the Committee, the proposals contained in the Government's White Paper on a [NHS] place complete control, the assessment of need, the whole of the local planning and the administration of the services, in the hands of the proposed Joint Authorities, ... composed of local authorities. There would be no direct contact

at any point between them and the voluntary hospitals to ensure the basis of partnership which has been referred to by successive Ministers of Health as an essential factor of the scheme. Any plan which would reduce the voluntary hospitals to a position of subservience to local authorities could only result in the lowering of standards and constitute an impediment to progress.

Fortunately, opportunities have been provided for consultation with the Minister of Health [Aneurin Bevan 1897–1960],[10] and the Committee have given their general support to the policy and action of the British Hospitals' Association [BHA]. It will be the policy of the [SHS] to maintain, at the highest possible standard, its Hospitals for the benefit of all seafarers who, from one cause or another, need to undergo hospital treatment when away from their home locality and who prefer to have their treatment among men of their own calling and to be looked after until they are ready to go to sea again.

Those who are in the special care of the Society are British seamen, Dominion and Colonial seamen, Indian and other Asiatic seamen, foreign seamen, seamen invalided from the Royal Navy, Dock and River workers in the port of London, women who are either seamen, i.e., nursing sisters and stewardesses, or the wives of seamen, and their children. For all these patients the Society will continue to provide special advantages not ordinarily to be found in landsmen's hospitals. Among such advantages may be mentioned: (*a*) Immediate admission by the Society's ambulance waiting on the quayside when a ship berths; (*b*) Longer retention in hospital and convalescent home, i.e., until the sailor is fit to return to sea; (*c*) Immediate admission for ailments which in most landsmen's hospitals would be referred for treatment at home; (*d*) Within the same group of Seamen's Hospitals special expert treatment is available for tropical diseases, tuberculosis, industrial injuries (including rehabilitation), venereal diseases and convalescence; (*e*) The Seamen's Hospitals are well acquainted with the methods of [MM] Offices, Consulates and Owners' Offices in dealing with seamen's affairs.

Furthermore, it must not be forgotten that there are other special activities in which the Society will continue to be engaged. Future progress in the study and treatment of tropical diseases, and postgraduate instruction in tropical medicine, will be frustrated without continued access to the tropical clinical material which is to be found collected together in the Society's Hospitals. The instruction of non-medical officers and crew in first aid and the rudiments of medical treatment and nursing care of the sick between ports could profitably be expanded at the Seamen's Hospitals, as also the endeavours which the Society has made to provide facilities for the postgraduate instruction of Ships' Doctors.

The Society looks forward to developing the already close collaboration which exists between the Port of London Health Committee and the Devonport Pathological Laboratories at the Dreadnought Hospital.[11]

Prelude to creation of the NHS

By 1946, the Second World War was fortunately an event of the past, and the Society was forced to look ahead with trepidation to the introduction of the NHS. The Report for this year was signed by Sir Ernest Murrant – the incoming Chairman:

> Shortly after the publication of the [NHS] Bill, the Committee, in accordance with the intention approved by the Governors … submitted a memorandum [to Bevan] asking that, within the general framework of the proposed Health Service, the Society's Hospitals shall continue to be Hospitals for Officers and Men of the [MM] of British and other nationalities in the Port of London. … the Minister's representative said that the Society had made out a strong case which was worthy of the Minister's careful consideration. He further agreed that in the best interests of seamen some special administrative co-ordination of the hospital arrangements for seamen was desirable, and that the detailed management of a hospital treating merchant seamen would be entrusted to a committee predominantly composed of persons with the special interests and experience necessary for the management of such a hospital.
>
> Upon the areas of the Regional Hospital Boards being announced, a further letter was addressed to the Minister's representative who replied that the Society's submissions would not fail to be dealt with when the appointment of Hospital Management Committees came to be actively considered. … Until [the 'appointed day' – 5 July 1948] the Seamen's Hospitals will continue [the Report reiterated] to depend upon voluntary contributions. Speaking at the Annual Court … last year [Murrant reminded his readership] Sir John Anderson [later 1st Viscount Waverley, 1882–1958][12] said: *"Those who by their contributions of money and service have hitherto maintained the Seamen's Hospitals, will be doing our seamen a great disservice if, at this juncture, they relax their generous efforts."*
>
> By way of reply to the many enquiries received from friends and supporters [the report continued], the Committee feel that they cannot do better than reproduce the following paragraphs written by the [BHA] explaining the significance of alterations made during the passage of the [NHS] Bill through Parliament:- 1. Observance of trusts in the redistribution of existing endowments. When redistributing the existing capital assets of the non-teaching hospitals, the Minister 'shall secure, so far as reasonably practicable, that the objects of the endowment and the observance if any conditions attached thereto, including any particular conditions intended to preserve the memory of any person or class of persons, are not prejudiced'. 2. Gifts made after 6th November, 1946, the date of the passing of the Act, to the existing governing body of a voluntary hospital or to trustees, will not be pooled when the Service comes into operation, but will be transferred to the appropriate new Management Committee so long as these gifts are made upon trusts which provide:- (a) For the administration of the property (i.e. gifts) as a capital fund separate from the general funds of the Hospital; or (b) For

> the application of the property (i.e. gifts) for some specific object distinct from the general purposes of the hospital and involving expenditure of a capital nature.
>
> The new Management Committee will continue to apply these moneys locally, according to the general or specific intention of the donor. Gifts made after the "appointed day." – Management Committees will be allowed to receive gifts and legacies of money of property and independently to administer such gifts as trustees on behalf of their hospital or group of hospitals. It will be unnecessary to make gifts to hospitals for general maintenance because this will be paid for by the State. But just as the State provision for the Fighting Services does not cover all the needs of the men in those Services (demonstrated by the existence of comforts and benevolent funds) so it is certain that the individual hospital in the Hospital Service will have needs not covered by the State payment.
>
> The Committee of Management therefore earnestly hope that good friends of the sailor will continue to ensure that members of the Merchant Navy who are patients of the Seamen's Hospitals will be abundantly supplied with all that they may need when they are laid up through illness of accident.[13]

At this point, the Chairman of the Society, together with his Deputy (Clifford Figg) and Treasurer (J C Nairne) wrote to Bevan, setting out the history and present state of the SHS and seeking clarification of envisaged plans for Seamen's Hospitals under the NHS.[14] This led to a discussion between the signatories of this letter (accompanied by the SHS Secretary, F A Lyon) and Mr Michael Reed – representing Bevan, on 8 July 1945; the proceedings are outlined in a subsequent memorandum.[15] Clearly there was already felt to be a distinct possibility of *fragmentation* of the SHS's 'Empire'.[16]

There was more about forthcoming implementation of the Act in the following Report (which stressed that although the 'Government [would] assume responsibility for the maintenance of the [SHS hospitals, it was hoped] that Governors and friends [would] continue their support by contributing to its Samaritan and Welfare Fund [set up in 1822]'):

> … the standard of the Society's hospitals, both as to personnel and equipment, will compare favourably with that of any other hospital entering the [NHS] on the Appointed Day … the Committee are able to forecast that, in their belief, it will not be necessary to ask the Ministry of Health for any financial assistance other than the customary payments for certain services rendered. … The six Seamen's Hospitals were found to be situated in the four Metropolitan Hospital Regions: the Dreadnought Hospital and the Angas Convalescent Home in the South East [SE], the [ADH] and the Tilbury Hospitals in the North East [NE], the [HTD] in the North West [NW] and King George's Sanatorium for Sailors in the South West [SW] Region.
>
> When the time came for Hospital Management Committees to be appointed, the Committee took advantage of the assurance previously

given by the Minister that he would further consider the Society's submissions that, in the best interests of seamen, some special administrative co-ordination of the hospital arrangements for seamen was desirable and that any management committee should be composed predominantly of persons with the special interests and experience necessary for the management of such hospitals.

The Minister approved the proposal of the [SE] Metropolitan Regional Board to appoint a Hospital Management Committee for the group of Seamen's Hospital comprising the Dreadnought Hospital and the Angas Convalescent Home. This Management Committee will [the Report continued] include members appointed after consultation with the National Maritime Board (comprising the [SF, NUS] and the Officers' Organisations), the [PLA], the Corporation of Trinity House and the [SHS]. The Minister subsequently agreed that the [*ADH*] was an integral part of the Dreadnought Hospital and decided that as such it would be controlled by the Management Committee appointed for the Dreadnought Hospital by the [SE] Metropolitan Regional Board. Mr. F. Arnold Baker, the Society's Deputy Chairman, [had] accepted the Regional Board's [RB] invitation to be Chairman of the new Management Committee.

King George's Sanatorium for Sailors [had] been grouped with King George V Sanatorium, Godalming, and the Surrey County Sanatorium, Milford.

The *Tilbury Hospital* [would] form one of a group of hospitals in South East Essex under the [NE] Metropolitan Regional Board. It [was] hoped that the new Tilbury Hospital House Committee [would] invite one or more representatives of the [SHS] to be of their number in order to maintain liaison with the Dreadnought Hospital in the best interest of seamen.

The [*HTD*] has been designated by the Minister as a teaching hospital in a group which includes University College Hospital [UCH] and which will be controlled by a new Board of Governors appointed by the Minister. It is expected that this Board will appoint a Committee to manage the [HTD] and that, in continued close liaison with the [LSHTM], the Hospital will be recognised as the Post Graduate Teaching Centre and Special Hospital for tropical diseases.

Urgent representations have been made to the Minister that steps should be taken immediately after the Appointed Day to increase the accommodation for In-Patients and to provide other necessary services for teaching purposes and for research.[17]

Transfer of the Society's hospitals to the NHS

The 1948 Report recorded the physical transfer of the Society's Hospitals (which were at the time 'free of all debt') into the 'hands of the Minister of Health in accordance with the provisions of the [NHS] Act'. This immediately resulted of course not only in *'fragmentation'* but a cessation of the core functions of the SHS. Sir Ernest Murrant ended his Annual Report, of a highly significant year in the history of the Society, with these lines:

> In flame beneath the tropics,
> In frost upon the floe,
> And jeopardy of every wind
> That does between them go.[18]

In the 1949 Report, Murrant reminded his readership of the *original* objectives of the SHS (as outlined in the Act of Incorporation – 1833 [Chapter 7]): '… for the charitable Relief of sick and distressed Seamen of all Nations in the Port of London, and for the providing them with Medical and Surgical Aid, Lodging, Support, and Clothing, until Convalescence, and until Employment could be again found for them in their meritorious Calling …'[19] Hostels for Seamen in the Port of London, [he emphasised], 'are immediately available to patients upon discharge (i.e. during the period of convalescence), the cost thereof being met from the Society's Samaritan Fund if private resources are insufficient'.

There was, he wrote, a real problem facing the *Voluntary Hospitals*, at that time, i.e. immediately after the introduction of the NHS; subscribers felt (not unnaturally) that the State had taken over management of these institutions, and therefore donations (had) declined markedly. Furthermore, the Ministry had (had) great difficulty in deciding what to do with the Seamen's Hospitals, and the Greenwich Hospital Authorities (who owned the *'Dreadnought'* premises) required clarification as to whether this hospital would continue to be used primarily by seamen.[20] As well as much discussion at SHS Management Committee meetings, a prolonged correspondence between the SHS and the Ministry of Health (much directed to the then Minister himself – Iain MacLeod – who had succeeded Bevan) resulted.[21]

Another issue related to transfer of *endowments*.[22] The sum total was that legal advice was sought and the word from Lincolns Inn was that it was 'not worthwhile to pursue the matter'. Counsel felt that *after* the introduction of the NHS Act in 1948, the sole objects left to the Charity were: 'provision of lodging support and clothing for sick and distressed seamen until convalescence, and until employment can be again found for them in their meritorious calling …'.[23]

Other post-war events

Royal visits

During 1946, HM Queen Mary (1867–1953) had visited the *Dreadnought* Hospital on 19 June, when she gave her permission for the library to bear her name. She had previously visited the ADH on 21 October 1938. Viscountess (later Countess) Mountbatten of Burma (1901–1960) had also visited the HTD at Portland Street on 2 July.[24] 1960 was marked by a visit to the *Dreadnought* Hospital (to the Annual Court of Governors) by HRH Princess Alexandra (1936–present), who had this to say: 'We owe so much to merchant seamen, not only for the essentials in daily life which we take for granted, but for our travels by sea and for the links which they help to forge between countries of the Commonwealth'.

Disposal of two of the Society's former hospitals

The 1948 Report alluded to:

> ... the sale of the former [HTD] premises at No. 25, Gordon Street, Endsleigh Gardens, W.C.1, [as a result] the loan granted from H.M. Treasury upon application of the Colonial Office [having been] repaid and part of the allocation received in 1919 was returned to the Joint Corporations of the British Red Cross Society and the Order of St. John of Jerusalem.

There was also news of the *Queen Alexandra Memorial Hospital, Marseilles* (which had once housed the sole SHS Hospital abroad); the building had been leased for three years, to the American Joint Distribution Committee, with an option to extend the tenancy for a further two years. A year later, it was recorded that the Society had completely 'opted out' of this venture:

> The Society has relinquished its leasehold and all other interests therein, and as a result a net sum of £21,895 3s. 5d. is brought to credit in the present Accounts. Thus terminates the Society's connection with the British hospital in Marseilles since 1928. In many respects this is to be regretted, but in the circumstances the Committee are satisfied that no better conclusion could have been arrived at. ...[25]

Other domestic matters

The year 1953 saw the dedication (by the Bishop of Southwark – the Rt Rev Bertrand Simpson) of a new Chapel – designed by H G C Spencely FRIBA, on 21 December (the previous one had been totally destroyed by enemy action in September 1940 [see above]).[26] In this year also, a new ambulance ('of the latest type [carrying] special lifting gear for use on board ship') was purchased for £2,100. The history of the safety of ships and well-being of seamen was referred to in a book of which the SHS had honourable mention.

The following Report alluded to an extension to the Nurses Home at ADH; largely because the ADH (lying in 'the heart of the dockland area') was 'abnormally remote from places of public recreation or entertainment'. An extension (at an estimated cost of £17,000) could not however 'be provided from funds made available by the Treasury to the [NHS]'.[27]

The 1961 report began with a sad announcement: the President, Captain Sir Ion Hamilton Benn Bt. (1863–1961) had died on 12 August of that year; he was succeeded by Sir Colin Anderson (1904–80).[28]

DENTAL CARE

The subject of dental care of seafarers (whilst in the Port of London for a limited period) was brought to the fore in the 1960 Report. The Society had spent £1,183 during the year to modernise the 'mechanical equipment in the dental surgeries at both the Dreadnought [Hospital] and [ADH]'. Four years later, this subject again came to the fore:

> An efficient dental service for seafarers has long been obstructed by the difficulty of making dentures with sufficient speed, and this has too often meant that a dental patient has had to rejoin his ship without efficient dentures (or even with none) and then to wait until he is next ashore for completion of the work. [This difficulty had been overcome by] making of dentures in a private dental laboratory and workshop near the Dreadnought Hospital. In view of the extreme importance to seafarers of this facility the Society has readily acceded to an appeal for help in financing such of the new arrangements as lie outside the scope of the [NHS].[29]

WINDING-UP OF THE DEVONPORT FUND

The 1955 Report contained an update on the Devonport Trust Fund which, the reader will recall, had been set up during the Great War (Chapter 20).

> … The Trustees of the First Viscount Devonport Trust Fund have decided that the initial object of that Trust has now been completed, that is to say, the erection of new buildings and/or the improvement of existing buildings at the Dreadnought Seamen's Hospital, Greenwich, as a memorial to the devotion of the men of the [MM] during the Great War, and therefore, in accordance with the original Agreement, the balance of the Fund should now be devoted to the general purposes of the [SHS] … the accounts of this Fund have consequently now been merged with those of the Society's general funds and the investments transferred to the Society's Trustees.[30]

A HOSTEL FOR PATIENTS' RELATIONS

The 1950 Report outlined the near completion (thanks largely to the Merchant Navy Welfare Board) of a hostel for *seriously* ill patients' relations. Numbers 29 to 32, King William Walk (which had been rebuilt after destruction by 'enemy action') had been leased to the Society by the Admiralty until 2024 (i.e. it was 'co-terminous with the lease of the Hospital itself'). The cost of the building was £10,000 (plus £2,000 for furniture), with an upkeep of £500 per annum. The following report indicated that this facility was completed, and in 1952 it was decided to name the new hostel 'Nairne House' as a memorial to the former Chairman of the Society (Sir Perceval Nairne) who had died in 1921 (Chapter 21).[31]

CARE OF THE ELDERLY (GERIATRIC) SEAFARER

The 1955 Report referred to this important topic, and the method being undertaken to address it:

> ... geriatric cases ... cannot remain as in-patients in a busy general hospital. It is thought that the number of such officers is not so large as to warrant the Society acquiring, equipping and staffing its own premises and advantage has therefore been taken of the homes managed by the Crossways Trust. By the investment of £5,000 in the Trust the Society will shortly be able to acquire five places in the Trust's two infirm homes, either at Ridgemead House, Englefield Green, Surrey, or at Grosvenor House, Kings Road, Brighton, Sussex. The Society has made itself responsible to the Crossways Trust for the weekly cost of maintenance of each patient, to which each officer will contribute according to his ability.[32]

The 1963 Report recorded that King George's Sanatorium for Sailors, originally opened as a sanatorium (*see* Chapter 20) was to become a *geriatric* hospital until it closed in 1987:

> In July, 1963 the King George's Sanatorium for Sailors [built by the Society at Bramshott Place, Liphook, Hampshire, in 1921 with funds collected by the first Earl of Inchcape – see Chapter 20] was designated by the Minister as a *geriatric* [my italics] hospital. The Society cannot help regretting that the march of time has swept away another of its former special hospitals, but is glad to have received assurance that satisfactory alternative accommodation is provided for seafarers suffering from tuberculosis.[33]

Extension of facilities

The 1958 Report referred to the fact that the 1833 Act of Incorporation (Chapter 7) did not provide for the 'benefit to seamen who by reason of permanent incapacity or old age could never again find employment in their meritorious calling, or their widows or immediate dependents'. As a result, the provisions of the Charity were extended:

> The body corporate the Trustees of the [SHS] shall apply the clear yearly income of the General Funds and Endowments and at their discretion the capital of the General Funds of the said Charity for the charitable relief of seamen of all nations in the Port of London or other ports or havens in Great Britain or Northern Ireland to which seafaring persons resort and their immediate dependents (including widows of such deceased seamen) who from sickness, misfortune or age are in need of assistance and for providing them with medical and surgical aid, lodging, support and clothing.[34]

Dreadnought Wing, Walmer

In 1959, the Annual Report, together with many subsequent ones, contained news of a new initiative:

> The Committee have always been persuaded of the merit of co-operation between charities operating in the same field, and they have therefore welcomed the opportunity which has presented itself in connection with the Trinity House Homes for Merchant Navy Officers at Walmer, Kent. These Homes, which were completed in 1958, are in the form of, at present, 14 single-storey cottages for married couples, widows and spinster daughters grouped about a central assembly hall and surrounding on three sides a lawn and terraced gardens with a view across common land to the sea. There remains to be provided however an *infirm wing* [my italics] to which the residents may be transferred when, on account of temporary illness or permanent infirmity, they can no longer look after themselves in the Homes and require nursing care.
>
> In consultation with the Trinity House, plans are therefore being prepared for a Dreadnought Wing to be added to the Homes at Walmer to which elderly and infirm Merchant Navy officers may be admitted from elsewhere as well as from the Homes themselves. The site would be provided by the Trinity House and the [Society] would erect thereon and equip a Dreadnought Wing [administered by a Dreadnought-Walmer Committee consisting of three representatives of the Trinity House and two from the SHS] for eight patients in the first instance, with possibility of future expansion, and separate accommodation for nursing staff. It is expected that the capital cost of this project would be in the region of £35,000 and then an annual expenditure of £5,000 [a sum which was to double in future years] would be required for its maintenance.

This new wing was officially opened by the in-coming President (Anderson) on 20 July 1962, in the presence of the Deputy Master and many Elder Brethren of The Trinity House.[35]

Future of the *Dreadnought* (the 'flagship') Hospital becomes increasingly gloomy

Shortly after introduction of the NHS on the 'appointed day' in July 1948 (see above) it became clear that the Ministry of Health had accepted a *new* lease (for 71½ years from 24 June 1953) in respect of the Dreadnought Hospital and 'additional premises', i.e. the Devonport Nurses' Home and Pathological laboratories at Greenwich, without reference to the SHS. This too resulted in an exchange of letters between the SHS Chairman (E H Murrant) and the then Minister of Health (the Rt Hon Iain McLeod, MP. The point at issue was, had the Ministry acted illegally in appropriating non-hospital property which had resulted from *voluntary* (charity) funds – i.e. the *'Devonport appeal'*)? Murrant challenged the Minister 'on moral grounds [and possibly] on legal grounds as well'.[36] The SHS ultimately 'let the matter rest for the time being' but were clearly not in agreement with the Minister's views on the matter! In fact, Murrant concluded his final letter: 'with a formal protest and dissent from [the Minister's] ruling'.[37]

The 1962 Report (i.e. fourteen years after implementation of the 1946 Act) contained the following statement; passage of time would, however, show this to be totally irrelevant:

> The Minister of Health's Ten-Year-Plan for the Hospital Service as yet makes no specific proposals for the Seamen's Group of Hospitals but there is nevertheless a possibility that, in due course, the Dreadnought may be moved nearer to the focus of shipping in the Royal Docks on the north side of the Thames. Should this happen, and since it is essential for the Society to remain hand in hand with the Seamen's Hospitals, particularly for the perpetuation of the important 'Nairne House' ... then money may be needed not only for the re-creation of these unique facilities and for the special distinctions that the Society has been able to confer on the Chapels and the Nurses' Homes of the Seamen's Hospitals, but also to provide a new Headquarters for the Society itself.
>
> For these purposes the Committee of Management intends to set aside annually such sums as it can afford from its General Funds, and once again the Society will seek and welcome help from all those whose generosity in the past has forged so powerful an instrument for the succour of sick and distressed seamen. It is the Society's special function to ensure that as far as possible the high standards of the past shall suffer no diminution in the present or the future, and that the means to meet peculiar requirements of the Merchant Navies of the world shall be preserved so far as is possible in the Seamen's Hospital of the years to come.[38]

The uncertainty concerning the future of the Society's hospitals had a very unstabling effect at this time. In order to finance a move to St Thomas's Hospital (should the necessity arise), the *Development Fund* was increased each year, and by 1985 stood at £800,000.

In 1968 (now 20 years after introduction of the NHS), the Ministry of Health issued a 'Green Paper' which received careful consideration by the SHS Committee of Management. Negotiations with the Greenwich and Bexley *Area Health Authority* on the future rôle of the *Dreadnought* Hospital had by then been exceedingly protracted; much discussion centred on the *location* of the hospital, its consultant cover, and number of beds. While initial responses seemed on the whole favourable, news from the Ministry became increasingly gloomy regarding the future of the *Dreadnought* Hospital. It was now considered timely that a removal of medical facilities to St Thomas's Hospital was the only viable option open (*see* Chapter 25).[39]

In 1971, a Working Party was set up to examine and, should it be found necessary, to re-define, the objectives of the SHS in the light of the changing circumstances (Chapter 24). Regarding this, the 1972 Report commented:

> ... as expected, [the] investigations [of the Working Party have] confirmed that social conditions, insofar as they affect the seafarer, have very greatly changed since the Society's foundation [in 1821], nevertheless it would appear that the original and present purposes of the

> [Society] are, in fact, still appropriate, but that new and realistic action should be taken ... to promote them. How such action may best be determined itself poses a new set of problems, having regard, for example, to the size, shape, and speed of modern ships and to the new methods of cargo handling, all of which affect the overall numbers, average age and length of service of the seafaring community. It is not easy even for those most deeply involved in the Shipping Industry to foresee precisely the likely conditions of an active seaman's life in, say, ten years time [i.e. the early 1980s], still less to forecast the probabilities of health and hospital requirements and hence the likelihood or nature of demands which might be made upon such an organisation as ours.[40]

By 1973, the future strategy, and fate, of the *Dreadnought* therefore hung very much in the balance:

> ... because the Shipping Industry ... is going through a period of re-organisation and, until it is known more clearly what the wind of change will do to the Merchant Navy, it is difficult to decide how best to set the Society's sails. We shall, of course, [the 1973 Report assured its readership] continue to the utmost of our ability to improve and expand what we are already doing, and it was for this reason that the Committee [has taken] steps ... to increase the flow of annual income.
>
> While examining the practical possibilities open to us, we have, ... become increasingly preoccupied with the very centre of our original interest, the *Dreadnought* [my italics] Hospital. We have watched with increasing concern, the continued erosion of the great group of Hospitals which this Society founded, expanded, and managed from 1821 until 1948. Under the administration of the [NHS] it is ... inevitable that special considerations, even apparently for seafarers in a maritime nation, should be at risk in the tidal wave of the national enterprise, but it has meant that one by one the Seamen's Hospitals of the former Group have disappeared.
>
> The most recent to go, as from 1st April 1974, have been the [ADH] and the Angas Convalescent Home and the only Hospital now left is the *Dreadnought* [my italics], which is itself seeking proper recognition from the Secretary of State for Social Services as an essential factor in the health of the Port of London of not only our own Merchant Navy, but of other Merchant Navies who use the Port of London. The current reorganisation of the [NHS] could strand the Dreadnought, or reduce her to a hulk, and only the urgent and valid representations of all those involved in the shipping industry (supported by ourselves) will keep her afloat.
>
> These representations have been and are continuing to be made, and we must hope that the absolutely essential nature of a hospital specifically maintained for the highly individual needs of the seafarers will once more be recognised and safeguarded for the future. This matter is so important that for the present it is necessary that it should take first priority in all our efforts and in all our plans.[41]

In 1974, however, the Chairman was to record this somewhat depressing 'message':

> Despite the hope which I expressed last year that I should now be able to report that 1974 had assured the settled security of the *Dreadnought* [my italics] Hospital, which will always be our principal concern … this has not yet proved to be the case. Notwithstanding all our endeavours in support of the Shipping Industry and the representations which the National Maritime Board has made to the Area Health Authority [AHA], into whose control the Hospital has passed, it is still not known when a decision on this vitally important matter will be reached.
>
> From 1st April [1974], the very considerable re-organisation of the [NHS] seemed likely to produce problems of personnel and management which might affect the work of the Dreadnought because of the disbandment of the former Seamen's Hospital Management Committee. This meant the loss of all its accumulated expertise in control of the Hospital's specialised facilities for seamen, and accordingly there seemed to be no alternative but to take precautionary measures for "watch and ward".
>
> The Society therefore set up a special Dreadnought Advisory Sub-Committee (to which were recruited members of the dispersed Management Committee and the Medical Staff), whose function is designed not only to safeguard existing Hospital services for seamen, but also to provide a forum where opinions and advice from all sections of the Shipping Industry could be collated for the assistance of the [AHA].
>
> This Sub-Committee … has been particularly fortunate in its liaison with the [BSF] (now to be known as the General Council of British Shipping), which has undertaken a widespread and successful campaign to inform every seaman of the facilities specifically designed for his peculiar needs and offered by the Dreadnought Hospital. As a direct result, there has been a notable increase in applications from seafarers for examination and treatment. The Sub-Committee has also secured valuable representation on the local Community Health Council.
>
> The Shipping Industry is itself being re-structured, not only from a career point of view but also with particular regard to health and welfare; and the Dreadnought Hospital, with all its national and international prestige, has, and will always have, as important a role to play as ever. And we, with our friends and supporters, will continue to discharge the special function for which we were originally founded, namely as the [SHS].[42]

Of course, justification for continuation of services in the *Dreadnought* depended to what extent it was used, and seafarers obviously took first priority. Collection of in-patient and out-patient statistics therefore became a matter of crucial importance. Table 22.1 contains annual figures for 'new patients' and 'others' from 1976 until 1979, geriatric cases being excluded from this analysis. In the quarter ending 30 June 1977, the proportion of seafarers admitted was 75.4%. In the following years,

Table 22.1: Annual attendance (excluding geriatrics) at the *Dreadnought* Hospital 1976–9.

Year	*Casualty & Out-patient*		*Rehabilitation Department*	
	New	*Others*	*New*	*Others*
1976	10,447	23,267	1,640	17,566
1977	11,013	23,810	1,710	18,793
1978	6,998	13,251	1,911	22,790
1979	6,223	14,388	1,896	23,990

the proportion fluctuated between 76 and 86%. The bed occupancy rate however, varied between 54% and 76%. It is clear that during this short period, both the attendance-rate and bed occupancy figures showed a steady decline.[43]

References and notes

1 Annual Report 120: 10–12; Anonymous. *Ministry of Home Security: air raids: what you must know, what you must do.* London: HM Stationery Office 1940: 65; Anonymous. *The War Office: Resuscitation equipment, organization, training and procedures* London: HM Stationery Office 1941: 56; Anonymous. *Fire protection: for the guidance of occupiers of factories and other business premises* London: HM Stationery Office 1942: 90. P Ziegler *London at War 1939–1945* London Sinclair-Stevenson 1995: 372. G C Cook, A J Webb. The Albert Dock Hospital, London: the original site (in 1899) of tropical medicine as a new discipline. *Acta Trop* 2001; 79: 249–255.

2 *Op cit.* See note 1 above (Reports): 121: 9–11.

3 *Ibid.* 122: 9–11.

4 *Ibid.* 123: 8–10.

5 *Ibid.* 124: 8–9.

6 *Op cit.* See notes 1 & 2 above; P Kemp. Boyle, William Henry Dudley, twelfth earl of Cork and twelfth earl of Orrery (1873–1967). In: H C G Matthew, B Harrison (eds). *Oxford Dictionary of National Biography*. Oxford: Oxford University Press 2004; 7: 114–5.

7 **Walter Edward Guinness**, first Baron Moyne (1880–1944) was the third son of the first Earl of Iveagh (1847–1916). He became MP for Bury St Edmunds after service in the Suffolk Hussars. After several senior political appointments, he became, in 1944, Resident Minister in Cairo. His assassination on 6 November 1944 by two members of the Fighters for Israel's freedom (previously the Stern gang) was counter-productive because it persuaded Winston Churchill to postpone creation of the Jewish state, and seriously damaged the Zionist cause. [*See also:* Anonymous. *Times, Lond* 1944; 7 November: 6; Moyne, M Brodie. Guinness, Walter Edward, first Baron Moyne (1880–1944). In: H C G Matthew, B Harrison (eds). *Oxford Dictionary of National Biography*. Oxford: Oxford University Press 2004; 24: 214–6].

8 *Op cit.* See note 5 above. See also: Anonymous. Lord Moyne shot: death in Cairo after attack: assailants caught. *Times, Lond* 1944; 7 November: 4.

9 *Op cit.* See note 3 above.

10 **Aneurin Bevan** (1897–1960) was Labour MP for the Ebbw Vale Division of Monmouthshire from 1929 until his death, and Labour Minister of Health in Attlee's government from 1945 until 1948. He was the architect of the National Health Service Act (1946). [*See also:*

M Foot. *Aneurin Bevan 1897–1960.* London: Victor Gollancz 1997: 634; D Smith. Bevan, Aneurin (Nye) (1897–1960). In: H C G Matthew, B Harrison (eds). *Oxford Dictionary of National Biography.* Oxford: Oxford University Press 2004; 5: 566–73].

11 *Op cit.* See note 1 above (Reports) 123.

12 **John Anderson** (1882–1958) OM GCB GCIE GCSI was a civil servant and politician. He had the reputation of being the greatest administrator of his age. He was a member of Churchill's War Cabinet. [*See also:* G C Peden. Anderson, John, first Viscount Waverley (1882–1958) In: H C G Matthew, B Harrison (eds). *Oxford Dictionary of National Biography.* Oxford: Oxford University Press 2004; 2: 52–6].

13 *Op cit.* See note 1 above (Reports): 9–11. [*See also*: SHS Council of Management Minutes: 21: 26–7, 121–2, 150–1, 160, 166].

14 E H Murrant, C Figg. J C Nairne to A Bevan. *National Health Service. Hospitals for Merchant Seamen in the Port of London.* 1946; 12 June: 3 [SHS Archive].

15 *Seamen's Hospital Society. National Health Service Bill. Memorandum of a meeting held on 8 July 1945*: 2 [SHS Archive]. [See also: *Op cit.* note 13 above (Minutes): 178].

16 *Op cit.* See note 13 above (Minutes): 225.

17 *Op cit.* See note 1 above (Reports): 127.

18 *Ibid.* 128: 4–7.

19 *Ibid.* 129: 4–6.

20 *Op cit.* See note 13 above (Minutes) 22: 56–7, 100; [See also: *Dreadnought Seamen's Hospital, Greenwich – lease from the Admiralty. National Health Service Act 1946*: Memo of meeting held on 28 July 1946: 2 (SHS Archive)].

21 F A Lyon to R F Tyas (Ministry of Health). *National Health Service Act. The Group of Seamen's Hospitals: Metropolitan Regional Hospital Boards.* 1948: 10 February: 2 [SHS Archive]; [See also: *Op cit.* See note 13 above (Minutes): 22: 146–7, 240–241].

22 *National Health Service Act, 1946. Transfer of Endowments Memo.* 1948; 8 May: 2 [SHS Archive]. [See also: F A Lyon (Ref 7/170) memo 1949: 21 May: 2 (SHS Archive); F A Lyon Memo 1948; 9 December: 4 (SHS Archive)].

23 F A Lyon. *Case to Counsel* 1954: 28 October: 2. [*See also*: J L Arnold. *Opinion* 1954; 30 November: 3 (SHS archive)].

24 G C Cook. *From the Greenwich Hulks to Old St Pancras: a history of tropical disease in London* London: Athlone Press: 1992: 281.

25 *Op cit.* See note 1 above (Reports): 131. [*Op cit.* See note 13 above (Minutes): 22: 1].

26 *Op cit.* See note 1 above (Reports): 133: 4–6. [*See also: Order of Service for the dedication of the Chapel of the Dreadnought Seamen's Hospital Greenwich on Monday, 21st December 1953*: 8 [SHS archive].

27 *Op cit.* See note 1 above (Reports): 135: 4–6; '*Seafarers and their ships*'. H M Stationery Office. 1955.

28 *Op cit.* See note 1 above (Reports): 141 and 142: 5–7.

29 *Ibid.* 1960: 4–7; 145: 4–7.

30 *Ibid.* 1955: 136: 4–6.

31 *Ibid.* 1950: 4–7; 132: 4–6; 133: 4–6.

32 *Ibid.* 156. [*See also*: *Op cit.* See note 13 above (Minutes) 24: 566].

33 *Ibid.* 143: 4–7.

34 *Ibid.* 138: 4–7.

35 Ibid (1959): 4–7; 1962: 4–7. [See also: *Op cit.* See note 13 above (Minutes): 23: 2–4, 7–8, 12–13, 16–17, 18, 27, 29–30, 36–7, 40–1, 43, 48, 51–2, 56, 57, 64, 66, 69–70, 78, 79, 100, 105, 113, 126, 132, 142, 146, 158–9, 175, 180, 187, 192, 209, 239–40, 248, 273, 282; 24: 340, 360, 382, 387, 404, 444, 460–1, 492, 495, 497; 25: 608, 615, 622, 634, 639, 661, 662, 739, 740, 747, 753, 761, 772, 789, 801, 812, 824, 833, 840, 850, 863, 873–4].

36 E H Murrant to I N MacLeod. *Dreadnought Seamen's Hospital, Greenwich. New lease from the Admiralty.* 1954; 17 November: 2; I MacLeod to E H Murrant 1954; 10 December: 1; E H Murrant to I MacLeod 1954; 13 December: 1; E H Murrant to I MacLeod 1955; 21 January: 2; I MacLeod to E H Murrant 1955; 10 March: 1; E H Murrant to I MacLeod 1955; 24 March: 1; I MacLeod to E H Murrant 1955; 29 March: 1. [SHS Archive].

37 G C Cook. Transfer of hospitals and 'additional premeses' to the state: questionable morality in the implementation of the National Health Service Act (1946). *Postgrad Med J* 2004; 80: 716–19.

38 *Op cit.* See note 35 above.

39 *Op cit.* See note 13 above (Minutes). 23: 250–251, 263; 24: 498, 510, 517–8, 567–8, 577–8; 25: 598, 613, 620–1, 631–3, 638–9, 646, 663, 689–90, 698, 707, 714–5, 730, 747–8, 754–6, 762–3, 768, 773, 790–2, 798, 804, 805, 815, 824–5, 833–4, 841–3, 849, 851.

40 *Op cit.* See note 1 above (Reports): 132: 8–9.

41 *Ibid.* 133: 7–9.

42 *Ibid.* 134: 7–9.

43 *Op cit.* See note 13 above (Minutes). 25: 613, 621, 639, 646, 653, 690, 699, 715, 730, 737, 748, 763, 792–3, 804, 816, 834.

Chapter 23

Disease(s) at the Society's Hospitals in the latter years of the twentieth century

In the twentieth century, diseases encountered by the Society tended to be less 'exotic' than had been the case in its early years. The 'germ-theory' of disease had become well established in the early part of the century, and antimicrobials (beginning with the sulphonamides, and from the 1940s onwards, antibiotics) were later introduced. However, as in former years, the disease pattern at the Society's hospitals was dominated by sexually-transmitted (or venereal [VD]) disease, and tuberculosis, both entities receiving numerous entries in the Committee of Management minute books. Successive Annual Reports give details of the numbers of patients undergoing treatment at the various SHS hospitals and dispensaries; that for 1929 records the largest number ever managed by the Society (Table 23.1).[1]

Table 23.1: Numbers of patients undergoing treatment at the Society's establishments in 1929.

	In- Patients	*Out- Patients*	*Total*
Dreadnought Hospital	2,881	12,910	15,791
Albert Dock Hospital	663	6,772	7,435
Hospital for Tropical Diseases	756	782	1,538
Tilbury Hospital	1,265	5,484	6,749
Queen Alexandra Memorial Hospital, Marseilles	295	–	295
King George's Sanatorium	93	–	93
Angas Convalescent Home	472	–	472
East India Dock Dispensary	–	661	661
Total	6,425	26,609	33,034

Venereal (or sexually transmitted) disease(s)

A centre for the treatment of VD was established at the *Dreadnought* and was opened on 1 January 1917; this had resulted from co-operation between the Society, 'the Local Government Board, and the London County Council [LCC]'. Shortly afterwards, in March of that year, a similar facility was opened at the ADH.[2]

On 14 December 1939, 'the Director of the *Dreadnought* VD Clinic – P[ercival] P Cole [FRCS] – made a recommendation to the Committee of Management [already approved by the Ministry of Health]' to re-open beds for 'ambulent VD cases' on the Ranlett floor to a maximum of 27 (thus increasing the number of emergency beds to 180). This move would, it was minuted, 'enable the [SHS] to represent to the [LCC] that there should be no reduction in their V.D. grant of £4,750 for the year ending 31st March 1941'. On 14 March of the following year, the Committee again addressed this matter, and the Society's Secretary 'was authorised to inform the [LCC] that the Board was willing to enter [into such an] Agreement ... on the lines [of that] operating in respect of the year 1939, it being understood that the amount of the [proposed] provisional grant ... in respect of the facilities provided at the *Dreadnought* Hospital was £5,400 and for the [ADH], £2,140'. On 18 July of that year, a further minute recorded that the LCC had reduced 'the grant for the year 1939/40 by £550, to £4,850'; this was however, considered not unreasonable, because 27 of the VD beds had been temporarily closed between 1 September and 31 December 1939.[3]

In March 1941, a suggestion for treating Dutch VD cases was broached; the Society had 'received through the [LCC]' an application from the Netherlands Shipping and Trading Committee. In September, the LCC allowance was further reduced 'from £5,400 to £4,050'; this again was based on a 'reduction in the amount of work done'. And in March 1942 'it was decided to renew ... agreements with the [LCC] for the year ending 31st March 1943, subject to the conditions [stated in a letter from the Clerk of LCC that] the amount of the provisional grants [were] the same as for the previous year ...'.[4] Two months later it was decided to 'renew the agreement with the [LCC] for the year ending 31st March 1944, subject to conditions being maintained at: the *Dreadnought* Hospital – at £5,000 and the [ADH] £2,500'. A further renewal for the year 1944/45 was made, provided that it be maintained at £5,000 (for the *Dreadnought*), and £2,500 (for the ADH).

In August 1942, the same Committee decided to purchase an Electric Incubator for the VD clinic at a cost of £21; the reason was that 'specimens [in the incubator] were being rendered useless' because gas was being 'cut off upon each air raid alert'.[5] In late 1943, the Management Committee authorised '... the Secretary to agree to the Essex County Council's ... request to establish and operate, at no expense to the Society, a male Out-patient V.D. Clinic in the grounds of the *Tilbury* Hospital, [while] reserving the right to reconsider the position at the end of hostilities'.[6]

VD propaganda

Earlier that year (1943), the LCC requested the display of 'Ministry of Health VD Propaganda Posters in the V.D. Clinic'; Cole (see above), with the co-operation of the SHS Secretary, had already made arrangements for these to be on view in other parts of the *Dreadnought* as well. However, the Committee of Management objected to this idea, possibly because the London Port Welfare Committee 'had decided against the display of posters on ships and had agreed that it would be best for distribution to be effected through the Port Health Authority [PHA]'.[7]

Tuberculosis

Mycobacterium tuberculosis infection had for many decades been more common in seafarers than 'landsmen' (*see* Chapters 11 and 16). The SHS had had experience with 'open-air' treatment in the early days of the twentieth century, and had of course opened a sanatorium for sailors in 1920. Now therefore this disease (streptomycin was not available until 1944) assumed a far higher profile in the annals of the Society – largely because several other infections had been brought under control.

Management of *M. tuberculosis* infection is given detailed (in-depth) coverage in this chapter because, apart from the attention given to 'open air' treatment in the early twentieth century, this important disease had hitherto received less attention than the emphasis that it warranted in the Society's annals.[8] At a meeting of the Management Committee in March 1942, the following was minuted:

> *Joint Sub Committee – Pulmonary Tuberculosis among Merchant Seamen.* At a [previous] meeting … it had been agreed that Dr. [Charles] Sundell [MRCP] and Dr. [Alexander] Wingfield [FRCP] should draw up a comprehensive memorandum on this subject. At their request the Secretary had prepared a preliminary draft for their consideration. This … had been considered by the Committee at Lord Cork [the SHS Deputy Chairman]'s request and had been approved, (subject to amendment by the doctors) for submission to the Board and further consideration by the Joint Sub-Committee … .[9]

The content of this draft memorandum is as follows:-

> PULMONARY TUBERCULOSIS AMONG MERCHANT SEAMEN …
> *Nature and Extent of the Problem.* There are about ¼ million actual cases of pulmonary tuberculosis in the British Isles and of these about 1,500 between the ages of 15 and 50 die each month. In spite of this the total number is kept up by a steady flow of recruits. Under war time conditions the disease shows a tendency to increase. The surest means of conquering tuberculosis lies in the detection in its earliest stages before it has become infectious. Accurate statistics are not available for recent years but the mortality has risen, the increase being 6% in the first year of the war and 10% in the second.[10]
>
> Although no figures are available to show the number of merchant seamen notified annually as suffering from *pulmonary tuberculosis* [my italics], nor the proportion of this number to the total personnel of the [MM], there are some statistics showing that the annual death rate from this disease is among the highest of the causes of death among seamen. For England and Wales in the years 1930–32 tuberculosis was the cause of 20% of all deaths notified in seamen. …
>
> The experience of the [SHS] over a long period, both at its Hospitals and at its King George's Sanatorium for Sailors [KGSS] is that seamen do not present themselves for treatment until the disease has taken so

> strong a hold on them that prolonged treatment is required. The three main reasons for this are:
>
> a) lack of facilities for detection and control of the disease in its earliest stages …
> b) the overwhelming anxiety of the sailor lest during his treatment his wife and children should be left quite inadequately provided for and dependent upon Public Assistance, and
> c) long deep-sea voyages without any medical attention and the seaman's disinclination to undergo prolonged treatment in a foreign port.
>
> It is certain therefore that during the time they are experiencing ill health which causes them ultimately to seek diagnosis and treatment, these seamen are a grave source of infection menacing many hundreds of their fellows in the restricted quarters on board ship.
>
> The evil effects are obvious upon the man power of the [MM], upon the social and economic circumstances of the individual and upon the finances of the Sanatoria and Hospitals providing treatment as well as upon the pockets of the shipowners who have to pay the cost of maintenance and treatment in foreign ports.

Thus, the magnitude of the problem in the seafaring community had to some extent been delineated. The next problem was what was to be done about it!

> *Detection of Symptomless Tuberculosis* … The first step towards the remedy of this state of affairs is by the detection of tuberculosis *before* [my italics] it produces symptoms. This can best be done by X-ray examination. For this purpose full-size X-ray films cannot be used for both practical and economic reasons and the appropriate procedure is that of miniature-radio-photography [MRP] as practised with proved results particularly by the Royal Navy, Royal Air Force and the Australian Army. By this means very large numbers of men can be examined at a single session and the small number requiring full-size X-ray films can be re-examined on the same day.[11]
>
> The difference between the application of such an examination to one of the Services and to those in civilian employment is fully appreciated, as are also the practical difficulties peculiar to the [MM]. The necessity for conquering tuberculosis in a group of the community whose conditions of labour (more especially in war time) are so favourable to its wide and fatal development, is so great and so urgent however that the following suggestions are submitted for earnest consideration. …

Then came sound advice on how the SHS and other maritime authorities should deal with the problem:

> *Practical Problems & Suggested Solutions* … Submission to examination by [MRP] cannot at present be anything but voluntary among 'civilian'

> workers, but it is suggested that such examinations could be included in the routine examinations by the Shipping Federation [SF], to the other parts of which no objection is raised. Emphasis should be laid upon the protection of the *whole crew* [my italics] against infection rather than on the suspension of the individual from his normal earning capacity. Although all the population do not live under conditions which render one man such a menace of infection to so many fellow-workers, the Trades Union Congress [TUC] in September 1941 passed resolutions in favour of x-ray examinations for young workers. It is true that some men would be lost to the [MM] but most of them could soon be restored to working capacity if not at sea then on land. Undetected and untreated, these men would not only be lost to the nation but would first be a danger and later a liability.
>
> Effective control would entail the institution of a medical record for each man. This would appear to differentiate the merchant seaman from other workers, but a strong argument in its favour is that the migratory character of a sailor's employment deprives him of regular contact with a panel practitioner or family doctor to whom landsmen have continuous access. Such a record could be incorporated in the seaman's continuous discharge book and would, it is thought, be valuable to the doctors attached to the Seamen's National Approved Society [SNAS] in various ports. …
>
> In the Port of London there are five centres for signing on crews and although at present there are no residential facilities for men awaiting the results of the suggested examination it should be possible to provide a mobile apparatus by which means the waiting period could be substantially reduced and travelling difficulties minimised. …
>
> To be effective, the detection of symptomless tuberculosis would have to be on a national scale, that is to say there would have to be [MRP] facilities in each principal port. In addition to the capital cost of the apparatus, there would be needed a developing and reporting centre staffed by radiographic technicians, clerks and a radiologist and physician to interpret the films. The cost would admittedly be high but large savings would be made in the expenditure on institutional treatment and sickness and disability benefits. (It may be pertinent to note here the considerable financial benefit which the [SF] and the P.I. Associations have derived from the organised and controlled treatment of industrial injuries at the Society's [ADH] Fracture Clinic and Rehabilitation Centre [see below]).

This memorandum ended by enumerating various problems which the authors considered specific to the sailor:

> *Special Conditions of Seamen's Employment.* … The confined atmosphere and restricted living space, the lack of amenities and opportunity for exercise and recreation as compared with landsmen expose seamen to dangers from infection greater than those to which workers ashore are

> subject. It is therefore suggested that *Pulmonary Tuberculosis* [my italics] should be included in the Schedule of Industrial Diseases for Merchant Seamen.

This draft memorandum was signed by:-

I. HAMILTON BENN, Chairman	C.E. SUNDELL, M.D., Physician
CORK & ORRERY, Deputy Chairman Committee of Management, Seamen's Hospital Society	A. WINGFIELD, M.D., Asst. Physician. Honorary Med. Staff

The Management committee minute (see above) continued:

> The Secretary had reported an interview on 4th March with Mr. Evans, Secretary to The Royal Seamen's Pension Fund who, while being in agreement with the preliminary draft memorandum, had expressed the view that, notwithstanding the evidence published on [MRP] by the [RN] from Chatham, it was desirable to take advantage of the facilities granted by the Shipping Federation [SF] and The National Union of Seamen [NUS] to make a series of examinations of Merchant Seamen on a purely scientific basis: Mr Evans felt that the case would not carry sufficient weight with the Shipping Industry without the statistics which would thus be obtained. It had therefore been recommended that in view of the gravity of the problem application should be made to King George's Fund for Sailors [KGFS] for a grant from the War Fund to meet the cost of a mobile [MRP] unit for this purpose, if priority facilities for its purchase could be obtained from the Ministry of Health, so that the Society could undertake this research.

The Draft which had already been approved by Sundell and Wingfield had been circulated before the Meeting, and the Secretary was therefore instructed to take the action recommended above. This memorandum was followed by another compiled by Mr H E (later Sir Hugh) Griffiths, FRCS (1891–1961), reiterating the fact that tuberculosis should be considered an *occupational* disease amongst Merchant Seamen, and therefore added to Section iii of the Workmen's Compensation Act (1925). These two memoranda formed the basis of a letter to *The Times*. In an attempt to improve matters, Mr [CS] Anderson had been invited to compile a statement to the [SF] 'with a view to its reaching the National Maritime Board (which consisted of representatives of the [SF] and also the Liverpool Steamship Association but none from Government) and the Interdepartmental Committee on the Health of the [MM].[12]

This minute ended:

> [KGFS] had decided to make a grant of £2,500 from the War Fund to the [SHS] 'for the purpose of taking steps as they considered necessary for combatting [sic] the spreading of tuberculosis among Merchant Seamen'.

> This was to be interpreted that the grant was available for the purchase of a transportable [MRP] unit for the purpose of examining on a purely scientific basis a series of 2,000 or more consecutive seamen as had been agreed by the [SF] and the [NUS]. It had been agreed that the best and quickest method of obtaining such an apparatus would be through the Medical Research Council [MRC] which had already ordered one unit and instructions had been given for this to be done.

Early detection, and Involvement of the National Union of Seamen (NUS)

A subsequent meeting (on 14 May 1942) decided that 'the Secretary, Dr [Alec] Wingfield and Dr J. E. Wood' should attend a meeting of the *National Association for the Prevention of Tuberculosis* in early June to present the views of the SHS. This raised the important issue of the value or otherwise, of MRP in the detection of early pulmonary tuberculosis; the radiological adviser to the RAF, Wing Commander R R Trail FRCP (1894–1971) was asked for his opinion in the light of his experience of some 30,000 cases.

Trail reported favourably on the Westinghouse apparatus (used by the RAF) which it was hoped 'could be delivered from America in about eight weeks'. The Joint Sub-Committee reported to a meeting held on 18 June 1942, when 'the Board noted with satisfaction the third leader in *The Times* ...'. This was followed by a letter signed by the President (Lord Moyne [1880-1944]) pointing out the enormous expense involved in the resulting 'scientific research'. At a meeting on 16 July, a report from the Joint Sub-Committee was received. The logistics (and necessary manpower) to augment mass radiography received in-depth coverage, but the major source of concern centred on the way the Union would respond. Detection of 'Tuberculosis in any individual case [would of necessity] place it in the position of contravening the 1930 Public Health (T.B.) Regulations' – 'every medical officer who shall become aware ... (of T.B.) ... must notify [the disease]'. The meeting agreed with Sundell, Wingfield, and the Secretary that they 'should seek a further conference with Mr [Charles] Jarman [1893–1947], [Acting] General Secretary of the [NUS]'.[13]

Site of involvement, and method(s) of management

Subsequent annual reports from the SHS Sanatorium concentrated on the site of involvement, as well as the *management* of *pulmonary* cases. Whereas in the majority, the lungs were affected, the larynx, joints (including the vertebral column), genitourinary system (including the epididymis), rectum and peritoneum, all accounted for significant disease.

Artificial pneumothorax was at that time the most usual form of management of pulmonary disease; other procedures were: thoracoscopy, phrenic avulsion/crush and thoracoplasty. Mean length of treatment seems to have varied between 200 and 400 days.

Criteria for selection for treatment at the SHS sanatorium

The LCC's tuberculosis officer requested details of the SHS policy regarding admission to their sanatorium; there were in fact three categories of sanatoria:

> Dr C.E. Sundell had stated that during the past 20 years he had acted on the principle of admitting to Bramshott all seamen provided that they could stand the journey thither. He referred to the Ministry of Health Circular 72/T which had been issued more than once to all County and County Borough Councils urging them to send sailors to [KGSS]. At Dr. Sundell's suggestion it was agreed that this matter be discussed by the Sanatorium Medical Council and a report received from them.[14]

The next positive move was the presentation of a statement on the patients currently undergoing treatment at Bramshott by Dr J E Wood MRCS LRCP (*see* Chapter 24), medical superintendent at the KGSS:

> Mr C.S. Anderson had instructed the Secretary to report that in his opinion any tubercular seamen who expressed the wish to go to Bramshott rather than to any other sanatorium had the right to admission to [KGSS]. After considerable discussion, it was decided that so long as beds at Bramshott were occupied by patients who were *not* [my italics] merchant seamen (on 23rd July these numbered 50 out of the total of 75 occupied) there did not arise the question of departure from the Board's existing policy, as carried out by Dr. Sundell, since 1921 Physician in charge of Phthisical patients [see above], that any tuberculous merchant seaman preferring to go there should be admitted to Bramshott and that any seaman In-patient at the Dreadnought Hospital should, upon notification as suffering from tubercle, be transferred forthwith to Bramshott if he so desired, unless in the opinion of the Honorary Physician he were unable to stand the journey thither by ambulance. With regard to Dr Sundell's suggestion that the matter be discussed by the Sanatorium Medical Council, the Board considered that as he had been in charge of the phthisical patients since 1921, his professional advice was sufficient to enable the Board to determine what their policy should be at the present time. The Board wished to know from Dr Wood how many of the 75 patients under treatment on 23rd July fell into each of the . . . categories referred to by ... Wingfield.
>
> In view of the abnormality of present war conditions (e.g., the considerable number of Royal Navy Ratings under treatment at Bramshott) it was not considered desirable or necessary formally to acquaint the L.C.C. Officer who had raised the question with the Board's affirmation of the policy and general practice which had obtained since the opening of the Sanatorium which was in accord with the Ministry of Health Circular 72/T.

The foregoing matters were brought to the attention of a meeting in September 1942. On the matter of 'active tubercle' being demonstrated by mass radiography,

Jarman 'expressed his willingness to receive formal representations as to certain legal difficulties which the Joint Sub-Committee had considered might arise if, under the present agreement with the Union and the [SF], the doctor who detected active [disease] in a seaman failed to notify the appropriate T.B. Officer or the man himself'. In *summary*, Jarman 'hoped that a scheme might be brought into operation whereby a seaman [who had been advised to undergo further investigation at the *Dreadnought* Hospital] would receive a grant through King George's Fund for Sailors [KGFS] for the maintenance of his dependents'. On the matter of criteria for admission to Bramshott, it was made clear that there would be no departure from the Society's present strategy (see above).[15]

THE ROLE OF MINIATURE-RADIO-PHOTOGRAPHY (MRP)

The position regarding MRP was summarised at a subsequent meeting of the Management Committee:

> *Tuberculosis – Miniature X-Ray Photography*. Mr Baker had reported that he and Dr Sundell, with the Secretary, had had a most cordial meeting with Mr Snedden and Mr Jarman on the 15th September. The latter had recognised that a medical practitioner, on becoming aware of Pulmonary Tuberculosis, had a statutory obligation to notify it to the T.B. Officer, and had also a recognised professional obligation to inform the patient of his infection and to refrain from informing anyone else. It had therefore been decided that the seaman's Discharge Book Number should be recorded upon his Miniature X-Ray Serial Card. The Reserve Pool Doctor would then be informed of the Discharge Book Numbers of those men in whom abnormality was suspected and he would advise the men in their own best interests to report to the *Dreadnought* [my italics] Hospital, Greenwich for further investigation. Mr Jarman hoped that a scheme might be brought into operation whereby a seaman so reporting for investigation would receive a grant through the [KGFS] for the maintenance of his dependents. The Board confirmed Mr Baker's undertaking that the Society would bear the cost of the man's investigation and hospital maintenance.
>
> This was considered to be very satisfactory and to offer further opportunity of discussion as to the method and manner in which seamen, showing abnormality in the miniature photographs, could be induced to undergo a further and complete investigation at the *Dreadnought* [my italics] Hospital.[16]

The Committee also considered a *Report* [on MRP] *of the Medical Research Council's Committee on Tuberculosis in wartime:*

> Dr Davies had referred to the observation of the Technical Sub-Committee that the correct interpretation of the miniature radiograph required the highest radiological skill and it had been agreed that Dr. White Phillips, Radiologist to the *Dreadnought* [my italics] Hospital, should be invited to give his advice upon all matters connected with miniature radiography,

or, failing him, Dr Mather Cordiner, Radiologist to the [HTD]. A matter on which the Radiologist's advice was immediately required was on the assembling and training of a team to carry out the mass radiographic examinations of seamen.

Sir Ion Hamilton Benn [1863–1961, SHS Chairman] had said that it would be desirable that ... Baker and ... Sundell, being in consultation with the [SF] and the [NUS], should have a personal interview with Sir Wilson Jameson [1885–1962, the Chief Medical Officer][17] to discuss how far and ... soon the recommendations contained in the Report would be applicable to the [MM] and if they would in any way affect the Society's project.[18]

SUPPORT FOR MRP

A Sub-Committee (consisting of Anderson, Mr F S A Baker, Sundell and Wingfield) met twice in the latter part of 1944 to discuss the merits or otherwise of MRP; on the latter occasion, White Phillips and Wood were also present (by invitation):

> The Sub-Committee [was] indebted to ... Wingfield for a report based on the examination of 1151 routine chest x-rays taken at the *Dreadnought* [my italics] Hospital in a period of 2¾ years. Since the main object of the investigation was to ascertain the incidence of *unsuspected* tuberculosis amongst seamen:
>
> i) films relating to 121 landsmen were discarded and the effective total thereby reduced to 1030, and
> ii) patients in whom tuberculosis had been previously diagnosed and where presenting symptoms were of lung disease had been excluded from the final total. Among [the] 1030 cases, 167 were found to have abnormalities of the lungs which appeared to be due to the tuberculosis, and these had been classified according to the Ministry of Health standard classification.
>
> The final pertinent analysis [demonstrated] that 1030 chest x-rays of Seamen had revealed 10 patients suffering from active post-primary tuberculosis in the absence of symptoms, i.e. 0.97%. There were also 41 cases of in-active post-primary tuberculosis ..., i.e. almost all had called for intensive investigation before it could be said with any confidence that the disease was *inactive* [my italics]. Even so it was not possible to be certain that the disease might not become active in the future if these patients came under excessive strain. ...
>
> THE SUB-COMMITTEE THEREFORE REPORTED THAT DR. WINGFIELD'S INVESTIGATION APPEARED TO LEAD TO THE CONCLUSION THAT ABOUT 1 IN EVERY 100 BRITISH SEAMEN IN THE MERCANTILE MARINE MAY BE SUFFERING FROM TUBERCULOSIS WITHOUT EXHIBITING ANY SYMPTOMS, AND THEREFORE INCAPABLE OF DETECTION EXCEPT BY X-RAYS. 4% OF THE CASES INVESTIGATED HAD BEEN FOUND TO BE CASES OF INACTIVE POST-PRIMARY TUBERCULOSIS. THE SUB-

COMMITTEE RECOMMENDED THAT THIS FINDING BE REPORTED TO THE SECRETARIES OF THE NATIONAL MARITIME BOARD AND THE MINISTRY OF WAR TRANSPORT ACCOMPANIED BY AN ASSURANCE THAT THE [SOCIETY] WOULD GIVE EVERY ASSISTANCE WITHIN ITS POWER TO THE ACTION WHICH THOSE BODIES MIGHT SUGGEST.

The Westinghouse … Unit had [by] now arrived from America. When the apparatus was ordered in May 1942, the intention was that it should be housed in two vehicles so as to form a completely mobile unit. Scientific developments since that date and acute difficulties in obtaining a whole-time professional 'director' to take charge of it, now led the Sub-Committee to the conclusion that this method was unsuitable and impracticable. There remained the question as to whether it should be:

a) Set up at the *Dreadnought* [my italics] Hospital, Greenwich, in which case arrangements would have to be made for seamen to be transported from the [MM] Medical Examining Centres in the Port of London, or
b) Locating it for certain periods at one or other of such Centres, in which case there would arise the question of accommodation on a considerable scale. This would have the disadvantage that the technical team of five … would not be under continuous supervision and that their work might be intermittent.

As to the cost of operating the Unit, it was estimated that this would amount to £3,000 per annum by way of salaries to the specially trained whole-time technical staff, and remuneration to the panel of members of the Society's Medical Staff. The £3,000 per annum excluded any allowance for rent, materials used, or depreciation.

... Wingfield had suggested that if the Unit were placed at the *Dreadnought* [my italics] Hospital, and the number of seamen photographed did not keep it working at normal pressure, consideration might be given to the question of making arrangements with the public health authorities and local practitioners which would ensure full-time utilisation of the plant and … reduce the unit cost of the examination of seamen.

The attention of the meeting had been drawn to the circular issued by the Ministry of Health cautioning employers of labour against instituting mass radiography examinations with apparatus and upon lines not in conformity with those approved by the Ministry.[19]

The full co-operation of the [SF] and its examining doctors and of the [NUS] would be essential, and the Sub-Committee held the view that the board should press these bodies for an indication as to what steps they proposed to take to deal with the problem, and how far they wished the [SHS] to assist them.

The Board approved the recommendation of the Sub-Committee which was supported by a letter dated 12th December from … Anderson.[20]

Future of the Sanatorium

Little more was heard of tuberculosis until March 1956 when the future of KGSS (since 1948 a component of the NHS) came to the fore:

> The Secretary reported that the South-West Metropolitan Regional Hospital Board [SWMRHB] were considering using the whole or part of [KGSS] for the treatment of cases other than those of *pulmonary tuberculosis* [my italics].
>
> In July last ... Lyon [the SHS Secretary] had had reason to suspect that some such proposal was in the air and at the same moment he had been informed that the architect was ready to draw up a detailed specification and bills of quantities for the new recreation building. He had therefore stopped this and said that the Society could not accept responsibility for any further expenditure on this project until further notice. Mr Nairne [the SHS Chairman] thought that this had been very prudent and the Secretary's action was CONFIRMED.
>
> [The minute continued] It was symptomatic of the general decline in the incidence of tuberculosis throughout the country that during the previous 2½ years the average number of merchant seamen under treatment in the 80 available beds at Bramshott had been about 40 daily, although this number had been even lower during the past 6 months. An analogous decline had been experienced in the calls upon the transit T.B. beds at the *Dreadnought* [my italics] Hospital and it was now found that a seaman could be transferred to a sanatorium near his own home without undue delay. In effect, although a unit of fully-staffed beds in a single sanatorium was still needed for treatment of tuberculous officers and men of the [MM], only 40 instead of 80 beds were required.
>
> On the 24th September ... Lyon had been invited by the Chairman of the Godalming, Milford, Liphook Hospital Management Committee [GMLHMC] to meet him at Bramshott to hear the Regional Board [RB]'s proposals. On behalf of the Society, ... Lyon had supported the Seamen's Hospitals Management Committee in their opposition to the total extinction of [KGSS] and the consequent dispersal of 40 T.B. seafarers elsewhere. The [RB]'s decision would probably be known after a further meeting on 12th October.
>
> Whether Bramshott were to be used wholly for some purpose other than that for which it was created, or whether half of it would still be retained for the treatment of T.B. seafarers, the Sub-Committee unanimously RECOMMENDED THAT the Society's proposal to spend £6,000 on a new recreation building there be deferred sine die.
>
> ... Lyon reported that the [GMLHMC] had decided to recommend to the [SWMRHB] that one half of [KGSS] i.e. about 40 beds should continue to be used for the admission of officers and seamen of the [MM]. ... Wingfield was of the opinion that there might be a further decline in the incidence of pulmonary tuberculosis with the effect that the number of beds required for M.M. patients would be progressively

fewer. The RECOMMENDATION of the Finance & General Purposes Sub-Committee was therefore APPROVED.

The Secretary [Lyon] had been asked by the [GMLHMC] if the Society were prepared to meet architect's fees for work already done to the amount of £252.5.1.. … Lyon had replied that as the Society felt obliged to defer further consideration of the project sine die by reason of the decision of the [SWMRHB], it was hoped that these fees would be met by the [RB]. This reply was CONFIRMED.[21]

Malaria

The HTD at Endsleigh Gardens had been closed since the outbreak of World War II on 3 September 1939; the *tropical* facilities had thereafter been relocated to the *Dreadnought* Hospital itself until 1944 (*see* Chapter 25), and there was *not* an 'enquiry-line' there on advice with respect to 'tropical' infections. The following minute, which is relevant in this context, refers to a meeting in November 1942; it is clear that the HTD staff were jealous of preserving their 'empire', as their successors are today:

> … The Secretary [Lyon] had reported a telephone enquiry from Professor Johnston, the Sector Hospital Officer, Sector 10, on behalf of Professor [FR] Fraser [FRCP] of the Ministry of Health, as to the number of cases of relapsing malaria seen in the past month. The number had been nine. The Secretary had understood that the object of the enquiry was to suggest that such cases should be transferred to Horton Hospital [Epsom] in order that Dr. Nicholl might observe the results of treating them with a new drug and comparing these results with the treatment by the same drug of cases of induced malaria. It [was] unanimously agreed that the transfer of such cases was *entirely undesirable* [my italics]. It did not appear that the Ministry had any power to order such transfers and the Committee of Management would not agree to Merchant Seamen being transferred. Sir Philip Manson-Bahr [FRCP] had recalled that the investigation of the effect of new drugs upon tropical diseases had always been investigated at the [HTD] and ... Wingfield had reported that he had recently carried out an investigation of this nature at the *Dreadnought* [my italics] Hospital for Dr. Warrington Yorke [FRCP] of Liverpool.
>
> The Secretary had [therefore] been instructed to inform … Johnston that the transfer of such cases … was considered undesirable and would not be approved, but that the Staff would be very ready to carry out investigations in collaboration with ... Nicholl. If it were desired to appoint or transfer ad hoc personnel to the *Dreadnought* [my italics] Laboratories this would be agreeable, and the Committee of Management would consider it proper, if it were necessary, to meet any expenditure from their funds which are available for tropical diseases among patients in their care.
>
> [This minute ended:] The Secretary reported that he had received no reply to his letter to … Johnston dated 22nd October 1942.[22]

Treatment of fractures

The 1930 Report referred to this matter, which was an important one in the development of the '*new*' ADH:

> During the past year a Committee, on which the [SHS] was represented, considered the important question of the treatment of fracture cases after their first care in hospital. A great many of these cases need special treatment by way of graduated exercises, under constant and expert supervision, to render them fit to resume work; but very little [had] been done in this way in England. The result is that many such cases remain on the sick list, drawing compensation pay for many weeks and even months without being able to resume their old occupation.
>
> The Committee came to the conclusion that … special treatment was highly desirable, and they hoped that the [Society] might be able to provide opportunities for an experiment in a small way; it being understood, however, that the patients would have to be *in-patients* [my italics] and that there would have to be ample space for workshops and equipment, also space for work and exercises in the open air, and that the whole unit would have to be under the supervision of an expert medical man.
>
> The Board of Management … came to the conclusion that, faced as they were with a very large capital expenditure for the reconstruction of the *Dreadnought* [my italics], and in view of the financial depression in the country, they could not at the present time undertake any further responsibilities, however desirable they might be. They hoped to reconsider the matter at a later date.[23]

Weil's disease (leptospirosis)

A Board of Management minute, in April 1940 refers to this infection – caused by a bacterium (*Leptospira* spp) spread to humans via rat's urine – which was then notoriously common in sewer-workers:

> *Treatment of … Weil's Disease.*
>
> In normal times the [HTD] had treated cases of Weil's Disease among employees of Messrs Mowlem engaged in sewer work. Messrs C.T. Roberts & Co., of 31, High Holborn who now had the sewer contract for London had enquired whether the Society could continue to give such treatment. In view of the fact that over an extended period the Devonport Pathological Laboratories [Chapter 20] had carried out tests for the [PLA] upon rats which were carriers of Weil's Disease, the Committee had agreed, upon the recommendation of ... Sundell, that cases of Weil's Disease (which had numbered 7 or 8 annually) might be admitted to the *Dreadnought* [my italics] Hospital.

This minute ended: It was reported that in the event Messrs Mowlem were retaining the sewer contract for the [LCC] and the Secretary was in correspondence with Messrs Mowlem on the question of payment for services which might be rendered to their employees requiring treatment for or suspected to be suffering from this Disease.[24]

Scabies

Scabies ('the itch') caused by a small ectoparasite had always been a problem in the seafarer; it had assumed enormous significance in the hospital-ship days (*see* Chapter 11). In 1942, the Medical Officer to the PLA, Dr Morgan, in conjunction with Drs Erskine (Dermatologist) and Davies (Pathologist) (*see* Chapters 15 and 24) – both of whom were employed by the SHS – decided to launch a campaign to *eliminate* this tiresome infection from the MM; to this end, Morgan set up a bureau at 5, Church Passage, Guildhall, EC2 with the objectives of:

i) 'collection of information [on this infection] among seamen',
ii) to 'direct seamen to appropriate treatment centres',
iii) to 'arrange for the disinfestation of their clothing and bedding',
iv) to 'secure hospital treatment for complicated or stubborn cases' (which should be dealt with at the *Dreadnought* [my italics] Hospital),
v) to organise a follow-up system to ensure that cases are not lost sight of, and
vi) to 'arrange for the periodic inspection of ships that have been infested'.

It was recommended that beds for six crew and three officer in-patients (a 'Scabies Unit') should be reserved at the *Dreadnought* for this purpose, and 'At least one whole-time male attendant, trained in the appropriate treatment of scabies' would be required.

A subsequent minute (late in 1942), contained a request from the Greenwich Borough Council for the use of the *Dreadnought's* facilities for disinfestation of the *clothing* of men from the Borough's Gas Cleaning Station; the SHS Board of Management agreed to this on an out-patient basis, but only as a *war-time* measure. Five guineas monthly was the cost of this facility.[25]

Radiation–induced disease

An early victim of x-ray complications was 'Mr. A. Parsons, the Society's Radiographer, who had died as a result of X-ray dermatitis on the 15th June (1928)'. He had been employed by the *Dreadnought* Hospital since 1909 (having already worked at the Westminster Hospital). While he earned the distinction of being amongst the pioneers in this branch of science, the report continued: 'he also suffered [one of] the penalties of those who blaze the trail that others may follow in safety'.[26]

References and notes

1 Annual Report 109: 18.
2 *Op cit.* See note 1 above. 96: 16; 97: 11.
3 Committee of Management Minutes. 20: 30, 57, 92.
4 *Ibid.* 154–5; 206; 253.
5 *Ibid.* 291, 369–70.
6 *Ibid.* 424, 450.
7 *Ibid.* 385.
8 G C Cook. Early use of 'open-air' treatment for 'pulmonary phthisis at the Dreadnought Hospital, Greenwich, 1900-1905. *Postgrad Med J* 1999; 75: 326–7. [*See also*: I A Campbell, O-Bah-Sow. Pulmonary tuberculosis: diagnosis and treatment. *BMJ* 2006; 332: 1194–7].
9 *Op cit.* See note 3 above. 20: 247–50. [*See also*: *Op cit.* See note 1 above: 122: 9–10]. [For details of Cork & Orrery *see* Chapter 22.]
10 P Stocks. Vital statistics of the second year of the war. *Lancet* 1942; i: 189–91.
11 D Galbraith. Pulmonary tuberculosis in recruits: further experience in a survey by the method of miniature radiography. *BMJ* 1941; i: 699–701; J V Sparks. Some problems of miniature mass radiography. *BMJ* 1941; i: 917–20; W G C Fitzpatrick. Mass miniature photoradiography in the Royal Navy. *Proc Roy Soc Med* 1941; 34: 406–10. [*See also*: S H Graham, M Davies. Tuberculosis in recruits. *BMJ* 1941; i: 920–4].
12 I H Benn, Cork & Orrery, C E Sundell, A Wingfield.. X-ray diagnosis. *Times, Lond.* 1942; 4 April: 5. [*See also*: Anonymous. Parliament: tuberculosis. *Times, Lond.* 1942; 1 May: 8; Anonymous. Detection of tubercle. *Times, Lond.* 1942; 2 May: 5; Anonymous. Testing the average. *Times, Lond.* 1942; 15 May: 5; *Op cit.* See note 3 above: 258–9.]
13 *Op cit.* See note 3 above: 20: 266; 267; 277; 284–5; Anonymous. Health in the Merchant Navy. *Times, Lond.* 1942; 16 June: 5; Moyne. Merchant Seamen. *Ibid.* 19 June: 5. [For details of Moyne *see* Chapter 22.]
14 *Op cit.* See note 3 above: 20: 292–4.
15 *Ibid.* 299–300.
16 *Ibid.* 309–10.
17 **Sir [William] Wilson Jameson** GBE FRCP (1885–1962) was Dean and Professor of Public Health at the London School of Hygiene and Tropical Medicine. He was also Chief Medical Officer to the Ministries of Health and Education from 1940 until 1950. Jameson worked with the King Edward's Hospital Fund for London (1950–1960). [*See also*: N M Goodman. *Wilson Jameson: Architect of National Health* London: George Allen and Unwin 1970: 216; G E Godber. Jameson, Sir (William) Wilson (1885–1962) In: H C G Matthew, B Harrison (eds). *Oxford Dictionary of National Biography.* Oxford: Oxford University Press 2004; 29: 767–8].
18 *Op cit.* See note 3 above. 20: 320.
19 Anonymous. Mass radiography: a cautionary notice. *BMJ* 1944; ii: 350.
20 *Op cit.* See note 3 above. 20: 529–31.
21 *Ibid.* 22: 254–5.
22 *Ibid.* 320–1.
23 *Op cit.* See note 1 above. 110: 18.
24 *Op cit.* See note 3 above. 20: 63. [See also: G C Cook. *Tropical medicine: an illustrated history of the Pioneers*. London: Academic Press 2007 (in press).]
25 *Ibid.* 20: 260–261; 286.
26 *Op cit.* See note 1 above. 108: 15.

Chapter 24

The Society's staff in recent times

Several medical disciplines required strengthening during, and more importantly immediately after, the Second World War (1939–45). In particular, the HTD (formerly at Endsleigh Gardens) – which had been closed throughout those grim war years – was in urgent need of the addition of several first-class consultants to its staff. Another discipline which required attention was the rapidly developing speciality of thoracic surgery – at the King George's Sanatorium for Sailors (KGSS). The medical and surgical staff of the Tilbury Hospital also required expansion – especially in the field of orthopaedics. There were other 'gaps': for example, in ENT surgery and gynaecology.

Although the medical and surgical staffing during the years 1940–86 was competent, it perhaps lacked the lustre of former years. There was no one of the national/international stature of figures such as Roupell, Budd, Leach or Busk (*see* Chapter 12), and certainly no one to match the 'giants' brought in when the LSTM (in 1899) and LSCM (in 1906) were formed. However, they were all highly competent, and many produced useful literary contributions – some of which are listed in the references at the end of this chapter. The following pages thus do not contain comprehensive details of *every* medical member of the SHS institutions in recent times, but the most significant members of the medical staff receive coverage.

Non-medical staff

Table 24.1 gives details of the senior members of the non-medical staff from 1940, until closure of most of the SHS facilities in the late twentieth century. This chapter also summarises most of the new recruits to the SHS administrative staff during this period which, with the implementation of the NHS Act in 1948 proved to be one of a steady decline in the manifold activities of the SHS. The reigning monarch had served as Patron of the Society from its foundation in 1821; however, in 2000 HM Queen Elizabeth II herself decided to 'hand over' to the Duke of York from 1 January 2001. With few exceptions, the senior non-medical staff of the Society served for relatively short terms when compared with those halcyon days, in which the Society had been one of the greatest medical charities in the land.

Table 24.1: Non-medical staff of the Society (1940–present).

Patrons & Patronesses:	
19[40]–52	HM King George VI KG*†
19[40]–53	HM Queen Mary KG
1953–2000	HM Queen Elizabeth II KG
2001–present	HRH The Duke of York CVO ADC
Presidents:	
19[40]–41	Rt Hon Baron Lloyd of Dolobran GCSI GCIE DSO (1879–1941)*
1941–44	Rt Hon Lord Moyne PC DSO (1880–1944)
1946–48	Admiral of the Fleet, The Rt Hon 12th Earl of Cork and Orrery GCB GCVO (1873–1967)
1949–61	Captain Sir Ion Hamilton Benn Bt CB DSO TD RNVR (1863–1961)
1962–77	Sir Colin Anderson KBE (1904–80)
1978–82	Mr Anthony Benn OBE (?–?)
1982–2002	Rt Hon. Sir Patrick Nairne GCB MC (1921–present)
2002–present	Sir Brian Shaw (1933–present)
Chairmen, Committee of Management:	
19[40]– 46	Captain Sir Ion Hamilton Benn Bt CB DSO TD RNVR*
1946–67	Sir Ernest Murrant KCMG MBE
1967–71	Captain Guy Lydekker OBE DSC RN
1971–78	Mr Anthony Benn OBE
1978–83	Captain R Hart CBE DSO DSC RN
1983–97	Captain I B Taylor OBE
1997–2004	Captain D T Smith OBE RN
2004–present	Mr J D Guthrie
Secretaries (and Administrators):	
19[40]–61	F A Lyon OBE*
1961–74	D A C Price VRD
1974–88	A G McBride
1988–93	J Allen
1993–2001	Mrs M C O'Halloran
2002–present	P Coulson
Treasurers:	
19[40]–43	Col Sir Robert Williams Bt*
19[40]–66	J C Nairne†
1961–74	F A Lyon OBE
1966–71	A Benn
1971–96	D R Archer
1974–80	D A C Price
1997–98	B T Roberts
1998–2002	J C Jenkinson MVO
2002–present	G P Ellis
Hospital Secretaries/House governors:	
Dreadnought	D A C Price
ADH	D A C Price
Tilbury	G W Whyte
HTD	A A Hood MBE / R L Lloyd
KGSS	J E Wood

Table 24.1 – *continued*

Matrons:	
Dreadnought	M Foster Smith/C A Howard
ADH	H S Sheard / M Foster Smith / Q E E Ager
Tilbury	M K Ireland / C C Ross
HTD	M Hill
KGSS	A M Wootton
Angas	D Lewis / C Fraser / E M Smith

* See also Chapter 21.
[+]Square brackets = already in post in 1940.
[†] A memorial service for J Cyril Nairne (1880–1966) was held in the Chapel of St Peter, the *Dreadnought* Hospital on 14 April 1966.

Medical Staff

This chapter summarises the careers of many of the senior medical personnel who began their association with the Society during the period under review. Tables 24.2 to 24.6 summarise most senior appointments; junior posts are in most cases *not* recorded in the *Annual Reports*.

Table 24.2: *Dreadnought* medical staff (1940–48).*

Consulting Physicians:	
19[40]–48	Sir Gordon Holmes[+]
1948	C E Sundell[+]
Consulting Physician in Tropical Medicine:	
1941–48	Sir Philip Manson-Bahr[+]
Consulting Surgeons:	
19[40]–44	W Turner[†]
19[40]–48	(Sir) Ernest Rock Carling
1946–48	E T C Milligan
1947–48	P P Cole[+]
Consulting Dermatologists:	
19[40]–48	H MacCormac[†]
1964–48	D Erskine
Consulting Opthalmic Surgeon:	
19[40]–48	L V Cargill[†]
1947–48	R E Bickerton DSO
Consulting ENT Surgeon:	
19[40]–48	R Lake[+]
Consulting Gynaecologist:	
1946–48	K M K Duff[+]
Consulting Neurologist:	
19[40]–48	F M R Walshe[+]

Table 24.2 – *continued*

Consulting Pathologist:	
1945–48	A Davies
Physicians:	
19[40]–48	C E Sundell[+]
19[40]–45	A C Hampson[+]
1945–48	A Wingfield
Surgeons:	
19[40]–47	P P Cole[+]
19[40]–45	E T C Milligan
1946–48	D M Cooper
1946–48	S Power
Gynaecologists:	
19[40]–46	K M K Duff[+]
1946–47	J Howkins
Ophthalmic Surgeon:	
19[40]–47	R E Bickerton DSO
1947–48	L Lurie
ENT Surgeon (Laryngologist)	
19[40]–48	F Courtenay Mason[+]
Dermatologist:	
19[40]–48	D Erskine
Neurologist:	
1947–48	C Edwards
Physician in Tropical Medicine:	
1947–48	F Murgatroyd
Radiologist:	
19[40]–44	Martin Berry
1944–47	C White Phillips
1947–48	O F W Robinson
Director-in-charge of Department of Physical Medicine:	
19[40]–48	J Sainsbury
Director of Pathology:	
19[40]–45	A Davies
1947–48	G L Robinson
Anaesthetists:	
19[40]–	J R Hasler
19[40]–47	W W Mushin
19[40]–47	R A Beaver
1947–48	Miss A Openheim
1948–48	C G Townsend
Director of VD Clinic:	
19[40]–47	P P Cole[+]

* This hospital closed in 1986; [+] See also Chapter 21; [†] See also Chapter 15.

'Dreadnought' Hospital

MILLIGAN

Edward Thomas Campbell Milligan FRCS (1886–1972) was born at Waterloo, near Ballarat, Victoria, Australia, and educated at Ballarat College and Melbourne University – from which he qualified in 1910. Following junior appointments in Melbourne, Milligan moved to Europe in 1914 with a Field Ambulance of the Australian Expeditionary Force; he published articles on the surgical management of war wounds, 'shell shock', and blood transfusion. Following the Great War, Milligan settled in London. He passed the FRCS examination in 1919, and he was soon elected to the staff of St Mark's, the Croydon General, and the *Dreadnought* (in 1921). He specialised in ano-rectal (for example, he perfected the abdomino-perineal operation for rectal carcinoma) and genito-urinary diseases. In 1942, he was President of the Section of Proctology at the Royal Society of Medicine. Milligan was a staunch Methodist and intimately associated with Moral Rearmament. There were no children of his marriage. (see also: Chapter 21).[1]

ERSKINE

David Erskine qualified at Guy's Hospital (MRCS LRCP) in 1931. He subsequently abtained an MD (Lond.) and DPH. Erskine had been a Medical Officer in the venereology and dermatology departments of Guy's Hospital. He combined the specialities of *dermatology* and *venereology* and apart from the *Dreadnought* he was on the staff of St John's Hospital, Lewisham.[2] He was the author of a number of papers on venereology.

BICKERTON

Reginald Ernest Bickerton studied medicine at Liverpool, Berlin and Vienna, qualifying in (MB ChB) in 1895. Apart from the *Dreadnought* he was *ophthalmic surgeon* to several London hospitals.[3]

WINGFIELD

Alexander Louis Wingfield FRCP (1907–69) was born at Finchley, London and educated at St Paul's School and St Thomas's Hospital, graduating MB BS in 1932 and MD in 1934. After junior appointments at the Willesden General, the Royal Free and Brompton Hospitals he pursued a career in chest and cardiovascular diseases, and held registrar and senior registrar posts at King's College and the National Heart Hospitals. Although appointed consultant physician to the *Dreadnought* in 1939, his career there really took off following the war. During Army service, he was Lieutenant Colonel in charge of a medical division and physician to the EMS. From the end of the war until 1951 Wingfield was a chest physician at St Stephen's Hospital; in 1946, he was also consultant physician to the Willesden General Hospital (where he subsequently died) and honorary cardiologist to St Andrew's Hospital, Dollis Hill. Wingfield was a member of the Medical Society of London and became its President in 1963–4. He was deeply interested in the history of medicine and bibliography. There were two daughters of his marriage. Some of Wingfield's publications have been preserved in the SHS archive.[4]

DAVIES

Arthur Davies MRCP received his medical education at Westminster Hospital and after several junior appointments became Consultant Pathologist to the Society as well as to several East End hospitals including: Queen Mary's, Stratford; King George Hospital, Ilford; the Jewish Hospital and St John's, Lewisham. Davies was a prolific author.[5]

COOPER

Desmond Marriott Cooper FRCS (1909–62) qualified MB BS (Lond) from St Thomas's Hospital in 1933. He became surgeon to the *Dreadnought*, Miller General, Woolwich War Memorial and the Brook General hospitals and held those positions at the time of his premature death on 27 August 1962.[6]

POWER

Stephen May Power FRCS (1902–87) was born at Reading and educated at St Ignatius College and the London Hospital Medical School from which he graduated MB BS in 1925. Following junior appointments, he was appointed consultant surgeon to the Royal London Homeopathic Hospital (1936) and later to the *Dreadnought* and Eltham District Hospital. During the Second World War, Power served as Lieutenant-Colonel, mostly in India, with the RAMC. Most of his papers were centred on urology; he made significant contributions to prostate surgery. Power wrote three books: *Surgical technique* (1952), *Surgical Diagnosis* (1957), and *Surgeon at the Bedside* (1962).[7]

HOWKINS

John Howkins FRCS, FRCOG (1907-present) was educated at Shrewsbury School and the Middlesex Hospital, from which he qualified in 1932. He became a consultant surgeon in *gynaecology* to St Bartholomew's, Hampstead General, and the Royal Masonic Hospitals. During the Second World War he served with the RAFVR. Howkins was appointed gynaecologist to the *Dreadnought* Hospital (1946-69). He edited several texts devoted to gynaecological surgery.[8]

LURIE

Leonard Lurie DOMS was educated at the (Royal) London Hospital and subsequently became *ophthalmic surgeon* to several London hospitals including the *Dreadnought*.[9]

EDWARDS

Colin Campbell Edwards MRCP was educated at Sydney University. He became a consultant neurologist to several hospitals, including the Dreadnought and Tilbury Hospitals. Edwards was the author of several papers on neurological topics.[10]

ROBINSON (OLIVER)

Oliver Francis Waring Robinson TD DMRE received his medical training at Belfast and King's College London. After several junior appointments, he became Senior Radiologist at the *Dreadnought* and Tilbury Hospitals.[11]

ROBINSON (GEOFFREY)

Geoffrey Lawrence Robinson qualified from the (Royal) London Hospital in 1929. He subsequently became pathologist to the Devonport Laboratories.[12]

MASHIN

William Woolf Mashin FFA RCS studied medicine at the (Royal) London Hospital and qualified (MB BS) in 1932. He subsequently became Professor of Anaesthesiology at the Welsh National School of Medicine. Mashin was a prolific author on anaesthesia.[13]

Albert Dock Hospital

Table 24.3 summarises the senior medical staff of the ADH from 1940 until its closure.

HANSCHELL

Hother McCormick Hanschell qualified from St Bartholomew's Hospital in 1907. He subsequently had several appointments in Africa, and became a consulting physician to the ADH; he was also Director of Dermatology and of the VD clinic there.[14]

BOYDE

Harry Caine Boyde qualified from St Bartholomew's Hospital in 1925. He subsequently served in several hospitals in the East end of London, including the ADH.[15]

FREEMAN

Harry Freeman FRCS (1894–1949) was born at Braila, Romania but his parents moved to England when he was a child, and he was educated at schools in Hastings, Croydon and Battersea Polytechnic. Following this he attended King's College, and Westminster Hospital Medical School, qualifying MRCS LRCP in 1921. He settled into general practice at Dalston and after 10 years there, took the midwifery diploma of the Society of Apothecaries, and in 1941 became FRCS. During the Second World War, Freeman and his wife (also a doctor) took charge of the air-

Table 24.3: Albert Dock Hospital (ADH) medical staff (1940–48).*

Consulting Physicians:	
19[40]–48	G C Low+
1947–48	Sir Philip Manson-Bahr+
1947–48	H M Hanschell
Consulting Surgeons:	
19[40]–48	T Pomfret Kilner
1948	(Sir) Hugh Griffiths+
Consulting Dental Surgeon:	
19[40]–46	T H Vaughan
Physicians:	
19[40]–47	P H (later Sir Philip) Manson-Bahr+
1946–48	H C Boyde
1947–48	F Murgatroyd
First Assistant in Medicine:	
1946–48	H C Boyde
Physician (or Acting Casualty Medical Officer) with Charge of Out-Patients:	
19[40]–46	F Murgatroyd
1940–46	H C Boyde
Surgeons:	
19[40]–48	H E (later Sir Hugh) Griffiths+
19[40]–48	C Hope Carlton
Assistant Surgeons:	
19[40]–46	R E Norrish
1946–48	H Freeman
1946–48	P M Kelly
Radiologist:	
19[40]–48	F G Wood
Pathologist (part-time):	
19[40]–47	H M Hanschell
Director of VD Clinic:	
19[40]–47	H M Hanschell

* This hospital was latterly used for mentally handicapped patients and closed in 1994; + See also Chapter 21.

raid casualty centre of No 34 National Fire Service area in Holborn. Freeman also operated on air-raid casualties at the ADH – to which he was appointed assistant surgeon in 1946; in that year, he was also elected assistant surgeon at the National Temperance Hospital. Freeman studied gastroscopy under Herman Taylor.[16]

KELLY

Patrick Michael Kelly FRCS (1912–89) was born in Dublin – the son of Sir Patrick Kelly CIE, Commissioner of Police in Bombay – and educated at Clongowes Wood

College, Co. Kildare; Corpus Christi College, Cambridge; and St Thomas's Hospital, London. He qualified in 1937. After junior appointments at his teaching hospital, St George's and Guy's Hospitals he served as a Wing-Commander with the RAFVR in Wales and the Azores. Specialising in urology, he was appointed after the war to the St Helier Hospital and St Anthony's Hospital, Cheam. There was a son and two daughters of his marriage in 1939.[17]

NORRISH

Reginald Eric Norrish FRCS (1900–75) qualified from St Bartholomew's Hospital, MRCS LRCP in 1927; two years later he became FRCS and was appointed to the staff of the Royal Northern Hospital and 4th London Territorial Army Hospital. During the Second World War, Norrish served briefly in Northern Ireland, and in 1941 he was placed in charge of a surgical division in India and Burma, with the rank of Lieutenant-Colonel. Following the war, he was appointed surgeon to the City General Hospital, Stoke-on-Trent. There was a son and daughter from his marriage.[18]

Tilbury Hospital

Table 24.4 summarises senior medical appointments at the Tilbury Hospital from 1940 until its closure.

PLUMSTEAD

Charles Edward George Plumstead received his medical training at St George's Hospital, London and qualified in 1925. He became a Consultant Surgeon at the Tilbury Hospital, but was essentially a General Practitioner, his 'firm' being 'Pinching and Plumstead' of Gravesend.[19]

DICKINSON

John Roscoe Dickinson FRCS (1909–96) qualified in 1934; he had studied at Cambridge University and Guy's Hospital. He obtained the FRCS in 1939. He subsequently became a consultant *obstetrician and gynaecologist* to several hospitals, including Tilbury.[20]

SMALL

Hugh Alan Dugleby Small FRCS (1910–81). Born at Hastings, New Zealand, Small studied medicine at Otago University, Dunedin. On arrival in England, he occupied junior posts at Great Ormond Street and the Royal Cancer Hospitals. During the 1939–45 War, he served as a Squadron Leader in the RAF; following hostilities, he was appointed surgeon to the Tilbury; Queen Mary's, Stratford; Wood Green and Southgate, Chase Farm, Barnet General, and Royal Northern Hospitals. Although a general surgeon, he made peripheral vascular disease his *forte*. Small wrote a good deal, developed a technique for hernia repair, and 'described a method of excising the track of a branchial fistula'. He also took an important part

Table 24.4: Tilbury Hospital medical staff (1940–48).*

Consulting Physician in Tropical Medicine:	
19[40]–48	P H (later Sir Philip) Manson-Bahr+
19[40]–48	N H (later Sir Neil) Hamilton-Fairley+
Consulting Surgeon:	
1946–48	C G E Plumstead
Consulting Gynaecologist:	
1946–48	K M K Duff+
Consultant Physician:	
19[40]–48	C E Sundell+
Consultant Surgeons:	
19[40]–44	P P Cole+
19[40]–43	C J Pinching
19[40]–48	C G E Plumstead+
Consultant Gynaecologists:	
1946–48	K M K Duff
1948–48	J R Dickinson
Surgeon:	
1944–48	H A D Small
Orthopaedic Surgeon:	
1946–48	H Osmond-Clarke
Gynaecologist:	
1944–46	K Duff+
1946–47	J Howkins
Laryngologists:	
1945–47	E Carew-Shaw
1948–48	J Littlejohn
Neurologist:	
1947–48	C C Edwards
Dermatologist:	
1948–48	B Phillips
Radiologist:	
19[40]–48	G White Phillips

* This hospital closed in 1969; + see also Chapter 21.

in postgraduate medical training – mostly at the Royal Northern Hospital. Small travelled widely – in Italy, Sicily, Greece, Iraq and South America. He was twice married; there were two sons and a daughter of the first, and two daughters of the second.[21]

OSMOND-CLARKE

(Sir) Henry Osmond-Clarke KCVO FRCS (1905–86) was born at Brookeborough, County Fermanagh and educated at Clones High School and Trinity College, Dublin. He qualified in 1926 and held house appointments at Manchester and London. He pursued postgraduate education in Vienna, Bologna, New York, Boston, and London. Following this, Osmond-Clarke was appointed clinical tutor in orthopaedic surgery at Manchester Royal Infirmary and lecturer in orthopaedic surgical pathology at the University of Manchester. He was also appointed consultant orthopaedic surgeon to Crumpsall Hospital, Manchester, and Biddulph Grange Orthopaedic Hospital, Stoke-on-Trent. From 1941–46 Osmond-Clarke served in the RAF with the rank of Air Commodore; following the war, he moved to London and (probably as a result of Sir Reginald Watson-Jones' influence) was appointed consultant *orthopaedic surgeon* posts at the (Royal) London, Oldchurch, Black Notley, Tilbury and East Grinstead Hospitals. He was later appointed to King Edward VII Hospital for Officers, King Edward VII Convalescent Home, Osborne (Isle of Wight), and was civilian consultant in orthopaedics to the RAF. He subsequently advised on the development of orthopaedic services in Israel, India, and Persia. He was also Vice-President of the RCS, and President of the British Orthopaedic Association. He wrote *Half a century of Orthopaedic progress in Great Britain* (1951). There were two daughters of his marriage.[22]

CAREW-SHAW

Edward Carew-Shaw FRCS studied medicine at King's College London, St George's and St Thomas's Hospitals, qualifying in 1926; he obtained the FRCS in 1932. He subsequently had a distinguished career in *oto-rhino-laryngology*.[23]

LITTLEJOHN

James Littlejohn MBE studied medicine at King's College London and St George's Hospital. After junior appointments, he became Consultant *Ear, Nose and Throat* Surgeon to several hospitals, including the Tilbury Hospital.[24]

Hospital for Tropical Diseases

Table 24.5 summarises medical staff of the HTD following the Second World War. The HTD ceased being under the wing of the SHS when the NHS came into effect in 1948. Several 'specialist' physicians and a pathologist were appointed. During these years, the staff of the HTD expanded markedly – despite the peripatetic nature of the institution. Several 'specialist' physicians and a pathologist were appointed.

MURGATROYD

Frederick Murgatroyd FRCP (1902–51) was educated at Wallasey Grammar School and Liverpool University; the professor of tropical medicine at the Liverpool School – Warrington Yorke – directed him towards a 'tropical' career. In 1927, he was appointed assistant lecturer in protozoology, and two years later clinical patholo-

Table 24.5: Hospital for Tropical Diseases (HTD) medical staff (1940–48).*

Consulting Physicians:	
19[40]–48	G C Low
1947–48	(Sir) Philip Manson-Bahr[+]
Consulting Surgeons:	
19[40]–48	T Pomfret Kilner[+]
1947–48	(Sir) Archibald McIndoe[+]
Consulting Neurologist:	
19[40]–48	F M R Walshe OBE[+]
Consulting Gynaecologist:	
19[40)–46	V B Green-Armytage[+]
Consulting Cardiologist:	
19[40]–46	D Evan Bedford[+]
Consulting Physician for Diseases of the Chest:	
19[40]–46	F G Chandler
Physicians:	
19[40]–47	(Sir) Philip Manson-Bahr[+]
19[40]–48	(Sir) Neil Hamilton Fairley[+]
1946–51	F Murgatroyd
1948	Sir George McRobert
Assistant Physician:	
19[40]–46	F Murgatroyd
Surgeons:	
19[40]–47	(Sir) Archibald McIndoe[+]
19[40]–48	C Naunton Morgan[+]
1951–48	H R I Wolfe
Dermatologist:	
19[40]–46	J M H Macleod
Ophthalmic Surgeon:	
19[40]–48	Col W E O'G Kirkwan
ENT Surgeon:	
19[40]–46	W H Morris
Radiologist:	
19[40]–47	G R Mather Cordiner
Honorary Helminthogist:	
19[40]–46	R T Leiper FRS
Honorary Bacteriologist:	
19[40]–46	W W C Topley FRS
Anaesthetists:	
19[40]–48	C Langton Hewer
19[40]–48	J Truscott Hunter
Pathologist:	
19[48]–48	P H Martin

* Towards the end of the Second World War, this hospital moved from Greenwich to 23 Devonshire Street, and from there to 4 St Pancras Way in 1951, followed by University College Hospital in 1998; [+] see also Chapter 21.

gist. Following work on filariasis at the Liverpool School's laboratory at Freetown, Sierra Leone, he was appointed lecturer in tropical medicine (under Yorke) at the Royal Infirmary and, from 1936–7 he undertook trials of synthetic agents for trypanosomiasis at the MRC unit, the Gambia. Moving to London, Murgatroyd was appointed to a lectureship in tropical medicine at the LSHTM, and assistant physician to the HTD (at Endsleigh Gardens), ADH and *Dreadnought* hospitals, which were at that time under the SHS; Murgatroyd had first-hand experience of amoebiasis, filariasis, blackwater fever, Weil's disease, kala-azar and trypanosomiasis. By 1939 (when the Second World War started) he was a consultant physician to the Colonial Office and a member of the Typhus Diagnosis Panel of the Ministry of Health; as a result, he was appointed assistant director of pathology in West Africa, with the rank of lieutentant-colonel, RAMC. In 1944, he was one of the first to enter Belsen. In 1950, he succeeded to Fairley's chair at the LSHTM, and carried out much of the planning for the opening of the HTD at St Pancras in 1951. He died suddenly and unexpectedly in late 1951. There were no children of his marriage.[25]

McROBERT

Sir George (Reid) McRobert FRCP (1895–1976) was born and educated at Aberdeen. He became Professor of Physiology and Pharmacology in the University of Rangoon, Burma (1925) and Professor of Medicine in the University of Madras (1934). McRobert retired from the IMS in 1951 and was appointed consultant physician to the HTD; He was President of the RSTMH from 1861 to 1963.[26]

WOLFE

Herbert Robert Inglewood Wolfe FRCS (1907-1970) studied medicine at St Thomas's Hospital, London, and qualified in 1932; three years later he obtained the FRCS. Wolfe became consultant surgeon to UCH, the National Temperance Hospital and the HTD.[27]

King George's Sanatorium

Table 24.6 summarises the medical staff of KGSS. With the Sanatorium for Sailors well established, it was essential to have an experienced thoracic surgeon on the staff; the three who followed one another were: Tudor Edwards, Barrett and Siddons.

BARRETT

Norman Rupert Barrett CBE FRCS (1903–79) was born at Adelaide, Australia and educated at Eton, Trinity College, Cambridge, and St Thomas's Hospital. Following qualification in 1928 he was appointed to a Rockefeller Travelling Fellowship and spent time at the Mayo Clinic. In 1935, Barrett was elected to the staff of St Thomas's Hospital, and shortly afterwards to the Brompton Hospital. He often visited South Wales and became an authority on the treatment of pulmonary hydatidosis. During the 1939–45 war, Barrett served in the EMS, and in 1944 was appointed consultant thoracic surgeon to King Edward VII Sanatorium, Midhurst, and the Ministry of

Table 24.6: King George's Sanatorium for Sailors (KGSS) medical staff (1940–48).

Consulting Surgeon:	
1944–45	Sir Henry Gauvain
Physician:	
19[40]–48	C E Sundell
Surgeons:	
19[40]	Gilbert Smith
19[40]–44	Sir Henry Gauvain
Laryngologist:	
19[40]–48	F Courtenay Mason
Chest Surgeons:	
19[40]–45	A Tudor Edwards
1945–47	N R Barrett
1947–48	A H M Siddons
Medical Superintendent & Director/Physician Superintendent:	
19[40]–56	J E Wood

Pensions. He was a member of Council and subsequently Vice-President of the RCS. He was interested in medical history. There were two daughters of his marriage.[28]

SIDDONS

Arthur Harold Makins Siddons FRCS FRCP (1911–2001) was educated at Harrow; Jesus College, Cambridge, and St George's Hospital Medical School. He was appointed Consultant General and Thoracic Surgeon to St George's Hospital in 1948. From 1942–46 he served in the RAF Medical Branch. He married three times (all of his wives predeceased him); there was a son and daughter of his first marriage.[29]

WOOD

John Eric Wood qualified (MRCS LRCP) from the Royal London Hospital in 1918. He was Physician Superintendent of the KGSS.[30]

Angas Convalescent Home

The sole change in the staff of this establishment, according to the Society's Annual Reports, was that W E Cooke replaced R G Dingwall as Resident Medical Officer.

COOKE

William Ernest Cooke FRSCI studied medicine in Dublin and, becoming interested in tropical medicine, was appointed outpatient physician and superintendent at the Hospital for Tropical Diseases.[31]

References and notes

1 Anonymous. *BMJ* 1972: i: 186 & 317; Anonymous *Plarr's Lives 1965–73:* 246–7.

2 Anonymous. Erskine, David. *Medical Directory* London: J & A Churchill. 1960: 668. [*See also:* D Erskine. Venereal disease. *Practitioner* 1943; 151: 305–14; Difficulties in the successful treatment of the venereal disease patient. *Br J Ven Dis* 1945; 21: 47–60; Epidermophytosis. *Med Press* 1949: 357–61; Parasitic disease of the skin. *Med Press* 1960; 244: 328–32.

3 Anonymous. Bickerton, Reginald Ernest, DSO. *Medical Directory* London: J & A Churchill. 1940: 27. [*See also*: R E Bickerton: Gas injuries to the eye. *Proc Roy Soc Med* 1940; 33: 227–9].

4 Anonymous. *Lancet* 1969; ii: 1261; Anonymous. *BMJ* 1969; iv: 625; *Munks Roll 6:* 469–70. [*See also:* AL Wingfield. Hyperventilation tetany in tropical climates. *BMJ* 1941; i: 929–30; 4:4 – diamidino stilbene in treatment of kala-azar. *Ann Trop Med Parasit* 1941; 35: 55–8; The investigation and treatment of bronchitis in recruits. *Med Press Circ* 1942; 207; The diagnosis and treatment of primary atypical pneumonia. *Med Press Circ* 1945; 213: 132–4; Pulmonary tuberculosis in merchant seamen. *NAPT Bull* 1945: 21–23; Agranulocytosis in kala-azar and use of adrenalin. *Trans R Soc Trop Med Hyg* 1941; 34: 421–8].

5 Anonymous. Davies, Arthur. *Medical Directory* London: J & A Churchill 1950: 81 [*See also:* A Davies, A Wingfield: Agranulocytosis in kala azar and use of adrenalin. *Trans R Soc Trop Med Hyg* 1941; 34: 421–8].

6 Anonymous. Cooper, Desmond Marriott. *Plarr's Lives* 1952–64*:* 87.

7 [MDS]. S Power *BMJ* 1988; 296: 1009; Power, Stephen May *Plarr's Lives 1983–90:* 301–2.

8 Anonymous. Howkins, John. *Medical Directory* London: J & A Churchill 2001: 1818; Who's Who 2002: 1055.

9 Anonymous. Lurie, Leonard. *Medical Directory* London: J & A Churchill 1950: 144. L Lurie: Cataract extraction by expression. *Br J Ophthalmol* 1961; 45: 133–7.

10 Anonymous. Edwards, Colin Campbell. *Medical Directory* London: J & A Churchill 1950: 96.

11 Anonymous. Robinson, Oliver Francis Waring. *Medical Directory* London: J & A Churchill 195: 2045.

12 Anonymous. Robinson, Geoffrey Lawrence. *Medical Directory* London: J & A Churchill 1965: 2043. [*See also:* G L Robinson: Aerosols: new light on some problems of disinfection. *Br J Phys Med Ind Hyg* 1946; 9; 151–4; Penicillin in general practice. *Postgrad Med J* 1947; 23: 86–92; Hodgkin's disease confined to the jejunum. *Lancet* 1948; ii: 822–3; Scattered muscle necroses associated with post-traumatic uraemia. *Lancet* 1950; i: 799–801; The haemolysin of Bacterium coli. *J Gen Microbiol* 1951; 5: 788–92; Precipitation test in fulminating fibrinopenia. *BMJ*1956; i: 626–7; Perlmann's tumour of the kidney. *Br J Surg* 1957; 44: 620–3; Case reports: double-barrelled aorta with bacterial endarteritic vegetations. *Br Heart J* 1958; 20: 571–4; The laboratory diagnosis of human parasitic amoebae. *Trans R Soc Trop Med Hyg* 1968; 62: 285–94; Laboratory cultivation of some human parasitic amoeba. *J Gen Microbiol* 1968; 53: 69–79; The preparation of amoebic extracts and their testing by complement fixation against clinically proved sera. *Trans R Soc Trop Med Hyg* 1972; 66: 435–49; Acute bacterial endarteritis. *Br Heart J* 1951; 13: 106–8; Melioidosis in a diabetic. *Postgrad Med J* 1966; 42: 327–8; The size of *Dientamoeba fragilis* in culture. *Trans R Soc Trop Med Hyg* 1968; 62: 156–8; Filarial complement fixation test for pulmonary tropical ceosinophilia with Ascaris antigen. *J Clin Pathol* 1968; 21: 394–6].

13 Anonymous. Mushin, William Woolf. *Medical Directory*. London: J & A Churchill 1960: 1669. [*See also: W W Mushin*: Notes on anaesthesia for facio-maxillary surgery. *Postgrad Med J* 1940; 16: 245–6; Anaesthesia for major dental surgery: an alternative to the endotracheal method. *Lancet* 1941: i: 46–8; Heavy percain spinal anaesthesia: experience gained in a series of 420 cases. *BMJ* 1942; i: 139–43; Alteration in respiratory rhythm in surgical

anaesthesia. *Postgrad Med J* 1942; 18: 83–7; A new circle type of carbon-dioxide absorber. *Lancet* 1942; ii: 727].

14 Anonymous. Hanschell, Hother McCormick. *Medical Directory London:* J & A Churchill 1950: 144. [*See also:* H M Hanschell: Sulphanilamide in the treatment of chancroid. *Lancet 1938;* i: 886–8; Climatic bubo or lymphogranuloma inguinale. *Trans R Soc Trop Med Hyg* 1938; 31: 578–86].

15 Anonymous. Boyde, Harry Caine. *Medical Directory* London: J & A Churchill 1950: 37.

16 Anonymous. Mr Harry Freeman. *BMJ 1949; ii: 880; Plarr's Lives 1930–51: 303.* [*See also:* Freeman, H. Gastroscopy. *Br J Surg* 1944; 32: 303; Acute osteomyelitis of lumbar spine in an adult. *BMJ*; 1946; ii: 610].

17 Anonymous. P M Kelly. *BMJ* 1990; 300: 532; Kelly, Patrick Michael. *Plarr's Lives 1983–90: 186–7.*

18 *Plarr's Lives 1974–1982*: 297–8.

19 Anonymous. Plumstead, Charles George Edward. *Medical Directory* London: J & A Churchill 1948: 1975. [*See also*: Plumstead, C G E. Femoral thrombosis following influenza. *Lancet* 1927; i: 568].

20 Anonymous. Dickinson, John Roscoe. *Medical Directory* London: J & A Churchill 1950: 86; Anonymous. *BMJ* 1996; 313: 164–5; *Plarr's Lives 1991–1996*: 73.

21 Anonymous. Hugh Alan Dugleby Small. *Lancet 1981;* i: 228; [VJD]. H A D Small. *BMJ* 1981; 282: 394; *NZ Med J* 1981; 93: 162; *Plarr's Lives 1974–82*: 367–8.

22 Anonymous. *Times, Lond* 1986; 27 October: 18; Anonymous. *Daily Telegraph, Lond* 1986; 27 October; Anonymous. Henry Osmond-Clarke. *Lancet* 1986; ii: 1290; [OJV-J] Sir Henry Osmond-Clarke. *BMJ*1986; 293: 1247; Henry Osmond-Clarke *Plarr's Lives 1983–90:* 282–3.

23 Anonymous. Carew-Shaw, Edward FRCS (1901–1998) *Medical Directory* London: J & A Churchill 1950: 53. Anonymous. *BMJ* 1998; 317: 544; *Plarr's Lives 1997–2002*: 61.

24 Anonymous. Littlejohn, James. *Medical Directory* London: J & A Churchill 1965: 1387.

25 Anonymous. Frederick Murgatroyd. *Lancet* 1951; ii: 1229; Anonymous. Frederick Murgatroyd. *BMJ* 1951; ii: 1586–7; Anonymous. *JAMA* 1952; 148: 660; Anonymous. Murgatroyd, Frederick. *Munk's Roll* 5: 299–300.

26 Anonymous *Times, Lond* 1976: 10 June; Anonymous. George Reid McRobert. *Lancet* 1976; I: 1420–1; Anonymous. Colonel Sir George McRobert. *BMJ*1976; ii: 706; 889; G Wolstenholme, V Luniewska. McRobert, Sir George (Reid). *Munk's Roll* 7: 371–2.

27 Anonymous. Wolfe, Herbert Robert Ingleood. *Plarr's Lives 1965–1973:* 401–2; Anonymous. *Lancet* 1930; i; 479. [*See also*: Wolfe, HRI. Spontaneous subarachnoid haemorrhage. *Br J Surg* 1953; 40: 319–25.]

28 Anonymous. *Times, Lond* 1979; 19 November: 6; Anonymous. Norman R Barrett. *BMJ* 1979; i: 203; Anonymous. *Ann R Coll Surg Eng* 1979; 61: 414–5; Anonymous. Barrett, Norman Rupert. *Plarr's Lives 1974–82*: 19–20.

29 Anonymous. Siddons, Mr Arthur Harold Makins. *Medical Directory*: London: J & A Churchill 1999; 3619; *Who's Who 2000:* 1866.

30 Anonymous. Wood, John Eric. *Medical Directory*: London: J & A Churchill 1960: 2053. [*See also:* J E Wood: A note on heliotherapy in pulmonary tuberculosis. Lancet 1926; ii: 372–4; Tuberculosis in the merchant navy *BMJ* 1942; i: 716–8].

31 Anonymous. Cooke, William Ernest *Medical Directory* London: J & A Churchill 1965: 450; G C Cook. History of Tropical Medicine – William Ernest Cooke FRCSI (1879–1967) and his Asian tour of 1929–1930. *Acta Trop* 2006; 100: 1–10.

Chapter 25

The Society (and its tropical medicine component) in the twentieth and twenty-first centuries

Between 1821 and 1939, the Society's 'Empire' had expanded, and eventually every need of the seafarer in the MM – from physical to spiritual health – had been provided. However, two World Wars and, more importantly, the introduction of the NHS, sounded the virtual 'death knell' of this valuable organisation. One by one, the component parts declined and were finally phased out. The fate of several of the SHS establishments has been outlined in Chapter 22.

The *LSCM* (Chapter 19) never recovered after the Great War. Tentative plans were at that time evolved to amalgamate this institution with the LSTM; in July 1942, P P Cole (a surgeon at the *Dreadnought* Hospital and member of the teaching staff of the LSCM) (*see* Chapter 21) reported to the Management Committee that Colonel Parkinson of the LSHTM 'had cordially expressed himself favourable' to the idea. However, at a meeting later that year the 'Board of Management [of the LSHTM] decided that for the time being no action could be taken' on this matter.[1]

Shortly after this, the future of the ADH also had become increasingly uncertain (see below). Thus, at a Committee of Management meeting in April 1947, the Chairman (Benn) reported that 'the Dock Labour Corporation [was] anxious to acquire the [ADH] as their main centre for rehabilitation and treatment of dock workers ...'. That hospital would then be controlled by the Ministry of Transport instead of the Ministry of Health. He concluded that if the ADH became detached from the *Dreadnought* in the forthcoming NHS reshuffle, this option was worth pursuing – provided the *administration* of the ADH stayed with the SHS. Much later, in 1971, it was agreed to place a 'written inscription on Vellum' at the ADH in order to record, for posterity, that some of the work benches there had been used by Manson and his colleagues during the early days of 'tropical medicine'.[2]

In 1956, the future of *King George's Sanatorium for Sailors* (KGSS) had also been finally decided (*see* Chapters 22 and 23); the SW Metropolitan Regional Hospital Board (SWMRHB) had plans to convert the facilities there 'for the treatment of cases other than those of tuberculosis'. The problem there was 'that during the [previous] 2½ years the average number of merchant seamen undergoing treatment in the 80 available beds ... had averaged about 40 daily, although this number had been even lower during the [previous] 6 months'. Also, it had become much easier for seafarers with tuberculosis to be treated at a sanatorium nearer their home. This was associated with a general decline in the 'incidence of tuberculosis throughout the country'; hence, a mere 40 beds were required for tuberculosis sufferers.[3]

The SHS in the latter years of the twentieth century

Although a great deal of attention during and after the Second World War had been given to *tropical medicine* (the Society had of course been instrumental in launching this discipline), (see below) health of the seafarer had always been the *raison d'etre* of the SHS. A Society memorandum in 1946 signed by Sir Ernest Murrant (Chairman), Sir Clifford Figg (Deputy Chairman) and J Cyril Nairne (Treasurer) addressed to the Minister of Health, Aneurin Bevan (1897–1960;[4] *see* Chapter 22), outlined the history and potential problems posed by the NHS. After expressing the view that the 'Hospitals for Seamen [in the Port of London]' including 'the endowment funds and landed property' should be allowed to continue, the authors highlighted the overwhelming importance of this *specialist* expertise (which was *not* present in hospitals for landsmen) in caring for sailors of all nationalities. Between 1934–8 for example, 75% of the sailors admitted to SHS hospitals 'were not domiciled in Great Britain'; 'Indian, Colonial and foreign seamen [they continued would] not be contributors under the National Insurance scheme [and therefore would] not ordinarily be eligible for benefit under the [NHS]'.[5]

The SHS 'letterhead' at this time read:

> The Seamen's Hospitals. *South-East Metropolitan Regional Hospital Board* [SEMRB] *comprising* Dreadnought Seamen's Hospital, Greenwich; Albert Dock Seamen's Hospital, Alnwick Road, E.16; Angas Convalescent Home, Cudham, Kent; Port of London Isolation Hospital, Denton, Gravesend, Kent.

The dialogue continued with a discussion at the Ministry of Health the following month. Michael Reed representing the Minister, in a generally cordial encounter, admitted that 'there might be considerable difficulty [in allowing the ADH, the Angus Home, Cudham, and King George's Sanatorium for Sailors continuing in their present form] having regard to the administrative machinery of the [RHB's] operating in defined areas'. There seems, however, to have been only minimal change in the *status quo* until 1956–7; on 15 November 1956, J C Nairne (speaking at a Management Committee meeting) maintained that 'there was no certainty that the administrative pattern of the Seamen's Group of Hospitals would not be altered'. The Committee was apparently '... informed [at this meeting] of a suggestion that in the future development of St Alfege's Hospital, Greenwich, [would allow] accommodation ... for 150 seamen [thus] enabling the *Dreadnought* [my italics] Hospital to be closed'.[6]

In a letter to the Society dated 5 March 1957, the SEMRHB intimated (after an inspection of the *Dreadnought* [my italics] Hospital and ADH) that they had 'decided that the present time [was] not opportune to pursue this matter', but they were 'nevertheless concerned at the high cost of running the *Dreadnought* [my italics]

Hospital, especially now that the rental has been increased'. Discussion at that meeting centred on the possibility, in the event of the *Dreadnought* Hospital being closed, of expanding the ADH.[7]

Cost and practicality of retaining the Dreadnought Hospital

A major survey of 'beds required by Merchant Seamen in the Port of London' for the next five years was carried out in 1959. Owing to a steep decline in the number of in-patients at the *Dreadnought* and ADH, cost per bed had risen sharply. The reason(s) for the decline in numbers was complex, but criteria for assessing requirements during the following five years were summarised:

i) The … diminishing [absolute] numbers in the British Merchant Navy*…;
ii) Possible increase in in-port man-days of European seamen if this country were to join the EEC;
iii) Continuing requirement for Asiatic seamen;
iv) Future development (or otherwise) of the Port of London; and
v) The probability of increased availability of beds for British seafarers near their *home* ports, other than London.

Any *comprehensive* survey would, it was concluded, inevitably involve significant input from:

- The Board of Trade;
- The Ministry of Transport;
- The British Shipping Federation;
- The National Union of Seamen (NUS);
- The Merchant Navy & Airline Officers Association;
- The Port of London Authority; and
- The Chamber of Shipping of the United Kingdom.[8]

Towards the end of 1971, the SEMRHB indicated that on the statistical evidence provided by 'bed occupancy and length of stay', they had decided that both the *Dreadnought* Hospital and *Angas Convalescent Home* should be closed, and that 'hospital requirements for seafarers should be concentrated at the [ADH]'. The policy of RHBs and their relationship with Boards of Management, had been set out in a Government memorandum dated 1952. Not surprisingly the Committee of Management – especially its *medical* members – felt that 'this proposal could not possibly be entertained, …'; immediate reaction was to recommend the closure of the ADH (indeed, there was verbal evidence that the Ministry of Health had in mind a 'new District Hospital in the Albert Dock area'), and to keep the *Dreadnought* Hospital viable. With increased air transport, a 'National Hospital for

---

* The introduction of container ships in the 1960s heralded this decline in numbers. Although merchant ships still required crew, their numbers diminished sharply. Furthermore, many of the great Shipping Companies, which formerly had a close association with the SHS, and had slowly evolved over the previous century, were also in decline.

Seafarers', the precise location of which was of less importance, was an alternative line of thought.[9]

A detailed 'breakdown' of the 'Future of the Seamen's Hospitals Group' was presented to the Management Committee at a series of meetings held between 17 January 1973 and 17 April 1974, when the Chairman of the SEMRHB (Collard) spoke of his Committee's plans to close the ADH and *Angas Home* and to transfer the *Dreadnought* beds to the Royal Herbert Hospital [Woolwich]! This plan was, however, simply 'not acceptable' to the SHS! The *Angas Convalescent Home* would probably (he continued) be handed over to 'one of the Mental Hospital Groups within the Region' on 1 April 1974; convalescent seafarers would from that date be accommodated at St Mary's Convalescent Home, Cliftonville, Margate. It had now been agreed that the ADH should be closed in October 1974, and that the orthopaedic facilities should be transferred to the *Dreadnought*, where 'recreational and rehabilitation facilities' would be established on the Upper East Floor, and the kitchen transferred from the ground to the top floor. Continuation of the *Dreadnought School of Nursing* had already been approved by the General Nursing Council for 'at least another five years', whilst the work formerly carried out at the Pathological Laboratory was 'almost entirely done' in the Greenwich District Hospital.

Overall this was regarded as good news, in that the *Dreadnought* was now designated an *International Hospital for Seafarers*. However, at a subsequent meeting (on 21 November 1973), it was stated, again by Collard, that the Secretary of State for Social Services, Sir Keith (later Baron) Joseph (1918–94) had ruled that a decision on the future of the *Dreadnought* would have to be taken by the *new* Area Authority which would come into being on 1 April 1974! It was unlikely in Collard's view that a definitive decision on the future of the *Dreadnought* would be taken for 'three or four years'.

FUTURE OF THE DREADNOUGHT INCREASINGLY UNCERTAIN (see also Chapter 22)

At a meeting on 21 November 1973, the future of the *Dreadnought* was discussed further. The case for retention of the *Dreadnought* was made by a delegation representing the SEMRB, the NUS and the Shipping Industry to the Secretary of State for Social Services. Joseph noted the points raised, but 'could not give any assurance before the matter had been considered by the Area … and the [RH Authorities]'.

Collard felt at that time that 'as a matter of the very greatest urgency' there should be (i) 'an immediate approach by the Shipping Industry to the Area Health Authority', and (ii) a 'Society of Friends of the Dreadnought Hospital should be formed to work with the [SHS] and the Shipping Industry …'. A minute of a meeting on 17 April 1974 (at which there was representation from the Navy & Airline Officers' Association, the NUS, the British Shipping Federation, and the PLA)[10] records that from then on the *Dreadnought* lay under the aegis of the Greenwich and Bexley Area Health Authority (GBAHA).

CLOSURE OF THE DREADNOUGHT IN 1986

The Chairman of the Society (Captain I B Taylor) began his 1975 Report: 'The future of the Dreadnought Hospital remains unresolved'. After outlining deliberations of the GBAHA, he finished this section of his report with:

> It is not anticipated that any firm decision will be taken for some time to come. In the meantime, although most of our attention will be concentrated on keeping the Dreadnought afloat, we will continue to discharge all those other special functions for which the Society was founded.[11]

The following year, the Report seemed mildly more optimistic:

> ... the [National Maritime Board, NMB] (advised by the Dreadnought Advisory Sub-Committee) [had] met with the [GBAHA] on two occasions ... to discuss the future of the Dreadnought Hospital, as a result of which both parties were in agreement on the continuing need for the Dreadnought Hospital to serve as a National Hospital for the Treatment of Seamen, with a suggested bed availability of 110. A joint recommendation to this effect was forwarded ... to the South East Thames Regional Health Authority [SETRHA] for onward transmission to [Joseph], and a decision is now awaited.[12]

But by the next year (1977), a great deal of uncertainty remained:

> ... [Joseph] issued a Press statement regarding the Area Health Authority's proposals for Hospital Services within the Greenwich and Bexley Area, the last paragraph of which read:
>
> 'In addition my Department will take up with the appropriate organisations the question of the Dreadnought Seamen's Hospital with a view to relieving the Area Health Authority of the need to provide all or part of the costs of this hospital from its allocation.'

Taylor continued:

> I do not wish to make the following comment unkindly, but it seems to me that there must be something wrong with a 'system' which has become so unwieldy that nothing can be decided until every conceivable stone has been turned and every conceivable combination of circumstances has been evaluated. It is beginning to be self-defeating.[13]

The 1978 Report was infinitely more encouraging:

> It is ... with profound relief and great delight that I can now announce that, after further meetings and correspondence during the year under review, [Joseph] ... notified his decision that the Dreadnought should continue on its present site as a hospital for the treatment of seamen. Our thanks for this successful conclusion to what has been a long and time consuming campaign are due not only to the [NMB] ... but also to the members of the Dreadnought Advisory Committee ... and the Society's officers who provided the vital background information.[14]

On 11 December 1980, a crucial (albeit acrimonious) meeting between 'members of the [NMB] and the [GBAHA]' was held in the Board Room of the Devonport Annexe, King William Walk. Serious financial problems facing the Area Health Authority were first highlighted. Taylor reiterated that the 'Government had agreed [that the *Dreadnought*] should be recognised as the National Hospital for the treatment of seamen'. He reminded the meeting that 'staff morale at the hospital was now at a very low ebb' and that certain vacancies (including that of the pharmacist) remained unfilled – in some cases due to difficulty in recruitment! Further, he 'confirmed that the [NMB] were convinced of the need for a separate budget [for the *Dreadnought* – in order to maintain essential services, including a pharmacist] and would pursue this with [Joseph]'. The importance of the Casualty Department at the *Dreadnought* (seafarers had never required a letter of referral) was stressed by members of the NMB. NGJ Thompson (of the Area Health Authority) clearly stated that 'there was no intention to close the hospital and it would be included in the Area Strategic Plan for the … years 1981–1991, albeit at a reduced level'.[15]

The Chairman's thoughts were once again summarised in the Report for 1980:

> … there were ominous signs that even some of the essential services to the hospital were being severely restricted. These did not … escape the attention of the Society's *Dreadnought Advisory Sub-Committee* [my italics], and the [NMB] at their meeting with the Chairman and Officers of the [GBAHA] in December last which sought reassurance of the hospital's future. At the same time the [NMB] requested a further meeting with the Minister for Health and this was arranged for January 1981. At this meeting the Minister re-iterated his predecessor's decision regarding the Hospital and at his instigation investigations are now being undertaken to ensure that in line with economic strictures now obtaining at all hospitals, the Dreadnought shall remain a viable hospital for seafarers. The National Maritime Board, together with the Dreadnought Advisory Sub-Committee, will continue to closely monitor the affairs at Dreadnought.[16]

There was now clearly a great deal of dismay and more was to follow. There were so many unresolved issues (most of a financial nature) that a transfer of the medical care of seamen to another site seemed the *only* solution. In his 1981 Report, the Chairman was to write:

> The minister [of Health, addressing a delegation from the NMB] expressed sympathy with the [NMB]'s view that consideration might be given to the possibility of provision for seamen in a unit outside of the Greenwich District.[17]

A new venue for care of the seafarer?

The following year, the possibility of a new venue was further explored:

> It is now common knowledge that the [NMB], with the active support of this Society, has proposed to the Minister for Health that the hospital

> needs for seafarers could be better provided for in a separate unit at St. Thomas' Hospital. ... Should the Minister agree to the N.M.B.'s suggested transfer, the regret at the loss of tradition and world-wide renown of Dreadnought at Greenwich will, we hope, be more than offset by the excellence of treatment that can be provided by St. Thomas' Hospital in a separate wing that will continue to bear the name of *Dreadnought* [my italics].[18]

In May 1982, Taylor reported to the Management Committee that 'with other members of [NMB] he had attended a meeting (with officers of the DHSS and the West Lambeth Health Authority) to discuss the possible move of the *Dreadnought* Hospital to a Wing of St. Thomas' Hospital'.[19] There were certain difficulties associated with this plan, notably a loss of identity, and problems with finance; for example an 1860 Wing of St Thomas'[20] would have to be refurbished at a cost of £300,000!

By October 1983, Taylor was able to report that a total sum of £1,200,000 had been identified (for the transfer) 'through the [SETRHA], St. Thomas's Hospital, and the Minister'. The proposal for transfer was 'now in course of being put out for consultation [by both Health Authorities]'. The earliest date at which this could begin (Taylor continued) was unlikely to be before late 1984.[21]

There were however, further delays – due to protestations by the Greenwich Borough Council, the respective RH Authorities, and the NUS. The consultation machinery proved to be exceedingly slow, and Taylor reported in October 1983 that 'a decision would not be reached until May, 1985 at the earliest'. A further problem resulted from St Thomas's reluctance to take any of the *Dreadnought* staff on board. Ultimately the decision was taken by the Minister of Health himself. The 'imminent' Ministerial decision was, however, not to be forthcoming until 1986 – some three years later than anticipated. Taylor reported, in 1985:

> It is with great relief, after several years of disappointment, that I am able to report that the decision to transfer hospital services for seamen from Dreadnought to St. Thomas' Hospital has now been made. An official announcement of this was made by the Minister in November, 1985 and the date for transfer then set for *April 1986* [my italics]. However, as regulations precluded any action on necessary refurbishment for the new Unit at St. Thomas' Hospital until after the Minster had announced his decision, it was impossible to get this work completed in time for the planned April, 1986 transfer. ... The Unit is to be established in two wards in Block 6, into which patients have been admitted since April, 1986. The refurbishing of this block is expected to start in the autumn of 1986 with completion estimated for June, 1987. [This work was subsequently delayed for about a year]. This will include the provision of recreational and ancillary facilities for the exclusive use of seafarers, the cost of which has been underwritten by this Society. While the work is in progress the Unit will move in its entirety to similar wards in Block 8. ... Arrangements have been made for a Branch Office of the Society to be opened at the Marine Society's [*see* Chapter 5] premises in Lambeth

> Road, close to St. Thomas' Hospital in order to provide immediate and closer support for the Unit and its staff. [The following report however, indicated that this provision was *not* considered necessary]. Hostel facilities have also been organised by the Society and seamen patients' relatives have been able to make use of them. We are optimistic about the future; yet there is great regret in saying goodbye to the traditions of the *Dreadnought* [my italics] Hospital and, in particular, to members of staff there, many of whom had given long and devoted service to sick seafarers.[22]

FAREWELL TO THE DREADNOUGHT STAFF

By October 1983, the Committee seem to have accepted the demise of the *Dreadnought*, and began discussing the form of a parting gift to (redundant) members of the staff (with ≥ 5 years service). One suggestion was for a limited edition (250 prints) of a specially commissioned painting of the *Dreadnought* – the original of which would hang in the new (*Dreadnought*) unit at St Thomas's Hospital. Another was that the presentation should take the form of a piece of glassware. However, concern was expressed regarding expenditure – which might not be acceptable to the Charity Commissioners! Ultimately 300 prints of a painting by Ray Evans RA were produced, and framed – to be presented to members of the *Dreadnought* staff – who were apparently duly appreciative of this gesture.

Removal to St Thomas's Hospital at last

At a meeting of the Board of Management on 16 April 1986, Taylor reported that the *Dreadnought* Hospital had been closed on 31 March, 'although [there were still] a few Health Authority staff on site to maintain security, pending the removal of remaining items of furniture, equipment and stores' as well as security patrols. The patients together with certain 'items of furniture and equipment [together with the billiard table]' had been transferred to the *Dreadnought* Unit at St Thomas's Hospital (which contained 56 beds situated in two wards, plus 'an additional four beds on specialist wards, such as gynaecology'). 'For the time being [Taylor reported] the Chapel and Queen Mary's library had been left intact', and the building handed back to the Royal Naval College (from whom it had been on loan since 1870 – Chapter 13). Items of medical equipment, purchased by the Society, and *not* required by St Thomas's Hospital, had been given to the local District Health Authority.[23]

The Dreadnought Unit

The 1986 Report announced the opening of the *Dreadnought* Unit:

> This Unit became operational on 1st April, 1986 and, as expected has involved increased expenditure by the Society. The figure of £14,000 for the nine months, reflects recurring expenditure undertaken by the Society to provide additional administrative support, nearby hostel facilities and items of medical equipment specifically for the Unit.[24]

At St Thomas's, all was initially proceeding well (the unit administrator was Mrs Phil Lake – formerly a senior sister at the *Dreadnought*), with the exception that there was a lack of co-operation from the senior Orthopaedic Surgeon. Meanwhile, it was reported that the '[NMB] had been offered a seat on the Lambeth District Health Authority', and the 'General Council of British Shipping Medical Officer [was] to join the Medical and Surgical Committee at St Thomas' Hospital'. Publicity for the new unit was being organised by the General Council of British Shipping.

But publicity (or lack of it) coupled with delays, were to plague the project; Taylor later reported:

> The ... Unit has now [1988] been operational for two years and occupancy has risen, albeit slowly. Despite past efforts to publicise the excellent medical services available to seafarers, there is evidence to show that many remain unaware of the new arrangements and it is intended to undertake a further publicity exercise. Contrary to the optimism expressed last year, building works on the permanent home for the Unit are not yet completed and the latest date is now September, 1988.[25]

The following year the Report recorded:

> The ... Unit was finally housed in its permanent quarters in September. Although the wards are situated in the *old* [my italics] part of St. Thomas', the decoration is pleasant and the area is comfortable and friendly. The lounge area, incorporating the recreation facilities, has been refurbished to a very high standard. The overall effect is one of real identity within the Unit and to complete the Merchant navy connection, the Red Duster flies proudly from the flagpole overlooking the river.[26]

And, in 1989, Taylor wrote:

> The highlight of the year for the Dreadnought Unit was the *official* opening ceremony by His Royal Highness Prince Philip, the Duke of Edinburgh, K.G., K.T., O.M., G.B.E., on 20th July [1989]. Mr. J. Garnett, C.B.E., Chairman of the West Lambeth Health Authority presented His Royal Highness to members of the Society, representatives of the Shipping Industry and those members of St. Thomas' staff who have special responsibilities for the Unit. [HRH] toured both wards and the recreation area and spoke to many of the seafarer patients.[27]

Treatment at the new unit 'was available to serving seamen, retired seamen, to serving seamen's immediate dependents and those members of the staff of shipping company officers directly involved with seafarers and shipping movement'. 'Convalescent facilities at Springbok Rehabilitation Centre at Alfold, Surrey [it was recorded] would continue to be available to serving seamen only ...'.[28] Successive Reports then devoted a great deal of space to progress reports of the St Thomas's Unit. Standards of patient care seemed to be satisfactory; however, there was a problem of delay in admission (this apparently remained as recently as the 2000 Report). Also, the lift serving the unit (later rectified) recurrently gave cause for concern; initial lack of funds at St Thomas's, had led to a suggestion that this be solved by 'moving the unit down a floor'.

In April 1991, a new approach to funding within the NHS came into operation; despite verbal assurances to the contrary this 'had an adverse effect on the patient activity in the Unit'. *Dreadnought* funds were 'allocated to the Districts [of] residence of the patients instead of directly to the South East Thames Authority/St Thomas' as hitherto'; this resulted, not surprisingly, in many General Practitioners not referring seafarers to the Unit. After protests from the Director General of the Chamber of Shipping the *status quo ante* was restored in April 1992.

Other problems later arose from the merging of St Thomas' with Guy's Hospitals (as recommended in the Tomlinson Report of 1992), as well as internal changes within St Thomas's. *Somerset* Ward (which was undergoing refurbishment) was re-designated as a medical ward, and only 10 out of 28 beds were 'earmarked for sailors'; *Northumberland* Ward (named after the 4th Duke of Northumberland [1792–1865] (*see* Chapter 12), who had served as a midshipman on HMS *Caledonia* and subsequently became First Lord of the Admiralty) retained its 28 surgical beds. In order to solve some of these problems, a 'Dreadnought Liaison Sub Committee', comprised of St Thomas's staff and SHS members was formed in 1995; this used some of the Society's funds (> £12,000) to purchase text books for nurses and items of medical equipment.

The 1998 Report recorded that the unit was at that time 'spread over three locations at two hospital sites: *Somerset* Ward [for medical patients – had been opened in December 1995] and the 11th floor North Wing within St Thomas' Hospital for medical cases, and Guy's Hospital for orthopaedic patients'. *Dreadnought* patients who needed 'specialised nursing [were] treated in the Wards appropriate to their care and medical condition'. The number(s) of new patients treated in the unit in 1998 was averaging ≥ 2000 annually.

The 1999 Report recorded a distinct change of tack, i.e. the two wards for the exclusive use of seafarers (*Somerset* and *Northumberland*) no longer existed as a dedicated unit; instead, seafarers were 'now treated throughout Guys' and St Thomas' Hospitals according to their *clinical* needs'. As well as 'active seafarers and fishermen', dependents and retired seafarers were now able to use the service.[29]

The Society's involvement in Tropical Medicine

Coupled with this decline in the overall status of the Society, but many years before closure of the *Dreadnought* Hospital, was uncertainty about the future of *tropical medicine*, which since 1899 had been a major activity of the SHS. The SHS had of course been instrumental in founding this medical discipline; the LSTM had been launched at the ADH (Chapter 18). In 1939, the HTD (at Endsleigh Gardens) – the successor of the LSTM – had been forcibly closed; the building had been requisitioned and was occupied by the War Office from 19 June 1940.[30] In the early years of the war the *future* of the discipline received a great deal of attention; N H (later Sir Neil Hamilton) Fairley[31] outlined in detail the discussions which took place at that time.[32] After Frederick Murgatroyd (1902–51) had been called up for service with H.M. Forces, E W Cooke (who had been Medical Superintendent at the HTD) took his place at 'the Consultative Out-Patient Clinic' (two sessions weekly) at a salary of £250 per annum. This arrangement came to an end, however, on 10 May 1941 when the Endsleigh Gardens building was rendered unsafe after the explosion of a landmine.

The Out-Patient Clinic was then transferred to the LSTHM, while *clinical* material was made available (to post-graduates) at the *Dreadnought* Hospital, Greenwich.[33] Because the Society intended continuing with its *tropical* interests, it was authorised to send a communication to the 'Medical Officers of Ports, the Ministry of Shipping, the Shipping Federation [SF] and the Medical Superintendents of Shipping Lines' indicating that 'tropical disease [cases] among seamen, particularly Indian seamen' should be sent *pro tem* to the *Dreadnought* Hospital.[34]

A post-war tropical hospital

The next topic for consideration was the type of *tropical hospital* required after the 1939–45 war. In the 1920s, i.e. when the LSHTM was being erected, there had been calls for an 'attached' clinical institution; the idea of an '*Imperial* Hospital' in close proximity to the LSHTM was seriously discussed.[35] This possible development was largely a result of a possible phasing out, at that time, of the SHS's support for the HTD at Endsleigh Gardens. However, the Society decided to continue supporting the *clinical* aspects of tropical medicine (for the benefit of sailors from the tropics), and there was certainly no necessity for the second (The Ross Institute & Hospital for Tropical Diseases [RIHTD] – see Chapter 20) in existence at that time, at Putney) hospital also dealing with tropical diseases.

In early 1941, 'informal conversations' had begun between the Society, the Colonial Office, and the LSHTM; the Colonial Office, it transpired, at that time 'wished to establish [after the war] a *new* Tropical Diseases Hospital at Greenwich'. It should be noted that by this time the RIHTD (see above) had been closed, the 'preventive' facilities being absorbed into the LSHTM and the (limited) *clinical* ones into the SHS's Endsleigh Gardens Hospital (HTD).[36] It was felt by the SHS Committee that 'if such a scheme as envisaged by the Colonial Office were brought to fruition it would greatly enhance the prestige of the Society'.[37] The Society's 1941 Report thus declared:

> It has been agreed that the need for improving facilities for the study of tropical medicine in London, and for the training of overseas doctors and nurses in modern hospital practice, can best be met by working in co-operation with the [LSHTM] as a *centre* [my italics] for these purposes. Since the full development of the proposal to establish a really worthy Hospital and Centre at Greenwich will depend on the availability of additional sites adjacent to that already occupied by the Society, steps are now being taken to ensure the full co-operation of Government Departments concerned in framing a plan for the reservation and future development of suitable sites.[38]

The SHS Chairman (Moyne – *see* Chapter 22) 'had caused to be drawn up [in April 1941] a plan for the establishment of a tropical diseases hospital and centre [TDHC] at Greenwich …'. The scheme was accepted, in principle, by the SHS Committee who informed the Secretary of State 'of their willingness to participate in discussions based on his plan'.[39] The first meeting of a committee (with representatives from the India Office, the Foreign Office, the Ministry of Health, the Colonial Office, the MRC, and the LSHTM – in addition to the SHS) was on 12 November 1941 at the Colonial Office.[40] At the following meeting (on 3 December) 'a skeleton schedule of the requirements was agreed', and at a visit to the Greenwich site on 7 January the following year, it was agreed 'to obtain and examine a technical report as to whether the sites on the North and South sides of Romney Road [then leased by the Admiralty to the SHS] were sufficient to accommodate': (i) the *Dreadnought* Hospital; (ii) 'The Tropical Diseases or Officers Hospital (say 100 beds)' for 'Colonial and other Government officials from overseas', 'Employees of business firms and interests from overseas', 'Senior Officers of the Mercantile Marine', and 'Other persons requiring treatment for tropical diseases', (iii) the Devonport Pathological Laboratories, (iv) the Devonport Nurses Home, (v) administrative offices, and (vi) 'Stores, Workshops and garages'.[41]

The first 'hitch' arose when Manson-Bahr (a member of the Committee) 'felt responsible for the security of tenure of the [HTD] Staff as at the outbreak of war'; 'he [therefore] felt unable to associate himself with the approval given to the Memorandum'.[42] However, in May, he gave his backing to a resolution of the SHS Board: 'that, in our opinion the active Honorary Medical Staff ... and those members of the Consulting Staff of the [HTD] who have been appointed as such after a period of recognised service on the active staff ... shall be RECOMMENDED TO THE BOARD to join the staff of the Dreadnought Hospital to take charge of the Department of Tropical Diseases at the Dreadnought Hospital'.[43] At a subsequent meeting, Stanley Hamp FRIBA tabled plans for the proposed *Dreadnought* Seamen's & Imperial Tropical Diseases Hospital on this site.

Hamp favoured a strategy 'to reconstruct [using the extant foundations] as much of the buildings remaining, with new buildings to replace those destroyed by enemy action', rather than erect an 'entirely new building'. These plans were forwarded to the Colonial Office, while various avenues for funding were being explored.[44] In addition, it was decided to attempt to identify alternative hospital accommodation which, it was anticipated, would be required immediately hostilities ceased, to investigate and treat personnel from SE Asia with tropical diseases. At a meeting at the Colonial Office, the Chairman, Harold MacMillan (1894–1986), a future Prime Minister,[45] circulated to members of the Committee a resolution (supporting the Greenwich proposals in entirety) which if approved 'would enable him to take the matter up with the Secretary of State for the Colonies at an early date'. In May 1943, an architect from the Ministry of Works and Parliamentary Secretary for the Colonies inspected the site, and in January 1944, a memorandum (signed by Lyon, the SHS Secretary) was issued by the SHS; it contained the following:

> Upon the recommendation of a Committee set up by the Secretary of State for the Colonies, it has been decided by the Government that a Tropical Diseases Hospital and Centre shall be established at Greenwich as soon as possible after the war, where persons suffering from tropical diseases will receive the necessary specialised treatment, where clinical

> instruction will be given to post graduate medical students and where tropical nursing will be taught. While it is expected that the Government will make a financial contribution to this Scheme the necessary capital expenditure alone may be estimated at £500,000 and very considerable additions will be required to existing endowment funds towards the maintenance of hospital beds and for scientific research work.[46]

Emergence of a temporary plan

The Ministry of Works refused to allow the Endsleigh Gardens Hospital to be re-opened towards the end of the war, and the SHS became interested in April 1944 in a property (23 Devonshire Street, W1) as the site of a *temporary* HTD.[47] The *raison d'etre* for this change of tack is unclear, but was probably motivated by *urgency*, as the war seemed at this time to be nearing a successful conclusion. This property was, however, occupied at the time by the BBC 'under a tenancy agreement for the period of the war'; the matter was later resolved because Sir Charles Jeffries (1896–1972) found alternative accommodation for the BBC.

An interest free loan of £60,000 from the Treasury, which was 'engineered' by Jeffries enabled the 23 Devonshire premises to be purchased.[48] The following statement (preserved in the SHS archive) summarises the set up at that time:

> The temporary [HTD] of 40 beds at No. 23 Devonshire Street had been brought into being by the Society at the request of the Colonial Office ... to provide officer accommodation for sick persons from the tropics including civilian internees repatriated from Japanese hands. Simultaneously the Colonial Office had obtained from the Society a licence to recondition the Somerset Ward of 36 beds at the Dreadnought Hospital, Greenwich, for the same purpose. There were also some 10 beds (including, say, 4 in single rooms) at the [ADH]. These 86 beds had been considered as an integral whole for the purposes covered by the Colonial Secretary's request. Owing to delays beyond the Society's control, the number of beds now available at No. 23 was only 18, and would not be 40 until Oct 1946.

This memorandum continued:

> The existing arrangements for the treatment of tropical cases by Dr. Murgatroyd at Greenwich shall be continued only until all 40 beds are available at No. 23 Devonshire Street ... . As soon as 40 beds are available there, the Society's *tropical* [my italics] patients shall be concentrated at the [HTD], 23 Devonshire Street, and in 12 beds (including some private rooms) at the [ADH], from which general medical cases would, if necessary, be transferred to Greenwich. Arrangements for admission to the [HTD] or [ADH] to be at the discretion of the Secretary [HTD]. Tropical cases at Tilbury would be transferred to the [ADH]. If, during the leave season or at other times of pressure, there were tropical cases which could not wait for admission to the [HTD] or

> the [ADH], such cases to be received for admission to general medical beds at the Dreadnought Hospital. Facilities for teaching at *any* of the Society's Hospitals would [meanwhile] continue to be available to the [LSHTM] *at their request*.[49]

The 1945 SHS report brought news of this *new* 'home' for tropical medicine:

> ... After protracted negotiations, and subject to [numerous] delays, premises for the [HTD – which had been 're-established ... on 17th September' and in-patient accommodation from February 1946] have been acquired at No. 23, Devonshire Street. The purchase of the 79 years unexpired lease has been facilitated by a loan from H.M. Treasury, upon application by the Colonial Office, secured by the Society's asset of the former hospital building in Endsleigh Gardens which is still under requisition by the Ministry of Works.[50]

An alternative scheme to acquisition of 23 Devonshire Street had been suggested by Miss Darlow, Secretary to Jeffries. She suggested that 'hospital huts of a type used by the Forces [be erected] on the garden front of the Devonport Nurses Home'. Manson-Bahr opposed this scheme, and asserted that if this went ahead, 'he would be unable to give his services there'.[51]

Serious 'snags' at Devonshire Street were however, a lack of space for 'residential accommodation for nurses [together with the] absence of resident medical officers' or outpatient consulting rooms'.[52] Overall, this property proved totally inadequate, particularly as large numbers of Far-eastern prisoners of war would inevitably return with a multiplicity of tropical diseases. It should be emphasised, however, that this was envisaged as a *temporary* venue only. It seems clear that Manson-Bahr was unhappy with this plan and he gave a lecture to the Royal Society of Tropical Medicine and Hygiene on 'the design and construction of a model hospital for tropical diseases'. The Society, while supporting this venture, 'disclaimed any commitments of whatever nature or obligation, to relate the research [involved in the preparation of the paper] to the Society's plans for a Tropical Diseases Hospital and Centre'.[53] Meanwhile, Manson-Bahr and Sundell (Chapter 24) were pressing for the opening of a definitive 'Tropical Hospital at the earliest possible time'.

Further discussion on the permanent future of tropical medicine

Regarding the *future permanent* of tropical medicine at this time, a significant meeting was held on 5 January 1945; the Chairman and Secretary of the SHS met Sir Wilson Jameson (1885–1962)[54] and Sir Francis Fraser (1885–1964)[55] at the Ministry of Health. It was agreed 'that the *ultimate* [my italics] aim [was] to establish at Greenwich a Tropical Diseases Hospital & Centre [which would] fit in with the Ministry of Health's comprehensive scheme for post-graduate medical teaching at the University of London'. Fraser had in fact, doubted the necessity for opening this *temporary* HTD ('at ... 23, Devonshire Street'), but Manson-Bahr 'expressed concern lest London should be left [temporarily] less well equipped with facilities for teaching and research in tropical medicine and the treatment of tropical diseases than Liverpool, America ...., Canada ... and even Switzerland ...'. There seems to have been agreement with Davies (the SHS pathologist) that 'Greenwich was not too inaccessible [as far as availability of clinical material for teaching purposes was concerned]'.[56]

Renewed interest in a tropical centre in Bloomsbury

In March 1945, Fairley (see above) wrote another memorandum, which was duly considered by the Management Committee.[57] His main thrust was as follows:

> it would be desirable to establish on a site near the [LSHTM], London House and the Wellcome Institution a new 'Imperial Hospital for Diseases of the Tropics' providing for the treatment of persons living in the tropics, suffering from non-tropical as well as tropical complaints'. Whilst Lord Cork felt that the SHS should *not* put [any] further money into tropical medicine than 'was necessary to ensure our seamen patients [receive] the best treatment available', J C Nairne (supported by other members of the Committee) considered that 'participation in the Imperial Scheme offered the best chance of preserving independence both with regard to the [NHS] and as regards financial stability.

This meeting was generally supportive of Fairley's scheme, but felt that it would of necessity take many years to bring it to fruition; in the meantime, the SHS should develop tropical facilities 'to the fullest possible extent both at No. 23, Devonshire Street and at Greenwich'. Shortly before that meeting, a Sub-Committee had met on 22 February when it was decided that the Society should be 'associated with a Post-graduate teaching School, and [also] a Chair of Tropical Medicine'.[58]

Fraser (see above) also approved of Fairley's paper in principle, but warned that this 'should be related to the whole scheme for postgraduate education at university standard'. The view of the University of London ... was that there should be a large general hospital for post-graduate teaching in the *University City* surrounded by small specialist hospitals, e.g. one for tropical diseases. Although this strategy was still far off, Fraser 'advocated immediate enquiries being made as to the availability of a site within close reach of the University for an *Imperial* [my italics] hospital for diseases of the tropics ...'.[59] Also at that meeting, Jeffries was of the opinion that the 'Imperial hospital would be a Government commitment [rather than an SHS one] financially, but probably managed by the SHS, for a governing body upon which all interests would be represented'.

The emerging NHS comes into the equation

At a meeting of the Sub-Committee (appointed to consider this matter) on 16 April 1946, 'it [was] proposed that University College Hospital [UCH] should be associated with this project'.[60] However, there was clearly unease concerning intimate relationship with an *undergraduate t*eaching hospital (recommended by the architects of the NHS); there were worries about preservation of autonomy; e.g. the

Hospital should have its own Governing Body, 'which should in no way be subordinate to the Governing Body of [UCH]' and should 'be responsible either directly to the Minister of Health or to some Board other than that of a teaching hospital'. If these conditions were *not* met, the SHS 'would not be prepared to interest itself in a Tropical Hospital'. An inter-departmental committee meeting on 14 October 1946 resolved 'to forward to the Secretary of State for the Colonies a recommendation that the approval of His Majesty's Government be sought for the expenditure of £1,000,000 to erect on a site within the *University City* a Tropical Diseases Hospital & Centre ... to be associated with the [LSHTM], but having separate legal status and direct responsibility to the Minister of Health'.[61]

Clinical care of tropical cases

At a Committee of Management meeting on 21 May 1946, it was recalled that a decision had been reached in 1942 (i.e. four years before) 'that the active Honorary Medical Staff of the [HTD] should join the staff of the Dreadnought Hospital to take charge of the Department of Tropical Medicine at the Dreadnought Hospital'. It was felt that 'the Board should now give effect to this recommendation ... by affirming that all patients of the Society suffering from tropical diseases, whether admitted to the Dreadnought, Albert Dock, Tilbury or Tropical Disease Hospitals, shall be recognised as being within the Department of Tropical Diseases [and therefore] under the professional care of [one of] the Physicians in Tropical Medicine'.[62]

Further moves for a tropical hospital and centre in Central London

In May 1947, Lyon (on behalf of the Society) introduced a memorandum on the 'New Tropical Hospital and Centre'; it had already been decided, he wrote, by the Interdisciplinary Committee (which had met the previous October) that the new *permanent* centre should be situated 'within the curtilage of the University City ...' with 'legal entity as a Postgraduate Teaching Hospital [an institute of the British Postgraduate Medical Federation of the University of London] under its own Board of Governors responsible directly to the Minister of Health', and that a report on this 'long-term scheme' had been forwarded (by the Committee) to the Secretary of State for the Colonies indicating that the nature of the scheme 'would justify His Majesty's Government accepting overriding liability for the estimated cost of £1,000,000.[63] Fairley (see above) was clearly of the opinion that Britain was in serious danger of losing its position as the premier player in *clinical* tropical medicine.

The Parliamentary Under Secretary for the Colonies (Ivor Thomas, MP) had meanwhile asked Lyon to enquire as to whether as an 'immediate short-term project' the requirement for a *temporary* facility could be fulfilled on the vacant bombed site at the corner of Beaumont Street and Marylebone High Street; perhaps connected to the HTD in Devonshire Street by a corridor. This planned corridor was, however, rejected by the Ministry of Health on account of a shortage of steel and other materials.[64]

The urgency of the matter was in any event confirmed by the Chief Medical Officer (Jameson) who stressed that under the NHS Act (1946), the Ministry of Health (and *not* the Colonial Office) would be financially responsible for maintenance of the hospital accommodation. As a result, a 'Shadow Board of Governors' was recommended. Negotiations for the Beaumont Street site (which was a property owned by Howard de Walden Estates) were protracted and ultimately proved sterile.[65]

Continuing uncertainty and an unsatisfactory solution to the tropical medicine dilemma

Widespread uncertainty surrounding the future of *clinical* tropical medicine in London was to some extent brought to an end in March 1948 (i.e. shortly before the 'appointed day'); an SHS Minute refers to a letter (dated 17 February) from the Minister of Health (Aneurin Bevan [Chapter 22]) which announced his provisional decision, arrived at after consultation with the University of London and the 'four Metropolitan [RHBs]'; the 'following Hospitals should [the Minister ruled] comprise a teaching unit:– University College Hospital, the National Temperance Hospital [which was later omitted, and St Pancras Hospital substituted], and the [HTD] …'.[66]

In April 1951, the HTD thus moved from Devonshire Street to St Pancras Way and the '*new*' HTD (now a component of the NHS and not the SHS) was officially opened by HRH the Duchess of Kent on 24 May ('Empire Day') 1951. An extension, the Jordan Hospital[67] – with accommodation for 18 leprosy patients – was opened (under UCH) at Redhill, Surrey. This property was subsequently sold to the University of London for £91,000 (the agents being Maple & Co Ltd); this transaction was exceedingly protracted – perhaps due to solicitor delays, and completion took place in March 1948.[68]

Fraser apparently remained, however, firmly of the opinion that '… the *Tropical Diseases Hospital & Centre* [my italics] might at some future date enter the British Federation of Post-Graduate Institutes'.

Does the Society have a future rôle?

Although an important rôle in the *health care* of seafarers seemed secured after the transfer of *clinical* facilities from the *Dreadnought* to St Thomas's, the status of the SHS itself had by now been seriously eroded and had constantly been under discussion throughout the previous decade. During these years, the SHS Committee and officers had been seriously 'tied up' with the future, and removal to St Thomas's Hospital (see above). Major problems resulted from the declining number of merchant seamen worldwide, and concern as to whether the Society was 'fulfilling its original purposes and objectives'? For example, '… even the Industry [did not know] which way it was going or how many men would eventually be employed', a theme which had been highlighted in a lecture delivered by the Docks Manager for Tilbury Docks, in 1970.[69]

In order to delineate the future direction of the SHS, a working party had been set up as early as 1973 'to find out, if possible, what other Societies concerned with the welfare of seamen were doing'. In summary, the recommendations to the Management Committee were: (i) 'no winding up of the Society's affairs', (ii) a continuing 'Samaritan role', (iii) setting up of a 'clearing house' (a matter which was the subject of much further discussion), (iv) 'support of research into problems of *alienation* and other allied questions …', and (v) a review of expenditure (including that on 'bricks and mortar') and the use of capital funds. In the ensuing discussion, it was generally felt that the Society was underestimating *publicity* of its ongoing activities. At a future meeting, a greater rôle in the 'field of preventative medicine' was suggested – an idea which originated from Dr R Hope, Director of the *Seafarers Education Service*, and Chairman of the Committee of *The Marine Society*. The 'Sealife Programme' (which aimed to examine 'future requirements of the Shipping Industry, both in terms of manpower and welfare') also received support from the Committee – especially its *welfare* aspect. The question of 'organising Medical Training Courses for Ships Officers [similar to those organised many years before] at the [ADH], mainly for Officers of Shell, B.P. and Esso tankers' was another suggestion – which apparently received enthusiastic support from the *Dreadnought* Medical Committee.

In December 1978 (i.e. eight years before closure of the *Dreadnought*), the *future* of the Society had received further 'in-depth' coverage. Purchase of 'medical and other equipment' at the *Dreadnought* – which the Area Health Authority had refused to provide (on account of expense) was the first recommendation of this working party. The possibility (subsequently approved) of 'sponsoring a symposium [at the *Dreadnought*] to bring together … Doctors or Medical Officers from Shipping Companies of other maritime nations, to discuss [with the medical staff of the *Dreadnought]* health matters concerning seafarers in general' was another suggestion. On the question of convalescence, owing to the Minister of Health's opposition to a prolonged period (leading to 100% fitness with immediate return to active service) it was suggested (and subsequently approved) that financial support be given to the convalescent facilities at the Springbok Centre. However, welfare was an area where there were 'many overlapping charities and other organisations', and it was generally agreed that whereas the SHS was satisfactorily covering this (see below), it might be appropriate to discuss the 'future role of the *Dreadnought* within the framework of the GBAHA'. The vast problem of geriatric care of the seafarer was also addressed; the GBAHA were adamant that it was impossible to 'accept seamen patients from outside the Greenwich and Bexley area'.[70]

In the field of medical research, the SHS had received in late 1980 an application from Dr G L Robinson (a former pathologist) and Mr P G Sargeaunt (chief technician) for research funding for a 5-year project involving amoebiasis. After discussion at a Committee Meeting, it was agreed (probably incorrectly) that the project had 'no relevance to the particular needs of seamen and it would be inappropriate for this Charity … to provide financial support!'[71]

Welfare requirements of Merchant Seamen and their dependents in the 21st century

The 1988 Report pursued the theme (previously discussed) of 'present day *welfare* [my italics] needs of seamen and their immediate families':

> [A] survey [failed to] highlight any area of the welfare spectrum which was not already covered, nor did it identify any new or wider role into which the Society could charitably extend its endeavours. The research did indicate [however] that many seafarers and their families feel there is a need for more counselling and advice support for the Merchant Navy, and what might be required is a *central information organisation* [my italics] to which they can turn for direction to the many services already available to them. It [was] considered impracticable for the Society to finance and sustain such an organisation on its own and these findings have thus been shared with other Maritime Charities with a view to determining what further co-operation and co-ordination between us is possible.[72]

The following Report enlarged upon this theme:

> In furtherance of our earlier research ..., the Society has supported the generation of, and is to participate in, discussions with the other principal charities under the auspices of the Merchant Navy Welfare Board about matters of common interest and the ways in which seafarers and their families can be made aware of the services available to them. ... In addition to our active support for the Dreadnought Unit [at St Thomas's] and continued efforts to publicise its availability, enquiries cover the call of, and availability of, convalescence facilities following hospital treatment, appropriate medical research, health care – diet/weight reduction, exercise, drug abuse, hazard of smoking and the care of the problem drinker. Much remains to be done.[73]

A GRANT-PROVIDING FUNCTION

In addition to funding the *Dreadnought* Unit, the SHS continued to be a major grant-giving organisation. In 1996, for example, it paid 'over £47,000 ... to support 154 individual applicants, as well as £196,751 to organisations which [cared] for seafarers. In 1998, a total of £251,904 was spent on grants to institutions, and during that year £150,000 was donated to the Sir Gabriel Woods Mariners Home in Greenock to care for mariners suffering from Korsakoff's Syndrome,* an

---

* This disease, which is a result of excessive alcohol consumption over a prolonged time-period, is characterised by polyneuropathy, confabulation, and memory gaps. It was first described by Magnus Huss (1807–90) a Swedish physician. The classical description of the syndrome is due to the Russian neuro-psychiatrist, Sergei Segeivich Korsakov (1854–1900) in 1887. Vitamin B_1 (thiamine) is of value in treatment. [*See also*: A Sebastian. *A Dictionary of the History of Medicine* London: Parthenon Publishing Group Ltd 1999: 449].

'alcohol-related [illness with features similar to] Alzheimer's Disease'.[74] Examples of bodies in receipt of welfare-related assistance were: Queen Victoria's Rest, the Royal Alfred Seafarers' Society, and the Merchant Navy War Memorial Society at Springbok.

'ADVICE LINE'

In 1994, a new strategy, the Seafarer's Benefits Advice Line (telephone no: 0845 7413318, run in partnership with the National Association of Citizens' Advice Bureaux) was set up; the principal object was to 'provide free, confidential (telephone) welfare rights advice to non-working and retired seafarers, fishermen, their dependents, and the agencies which deal with them'. This service was immediately available 'throughout Great Britain, offering advice and assistance on subjects such as pension entitlements, income support, housing benefit, Social Fund and DSS regulations, and in addition offering debt counselling, case work in pursuing benefit claims, and benefit checks to calculate the caller's entitlement to benefits'. This project was formally launched by the Rt Hon John Prescott, MP (1938–present) on 24 September 1996.[75]

Alterations to the 1833 Act of Incorporation (see Chapter 7)

The Act of Incorporation, under which the SHS had operated for the greater part of two centuries was modified by Parliament (coming into effect on 29 January 1999) in 1998: the Committee of Management was renamed the General Committee; the Finance and General Purposes Sub-Committee became the 'Seal, Finance and General Purposes Sub-Committee'; and, one year from its adoption, one-third of Trustees now retire by rotation, whilst the Chairman and Treasurer are appointed every three years.[76]

Anniversaries, and the Society today

The eighth of March 1971 marked the 150th anniversary of the foundation of the Society; to commemorate this event, preparations for official events began in early 1970. The venue was the Royal Naval College, Greenwich, and the guest of honour was HRH the Duke of Edinburgh (1921–present). A service was held in the Royal Naval Chapel, and the Annual Court of Governors met in Trident Hall. There was a luncheon party with friends and benefactors in the Devonport Nurse's Home for the Society's Committee of Management, and the Hospital Management Committee of the Group of Seamen's Hospitals. The 175th anniversary was marked by a luncheon at Watermen's Hall on 22 March 1996.[77]

The Chairman's Report to mark the end of the second millennium (2000), compiled by Captain David Smith OBE, listed the Society's major initiatives, in addition to those already mentioned: the *Seafarers Medical Care Review*, redevelopment of the *Royal Alfred Seafarers' Home* (at Banstead), co-operation with the *Merchant Navy Welfare Board*, and an internal *Management Review*. The *property portfolio* had by then [he recalled] been almost entirely liquefied.[78]

A new rôle for the Dreadnought buildings

The *Dreadnought* Hospital (the 'flagship' of the SHS) lay empty for a decade and more; after a great deal of uncertainty and politicising it has 'resurfaced' as the Library and Technological Centre of the University of Greenwich.[79] The Devonport buildings now house residential and student union facilities for the University.

References and notes

1 Committee of Management Minutes: 20: 285–6, 331.
2 *Ibid.* 22: 37; 24: 365.
3 *Ibid.* 22: 254–5.
4 **Aneurin Bevan** (see Chapter 22).
5 E H Murrant, C Figg, J C Nairne to A Bevan. 1946; 12 June: 3. *Memorandum: National Health Service: Hospitals for Merchant Seamen in the Port of London* [SHS Archive].
6 *Memorandum: Seamen's Hospital Society: the National Health Service Bill.* 1946: 13 July: 2 [SHS Archive].
7 *Op cit.* See note 1 above. 22: 260–1.
8 *Ibid.* 24: 307–9, 332, 339; [*See also*: Anonymous. The P. & O. Steam Navigation Company: from the days of sail – to turbo-electric liners. *SHS Quart Mag* 1934; 6 (3) 13–14; Anonymous. The Orient line to Australia: over eighty years of steady progress. *Ibid* 1954: 6 (4): 18–20; Anonymous. The Royal Mail Line to South America: the first Ocean-going postmen. *Ibid* 1935; 7(1): 16–17; Anonymous. The Cunard White Star Line: the largest fleet on the North Atlantic. *Ibid* 1935; 7(2): 21–23; Anonymous. The Union Castle Line: how the Crimean War caused the birth of a great mail service. *Ibid.* 1935; 7(3): 18–20; Anonymous. The "B.I.": the world's greatest merchant fleet. *Ibid.* 1935; 7(4): 20–22; Anonymous. *The Blue Funnel Line: eighty-four years with the China boats. Ibid.* 1936; 8(1): 22–24; Anonymous. The Elder Dempster Lines: humanitarian reasons founded this company. *Ibid.* 1936; 8(2): 20–22. [H.E.H.] "The Clan Line in the Great War" by Sir Archibald Hard. *Ibid.* 1936; 8(3): 19; Anonymous. The Clan Line: pioneers of the cargo fleets. *Ibid.* 1926; 8(3): 17–18; Anonymous. The New Zealand shipping Company: sheep farmers helped to establish this line. *Ibid.* 1936; 8(4): 21–22; Anonymous. The Lamport and Holt Line: trading with Latin America. *Ibid.* 1937; 9(2): 21–22; Anonymous. The Canadian Pacific: solving the North West Passage problem. *Ibid.* 1937; 9(1): 21–22; B Cable. A hundred years of the P. & O., 1837–1937. *Ibid.* 1937; 9(4): 9–11].
9 *Ibid.* 390–3, 398, 425; [*See also*: *Memorandum: The Relationship between Regional Hospital Boards and Boards of Management* (R.H.B.[S] [52]17) 1952; 19 June: 6. (SHS Archive)].
10 *Op cit.* See note 1 above. 24: 428–9, 440–1, 446, 455–6, 467–71, 478.
11 Annual Report: 155: 7–9.
12 *Ibid.* 156: 7–8.
13 *Ibid.* 157: 7–9.
14 *Ibid.* 158: 7–9.
15 *Dreadnought Seamen's Hospital: notes of a meeting held on 11 December 1980*: 7 [SHS Archive].
16 *Op cit.* See note 11 above: 160: 7–9.
17 *Ibid.* 161: 9–11.
18 *Ibid.* 162: 9–11.

19 *Op cit*. See note 1 above. 25: 754–6.
20 E M McInnes. St Thomas' Hospital London: George Allen and Unwin Ltd 1963: 230; G C Cook. Henry Currey FRIBA (1820–1900): leading Victorian hospital architect and early exponent of the 'pavilion principle'. *Postgrad Med J* 2002: 78: 352–59.
21 *Op cit*. See note 1 above. 25: 790–2, 815, 824–6, 833–4, 841–3, 851.
22 *Op cit*. See note 11 above: 165: 9–11.
23 *Op cit*. See note 1 above. 25: 800, 803–4, 814, 850, 874.
24 *Op cit*. See note 11 above: 166: 9–11.
25 *Ibid*. 167: 9–10.
26 *Ibid*. 168: 9–10.
27 *Ibid*. 169: 9–10.
28 *Op cit*. See note 1 above. 25: 893–6; [*See also*: *Op cit*. *see* note 11 above: 166].
29 *Op cit*. See note 11 above: 170: 9–10; 171: 9–10; 172: 9–10; 173: 9–10; 175: 9–11; 176: 11–13; 177: 11–13; 178: 11–14; 179: 11–15; 180: 3–6.
30 *Op cit*. See note 1 above. 20: 93; 21: 47–48, 69, 151. [*See also*: AN AGREEMENT made the twenty-fourth day of October 1940 BETWEEN the Seamen's Hospital Society of Greenwich, S.E.10 of the one part and HIS MAJESTY'S PRINCIPAL SECRETARY OF STATE FOR THE WAR DEPARTMENT ... WHEREAS The Department has taken possession of The Hospital for Tropical Diseases, 25 Gordon Street, London, W.C.1. ... (SHS Archive)].
31 **Sir Neil Hamilton Fairley** (see Chapter 21).
32 Fairley N H. The Hospital for Tropical diseases (U.C.H.), London. *Univ Coll Hosp Mag* 1952; 37: 114–8.
33 *Ibid*. [*See also*: G C Cook. History of tropical medicine – William Ernest Cooke (1879–1967) and his Asian tour of 1929–1930. *Acta Tropica* 2006; 100: 1–10].
34 *Op cit*. See note 1 above: 20: 98, 129.
35 A May. *London School of Hygiene and Tropical Medicine 1899–1999* London: London School of Hygiene & Tropical Medicine 1999: 40.
36 G C Cook. A difficult metamorphosis: the incorporation of the Ross Institute & Hospital for Tropical Diseases into the London School of Hygiene and Tropical Medicine. *Med Hist* 2001; 45: 483–506.
37 *Op cit*. See note 1 above: 20: 147.
38 *Op cit*. See note 11 above 121:
39 *Op cit*. See note 1 above: 20: 160–1.
40 *Ibid*. 217, 223–4.
41 *Ibid*. 231, 239.
42 *Ibid*. 259–60.
43 *Ibid*. 267–8.
44 *Ibid*. 269–70, 275.
45 **(Maurice) Harold MacMillan**, first earl of Stockton MP OM FRS (1894–1986) was British Prime Minister and First Lord of the Treasury (1957–63). He had been educated at Eton and Balliol College, Oxford. MacMillan was Parliamentary Under-Secretary of State for the Colonies in 1942. [*See also*: H C G Matthew. Macmillan, (Maurice) Harold, first earl of Stockton (1894–1986). In: H C G Matthew, B Harrison (eds). *Oxford Dictionary of National Biography*. Oxford: Oxford University Press 2004; 35: 879–96].
46 *Op cit*. See note 1 above: 20: 378. [*See also*: In: *SHS Memorandum: 'Post-war plans'* 1944; January: 7 (SHS Archive)].
47 *Op cit*. See note 11 above 124.
48 *Op cit*. See note 1 above: 21: 13–14, 19–20.

49 *Memorandum:* C E Sundell, P Manson-Bahr, N Hamilton Fairley, A Wingfield, F Murgatroyd. *Seamen's Hospital Society*: Thursday, 30th May, 1946: 3 [SHS Archive].
50 *Op cit.* See note 1 above: 21: 496.
51 *Ibid.* 506.
52 *Ibid.* 20: 458–9, 466; 495–6, 500, 530–1; 21: 184.
53 *Ibid.* 470–1.
54 **Sir (William) Wilson Jameson** GBE FRCP (1886–1962) was Dean and Professor of Public Heath at the London School of Hygiene and Tropical Medicine from 1931–1946. He was Chief Medical Officer to the Ministries of Health and Education from 1940 until 1950. [*See also*: N M Goodman. *Wilson Jameson: architect of National Health.* London: George Allen and Unwin 1970: 216; G E Godber. Jameson, Sir (William) Wilson (1885–1962) In: H C G Matthew, B Harrison (eds). *Oxford Dictionary of National Biography.* Oxford: Oxford University Press 2004; 29: 767–8].
55 **Sir Francis Richard Fraser** FRCP (1855–1964) was Director of the British Post-graduate Medical Federation from 1945 until 1960. He had formerly held Chairs of Medicine at the (Royal) Postgraduate Medical School and St Bartholomew's Hospital, and had been Director-General of the EMS. [*See also*: J McMichael. Fraser, Sir Francis Richard (1885–1964) In: H C G Matthew, B Harrison (eds). *Oxford Dictionary of National Biography.* Oxford: Oxford University Press 2004; 20: 831–3].
56 *Op cit.* See note 1 above: 21: 6–8. [*See also:* G C Cook. *John MacAlister's other vision: a history of the Fellowship of Postgraduate Medicine*. Oxford: Radcliffe Publishing 2005.]
57 *Op cit.* See note 1 above: 21: 23–4.
58 *Ibid.* 25.
59 *Ibid.* 32–3.
60 *Ibid.* 156.
61 *Ibid.* 208. [*See also*: *Op cit.* See note 1 above: 22: 12–13].
62 *Ibid.* 22: 160–1. [*See also: Memorandum* note 63 below].
63 F A Lyon. *Memorandum: 'New Tropical Hospital and Centre'* 1947: 20 May: 2 [SHS Archive].
64 *Op cit.* See note 1 above 22.
65 *Ibid.* 85.
66 *Ibid.* 135–6, 147–8.
67 G C Cook. *From the Greenwich hulks to Old St Pancras: a history of tropical disease in London* London: Athlone Press 1992: 287–99.
68 *Op cit.* See note 43 above.
69 P Padget. The development and achievement of Tilbury Container Port. *Port of London* 1970: 302–307.
70 *Op cit.* See note 1 above. 24: 400–1, 411, 415–6, 421, 430–2, 441–2, 474–5, 478–9, 490, 497, 517, 525–6, 536, 546, 555, 566, 577; 25: 598, 605, 613, 620, 631, 638, 646, 652–3, 662–3, 671–2, 688–90, 697–8, 707, 714, 723, 730, 740, 747–8, 754, 762.
71 *Ibid.* 25: 717–8, 878.
72 *Op cit.* See note 11 above: 168.
73 *Ibid.* 169:
74 *Ibid.* 176–180.
75 *Ibid.* 174–178.
76 *Ibid.* 178. [*See also*: F W W McCombe to F A Lyon. *County – London; Plan – Greenwich; Seamen's Hospital Society* 1958; 30 May: 2; F A Lyon to F W W McCombe 1958; 20 June: 1. (SHS Archive)].
77 Luncheon: Watermen's Hall 22 March 1996 [SHS Archive].
78 *Op cit.* See note 11 above: 180.

79 G C Cook. Changing rôle(s) for the Royal Hospital, Greenwich. *Hist Hosp* 2001; 22: 35–46. [*See also*: Anonymous. *Private Eye* 1997 (no 933): 19 September: 15; A Thomson. Bond issue secures Greenwich future. *THES* 1993; 9 October: 5; Anonymous. Greenwich Forum. *Times, Lond* 1998; 9 October: 26].

Appendix I

The Board of Management Minute Books, and their dates

1 8 March 1821 – 2 October 1824.
2 8 October 1824 – 18 December 1829.
3 2 January 1830 – 25 July 1834.
4 1 August 1834 – 30 May 1840.
5 5 June 1840 – 13 February 1846.
6 20 February 1846 – 29 November 1851.
7 5 December 1851 – 14 May 1858.
8 29 May 1858 – 8 March 1867.
9 15 March 1867 – 14 July 1876.
10 28 July 1876 – 22 June 1883.
11 13 July 1883 – 28 March 1890.
12 11 April 1890 – 9 July 1897.
13 13 August 1897 – 8 May 1903.
14 22 May 1903 – 14 July 1910.
15 11 August 1910 – 11 July 1918.
16 8 August 1918 – 9 June 1924.
17 14 July 1924 – 8 October 1930.
18 12 November 1930 – 12 December 1935.
19 16 January 1936 – 17 August 1939.
20 14 September 1939 – 14 December 1944.
21 18 January 1945 – 17 December 1946.
22 21 January 1947 – 19 November 1959.
23 7 April 1960 – 18 September 1969.
24 19 November 1969 – 17 November 1976.
25 19 January 1977 – 15 January 1986.

Appendix II

Appeal notice issued after the Public Meeting on 8 March 1821

SEAMEN'S HOSPITAL.

THE Committee for managing the Funds subscribed in the winter of 1817-18, for the Relief of the Distressed and Destitute Seamen, who were found in such numbers in our streets, having ascertained, by sad experience, "that "there are in the course of the year, in the Port of London, from 700 to 800 "sick and diseased seamen, destitute of medical or surgical aid," and recommended, upon closing that establishment, that a permanent hospital should be provided, for the purpose of administering to their relief; a Public Meeting was held on the 8th instant, at which it was determined that a PERMANENT FLOATING HOSPITAL should be established on the River Thames; and a Provisional Committee was appointed, "for framing rules and regulations for the "government of the Hospital, with authority to fix a day for the General "Meeting of Subscribers, for the election of a Committee for the promotion and "management of the interests and concerns of the Charity."

As the extent of the Plan must depend upon the amount of the Funds contributed, the Provisional Committee are desirous of drawing the serious attention of the Public to the motives and object of the intended establishment, and anxiously solicit the favor of their early Subscriptions for its support.

Seamen, from their peculiar character, and the nature of their avocations, are almost universally strangers to the ordinary modes of obtaining relief in periods of sickness, particularly on their arrival at a port to which they do not belong; and, therefore, notwithstanding that the utmost relief is afforded by the various excellent hospitals and medical Institutions in and about the metropolis, consistently with their means, and with the rules by which they are governed, those Institutions are, from the circumstances above-mentioned, not sufficiently available to the wants of this meritorious but unprotected class of men.

Indeed, it is unfortunately but too well known, that many perish in our streets, through want of friends to whom to apply for admittance to these Institutions. To avert such miseries in future, by facilitating the admission of the friendless and unrecommended, immediately upon their application, in all cases requiring medical or surgical assistance; and thus to rescue these unfortunate beings from wretched and untimely deaths, is the object of the proposed Establishment.

The Hospital will be formed on board the ship Grampus, (a two-decker) which has been liberally presented by His Majesty's Government for the purpose; a naval surgeon will reside on board; it will also be attended by visiting physicians and surgeons, who have kindly offered their gratuitous services, and will be rendered as congenial as possible to the feelings of the individuals for whose benefit it is intended.

The Committee beg to express the satisfaction they feel in laying before the public, the following list of Noblemen and Gentlemen who have already signified their willingness to become Vice-Presidents; and also in making known the liberal manner in which the Public Companies have answered the application made to them; not only as affording an important addition to the Funds, but as sanctioning the opinion which has been formed of the necessity of such an Institution as the proposed Hospital.

PATRON, HIS MOST GRACIOUS MAJESTY THE KING.

VICE-PRESIDENTS:

Right Rev. Lord Bishop of Durham
Right Rev. Lord Bishop of Chester
His Grace the Duke of Bedford
The Right Hon. Earl Spencer
The Right Hon. Earl Bathurst
The Right Hon. Earl Darnley
The Right Hon. Earl of Aberdeen
The Right Hon. Earl of Hardwicke
The Right Hon. Earl of Liverpool
Right Hon. Lord Viscount Melville
Right Hon. Lord Viscount Torrington
Right Hon. Lord Ellenborough
The Right Hon. Lord Calthorpe
Alexander Baring, Esq. M.P.
John William Buckle, Esq.
Captain Joseph Cotton
Sir John William Lubbock, Bart.
William Manning, Esq.
W.T. Money, Esq. M.P.
Thomas Reid, Esq.
Thomas Wilson, Esq. M.P.
W. Williams, Esq. M.P. Treasurer.

PROVISIONAL COMMITTEE.

Sir John William Lubbock, Bart.
Aaron Chapman, Esq.
Captain C. C. Owen, R.N.
John Deacon, Esq.
J. W. Buckle, Esq.
George Lyall, Esq.

	Donations.			Annual Subscriptions.		
	£.	s.	d.	£.	s.	d.
His Most Gracious Majesty the KING	105	0	0	105	0	0
His Royal Highness Prince Leopold	50	0	0			
The Corporation of the Trinity House	200	0	0			
The Honorable the East India Company	105	0	0			
The Royal Exchange Assurance Company	105	0	0			
The London Assurance Company	105	0	0			
The Gov. and Company of the Bank of England	100	0	0			
The West India Dock Company	52	10	0			
The Right Hon. Earl Spencer	50	0	0			
The Right Hon. Earl Darnley				10	10	0
The Right Hon. Earl of Rocksavage	10	10	0			
The Right Rev. Lord Bishop of Chester	10	10	0			
The Right Hon. Lord Ellenborough	10	10	0	10	10	0
The Right Hon. Lord Arden	10	10	0			
The Right Hon. Viscount Torrington	10	0	0	2	2	0
Rear-Admiral Sir Edw. Codrington	5	5	0	2	2	0
The Rev. Sir S. C. Jervoise, Bart.	21	0	0			
Sir J. W. Lubbock, bart.	10	10	0	2	2	0
Stewart Marjoribanks, Esq. M.P.	10	10	0			
William Taylor Money, Esq. M. P.	10	10	0			
William Wilberforce, Esq. M. P,	10	10	0			
Thomas Wilson, Esq. M. P.	21	0	0	2	2	0
William Williams, Esq. M. P.	21	0	0	2	2	0
Rear-Admiral Spranger	5	0	0			
Rear Admiral Lake	2	2	0	1	1	0
Rear-Admiral West	2	2	0	1	1	0
Captain George Acklom, R. N.				2	2	0
Captain W. Bathurst, R. N.				1	1	0
Captain Bowles, R. N.				1	1	0
Captain Dillon, R. N.				1	1	0
Captain Digby, R. N.	10	0	0	1	1	0
Captain C. C. Owen, R. N.	10	10	0	1	1	0
Captain Nurse, R. N.				1	1	0
Captain Richbell, R. N.				1	1	0
Captain J. Shaw R. N.				1	1	0
Captain William Young, R. N.	10	10	0			
Captain Gooch, H. C. S.	10	10	0			
Captain Loch, H. C. S.	10	10	0			
Captain Lockner, H. C. S.	10	10	0			
James Alley, Esq.				1	1	0
John Blackett, Esq.	10	10	0	2	2	0
Mrs. Bish, Sen.	10	10	0			
Aaron Chapman, Esq.	10	10	0	1	1	0
Jonathan Chapman, Esq.	10	10	0	1	1	0
Wm. Curling, Esq.	10	10	0			
Duncan Campbell, Esq.	10	10	0			
Joseph Dowson, jun. Esq.	10	10	0			
John Drinkald, jun. Esq.	10	10	0	2	2	0
Charles Francis, Esq.	10	10	0	1	1	0
Halifax Mills, Esq.				10	10	0
Patrick Home, Esq.	5	5	0	1	1	0
George Joad, Esq.	10	10	0			
W. G. Key, Esq.				1	1	0
George Lyall, Esq.	10	10	0	1	1	0
A Lady	0	10	6			
Arch. Marjoribanks, Esq.	10	10	0			
J. C. Reeve, Esq.				1	1	0
Matthias Robinson Esq.	1	1	0	1	1	0
Messrs Thomas Sturge and Sons	15	15	0	3	3	0

Instructions to personnel on the last of the Hospital-ships

INSTRUCTIONS
TO
PATIENTS & OTHERS

Every Man in the Working Party or Convalescent, able to make himself useful, is to obey such Orders and Directions as may be given him by the Officers, and to use his best endeavours to perform the Duty required of him. Upon these conditions, and compliance with the Rules of the Ship, he will ensure to himself the favor and encouragement of the Committee; and a contrary line of Conduct will cause him to be expelled, as undeserving their protection, and a mark placed against his Name which will prevent his being received again in case of future illness.

As Cleanliness is of the utmost importance, every Man will be required to keep himself and his Clothes clean, to be shaved not less than twice every week, and to keep his hair at all times cut, clean, and in order; and to bear in mind, that he is expected to repair his Clothes, and is not to be seen at any time with them torn or out of repair.

All complaints, relative to Provisions, or any other grievances, are to be made in a respectful manner to the Superintendent, who will immediately inquire into them.

The Decks are to be swept, or otherwise cleaned, directly after Meals, and no Man is, on any account, to spit about the Decks, or to throw bones or dirt, of any description, about the Ship.

As the Water Closets have been frequently out of order, by improper things being put down them, any Patient injuring them in this or any other manner, will be immediately dismissed.

Men, in the Working Party, will, by applying to the Superintendent, have leave to seek for employment; but they must return on Board again by Four o'Clock during Winter, and Six during Summer, otherwise they will be considered discharged.

Should any Man, on Surgeon's leave, remain on Shore all Night, without having the Superintendent's and Surgeon's permission to do so, he will be dismissed the Ship.

No Smoking to be allowed in the Ship.

No Patients to open or shut the Ports without permission from the Surgeon or Nurse.

Patients on no account to go into those Wards to which they do not belong.

The Patients are to retire to their Beds at Eight o'Clock in Winter, and Nine o'Clock during the Summer, and are not to talk or make any noise afterwards.

Patients capable of rendering assistance are expected to do so to those who are too weak to help themselves.

Patients are desired to comply with the Orders of the Medical Officers and Nurses.

Patients are particularly requested, if they see any thing improper going on in the Wards, to make the same known to the Superintendent or Surgeon; and if the Orders of the Surgeon have been neglected by the Nurses, to report such neglect to the Surgeon.

No Swearing or improper language to be made use of by the Patients, on pain of expulsion.

No Person to bring Wine, Spirits, or Beer, on board, without leave from the Superintendent.

The Patients are not to be admitted into the Galley.

No Person, in the service of the Seamen's Hospital, is allowed, on any account to receive money, directly or indirectly, from the Patients or their Friends, or to supply the Patients with any article whatever, without permission from the Superintendent or Surgeon.

All Patients capable, are desired to attend Prayers Morning and Evening, and Divine Service on Sundays.

Patients at any time desirous of receiving spiritual consolation, are to make their wishes known to the Superintendent who will send for the Chaplain, or any other Minister to visit them

Patients who may be in too weak a state to write to their relations or friends, will have the same done for them, on applying to the Superintendent.

Patients who may receive Wages, or any other monies or property while under the care of this Charity, are advised to leave the same for security in the hands of the Superintendent; and if they are desirous of making their Wills, or otherwise to dispose of their Property, they will be furnished with regular Forms, by applying to the Superintendent, who will attend to their wishes in filling up the same, and see that they are duly witnessed.

BY ORDER OF THE COMMITTEE OF MANAGEMENT,

JANUARY, 1857.

S. KEMBALL COOK, Secretary.

Appendix IV

Log of the *Dreadnought* 1865–68

The Society's archive contains extracts from the log of the last of the Hospital-ships – HMS *Caledonia* (renamed) HMS *Dreadnought*, the Society's clinical base between 1857 and 1870. The following entries are those for four days during the period 1865–68:

Monday 2nd Jany 1865
AM„ Light Wind Frost & Fog – At 12.30„ M Cook ret^{d} at 8„.2/2. In the Well „ at 8„10. The Ass^{t}Surgeon went on shore and ret^{d} at 9„ 0„ at 9„ 0„ the – Chaplain came and went on Shore at 12„ 50„ at 10.30 Mr Cook went on shore.

PM„ at 12„ 30 the Rev^{d} C Von Bulou visited the Foreign Patients and went on Shore at 2„40„ at 2„0„ sent the body of Joss Barazarda on shore for Interment. In charge of Z M "Harrington„, who reported that the burial at 3„ 30„ at „3„ 15„ the Super^{dent} read the Prayers at 3„ 45„ the Ass^{t} Surgeon went on Shore „ at 4„ 0„ Dr Ward„ visited His Patients (32) and went on Shore at 4„ 30„ Rec^{d} 200lbs Bread„.

[On this day, there were 9 admissions and 11 discharges, leaving 181 on board, of whom 173 were victualled.]

Thursday 19th Jany 1865
AM„ Light Wind„ with fog at 8„ 4 Inc in the Well „ 'at 9.0. Super^{dent} read prayers'. PM. "at 2„0 sent the bodies of William Waldens and Charles-Johnston on Shore for Interment in charge of Z M Stankey who reported the burial at 3„30." "at 2„ 15„ the Chaplain came and went on shore at 4„ 0„" "at 6„ 0„ the Ass^{t} Physician Retnd" "at 8„30 the Ass^{t} Surgeon went on Shore", at 9„ 20, the Sup^{d} went on Shore and … at 9.50." "Rec^{d} 200 lbs Bread 210 Bry "40 lb. mutton" "1120 lb Potatoes "1/6 Greens".

[On this day, there were 4 admissions and two discharges leaving 191 on board, of whom 187 were victualled.]

Wednesday 15th April 1868
AM. Light wind and fine. At 2.45„ the Ass^{t} Phys^{n} returned "At 8-0 6½ [?] in the Well.

At 9-0„ Dr Ward visited his patients (24) left at 9-35. At 9-10, the chaplain came and left at 11.50. At 11.50 the Ass^{t} Surgeon left and retnd at 1.20pm. At 2.10 Mr Littleton left and retnd at Midnight. At 2.55, the Chaplain came and left at 4-50. At 3-45, the Superintendent left and ret^{d} at 5.15. The Surgeon reported J^{d} Christie & F Coyne "watchmen on Surgical Deck„ J Dyden & E Dixon Watchmen on Med^{l} Deck Rec^{d} 160 lbs Bread, 9 Galls Porter."

[On this day, there were 6 admissions and 7 discharges; there were 158 on board and 153 were victualled.]

Thursday 30 April 1868

AM. Fresh Breeze and fine. "at 7-40 Departed this Life Daniel McCarty." At 8-7 [?] in the well. At 9-0 Dr Barnes visited his patients (28) & left at 9-25. At 9-0 the Chaplain came and left at 12-11. At 10-11 the Surgeon left and ret^{d} at 4.15. At 11.20 the Superintendent left and ret^{d} at 1-50. At 1-15 the Ass^{t} Physician left". At 3.10 the Chaplain came and left at 4.00. At 4.50 the surgeon left.

Rec^{d} 160 lbs Bread – "85 lbs Beef" – 5lbs Mutton "336 lbs Potatoes".

[There were 3 admissions and 6 discharges this day, leaving 157 patients on board. 155 were victualled.]

Index

List of abbreviations:

ADH	Albert Dock Hospital
CRDS	Committee for the Relief of (distressed) Destitute Seamen
HTD	Hospital for Tropical Diseases
LSCM	London School of Clinical Medicine
LSTM	London School of Tropical Medicine
KGSS	King George's Sanitorium for Sailors
SHS	Seamen's Hospital Society

Page numbers in *italics* refer to illustrations.